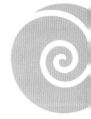

Contents

Contents

NURSING
PRACTICE AND
HEALTH CARE

NURSING PRACTICE AND HEALTH CARE

5th Edition

Edited by

Sue Hinchliff RN RNT BA MSc, Consultant to the Nursing and Midwifery Council; Consultant to the Royal College of Nursing Accreditation Unit; Nurse Advisor to THET; Visiting Professor in Nursing and Nursing Education to London South Bank University

Sue Norman RN BEd (Hons) RNT NDNCert Hon DSc, previously Chief Executive/Registrar, United Kingdom Central Council for Nursing, Midwifery and Health Visitors; Visiting Professor in Nursing Policy and Development to London South Bank University

Jane Schober MN RN DipN (Lond) DipN Ed RNT RCNT, Principal Lecturer, School of Nursing and Midwifery, De Montfort University, Leicester

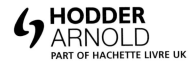

HODDER ARNOLD
PART OF HACHETTE LIVRE UK

First published in Great Britain in 1989 by Hodder Arnold
Second edition 1993
Third edition 1998
Fourth edition 2003
This fifth edition published in 2008 by
Hodder Arnold, an imprint of Hodder Education, part of Hachette Livre UK
338 Euston Road, London NW1 3BH

www.hoddereducation.com

Hachette Livre UK's policy is to use papers that are natural, renewable and recyclable products and made from wood grown in sustainable forests. The logging and manufacturing processes are expected to conform to the environmental regulations of the country of origin.

Whilst the advice and information in this book are believed to be true and accurate at the date of going to press, neither the authors nor the publisher can accept any legal responsibility or liability for any errors or omissions that may be made. In particular (but without limiting the generality of the preceding disclaimer) every effort has been made to check drug dosages; however it is still possible that errors have been missed. Furthermore, dosage schedules are constantly being revised and new side-effects recognised. For these reasons the reader is strongly urged to consult the drug companies' printed instructions before administering any of the drugs recommended in this book.

British Library Cataloguing in Publication Data
A catalogue record for this book is available from the British Library

Library of Congress Cataloging-in-Publication Data
A catalog record for this book is available from the Library of Congress

ISBN   978 0 340 92888 2

1 2 3 4 5 6 7 8 9 10

Commissioning Editor:	Joanna Koster/Naomi Wilkinson
Production Controller:	Andre Sim
Project Editor:	Clare Patterson
Cover Designer:	Laura De Grasse
Artwork:	Charon Tec Ltd.
Index:	Dr Laurence Errington

Typeset in 10.5/12.5 Gillsans by Charon Tec Ltd., A Macmillan Company.
Printed and bound in Italy

What do you think about this book? Or any other Hodder Arnold title?
Please visit our website: www.hoddereducation.com

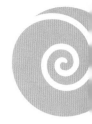

Contributors

Angela Barry RN
Student Midwife, City University, London, UK

Ruth Beretta RN DipN BSc (Hons) MA MSc RNT
Curriculum Area Manager, Social Science, Social Work and Health Professions, Cornwall College, Cornwall, UK

June Clark DBE PhD RN FRCN
Professor Emeritus, Swansea University, Swansea, UK

Rosemary Cook CBE MSc PGDip (Applied Social Research) RGN PN Cert
Director, Queen's Nursing Institute, London, UK

Sue Davies PhD MSc BSc RGN RHV
Visiting Reader, School of Nursing and Midwifery, University of Sheffield, Sheffield, UK

Christine Eberhardie TD MSc RN RNT FHEA Cert HSM
Honorary Principal Lecturer in Nursing, Faculty of Health and Social Care Sciences, Kingston University and St George's, University of London, London, UK

Jacqueline Elton MA BSc (Hons) RN
Matron, Directorate of Medical and ED Services, University Hospitals of Leicester NHS Trust, Leicester, UK

Judith Evans BA MInstLM RN
Matron, Cardio-Respiratory Directorate, University Hospitals of Leicester NHS Trust, Leicester, UK

John Fowler PhD MA BA RGN RMN DipN RCNT Cert Ed RNT
Principal Lecturer, School of Nursing and Midwifery, De Montfort University, Leicester, UK

Paul Gibbons RN DipN Diploma in Philosophy and Health Care
Health Care Governance Consultant, North Yorkshire

Catherine Lawrence MSc BSc (Lon) RSCN Dip N(Lon) Dip N Ed(Lon)
Principal Lecturer in the Department of Children's Nursing, London South Bank University, London, UK

Jacqueline McKenna RN DipN MMedSci
Director of Nursing and Strategic Planning, Medway NHS Foundation Trust, Gillingham, UK

Mike Nolan BEd MA MSc PhD RGN RMN
Professor of Gerontological Nursing, Sheffield Institute for Studies on Ageing, School of Medicine and Biomedical Sciences, University of Sheffield, Sheffield, UK

James Partridge OBE DSc (Hon) FRCSEd (Hon) MSc MA
Chief Executive, Changing Faces, London, UK

Hayley Reading BA (Hons) Dip IC RN
Matron, Directorate of Medical and ED Services, University Hospitals of Leicester NHS Trust, Leicester, UK

Contributors

Nick Salter RNA MA BSc (Hons) Dip N Cert Ed HEA (Fellow)
Principal Lecturer, Adult Nursing, School of Nursing and Midwifery, De Montfort University, Leicester, UK

Susan Savage MSc BNURS (Hons) RN RSCPHN-HV
PCT Executive Nurse, Heywood, Middleton and Rochdale Primary Care Trust, Rochdale, UK

Jane Schober MN RN DipNEd DipN Lond RCNT RNT
Principal Lecturer, School of Nursing and Midwifery, De Montfort University, Leicester, UK

Marcelle de Sousa RSCN RGN BSc (Hons) MA
Adolescent Nurse Specialist, UCL Hospitals NHS Foundation Trust, London, UK

Penny Tremayne MSc PGDip (Ed) BSc (Hons) DipNS RGN
Senior Lecturer, School of Nursing and Midwifery, De Montfort University, Leicester, UK

Caroline Woolrich RN
Advice Centre Professional Adviser, Nursing and Midwifery Council, London, UK

Stephen G Wright FRCN, MBE
Faculty of Health, Medical Sciences and Social Care, University of Cumbria Carlisle; and Chair, the Sacred Space Foundation, Sparket, UK

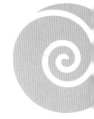

Foreword

Good health is probably one of the most precious personal assets that an individual can possess. Like much in life, we take it for granted until our health, or that of our family or friends, is compromised in some way. As a reader of this successful and important textbook, you will be somewhere on your journey towards or returning to gaining a licence to practise as a registered nurse and therefore in a position to make a difference to people's health and well-being.

I have had the privilege to witness the enormous positive contribution that nurses and nursing make to the lives of individuals, families and communities nationally and internationally. Challenges to health, not least lifestyle, longevity and enduring illnesses, are constantly emerging and changing. Meeting these challenges demands development of knowledge and practice based on evidence and skills, while maintaining the humanity and compassion that are at the heart of nursing care. This book makes a significant contribution to that development.

We are fortunate in the UK to have strong professional self-regulation made explicit in the NMC Code (2008), which sets out standards of conduct, performance and ethics for nurses and midwives. These standards are a pledge to the public as a statement of what can be expected of qualified nurses and midwives, and they articulate the values that underpin nursing and midwifery education and practice. That's why this book is important – it is the first in which the 2008 NMC Code forms a major theme throughout.

Public and patient involvement and the importance of the patient experience are now key features of health care development, and I am delighted to see that the first chapter of this book is written by a patient about his experience and expectations of nursing. Equally important is the chapter that follows on the perspective of someone who is experiencing what it is like learning to become a nurse. These first two chapters followed by Professor Dame June Clark's chapter on the essence of nursing set the tone for a text that helps to create a practical, academically robust and highly relevant foundation for current and future nursing practice – one of the best careers in the world.

I hope you enjoy your journey.

Christine Hancock

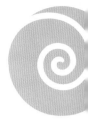

Preface

As we prepared this fifth edition of *Nursing Practice and Health Care*, we reflected on the changes that have taken place in the NHS, health care and nursing in the years since we commissioned and edited the first edition, which was published in 1989.

Back then, there was no NHS Plan, no targets and no NHS trusts – foundation or otherwise; competencies for practice were just starting to be used in nurse education; there were national boards to oversee nurse education, and the United Kingdom Central Council for Nursing, Midwifery and Health Visiting (UKCC) – the predecessor to the Nursing and Midwifery Council (NMC) – was developing a new approach to nurse education called Project 2000.

Since then, nursing has become increasingly complex, more evidence-based, more confident of its place within higher education and – while focusing on working with the multiprofessional team – more sure of its role in delivering seamless 24-hour high-quality care with the patient right at its centre.

This text has always sought to be a companion on the student's journey towards being an accountable professional, licensed to practise thoughtful and compassionate nursing care. Its success in this is evidenced by the publication of this fifth edition.

We have undertaken a thorough review of all the chapters of this core text since the previous edition was published in 2003. That fourth edition had a particular emphasis on the 2002 version of the NMC Code, the ways in which it underpinned the practice of nursing and its importance in helping students to become accountable licensed practitioners. We set out to help nurses to view the NMC Code positively as a set of principles to guide practice rather than a stick with which to challenge poor conduct. One of the most significant changes to take place recently during the preparation of this fifth edition has been the publication in April 2008 of the latest version of the NMC Code.

In this edition, for ease of use, we have divided the text into five parts:

1 Perspectives on nursing
2 Learning nursing
3 Practising nursing
4 Key aspects of care
5 Professional support and development

One of the student reviewers of the fourth edition suggested that we start the book with a user's view, a student's view and an expert practitioner's view of what nursing is, and so we commissioned the three chapters in Part 1, where we would advise readers to start. We do hope you enjoy this innovative section.

We realised that, after this, readers are likely to dip in and out of the text as their particular programme or learning needs dictate, and so we have tried to ensure that throughout there are common themes that help to give a consistent structure to the whole. These include:

- the NMC standards of proficiency that are expected of students;
- patient-centredness and a firm grounding in practice;
- a multiprofessional approach to care;
- a UK-wide perspective, so readers in any of the four countries that make up the UK will find the text relevant to them;

- addressing quality issues;
- promoting and maintaining health;
- exploring where the NMC Code (2008) applies;
- the challenges and excitement of nursing care;
- any changes in disease patterns;
- diversity and cultural issues;
- relevant ethical and legal issues.

Alongside the themes, authors have been asked to incorporate common features in the chapters after Part 1 to aid learning, such as:

- bulleted intended learning outcomes;
- patient scenarios;
- reflective points and some commentary;
- explanation of terms that might not be familiar;
- relevant, recent annotated suggestions for further reading;
- useful addresses and websites.

Whether you are using this text as a student nurse at diploma or degree level, as a lecturer-practitioner while undertaking continuing professional development, or as nurse on a post-registration programme of some kind, we hope that you find it easy to read, interesting, thought-provoking and an essential guide to your learning.

Readers should note that the views expressed are those of the contributors and are not necessarily those of the editors.

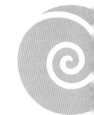

How to use this book

The fifth edition of this very popular textbook is designed as an essential resource for those studying nursing and preparing for registration. Here are some suggestions to help you use the book effectively.

A key advantage of this textbook is that it may be used sequentially or, as is more likely, a text you may dip in and out of. The themes and topics within the text may form the core to some of the modules you study or they may support ongoing themes throughout your programme. A textbook such as this will inevitably contain some overlap and repetition as different authors discuss and analyse, for example, the NMC Code in relation to their topic area. This adds to the comprehensiveness and breadth of the text as a range of patient groups and professional themes are featured.

Use this book to aid your studies by:

- Locating your topic or themes in the contents list and index.
- Using the introduction in each chapter to gain an overview of the aim and content of the chapter.
- Using the reflection points to explore and review key issues and discuss implications for practice with colleagues and peers.
- Referring to the areas where cross-referencing to another chapter is detailed as a means of broadening your reading.
- Using summaries and conclusions to focus on outcomes and key arguments.
- Referring to the three appendices to substantiate the content of the NMC Code, the NMC standards and the NMC guide for students of nursing and midwifery.
- Reading the papers/texts within the further reading section, in each chapter, to support the topic.
- Using the web site references to access current data.

Enjoy using this book!

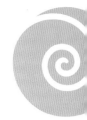

Acknowledgements

Chapter 6 (Principles of professional practice) is based on chapter 2 from the previous edition which was written by Norma Fryer; it has been revised and updated for this current edition by Caroline Woolrich.

Chapter 15 (The needs of children) is based on chapter 8 from the previous edition which was written by Cathy Lawrence, Faith Gibson and Judy Zur; it has been revised and updated for this current edition by Cathy Lawrence.

PART I

Perspectives on nursing

Receiving nursing: a patient reflects on his journey

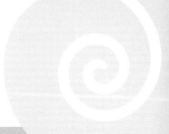

James Partridge

It is very fitting that the latest edition of this highly regarded textbook should start with a patient's perspective, because in the UK and, I think, in other countries too, the concept of a 'patient-led health care system' is now accepted as best practice: patients can be, and should be, guiding all health care practice in alliance with the professionals who care for us.

The opportunities that are open for a recently qualified nurse are amazingly different from what they were 20 years ago. Nurses are now recognised as highly specialised practitioners. Actually, I think it was ever thus, but nurses were not recognised as being so. Without nurses, most of today's increasingly complex medical and surgical interventions could not be attempted – neither could palliative and long-term care be provided. Nurses are now working as equals, in theory at least and often in practice too, in multiprofessional teams with medics, physiotherapists, dieticians and many others. This ethos will become more and more accepted as the training of the next generation of health care professionals proceeds – with patients recognised as equal partners too.

It is a privilege to be asked to write this introductory chapter in a nurses' textbook, but I am conscious that, although I have received a wide range of nursing care, I cannot possibly give a full picture of what nursing today is about in so many different locations in health care. I hope, however, to be able to reflect on some of what some patients experience.

A journey into the unknown

I often liken a patient's entry into the health care system as the start of a journey, which very rarely has a joyful holiday feel to it – perhaps the exception is midwifery. Most of us are making the journey unplanned, unprepared and unsure; it is not one that most of us choose to take, because of its perils and uncertainties.

It is a weird journey – not a magical mystery tour either – into places where strange foreign customs are met, such as the bedpan routine and the white-coated hierarchy, where a foreign language full of very long words (that, in the case of drugs and infections, are not even in a dictionary – or, at least, not a dictionary that one tends to carry around) is spoken, and for which the traveller has rarely been given a Lonely Planet guidebook. But, unlike the package holiday deal, lonely it can certainly be.

In most parts of today's health care system, the doctor or surgeon sees him- or herself as the chief of the tour-operating company or the aeroplane's pilot, sealed behind a locked door or protected by junior staff, secretaries and nurses from too much contact with the 'passengers'. Change is happening, but slowly, not least because of the fear of 'passengers' suing over faulty information or failure to stick to lift-off (appointment) times. The physiotherapists and other therapists usually have the skills to ensure that you are physically as fit as possible to make a smooth ending to the journey to return to your community – they're like personal fitness trainers and sports psychologists.

What role do nurses play in the patient's journey? It seems to me that the nurse's role is typically a multi-tasking one, a subtle blend of TLC giver, translator and interpreter, companion, map reader/route finder, advance party, bag carrier, counsellor, pain and stress reliever, advocate with the pilot, and perhaps many more.

Let me try to illustrate with a little of my own journey.

Setting out

As a child and teenager, I had been required to visit old people in hospital and had had one minor operation, but I was definitely totally unprepared for my journey – and how reliant I would become on nurses in the process.

Shortly after my eighteenth birthday, I turned over a Landrover on a bend of a deserted road in Wales at about 30 mph – it blew up as the sparks ignited the petrol tank underneath the driver's seat. I was the driver – and the last one out. Four others got out largely unscathed – and I imagined that I was just singed. But I was aware of the ghastly smell of burning clothes and flesh – and that my face was swelling fast and going numb. People stood around, unsure what to do. The car behind stopped, and one of the passengers knew exactly what had to be done – a woman who just happened to have been trained as a nurse.

She covered my face with a clean cloth and wrapped me in her huge white fur coat. Her car became my ambulance to the nearest hospital, and from there I was rushed, sirens blaring, to a bigger one with a specialist burns unit. Gentle hands removed my clothes, careful not to cause any more pain, injections and blood transfusions – and a gentle voice asking 'Can you see us?'

'Yes, a bit blurred, but yes . . .' and then I was out.

It may be over 35 years ago but I can still recall my first conscious moments many hours later – a nurse saying 'You're OK, keep calm' and my whispering 'Where am I? Can I get up? What have I done? When will I be able to see?' Questions, questions – all gently answered with just enough information to keep my spirits up and with none to make me worried. Not being able to see was a hurdle for me, but the nurses communicated beautifully – visitors' timings, food, bowel movements (translation, please), surgeons, blood tests, injections for pain, infection and everything (pause for pin-cushion black humour) – and as I was totally incapacitated they tended to my every need, washing, feeding . . . From a highly self-reliant person, in just 24 hours I had become completely dependent, and I did not like it a single bit.

After 3 days on the critical list, my body gradually started to heal – nearly 40 per cent burns, much of them third degree, especially to my face, hands and right leg, do not heal quickly, I discovered. 'Maybe 3 weeks, maybe a bit more' was the early estimation – I sensed it was an optimistic one, again designed to prevent my energy for the fight waning. I was transferred 10 days later in an ambulance to London, an excruciating 4-hour journey with a nurse at my side humouring me – and asking me for directions through Reading – ridiculous!

Settling in for the long haul

The next 3 months were to be a blur of operations, dressing changes, saline baths, pain, sedation, raging infection, barrier nursing, ghastly soft/liquid food and Complan – all conducted by a group of caring people I'd never met before. I came to trust the nurses of the burns unit of Queen Mary's Hospital, Roehampton, absolutely. The Sisters Pooley and Broughton, two male nurses, Fred and Duncan, strong and gentle, and a string of staff nurses and students (some very stunning with whom I could still flirt, even behind their masks – a great lesson, I realised later, after my face was revealed in the mirror).

They got to know me, to know how to help me deal with my pain and nausea, what I needed to keep sane and what would motivate me. And they got to know my parents and family too – informing them more honestly than me, I think, about my prospects and preparing them and me for the mirror moment. Trust was built and never confounded. An object lesson.

I knew I had to look in a mirror some time and, after 3 months, I was ready – or so I thought. With great care, the nurses timed the moment – I needed one of them close by but not too close, allowing me space and time to see the shocking mess that was my face – was it really me any more behind the oozing scabs, the reddened scars, the gross distortions around my eyes and mouth? I cried in the night, the night nurses knew.

My face's future became my great focus – oh yes, my legs were damaged too and I could not yet walk, but I would somehow. But was there any 'somehow' with a face like that? One of the nurses escorted me down the corridor to the restaurant a few weeks later on one of my early short walks – my first experience of hyper-self-consciousness feeling all eyes on me and yet none could bear to look me in the eye.

But the nurses did make eye-contact – and so did the lovely ward cleaner, Josie – and yet I doubt whether any of them really knew how incredibly vital that was for me; through it, they were asserting that they could still see 'me' and that they were willing to communicate, willing to look for me. How different I would find it outside, where people looked away instinctively. A little later, a small party of nurses took me to the local pub – terrifying for me but, as I was later to learn, pubs close to burns units get used to people looking like me – and one of the nurses had primed the barman – eye contact was made.

The other thing I remember was that, despite the fact that my nurses were all under pressure (although 'targets' hadn't been invented, time and motion studies certainly had been), many of them made time to talk to me. Not just about the technicalities, but allowing conversations about other things, normal things – from which would drop, as I suspect they knew, my real anxieties (behind my stoic exterior).

Moving on

Leaving that burns unit was a sad day – it was a cocoon in which I was totally accepted and to which I would make many return trips to pay tribute. But I knew I had to move on, to other wards to begin reconstructive surgery that would go on and on and on over the next 4 years, and I knew I had to try to get back into society too, to try to start my life up again.

And in this rehabilitation phase of my journey, nurses started to play a different role. Instead of me relying on them for physical and emotional support, now they became vital sources of information and knowledge that I could not get from anyone else, it seemed – or nobody appeared to have the time to explain and listen to my questions. What could reconstructive surgery offer? How long would it take? Why can't they just fix these scars? Why are they called 'hypertrophic'? (Could you spell that please?)

The nurses in the wards that I was now on were trained to carry me through the rehabilitation stage – here, the challenge is not so much one of survival but of battling through the various barriers I was now faced with, such as regaining strength and dexterity. Most of all, I was trying to rebuild my self-confidence and to discover that elusive self-esteem that had been so shattered by the discovery of my lost looks. I had traded on my looks in my first 18 years, but now they seemed bound to count against me for the rest of my life – little chance of intimate relationships, no chance of a proper job.

Twenty years after my hospitalisation, I commissioned a piece of research to explore how well nurses in burns care and maxillofacial surgery were prepared to help patients with their 'soft' psychosocial issues, as distinct from the 'hard' technical, physical and functional issues (Clarke and Cooper, 2000). It found that although nurses did appreciate that the psychosocial issues were often at the forefront of patients' needs, their capacity to provide a trained response was limited. I am glad to say that Changing Faces now provides training courses designed to change that skill deficit – and to get health care planning to recognise it and provide a biopsychosocial approach.

My reconstructive surgery lasted 4 years, 1 year of which was spent having a major tube pedicle raised on my back and transferred to my chin. This was a long period of frequent hospitalisation, and again nurses became the rocks on which I built my recovery. Even if the surgeons seemed distant and rather aloof, the nursing team counselled me through the anxious high-risk times. Pedicles were the approved method for moving large flaps of skin in those days (before microsurgery made free flaps possible), and they were fraught with problems, especially in the periods just before and after one end of the pedicle was moved and attached to another place – the blood supply had to be re-established somehow.

One of the most challenging parts of nursing, I think, is getting the balance right in talking about how a procedure has gone or about the prognosis or risks ahead. If you are too optimistic, patients can be disappointed; but if you are too pessimistic, you can demotivate a patient – and their family – quickly. I observed my medical and nursing team struggling with this everyday dialectic and, in the height of my anxiety, I frequently tried to second-guess their real views.

Patients (and families) today rightly expect, as I did then, to be thoroughly informed about the progress of their treatments and to be involved in decision-making. In the 1970s, such involvement was not so encouraged – and several of the senior nurses often took on a mediator/advocate role for me in discussion with my surgeon and his medical staff. It was hard to convince the latter sometimes that my knowing was in my own best interests and I applaud my nurses for helping me – old-school doctors in white coats can be very intimidating!

Wanting to be a citizen again

Mine was a rather exceptional journey, I recognise – an acute emergency followed by a very long rehabilitation phase. But the value I placed on nurses was never stronger than right towards the end of my journey as I was trying to throw off the 'patient' label and become a citizen again – not easy when many people I met asked me 'When are you going in [for more surgery] again?' – just as some still do, 30 years on!

By then, I had discovered the wonders of plastic surgery, but its limits too. I had come to realise and accept that my face would never be the same again, and that I had to mourn my lost looks. But what I found far more difficult was that there was nothing and nobody available to help me deal with living with my disfigurement every day, in public places, meeting strangers, making friends, getting work, dealing with staring and discrimination (I had already been turned away from a restaurant).

Some nurses, and a few other professionals too, seemed to understand my everyday struggle and were willing to be seen with me in the street and pubs. Perhaps without realising what they were doing, that allowed me to experiment with how to behave, in their company, not isolated and alone.

Ironically, the hospital was famous for its rehabilitation centre for limbless people – Douglas Bader had got his tin legs there. And I found myself thinking about what psychosocial rehabilitation could be provided for people like me with disfigurements, from accidents or – as some of my fellow patients had acquired theirs – from cleft lips and palates, cancer surgery, birthmarks or facial paralysis. One of the senior nurses in the burns ward gave me the opportunity to write an article in autumn 1974 in the *QM Hospital Magazine* expressing these views (I still have a copy) – the real origin of Changing Faces.

Patients can be trying too

Nurses care for patients in so many different situations – and I am sure bring other assets to make their journeys more successful and less daunting. Sometimes too, patients are not as motivated as I was – nor do they always want to make decisions. In the case of serious terminal illness, patients lose their capacity to do even the most mundane things, relying on nurses to do virtually everything – indeed, almost fearing that they might do things wrongly even though they are able to do them – 'pyjama-induced paralysis', as it has been called.

Patients can also become tiresome, complaining about many little things – not the self-reliant 'expert patients' that are now revered. But most patients have a reason for their complaints, not least because we all have to put up with much indignity – being so physically close to other patients, hearing and smelling . . . It is not ideal. Nurses have to glean information too, often about parts of life that are otherwise private – and this can be humbling for both parties. Subtlety and tact are called for in spades. But firmness is too.

Summing up

Patients' journeys are made so much more dignified and civilised because of nurses. Nurses are the front line in all health care – the first human face that many patients see or sometimes only hear or feel, the first voice that gives them information, crucial to their map-referencing and reorientation. Nurses are vital companions on the journey ahead – playing many roles, TLC givers, translators, map readers, counsellors, stress relievers and advocates, with the pilot among them.

Being 'nursed well' is a joy – in the acute stage, the feel of clean sheets, cool linen, soft hands, washed hair, gentle words of encouragement, favourite food (pink blancmange after operations was mine) make you feel special. And later on too, the wise counsel, firm assurance and safe hands of rehabilitation and palliation guide us carefully to our journey's end, whatever that may be. Not that I wish to go on my particular journey again!

Acknowledgements

I would like to dedicate this chapter to all the nurses of the plastics and burns wards of Queen Mary's Hospital, Roehampton, London SW15, 1970–75, and also thank Alison Bartlett, Rosanna Le Cheminant and Claire Marley, all nurses past or present, for their very helpful comments on earlier drafts.

References

Clarke A and Cooper C (2000). Psychosocial rehabilitation after disfiguring injury or disease: investigating the training needs of specialist nurses. *Journal of Advanced Nursing*, **33**, 1–9.

Further reading

Changing Faces. www.changingfaces.org.uk.
Information about the Changing Faces training courses and study days for health professionals.

Partridge J (1990). *Changing Faces: The Challenge of Facial Disfigurement*. London: Penguin.
Now available from www.changingfaces.org.uk.

Partridge J (2006). From burns unit to board room. *British Medical Journal*, **332**, 956–9.

2 Being a nurse

Angela Barry

First year: my shaky 'foundation'

This chapter is a personal view of the journey into nursing. As I write it I am coming to the end of my time as a student nurse, sufficiently near to reaching my objective to evaluate the whole student experience, but not so far beyond it that I have donned rose-tinted spectacles. With or without those spectacles, this account is written from an individual perspective – but one that has naturally been influenced by the stories and experiences of my fellow students. It is written with a student – or potential student – readership in mind. However, it is not designed as a 'how to survive the ward' guide; nor is it packed with tips about pacing your work, passing exams or handing in the perfectly crafted essay. This guidance exists formally and informally throughout the student world.

So why read this chapter? After all, this is a textbook – one that I also picked off the shelf and chose carefully, among a few others, at the start of my studies. Perhaps the answer lies in those very textbooks; or perhaps the point is that it does not. Among the books on anatomy and biology, ethics and communication skills and all the other subjects that leapt out from a 3-year curriculum, what was missing, for me, was a voice that said 'This is what it was like, the experience of being a student nurse – at least, this is what it was like for me.'

Of course, everyone who enters nursing does so from a unique standpoint. I was looking not for a template on which to model my attitude, but rather something to reassure me that my moments of doubt, my moments of certainty, and the range of emotions that I encountered in between, were all valid. From where I am now, I can see that every one of those feelings, correctly identified and considered in context, is an important part of the learning process. Further, the means by which we identify our feelings, and learn how to channel them usefully, is a thread that can run through coherent nursing practice. On day one, however, the terms 'reflection', 'empathy' and even 'enquiry' would have seemed a generous way of describing my contradictory thoughts and my rather random attempts to clarify them. It is participation in the course itself that has furnished me with the tools to unpick and reframe my earlier feelings and to make sense of much of what happened next.

When I review my first few days and weeks as a student nurse, I see a universe that had shrunk to a single point of focus, only to be renewed and expanded by the 3 years that followed. That initial point of focus was myself, a fact to which I was almost completely blind. Like many of my colleagues, I am a mature student. The average age for joining the profession is currently mid-thirties, and this situation is by no means exclusive to the study of nursing. However, I have come to believe that for many who, as adults, choose a traditionally vocational course – such as nursing – the beginning of their chosen studies can also feel like the culmination of an earlier journey.

It took some years of stripping away the barriers to becoming a nurse, many of them self-imposed, before I finally found myself walking through the doors of a university. Some barriers were simple to identify – growing family, money and current career all featured and are easy for others to recognise, if not necessarily to empathise with. What were more difficult to reconcile were the issues concerning status, self-image and denial. I had to consider the prospect of becoming very 'junior' once more, taking instructions from others, quite probably much younger than myself, and being perceived, correctly, as a 'learner'. Ironically, with every year that passed, these difficulties appeared less and less important when compared with the damage that not acting on my instincts was starting to inflict. The fact remained that no amount of logic, or application of intellect, could remove the fundamental draw that nursing had always held for me. No matter how unfashionably self-regarding it was to think in terms of a 'calling' to a career, and no matter how much I dismissed my rather too comfortable 'dilemma', there was nursing, snapping at my heels and whispering in my ear.

I was eventually to concede that, if I did not act soon, it really would be too late. The prospect of looking back on a working life that had not encompassed my one constant ambition seemed too pathetic to contemplate. Entering nursing for me was a process of stripping away objections rather than building up a rationale, a process that I now recognise as common to many of my student colleagues. Some of us really do start out not so much with the enthusiasm of the single-minded, but with the acceptance that comes after a period of struggle with our instincts and counter-instincts. Looking back, it is hardly surprising that such an introspective progression meant that, by the time I started university, I had refined the whole of nursing into that single point of focus, a personal quest, with myself firmly at the centre. But at the centre of what, I had no idea.

Nor did that situation resolve itself overnight. Initially, getting to grips with the practicalities of a 3-year timetable, and attempting to formulate a picture of all that needed to be achieved, provided plenty of food for thought. From the outset we were taught the concepts of reflection and reflective practice and introduced to models of self-assessment to assist in this. We learned that, although, necessarily, there was a practical division between our academic learning and the learning acquired through our placements, reflection would provide the vital bridge and feedback mechanism between the two. In this way, nursing knowledge and nursing skills would achieve symbiosis, leading to personal practice that was greater than the sum of these component parts. I remember, quite clearly, being airily dismissive of the entire construct while cosily ensconced in the early, academic weeks of my foundation year. Then I had my first placement.

It would be fair to say that the university prepared us very thoroughly for our initial spell in a ward environment. We had been drilled extensively in a number of basic tasks to ensure that we had something practical to offer. The NMC Code (2004, updated 2008) had been mandatory reading, and our first essay was designed to demonstrate our understanding of its requirements. Additionally, in class, we had been given the space and time to explore any anxieties that our prospective placements had highlighted, for example the role of mentorship, our status as supernumerary, and so on. I was, I felt, ready for whatever would come my way.

The first task I was assigned on arriving at the ward was to assist a male patient who wished to take a shower. Anxious to impress, my head was full of all we had been taught – creating a hazard-free environment, ensuring the correct temperature, maintaining dignity and privacy – in fact, everything but the issue that presented itself. What I had not anticipated was the uninhibited way in which the patient undressed himself in my presence and then, without hesitation, directed the help he needed from me with this personal task. I had been wearing a nurse's uniform for 1 hour at this point, a detail of which the patient was unaware. That uniform did two closely linked things. It overrode for the patient the fact that I was previously unknown to him, and it acted as a visible manifestation of my profession and consequently my 'professionalism'. He therefore did not question my fitness to carry out a usually private act, such as washing him. His trust was immediate and, since I was a stranger, wholly invested in the generic of the uniform. It was an acknowledged symbol of an ethical, regulated, skilled and accountable profession and I was tacitly expected to embody these characteristics.

This was a timely lesson on my first day. Nursing wasn't all about me, my self-image or my personal mission. My training could not simply comprise the fragmented acquisition of a range of academic and practical skills, interpreted by me and applied in isolation. The different aspects of my learning needed to inform each other, to be placed in context or be rendered useless in the face of a real, live patient. This 'reflection' I had heard so much about suddenly seemed to make sense.

It is difficult to convey accurately the impact of what for me was a truly revelatory moment. The account I am writing confers the double-edged benefits of hindsight over what happened next. Without qualification, it could suggest that I immediately set myself a series of logical questions to assist in a personal reappraisal of the meaning of 'nursing' and my part in it. This, I have to record, is nonsense. What actually occurred was that I entered a period of sporadic, interior freefall throughout my first placement and beyond, using the roots and branches of the tasks I had learnt to provide the occasional toehold or an intermittent sense of tenuous stability.

It occurred to me, even as I wrote the preceding paragraph, that as one writes about reflection, one inevitably reflects. For example, I had never considered, until the moment in which that last sentence took shape, the possibility that the emphatic teaching of those basic tasks by the university was more than just a means of making us useful, or making us feel useful. Perhaps educational bodies are only too aware of the need that first-year students have for something practical to hold on to.

Gradually, over time, I now realise that I started to seek out answers before having clearly identified the questions. This, of course, did not invalidate the questions, particularly when they were confined to a repetitive inner dialogue and not for general consumption. However, it does acknowledge the difficulty in refining a mass of conflicting, personal thoughts into a tidy common coinage, while retaining an overall sense of the confusion that lies behind them. To summarise, I had focused on my personal relationship with nursing to the exclusion of any identifiable, external context. For example, what was required of a nurse and by whom? Who set the agenda, on the ward, in the school, nationally?

I had been metaphorically turned inside-out. The trigger for this shift was, indeed, as simple as that first encounter with a patient. Nonetheless, it took several stages of reflection and the acquisition of greater experience before I could link some of my ensuing lines of enquiry, and some of my subsequent choices, to that moment.

I began by discussing the experience with my mentor. That sounds straightforward enough, but two issues stood in the way. First was my inability at that stage in my training to concede that mentoring was really necessary. After all, hadn't I already taken the difficult decision to become a nurse? For goodness sake, I had the NMC Code and some textbooks – what else could I possibly need? Second was my confusion over what had actually taken place. The patient had been washed to his satisfaction, we had exchanged some pleasant dialogue and I had returned him successfully to his bedside. He had been completely unaware of the train of thought that his trusting actions had provoked – this train of thought being nothing more at that point than a series of unlabelled, inner responses.

On the first issue, my attitude to mentoring: I went into the initial meeting with my mentor, pushing before me every barrier that my complacency and arrogance had set up. In terms of being mentored, my personal Rome was not to be built in a day, and these negative aspects have continued to surface, from time to time, right up to the present. On the second issue, the incident in question: clearly it would not have been sufficient for me to sit down and announce to my mentor that a male patient had removed his clothes and that 'I had some feelings about this'. In preparing for the meeting I decided that I needed to pin down exactly what I had felt, what those thoughts and feelings had revealed and what I should consider doing next. In other words, I had begun to reflect.

By the time I met formally with my mentor, reflection had helped me to deconstruct, and therefore to relate, what had happened. I was able to say that the incident had usefully illustrated for me the automatic expectations associated with a nursing uniform, and the corresponding responsibility to meet those expectations. It had also underlined that safe nursing practice was not just about physical tasks and practically based health and safety precautions; it was also about recognising situations where abuse may occur – staff-to-client, client-to-staff, staff-to-staff – through the trust that is placed in the visible, but arguably superficial, symbols of professionalism, such as a uniform.

My early, tentative moves towards turning my focus outwards arose directly from this meeting and began with a look at how the ward 'philosophy' could be related to my reflection. Perhaps, my mentor suggested rather tactfully, I was not the first person to have had these thoughts. The ward, in common with the rest of the hospital, used a well-known model of nursing as the framework for care delivery. It is not necessary to describe the features of the model in question, except to note that, like most nursing models in current practice, it is thought to have both its relative strengths and weaknesses. In an attempt to provide a more holistic basis for reflection and care, the ward philosophy sought to develop nursing practice beyond a simple synopsis of the main features of the model. The expanded scope of the philosophy clearly responded to some limitations in the hospital's model of choice and sought to redress these by introducing elements based on staff group reflection, some of it qualitative and some of it based on practical empirical outcomes. For example, pertinent to my own experience and the resulting reflections concerning potential abuse, there was a section describing how, when people are unwell, they can lack their usual discretionary powers and may, as a consequence, become vulnerable. It went on to detail how such vulnerability could be manifested and the corresponding behaviours expected of a staff member in such an event. Because these behaviours were tailored specifically to the real-life, built environment of the ward, as well as to its primary medical specialism, they appeared persuasive and to have integrity.

The existence of a documented and accessible philosophy demonstrated to me that the nurses on the ward were not working in isolation. They were not self-consciously 'being nurses', a position that I was in danger of adopting. Rather, they were nursing as part of a coherent structure, which in turn, as I gradually came to learn, reflected the priorities of a number of ever larger structures – the hospital, the strategic health authority, the nursing profession, and so on.

Reflection is often described as a cyclical process (e.g. see Bulman and Schutz, 2004). I have returned to this early experience, and my attempts to make sense of it, several times during the course of my training. Inevitably, with each layer of refinement, something about the initial 'gut' reaction is lost. However, I still view it as the catalyst that prompted me to consider what it means to provide and manage fundamental, human care within an ethical framework.

For some reading this chapter, it will have been precisely those considerations that drew them to the profession of nursing in the first place. Others, in choosing nursing as a career, will have achieved a tidy balance between internal and external drivers. But only a few will pass through their training without experiencing at least one moment when their preconceptions are turned upside-down and revealed, possibly for the first time, as preconceptions.

By the time I returned to university I had started to identify the lines of enquiry that I wished to follow. Prompted by being back in the classroom, I began by asking myself whether I was being taught correctly, as opposed to 'learning' correctly, and by what yardstick this was measured. Another example of my arrogance? Perhaps, but please bear with me! These questions should not be misinterpreted. Currently, and indeed for some time, there has been debate within the nursing profession concerning the need to move away from teaching-centred to learning-centred models of nursing education. Today's students of nursing are being educated in a health care climate of growing complexity and innovation. This should be reflected formally, within university curricula, and also in the establishment of a common approach to learning, shared by educators and students alike. The general move towards enquiry-based learning supports the necessary shift in emphasis away from the passive acquisition of knowledge but arguably needs to be augmented by other, innovative methods of teaching. The increasing availability of information and communication technology to support learning is also driving this change.

You will doubtless form a view on this, as I have done, as you pass through your training. Indeed, you may conclude that how you strike a balance between 'being taught' and 'learning' will prefigure the sort of nurse that you will become. If this line of thought or enquiry should appeal to you, then a publication that has been very useful to me is *Professional Learning in Nursing* (Spouse, 2003). However, at the time that I was piecing together my lines of enquiry, the question of 'correct teaching' related solely to the standard and content of what I was being taught. I had done no research whatsoever before applying to a school of nursing, and my ignorance seems staggering to me now. For all I knew about the accountability, performance or relative quality of the school I was attending, the teaching staff could have been handing out leaflets from the back of a barrow while writing tomorrow's lecture. Clearly, as my recent ward experience had shown, this tunnel vision approach to learning was not going to allow me to make the most of my opportunities.

As luck would have it (or was it simply well-considered timing?), one of the first lectures on our return to the classroom concerned the governance structure of the university and the school of nursing. We were told that a steady flow of student representatives was needed for the various committees, sub-committees and working groups responsible for the standard of education and the quality of practice experience offered by the school and its partner trusts. The lecture, as well as being informative, was a recruitment drive for student volunteers. I put up my hand, alongside many others, and the subsequent attachment to a committee has been both interesting and illuminating.

I discovered that, far from operating in a vacuum, the school was subject to a continuous cycle of rigorous internal and external audit, designed to promote professional education and protect the public. Every aspect of the curriculum, indeed the curriculum itself, was scrutinised at intervals by professional and regulatory bodies, including government representatives and the NMC. The activities of the school, including those relating to student practice placements, were evaluated against a stringent set of quality standards. Supporting evidence was required to establish the relative effectiveness of the school and to demonstrate that policy was translated into practice. This evidence included documentation, interviews with staff and students and feedback pro forma. I learned that mentor support, student assessment in practice and theory, link lecturer support and quality of teaching were just a few of the factors considered in detail.

Membership of a committee does not appeal to everyone. It would, of course, be possible to unpick the workings of most schools, and their place in the wider academic and professional world, by looking at their websites or reading their literature. But if you sense that you would enjoy a more three-dimensional look at your place of training, or would seek to influence the future direction that it takes, then I recommend finding out about your local committee structure and your possible place on it.

Second year: our house in order?

It has proven to be less straightforward for me to make practical sense of the prevailing national agenda. Since this chapter represents a wholly personal perspective, I do not propose to write in depth about the consecutive government public health White Papers that have effectively book-ended the period of my training. It will be an essential part of your training to get to grips with the laudable intentions of these papers and to attempt to marry the everyday reality of nursing with the priorities and aspirations they espouse. For me, as I will describe, this exercise led to some conflict, most noticeably during my placement with a team of community nurses.

While working in the community, I began to evaluate how the contemporary national agenda related to the patients I visited, and to what extent it impacted on their physical and psychosocial well-being. The placement was an opportunity to set in context the knowledge that I had acquired in school about public health and the delivery of health-related services outside a standard, clinical environment. I came to realise that many of the issues I was encountering in the community, and the corresponding range of multiprofessional care designed to respond to these issues, could be linked to the public health White Papers *Saving Lives: Our Healthier Nation* (DH, 1999), *Choosing Health: Making Choices Easier* (DH, 2004) and *Our Health, Our Care, Our Say: A New Direction for Community Services* (DH, 2006).

As a second-year student nurse, I was becoming aware that the manner and emphasis of the care I sought to provide was influenced, consciously and unconsciously, by the relative importance placed on 'health', a concept that incorporates promotion and prevention initiatives, and 'health care', which implies, in part, dealing with the consequences of individual life 'choices'. This shifting emphasis existed in my theoretical learning but more influentially in what I began to observe in practice within the community.

Although each White Paper concentrated on reducing the health inequalities that impede free choice, for example those caused by poor education, bad housing or social exclusion, the later papers placed an increased importance on the contributions that individual choices make to public health. In this, they reflected the direction of *A Patient's Guide to the NHS* (DH, 2001), which moved away from the earlier 'patients' charter' approach and underscored the responsibility of the individual to promote their own health. The White Papers set targets that highlighted preventability and excellent health standards for all, not just the 'privileged few', thereby placing a firm contemporary focus on 'health' rather than 'health care'. The government expects to see this emphasis as an integrated aspect of local health care delivery and describes the need to reorient the NHS to achieve this end. The targets are considered tough, but attainable by 2010 – provided, as the papers describe, that people, communities and government work together in partnership.

Health professionals practising today, and students within health disciplines, are working or learning beyond the chronological mid-point predicted for the achievement of these targets. Services are being provided to an increasingly better informed society, and one that has arguably become less tolerant of those who deviate from widely accepted standards – for example, smokers. But the concomitant changes required to eradicate health inequalities, and to facilitate unhindered choice for all, are lagging behind. Additionally, what of those who reject health standards that are set by others, or who grew up with certain expectations of 'health care' and have no wish to change their views later in life?

During my attachment to the community nursing team, I frequently encountered patients whose illnesses, if not a direct consequence of their lifestyle choices, were certainly exacerbated by them. The current health agenda, detailed across recent National Service Frameworks, sets prescriptive targets for a reduction in the 'four main killers' – cancer, coronary heart disease and stroke, accidents and mental illness. The composition of the multiprofessional community team to which I was attached reflected these priorities and offered services that were undoubtedly of potential benefit to many of the patients in the community. Often a suggestion to a patient that, for example, input from a smoking cessation nurse or a dietician could be useful was greeted with enthusiasm and willingly taken up. Occasionally, however, such suggestions were far from welcome and the patient would make it clear that their priorities lay elsewhere entirely.

My conversations with or about the latter group of patients provided good material for reflection during the second year of training. I reflected on the tension between delivering care that was driven by the extant requirements or aspirations of society, while at the same time attempting to respect the autonomy of individual patients. Respect for autonomy, we had been taught, was a requirement of the NMC Code and arose from the concept of basic, unassailable human rights. Many patients who declined additional health input were demonstrably aware of the impact that their smoking, or obesity, or alcohol intake was having on their life. There appeared to be no doubt that in opting not to conform to the advice of health professionals, they were doing so from a position of fully informed decision-making.

This was difficult. It was clear to me that, despite being aware of the potential consequences, some people, to use the language of the prevailing agenda, were 'making choices' that the health professions would not generally consider to be in their best interests. But surely we should have been more persuasive? Perhaps forced them to reconsider? After all, it was for their own good, wasn't it? That debate alone could occupy your entire period of training, particularly once you start to include the impact of cultural considerations and the fact that the majority of care is delivered to people in their own homes or the immediate local environment.

For me, reflection on this subject has been open-ended, since the wider I searched for an answer the more difficult the question became. Beneficence may be regarded by some as a superior principle to autonomy. There is, I think, great truth in the claim that acts that interfere with the autonomy of others are routinely justified by the assertion that such acts are for the benefit of those being interfered with.

I have continued to consider how this last reflection can be usefully applied when it is the drive of a national agenda that is interfering with the free choice or 'autonomy' of individuals. Throughout training, student nurses encounter many definitions of 'health', including those that question the possibility of any wholly autonomous standpoint. So the question is inevitably posed: in matters of health, to what extent can an individual ever exercise free choice? Although no answers were to be gained from my community placement, it was instrumental in stimulating an interesting strand of reflection that has followed me into my third and final year.

Third year: the key to the door

As the end of my training approaches the employment situation is looking noticeably different from the way it appeared at the outset. One advantage of being an older student is that I have seen the balance of supply and demand in the nursing profession alter several times during the course of my working life. Consequently, during the current period of reduced recruitment and cut-backs, I am able to retain a longer view of what the next few years will bring. I remain optimistic, and not simply as a result of understanding the ebb and flow of the employment tide.

My optimism also relates to some aspects of a nurse's training that do not appear under the subject headings of the curriculum. I have already described the blinkered way in which I embarked upon my training. If I had been asked during my foundation year what I wished to do upon achieving my qualification, my answer would certainly have been restricted to the pursuit of one or two specific nursing disciplines. I would have argued quite strongly that job satisfaction lay almost entirely in the subject matter, without giving any thought to the working environment or the method of delivery. A third-year ward placement changed all that.

When I received the details of the ward in question, I greeted the news neutrally. It was, as expected, a medical placement, since the specific learning module to which the placement was attached included a formal assessment of safe practice in drug administration. I had already undertaken several placements, including my elective placement, at the hospital concerned and had picked up a little information about the ward. Its specialist concerns were gastrointestinal conditions and rheumatology – interesting areas, but neither one related particularly to the direction I saw myself taking. The ward patient group closely represented the demography of the immediate location of the hospital, an area high on the social deprivation index with widespread street drinking and homelessness problems. Many patients were well known to the staff, having been on a cycle of admission, stabilisation and management, followed by readmission, over a number of years. I had heard, during my earlier placements at the hospital, that the workload on the ward was heavy, both practically and emotionally. I approached the placement with an open mind, but also with a sense of pragmatism. It was, I thought at one level, simply the next phase to be passed through.

What followed was an exhilarating and inspirational 10 weeks. The reasons for this were slow to unfold and were pieced together over time, largely through my attempts to describe to others just what had made the placement so special. The staff group was as diverse, and the access to resources as uncertain, as any other ward I had experienced. So just what was it that made my stay there so special? In summary, the ward was a testament to the power of good leadership, strong teamwork and the establishment of a common purpose.

As the ward went about its day-to-day business, there was no covert pecking order of tasks. What needed to be done was done, and by whoever was free and suitably qualified to undertake the job. That and a real commitment to that misused adage 'unconditional positive regard' were the simple twin concepts upon which the ward was built.

The sight of a senior nurse or ward sister washing a patient just admitted from the streets, making up the numbers when it came to stripping beds or feeding those who were very frail sent out extremely strong messages about the value of such tasks. Consequently, no health care assistant and no student ever felt that their roles were defined by what the qualified or senior staff did not care to do. All nursing actions had value, and that value was conferred by the priorities of the patients, rather than any notional hierarchy based on the relative complexity of the jobs to be completed.

Every morning, the senior nurse on duty would greet each patient and take a little time to exchange a few remarks that reinforced their individuality and tacitly demonstrated interest and respect. It is impossible to overstate the benefit that this had on a group that routinely included several people whose general status and condition had caused them to become marginalised in the wider world. It was also just one of several instances of leading by example, and setting a creditable benchmark for all staff to follow, which were the hallmarks of the ward.

The placement was, as predicted, physically very hard and every shift seemed to bring a different challenge. The nights were emotionally demanding. The ward could seem a very lonely environment for patients struggling with the confusion that accompanied withdrawal from alcohol or drugs. For the first time, I truly understood the expression 'to be beside yourself'. I also learnt some very profound lessons concerning what it is to be human, and the requirement of every nurse to identify and nurture that spark of humanity in people who are in a dark and possibly frightening place. The 'common purpose' of the ward was founded on this requirement and provided not only a unifying factor for the staff but also a great support for any students assigned to the ward. There is a sense of confidence to be gained from a workplace that sends out a consistent message, regardless of which member of staff is spoken to.

By the time the placement ended, my thoughts regarding what constituted job satisfaction had altered completely. My priorities are now concerned far more with finding a ward or working environment with an ethos similar to the one I have described. To start my nursing career in such a setting would seem to offer and encourage almost limitless possibilities.

In concluding this chapter, I am much less conscious of what I have written than of what I have not. I have certainly lived through quite concerted periods during which I have seriously questioned the wisdom of my decision to become a nurse. The fact that I have continued on the path is a testament to the very positive times during my training that have provided a counter-balance. In this account, I have deliberately avoided adhering solely to incidents that have been related to individual patients. In part, this is because I am aware that, as a student, my feelings and reflections are buffered by my limited accountability and restricted by my limited experience.

But I will share one last incident with you, the one to which I return each time I evaluate my fitness to enter the nursing profession. It is three in the morning. I am working alone in a dimly lit side-room, taking the observations of an elderly lady who has been drifting in and out of consciousness for several days. As I quietly count her respirations, she suddenly opens her eyes and clasps my hand with a strength that is quite unexpected. 'Nurse,' she says, 'Am I all right?' I am momentarily startled, but I immediately sense the multiple layers of what she is asking me. I feel out of my depth, I feel inadequate to the task. But, most of all, I feel privileged to be there and, as I answer, that is my starting point.

References

Bulman C and Schutz S (eds) (2004). *Reflective Practice in Nursing*, 3rd edn. Oxford: Blackwell.

Department of Health (DH) (1999). *Saving Lives: Our Healthier Nation*. London: HMSO.

Department of Health (DH) (2001). *A Patient's Guide to the NHS*. London: HMSO.

Department of Health (DH) (2004). *Choosing Health: Making Choices Easier*. London: HMSO.

Department of Health (DH) (2006). *Our Health, Our Care, Our Say: A New Direction for Community Services*. London: HMSO.

Nursing and Midwifery Council (NMC) (2008). *The Code: Standards of Conduct, Performance and Ethics for Nurses and Midwives*. London: Nursing and Midwifery Council.

Spouse J (2003). *Professional Learning in Nursing*. Oxford: Blackwell.

What is nursing?

June Clark

Introduction

It's a strange thing. Nursing is experienced at some time in their lives by almost everybody. Millions of people in every country in the world do it every day. The first chapter in this book has described one person's account of how it feels to experience nursing care; the second chapter gives the perceptions of someone who is just beginning to nurse. If you search the literature you will find thousands of books and articles that have tried to define or describe nursing. Few have managed to capture its richness and complexity. In 1859 Florence Nightingale wrote 'I use the word nursing for want of a better' and 'The very elements of nursing are all but unknown' (Nightingale, 1859).

Almost 150 years later nursing is still difficult to define and is still poorly understood.

Learning objectives

After studying this chapter you should be able to:

- give an account of what nursing involves;
- describe nursing accurately as you understand it now;
- evaluate a range of different definitions of nursing;
- state the value of nursing diagnoses;
- analyse the components of the 2003 Royal College of Nursing (RCN) definition of nursing;
- develop your own personal concept of nursing.

Defining nursing

Dictionary definitions of nursing don't help very much. Most begin with 'suckling an infant'. Those that refer to nursing as an occupation or profession do so in terms that are much more limited than 'real' nursing. For example, they talk about 'caring for the sick and injured' and 'assisting doctors'. As we shall see, nursing is concerned with health and healthy people as much as it is with sickness and sick people, and it includes coordinating care provided by a team of people, teaching (patients, their carers and other nurses), managing services, undertaking research and developing health policy, as well as providing hands-on care. Modern nurses would certainly reject the idea that nursing is primarily about 'assisting doctors'. The tenth edition of the *Concise Oxford Dictionary* has simply given up: it does not give a definition at all but merely lists 'nursing' as a derivative of the noun 'nurse'.

However, it is important to recognise that the question 'What is nursing?' is not the same as 'What is a nurse?'. The question 'What is a nurse?' is relatively easy to answer: in most countries a nurse is defined as a person who has undertaken a specific educational programme that entitles him or her to practise legally as a nurse in that particular country. In the UK, as in many other countries, the title 'registered nurse' is protected in law and may be used only by those who have so qualified. But just as not all teaching is done by teachers, so 'nursing' is done by many people – relatives, other informal carers and a variety of care assistants. Moreover, as we shall see later, the idea that 'nursing is what nurses do' dangerously limits our understanding.

Public perceptions may be similarly limited. The stereotypes begin early. Little girls still dress up in a uniform with a white apron and a frilly cap, while the little boys pretend to be doctors.

Some people still think that all male nurses are gay. Most people associate nursing with the physical tasks of keeping a sick person – usually a sick person in hospital – safe, comfortable, nourished and clean. Some see nursing as carrying out tasks associated with medical treatment. Although both of these things are indeed part of nursing practice, they are certainly not the whole picture.

How patients see nursing is in fact surprisingly difficult to discover. There are many anecdotal accounts, but there is not much research. Nurses' views, and nurses' views of patients' views, may not be the same as patients' views. A study undertaken by von Essen and Sjoden (2003) reviewed and confirmed the findings of several other studies that what patients thought was important about nursing differed considerably from nurses' views: while nurses emphasised the psychosocial aspects of caring, patients were more concerned with 'competent clinical know-how'. Darbyshire and Gordon (2005) recount an interview with a patient who praised the nurses because 'they were always there', but when the interviewer explained what else the nurses did the patient was stunned: 'I didn't know nurses did all that' she said.

Media portrayals are often less than helpful. In recent years some television programmes, such as *Casualty*, have tried to portray a more realistic image, but there are still examples of the traditional stereotypes of nurses as 'angel, battleaxe, handmaiden or whore' (Jinks and Bradley, 2003). There is a considerable literature that documents and analyses media images of nursing (e.g. Kalish and Kalish, 1987; Bridges, 1990; Darbyshire and Gordon, 2005).

Does it matter?

But does it matter? Do we really need to be able to define nursing – can't we just do it? Yes, it does matter, and we do need to be able to define it – or at least to be able to describe it accurately – for several reasons.

First, people have a right to know what they can expect from a professional nurse. The RCN says:

> *It is part of the social mandate of a profession to make clear to the public the nature of the service it offers . . . This is the basis of the relationship of trust between the profession and the public it serves and between the individual professional and the patient to whom the professional owes a 'duty of care'.*

(RCN, 2003)

Second, as the same document continues:

> *Governments and providers of health care have to ensure that that the most effective mix of staff is giving care in the most cost-effective way, and they need to utilise their major resource efficiently and effectively.*

(RCN, 2003)

In our present-day health care system, in which services are commissioned and provided through contracts, specifying exactly what is to be provided is very important. This specification enables the variety of providers to be monitored against key quality indicators and benchmarks.

It is not only the commissioners who have an interest in the specification of what services are to be provided and at what quality; as Darbyshire and Gordon (2005) point out: 'If the public does not understand the breadth and complexity of nursing work, it cannot fight for the social and financial resources that allow nurses to do that work.'

Similarly, 'If you can't name it, you can't control it, finance it, teach it, research it, or put it into public policy' (Clark and Lang, 1992).

This quotation refers to the importance of using standardised terminology to describe nursing and is discussed in more detail in Chapter 11.

The third, and perhaps most important, reason is the recognition that every nurse holds in her head what Henderson (1978) called 'a personal concept of nursing' – what it is, what it is for and how to do it. This personal concept – private because we rarely share it with other people – influences, or even determines, how each nurse practises. The purpose of this chapter is to help you to develop your own personal concept.

Reflection point 3.1

Stop and think for a moment about what your personal concept of nursing is. Has it changed from when you were at school? First thought about studying to be a nurse? From your first clinical placement?

It is likely that it will have changed and may well have become more complex rather than clearer. Don't worry about this. It will almost certainly change several times throughout your career – in fact I would worry if it stayed stagnant! It would be good to reflect on this from time to time and maybe keep your concepts so that you can look back on them later and trace the progress of your thinking.

Some classic definitions

Let's begin with what some other people have said.

Florence Nightingale

Florence Nightingale is recognised as the founder of modern nursing. In 1859 she published a little book called *Notes on Nursing: What It Is and What It Is Not*. It was written not as a textbook for nurses but 'simply to give hints for thoughts to women who have personal charge of the health of others' (Nightingale, 1859).

In this small book, and in other publications (she was a prolific writer), Nightingale set out her thoughts about nursing in ways that, more than a century later, and in spite of the enormous changes that have taken place in nursing and health care since then, still capture much of the essence of nursing. For example:

> *Experience teaches me that nursing and medicine must never be mixed up. It spoils both.*
>
> (Letter to Dr Henry Ackland, 1869)

> *Nature alone cures . . . And what nursing has to do in either case is to put the patient in the best position for nature to act upon him.*
>
> (Nightingale, 1859)

> *Every day sanitary knowledge, or the knowledge of nursing, or in other words, of how to put the constitution in such a state that it will have no disease, takes a higher place.*
>
> (Nightingale, 1859)

> *I use the word nursing for want of a better. It has been limited to signify little more than the administration of medicines and the application of poultices. It ought to signify the proper use of fresh air, light, warmth, cleanliness, quiet, and the proper selection and administration of diet – all at the least expense of vital power to the patient.*
>
> (Nightingale, 1859)

So, even in 1859, some important ideas about nursing were established:

- Nursing is different from, and not a sub-division of, medicine.
- Nursing focuses on the patient, not on the disease.
- Nursing is concerned with health, not only with sickness.
- Nursing is more than specific tasks.

Virginia Henderson

Probably the best known definition of nursing is the one developed a century later by Virginia Henderson. In 1960 this definition of nursing was adopted by the International Council of Nurses, and it is still the most widely and internationally used definition of nursing. The best known part of Henderson's definition is her description of 'the unique function of the nurse'

to assist the individual, sick or well, in the performance of those activities contributing to health or its recovery (or to peaceful death) that he would perform unaided if he had the necessary strength, will, or knowledge. And to do this in such a way as to help him gain independence as rapidly as possible.

(Henderson, 1960)

This definition, like that of Nightingale's, emphasises health and its recovery and facilitates independence and self-care. This part of Henderson's definition, which is the part usually quoted, refers to the nurse's *independent* function: 'This aspect of her work, this part of her function, she initiates and controls; of this she is master'.

However, this is only the first part of Henderson's definition. She continues:

In addition she helps the patient to carry out the therapeutic plan as initiated by the physician.

She also as a member of a team, helps others as they in turn help her, to plan and carry out the total program whether it be for the improvement of health, or recovery from illness, or support in death.

(Henderson, 1960)

This distinction between dependent, independent and interdependent practice is critical to understanding the complexity of nursing and its particular contribution within the multiprofessional health care team.

Like Nightingale, Henderson did not set out to define nursing. In a seminal article based on a lecture she gave in London in 1977, she reviewed other people's definitions and described her own as her own 'personal concept' (Henderson, 1978). Later, she wrote:

I would like to emphasis that I am not presenting my point of view as one with which I expect you to agree. Rather I would urge every nurse to develop her own concept, otherwise she is merely imitating others or acting under authority.

(Henderson, 1991)

Although Henderson's definition is still the most widely used, it has been criticised as limiting nursing to the physical care of individuals and not including families or communities, which are the focus of the care of community and public health nurses. It is true that nursing practice has changed and expanded a great deal since the 1960s, and much of the criticism is due to an exclusive concentration on the 'unique function' part of her definition, but, as Henderson points out, personal concepts develop over time and change as the result of experience. In 1991 she wrote: 'I do wish people would stop talking about that book as though my concept of nursing stopped developing over 20 years ago!' (Henderson, 1991).

Other perspectives

Meanwhile, by the early 1970s, thinking about nursing had moved on considerably, especially in the USA, where several nursing theorists (mainly nurse teachers) were trying to analyse the concept of nursing and to develop what have become known as 'nursing models', primarily to find ways of teaching about nursing to students. Some of these are described in more detail in Chapter 12. These 'grand theories' (e.g. Rogers' (1970) 'science of unitary man', Roy's (1970) 'adaptation theory', Orem's (1971) theory of 'self care deficits' and King's (1971) 'human interaction' theory), and the more operational 'practice theories' (e.g. Travelbee, 1966; Orlando, 1972; Roper *et al.*, 1985), are still sometimes used to help nurses to focus on the goals of their nursing care and to provide frameworks for patient assessment.

Another approach that began around this time focused on identifying and naming the conditions that nurses know about and treat – nursing diagnoses – which are analogous to the diseases that doctors know about and treat – medical diagnoses. In all disciplines, identifying, naming and classifying their 'phenomena of concern' is the first step in developing their knowledge base – for example, the development of the periodic table in chemistry, or the classification of species and varieties of plants in botany. In 1973 a conference was held in St Louis, Missouri, USA, to try to identify, define and classify a list of nursing diagnoses; 10 years later this became the North American Nursing Diagnosis Association (NANDA), which is now an international organisation (NANDA-I) with members in many countries. The NANDA-I taxonomy of nursing diagnoses is updated and published every 2 years (NANDA International, 2007) and is translated into several languages and used all over the world. Nurses in the UK have until now shied away from formally using the term 'nursing diagnoses' or the NANDA-I terminology – perhaps held back by the old-fashioned idea that 'only doctors diagnose'. The truth is that all professionals 'diagnose' their clients' problems in order to decide what to do to solve them; the only difference is in the type of 'problems' that they diagnose, which in turn depends upon their knowledge base. Peplau (1987) defined nursing diagnoses simply as 'the problems that nurses fix'. Now, however, the requirements for computerising patient information in electronic health records are forcing UK nurses to reconsider their approach (see Chapter 11), and the NANDA-I terminology is incorporated in the standardised terminology (Systematised Nomenclature of Medicine – Clinical Terms – better known as SNOMED-CT) that will in future be the required language for all electronic health information in the National Health Service (NHS).

In the USA, nursing (that is, what nurses are allowed and not allowed to do) is defined legally in each state's Nurse Practice Act. In 1972 the New York State Nurse Practice Act defined nursing as

diagnosing and treating human responses to actual or potential health problems through such services as case finding, health teaching, health counselling, and provision of care supportive to and restorative of life and wellbeing.

At about the same time, the American Nurses Association (ANA) used this definition as the basis for its work on developing Standards for Nursing Practice – work that was echoed a decade later in the UK. The first Standards (ANA, 1973) were:

1. *The collection of data about the health status of the client is systematic and continuous; the data are accessible, communicated and recorded*

2. *Nursing diagnoses are derived from the health status data*
3. *The plan of nursing care includes goals derived from the nursing diagnoses*
4. *The plan of nursing care includes priorities and the prescribed nursing approaches or measures to achieve the goals derived from the nursing diagnoses*
5. *Nursing actions provide for patient/client participation in health promotion, maintenance and restoration*
6. *Nursing actions assist the client/patient to maximise his health capabilities*
7. *The client/patient's progress or lack of progress towards goal achievement is determined by the client/patient and the nurse*
8. *The client/patient's progress or lack of progress towards goal achievement directs re-assessment, re-ordering of priorities, new goal setting and revision of the plan of nursing care.*

The exact wording of the ANA Standards has been updated several times since 1973, but the core remains unchanged. In 1980 the ANA published a seminal document entitled *Nursing: A Social Policy Statement* (ANA, 1980), which included the following definition of nursing: 'Nursing is the diagnosis and treatment of human responses to actual or potential health problems.'

The Standards and the 1980 definition maintain the four key concepts identified above in Nightingale's definition, but in addition they emphasise the process of clinical decision-making (diagnosis and treatment), which is the core of professional practice but had not been made explicit in earlier definitions. They also make explicit the distinction between nursing and medicine first expressed by Nightingale by identifying the knowledge domain of nursing as not the disease but the person's responses.

By 1997, 42 of the 51 states of the USA were using these concepts in their nursing legislation, and in 1987 the definition was incorporated into the definition used by the International Council of Nurses.

It is sometimes suggested that these definitions 'intellectualise' nursing and lead to a neglect of 'basic nursing care' – the part of nursing that Henderson called 'the unique function of the nurse'. Indeed, the media has used phrases such as 'too posh to wash' and 'too clever to care'. Some people have suggested that the use of the term 'basic' to describe this aspect of nursing care devalues it, and they prefer the term 'fundamental'.

In an effort to re-establish the value of this part of nursing, an initiative called *Essence of Care* in England and *Fundamentals of Care* in Wales is refocusing nurses' attention on aspects of care such as patients' nutrition, hygiene and comfort needs.

The Royal College of Nursing 'Defining Nursing' project

In 2003 the RCN began a project to develop a definition of nursing that could be used by nurses to:

- describe nursing to people who do not understand it;
- clarify their role in the multiprofessional health care team;
- influence the policy agenda at local and national level;
- develop educational curricula;
- identify areas where research is needed to strengthen the knowledge base of nursing;
- inform decisions about whether and how nursing work should be delegated to other personnel;
- support negotiations at the local and national levels on issues such as nurse staffing, skill mix and nurses' pay.

Until this time it had not been thought necessary, or even desirable, in the UK to develop a definition of nursing. Indeed, in 1999 the United Kingdom Central Council for Nursing, Midwifery and Health Visiting (UKCC) had said that it was sceptical about the usefulness of trying to arrive at a definition and had concluded that 'a definition of nursing would be too restrictive for the profession'.

By 2003, however, a number of factors were becoming important. Cost-containment measures and a shortage of registered nurses were leading to skill-mix changes in which work formerly undertaken by nurses was being transferred to lesser qualified (and therefore cheaper) staff. At the same time, nurses were also under pressure to take on work that was formerly undertaken by doctors. It was important to patient safety, as well as to nursing as a profession, to be able to distinguish between the role of the registered nurse and the equally valuable but different role of the health care assistant, and to identify the particular contribution of nursing to medical tasks. The final trigger was the UK government decision in 2001 that nursing care should be funded through the NHS and free of charge to the user at the point of delivery, while 'social care' should be provided through local authorities and therefore means tested – implementation of this policy required a definition that distinguished between the two.

The work was undertaken by a small steering group and included wide consultation with RCN members. The definition was derived from a values clarification exercise (Warfield and Manley, 1990) in which participants were asked to complete and think about the following sentences:

1. *I believe that the purpose of nursing is . . .*
2. *I believe that this purpose is achieved by . . .*
3. *I believe that nursing knowledge is about . . .*

Reflection point 3.2
Try to answer the three questions above for yourself.
Your answers may depend a lot on the experiences to which you have been exposed so far in your course – and there is no one correct answer.

You might have thought that the purpose of nursing is to improve the health of the local community or to help someone who is dying to achieve a 'good death', without pain or anxiety and surrounded by loved ones at home.

You might feel that this purpose could be achieved by nurses undertaking specialist education and the development of more nurse-led services.

You might think that nursing knowledge is about using knowledge and skills from a range of disciplines to inform solutions to complex patient problems and to develop clinical judgement.

The definition that emerged (RCN, 2003) is expressed in the form of a core supported by six defining characteristics, as shown in Figure 3.1 (page 26) and Box 3.1. It is important to recognise that nursing is the totality: although some parts are shared with other health care professions, the uniqueness of nursing lies in their combination. Nursing is rather like a cake – the uniqueness is not in the individual ingredients (e.g. flour, butter, sugar, milk, egg) but in the way they are combined and in the chemical changes that take place when they are cooked together (e.g. to produce pastry or a Victoria sponge).

The core: clinical judgement

Nursing is the use of clinical judgement in the provision of care to enable people to improve, maintain or recover health.

There are many ways of looking at nursing – as an activity, an occupation, a profession or an academic discipline. The most common approach to defining nursing is by describing 'what nurses

BOX 3.1 The RCN definition of nursing

Nursing is the use of clinical judgement in the provision of care to enable people to improve, maintain or recover health, to cope with health problems, and to achieve the best possible quality of life, whatever their disease or disability, until death.

It has the following defining characteristics:

- *A particular purpose*: to promote health, healing, growth and development, and to prevent disease, illness, injury and disability. When people become ill or disabled, the purpose of nursing is, in addition, to minimise distress and suffering and to enable people to understand and cope with their disease or disability, its treatment and its consequences. When death is inevitable, the purpose of nursing is to maintain the best possible quality of life until its end.
- *A particular mode of intervention*: nursing interventions are concerned with empowering people and helping them to achieve, maintain or recover independence. Nursing is an intellectual, physical, emotional and moral process that includes the identification of nursing needs; therapeutic interventions and personal care; information, education, advice and advocacy; and physical, emotional and spiritual support. In addition to direct patient care, nursing practice includes management, teaching, and policy and knowledge development.
- *A particular domain*: the specific domain of nursing is people's unique responses to and experience of health, illness, frailty, disability and health-related life events, in whatever environment or circumstances they find themselves. People's responses may be physiological, psychological, social, cultural or spiritual and are often a combination of all of these. The term 'people' includes individuals of all ages, families and communities, throughout the entire lifespan.
- *A particular focus*: the focus of nursing is the whole person and the human response rather than a particular aspect of the person or a particular pathological condition.
- *A particular value base*: nursing is based on ethical values that respect the dignity, autonomy and uniqueness of human beings, the privileged nurse–patient relationship, and the acceptance of personal accountability for decisions and actions. These values are expressed in written codes of ethics and supported by a system of professional regulation.
- *A commitment to partnership*: nurses work in partnership with patients, their relatives and other carers, and in collaboration with others as members of a multiprofessional team. Where appropriate, they will lead the team, prescribing, delegating and supervising the work of others; at other times, they will participate under the leadership of others. At all times, however, they remain personally and professionally accountable for their own decisions and actions.

Reproduced with kind permission of the Royal College of Nursing.

do' in terms of roles, functions and tasks. This approach sees nursing as a collection of activities – skilled activities that require some training and must be undertaken with care and compassion – but activities that are derived from the orders, decisions, purposes and knowledge base of other disciplines, usually medicine. This is the 'nursing as doing' model, which is the dominant stereotype of nursing held by the public, doctors and many nurses. This approach is inadequate because it limits the concept of nursing to hands-on care and because 'who does what', especially in health care, is determined by circumstances and changes over time. Many tasks now undertaken routinely by nurses were once the prerogative of doctors. There was a time when taking a patient's blood pressure was exclusively a medical task; for many years it has been a core nursing task; with the advent of electronic measuring devices it is becoming a task that may be delegated to a health care assistant; and many patients now routinely measure and monitor their own blood pressure. The shortage of doctors, whether in the UK because of EU regulations about maximum working hours, or in

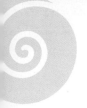
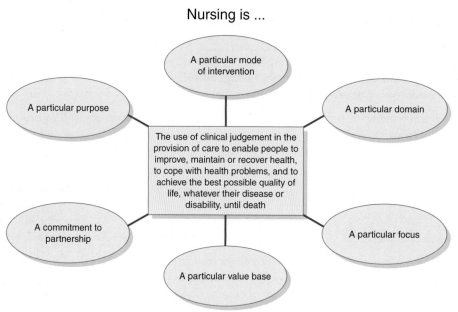

Figure 3.1 The RCN definition of nursing. Reproduced with kind permission of the Royal College of Nursing.

rural Africa because there are no doctors available, means that nurses take on complicated technical procedures, including surgery and the prescribing of drugs. With specific training and enough practice, almost anyone can do almost any task. Even very complex tasks can be achieved if they are broken down into small pieces.

In health care, however, this approach may be dangerous. For example, a person may learn the technique of measuring a patient's blood pressure, but they may not understand that a particular set of numbers indicates that the patient is unwell or at risk or may not be able to relate the blood pressure measurement to other observations or other factors relating to the particular individual in order to take action to prevent a life-threatening situation. The (true) story contained in Box 3.2 illustrates how this can happen.

This approach also negates the concept of nursing as an autonomous profession or as an academic discipline. If nursing can be reduced to a series of tasks, albeit requiring skill and undertaken with compassion in a caring relationship, then it follows that the nurse is no more than the agent of the person who has the knowledge and authority to decide whether and how the task is to be undertaken. This model of nursing is the basis of the image of the nurse as the 'doctor's handmaiden'. In this model nurses just need a strong stomach, a caring heart and a modicum of practical training. They do not need a university education, as other health professionals have, and they certainly do not need to know about things such as research and theory. The frontier is marked by a signpost that says: 'To knowledge: no nurses past this point'.

The alternative approach sees nursing as the decision-making that guides and determines the activities – the judgements about the nature of the presenting problem and the decisions about what should be done about it. This does not in any way underestimate or devalue the activities or tasks, or the degree of skill required to perform them, but it suggests that their rightness and their success depend fundamentally upon the thinking behind them. This approach focuses on

BOX 3.2 Tickbox nursing: the risks of the 'nursing is doing' model

A while ago my husband was admitted to an accident and emergency department with severe breathing difficulties. (It turned out to be late-onset asthma, but we didn't know that until some time later.) At the point of admission, his vital signs were recorded and he was given oxygen and salbutamol; within a short time he was feeling much better, and he was transferred to a ward. Soon it was time for the routine task of 'doing the obs'.

Nowadays, of course, this task is computerised, and because 'the machine does all the work' the task was, in this hospital, delegated to a health care assistant. She put the sensor on my husband's finger to measure his 'sats' (oxygenation saturation level) and wrote down on the bit of paper she was carrying the figure that appeared on the screen. I could see that the figure was considerably lower than that recorded at the point of admission – indeed, dangerously low. As the health care assistant was about to move on to the next patient, I pointed this out to her, saying that I didn't think the figure could be right, but what was she going to do about it? 'Oh', she said, 'I just write it down and then Staff Nurse charts it later. I expect the machine is broken.' She took the cart away and replaced it with another one, which did indeed give a more realistic recording.

I also asked her why she was writing down the results on a scrap of paper. 'Well, the doctor's doing his round,' she replied, 'so the notes are on the trolley. I'll give it to Staff Nurse and I expect she'll fill it in later.'

Note in particular:

- the use of information and communications technology (ICT) in nursing practice (see Chapter 11). This particular story illustrates the risks of the 'nursing as doing' model in relation to the use of ICT, but the principles apply equally to nurses undertaking, for example, tasks formerly undertaken by doctors;
- the risks to patient safety, both from the overreliance on hardware and from inadequate documentation.

'thinking nursing' as well as 'doing nursing'. This model is the core of all professional practice: the professional (the doctor, the nurse or the lawyer) uses their knowledge to understand the problems presented by the client and to identify ways of solving them. The core skill is the judgement that matches the knowledge base to the individual client's need – the process that in the health professions is usually called 'clinical judgement' or 'clinical decision-making'. It is this that distinguishes the practice of the qualified nurse from that of the health care assistant.

There is an extensive literature about clinical judgement, clinical reasoning and clinical decision-making. Some authors use these terms interchangeably, while others distinguish between 'judgements' as the assessment of situations and 'decisions' as choosing what to do about the situation (Thompson and Dowding, 2002). Clinical judgements are decisions about the status of the patient (individual or family) and the contextual situation affecting them based on findings and their interpretation, typically expressed as a diagnosis; clinical decisions are typically treatment decisions. In practice they are inextricably linked, as in the phrase 'diagnosis and treatment of . . .' or, in everyday language, 'What is the problem and what shall we do about it?'

There is also an extensive literature on the processes that people use in making judgements and decisions. Psychologists have developed several theoretical frameworks to analyse and explain the thinking processes that lead to the judgements and decisions. Hurst (1993) groups these into two categories: the 'information-processing system theory' developed by Newell and Simon (1972) and the 'stages model theory', of which there are many variants. However, in real life, decision-making is not always as clear-cut as these theories suggest. Benner showed that novice nurses and expert nurses use different thinking processes: while novice nurses needed a systematic structure to support their decision making, the expert nurse 'has an intuitive grasp of the situation and zeros in on the accurate region of the problem without wasteful consideration of a large range of unfruitful problem situations' (Benner, 1984).

Nurses talk about 'the nursing process' (see Chapter 11), but in fact the process is the same for all the clinical professions: what makes it 'nursing' is the nursing knowledge (as opposed to any other kind of knowledge) that is used. It is similar to the problem-solving process that most people use intuitively to manage the challenges of everyday life, but for clinical practice it is made systematic and formalised. The nursing process is simply the way that nurses structure their thinking in order to identify and solve their patients' problems. In clinical practice, judgements and decisions are shared with other people through documentation in patient records. Nurses whose personal concept of nursing is based on the 'nursing as doing' model often see documentation as a chore that they do only because they are told to. Nurses who see 'nursing as decision-making' recognise that documentation is important as the method of communicating their decision-making to others (see Chapter 11).

Since it was first formalised and introduced into nursing in the USA in the 1950s, the nursing process has been refined and developed. Pesut and Herman (1999) distinguish three generations, each influenced by the state of knowledge development available at the time. The first generation used a logical linear four-step process of assessment, planning, implementation and evaluation. In the 1970s, as the work of the ANA and NANDA (described above) and of scholars such as Gordon (1976) and Carnevali *et al.* (1984) developed, the significance of clinical reasoning and nursing diagnosis was recognised, and nursing diagnosis was included as a fifth stage to form the bridge between assessment and planning. Since the 1990s, the greater emphasis on outcomes and the development of computerised information systems has led to a third generation in which several more steps can be identified and the process is seen as interactive and iterative rather than linear. Nursing in the UK still uses the first-generation model and is only just beginning to consider the implications of computerised patient records (see Chapter 11).

A particular purpose

The purpose of nursing is to promote health, healing, growth and development, and to prevent disease, illness, injury, and disability. When people become ill or disabled, the purpose of nursing is, in addition, to minimise distress and suffering, and to enable people to understand and cope with their disease or disability, its treatment and its consequences. When death is inevitable, the purpose of nursing is to maintain the best possible quality of life until its end.

Nursing, like many other concepts, is often defined by it purpose. Although many people see nursing as being concerned primarily with caring for sick people, it has been clear from the days of Florence Nightingale that the goal of nursing is health – promoting, maintaining and restoring it. The respondents in the RCN values clarification exercise identified six key purposes:

- to promote and maintain health;
- to care for people when their health is compromised;
- to assist recovery;
- to facilitate independence;
- to meet needs;
- to improve/maintain well-being/quality of life.

Defining the purpose of nursing as 'health' requires us to think about what 'health' means. Health is even more complex and difficult to define than nursing, and the literature about its meaning is even larger than the literature that attempts to define nursing. The most famous definition is the one used in the constitution of the World Health Organization (WHO), which states that 'health is a state of complete physical, mental and social well-being and not merely the absence of disease or infirmity' (WHO, 1946).

The importance of this definition is its statement that health is 'not merely the absence of disease or infirmity'. This is an attempt to counter the 'negative' model of health, which assumes that health is the opposite of illness and illness is synonymous with the presence of disease. Although this model is rarely defended in intellectual argument, it is still the model that underpins our NHS, which is concerned mainly (in spite of recent attempts to reorient it) with the treatment and, to a lesser extent, the prevention of disease. It is also one of the differences between the disciplines of nursing and medicine: the knowledge base and most of the interventions of doctors are concerned mainly with the detection and modification of disease processes, whereas nursing, as we shall see, is concerned with the person rather than the disease. It is also argued that people can be healthy even when they are suffering from a disease (e.g. a healthy diabetic person).

This WHO definition, and in particular the phrase 'complete state', has often been criticised as an idealistic goal rather than a realistic proposition. Others argue that health cannot be defined as a state at all but must be seen as a process of continuous adjustment to the changing demands of living and of the changing meanings we give to life. This kind of definition draws on the concept of homeostasis – a state of balance – in which health is the state of balance that is maintained by the person's ability to respond to challenges (stressors). A model of nursing that uses these ideas is described later in this chapter. Modern definitions usually include the concept of functional ability and the ability to lead a socially and economically productive life, and to reach one's physical, psychological and social potential. The WHO describes the 'mission' of nursing as follows:

The mission of nursing in society is to help individuals, families, communities and groups to determine and achieve their physical and mental and social potential and to do so within the challenging context of the environment in which they live and work.

(Salvage, 1993)

One of the most attractive definitions of health is that of Katherine Mansfield:

By health I mean the power to live a full, adult breathing life in close contact with what I love – I want to be all that I am capable of becoming.

(Katherine Mansfield, quoted in Stead, 1977)

A particular mode of intervention

Nursing interventions are concerned with empowering people and helping them to achieve, maintain, or recover independence. Nursing is an intellectual, physical, emotional and moral process which includes the identification of nursing needs; therapeutic interventions and personal care; information, education, advice, and advocacy; and physical, emotional and spiritual support. In addition to direct patient care, nursing practice includes management, teaching, and policy and knowledge development.

This characteristic contains three key concepts: first, that nursing is concerned with enabling and empowering people towards independence; second, that nursing is a process that consists of more than just tasks; and third, that nursing is not limited to direct patient care.

The idea that nursing is concerned with enabling and empowering is visible in Florence Nightingale's writings but is expressed most explicitly in Virginia Henderson's words: '. . . to do those things that he would perform unaided if he had the necessary strength, will, or knowledge. And to do this in such a way as to help him gain independence as rapidly as possible.'

This idea conflicts with some of the common stereotypes of nursing as doing things 'to' or 'for' people. In her 'model' of nursing (which is described in Chapter 12), Dorothea Orem focused on the patient's need for 'self-care'. She identified three modes of nursing intervention: wholly compensatory care (where the nurse compensates entirely for the patient's inability to engage in self-care, e.g. when he is unconscious), partial compensatory care (where the nurse compensates partly, while encouraging the patient to do what he can), and supportive-educative care (where the nurse teaches and guides the patient towards self-care). Most people would agree that, in general, it requires more time and greater skill to teach a patient (e.g. following a stroke) to feed himself than simply to feed him. In a study in Belgium, in which the activities of nurses with patients who were unable to feed themselves, as recorded in the annual census of nursing activities, were analysed, changes in available staffing and skill mix affected the kind of care that the patients received: when the nursing workforce was reduced or diluted by lesser qualified staff, compensatory care was maintained, but supportive-educative care was greatly reduced (Evers *et al.*, 2000).

The range of activities undertaken by nurses is enormous. A research team based at the University of Iowa has developed a standardised classification of 514 interventions and more than 12 000 associated activities that nurses perform (McCloskey-Dochterman and Bulechek, 2004). An intervention is defined as 'any treatment, based upon clinical judgement and knowledge, that a nurse performs to enhance patient/client outcomes'. Each intervention has a standardised label and a definition and includes several activities that are at the more concrete level of action. For example, the intervention called 'bowel management' is defined as 'establishment and maintenance of a regular pattern of bowel elimination' and includes 18 activities ranging from teaching the patient about diet to insertion of rectal suppositories. As discussed in Chapter 11, documentation of nursing interventions using this kind of standardised terminology can make visible what nurses do, can provide for much more accurate care planning, and, when the data pertaining to many patients are aggregated for analysis, can provide the data required for identifying best practice, for allocating resources and for research.

The second concept is that nursing is far more than a collection of activities or tasks. Everyone recognises the technical aspects of nursing, but nursing is also:

- an intellectual activity because it involves using knowledge to make judgements and decisions;
- a social activity because it involves interaction with one or more other people;
- an emotional activity because it requires the practitioner to share the patient's experience and to work in partnership with them to agree and achieve common goals;
- a moral activity because it depends on a relationship of trust, in an environment where choices and decisions do not depend solely on scientific knowledge;
- a political activity because it involves the allocation of scarce resources in situations where demand may not equate with need and may exceed supply.

Third, nursing practice does not always involve direct patient care: 'In addition to direct patient care, nursing practice includes management, teaching, and policy and knowledge development.'

For example, the WHO identifies four functions of the nurse as

- providing and managing direct patient care;
- teaching patients, clients and other health personnel;
- acting as an effective member of a health care team;
- developing nursing practice based on critical thinking and research.

Anyone who is using nursing knowledge to make decisions to achieve nursing goals is engaging in nursing practice.

A particular domain

The specific domain of nursing is people's unique responses to and experience of health, illness, frailty, disability and health-related life-events in whatever environment or circumstances they find themselves. People's responses may be physiological, psychological, social, cultural or spiritual, and are often a combination of all of these. The term 'people' includes individuals of all ages, families and communities throughout the entire life span.

The term 'domain' originally referred to the piece of land, or the territory, for which a particular ruler was responsible. Just as the word 'territory' is no longer limited to a piece of land, so the word 'domain' is used to describe any kind of delineated area of responsibility. The 'domain of nursing' is what nurses are responsible for that is distinct from what other people are responsible for. We sometimes use the phrase 'scope of practice'. What we are responsible for depends on what we 'know about', and so the term 'knowledge domain' has come to mean the specific body of knowledge that a particular group (e.g. nursing) has that is distinct from the body of knowledge that another group (e.g. medicine) has.

Disciplines define themselves and distinguish themselves from other disciplines by their knowledge domain – what they 'know about'. However, nursing knowledge is a contested issue: What is it that nurses know about that other people do not and that enables them to do what they do? In the values clarification exercise described above, this was the question that nurses found most difficult to answer.

The answer to the question is important for two reasons:

- Having a distinct and organised knowledge base is one of the key characteristics of a profession. Although some people argue that the aspiration to professional status is merely selfish self-aggrandisement, most nurses value the concept of professionalism as being one of their most important attributes and one that is essential for enabling them to provide high-quality nursing care to patients.
- Of all the defining characteristics in the definition of nursing, this is the one that most distinguishes nursing from the other health care professions: it is the one that is unique to nursing and is therefore what makes nursing unique.

It is clear, both from the research literature and from observations of expert nursing practice, that nurses do have and do use a distinctive knowledge base, although it is not always well articulated, formulated or tested. Benner (1984) described nursing knowledge as 'embedded in clinical practice'.

Having a defined discipline-specific domain does not, of course, preclude developing collaborative knowledge; nor does it limit members of one discipline from using knowledge developed in another discipline. Professional practitioners draw on the knowledge of many other disciplines in addition to their own. Figure 3.2 shows how the knowledge bases of health care professionals overlap; the relative sizes of the unique area and the overlap areas vary according to the circumstances and the field of practice.

In health care, each profession's knowledge base includes discipline-specific knowledge about the particular conditions or problems that constitute the discipline's phenomena of concern, and the particular interventions that can be used to solve them. Doctors know about diseases (we call them 'medical diagnoses') and how to treat them; nurses know about conditions that some people call 'nursing problems' ('nursing diagnoses') and how to treat them.

Sometimes these responses (e.g. ineffective breathing pattern) are the results of a disease process (e.g. pneumonia), but they may also be responses to medical treatment (e.g. mechanical ventilation) or life events (e.g. sudden bad news). The conditions that nurses know about and treat most commonly relate to the following:

- a self-care deficit: the person's inability to manage the normal activities of daily living;
- a knowledge or motivational deficit: the person's lack of knowledge, understanding or will to behave in ways that are necessary to recover or improve health;
- physiological or psychological instability;
- pain or discomfort;
- an identified risk of any of the above.

One problem is that, at present, nursing has no universally agreed terminology to describe its 'phenomena of concern'. Standardised terminology is essential for articulating the knowledge base and testing it through research. This problem is discussed in more detail in Chapter 11.

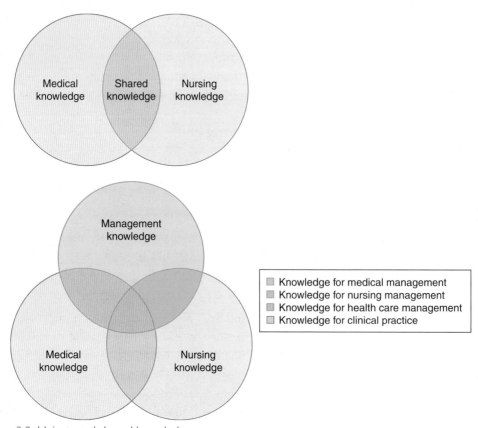

Figure 3.2 Unique and shared knowledge.

Philosophers have debated the nature of knowledge, different kinds of knowledge, and how knowledge is developed and used for centuries. In nursing, these issues have been discussed seriously only since the early 1960s, but since that time they have become an important part of efforts to understand the nature of nursing.

One of the most seminal papers was published by Carper in 1978. Carper identified four 'patterns of knowing' in nursing:

- Empirics: the science of nursing – scientific knowledge derived from empirical research.
- Aesthetics: the art of nursing – the creativity, intuition, and 'ways of working' that nurses use in their practice.
- Personal knowing: this is about knowing oneself and relates to the 'therapeutic use of self' in the way in which nurses relate to and interact with patients.
- Ethical knowing: 'the understanding of different philosophical positions about what is good, right, and wrong' (Carper, 1978).

Carper's analysis has been much discussed by other authors since 1978, but her distinction between the four patterns is still useful for helping us to think about the richness of nursing knowledge and the complexity of nursing practice.

Another important distinction is the difference between 'know-how' and 'know-that' (Polanyi, 1962). 'Know-how' knowledge is associated with personal experience, is usually unarticulated or is communicated by word of mouth, and is used directly in nursing practice. 'Know-that' knowledge is derived from theory and research, is usually communicated through the written word and formal education programmes, and is used for describing, predicting and prescribing nursing practice. 'Know-how' knowledge is sometimes related to the 'art' of nursing, and 'know-that' to the science. In the UK, perhaps more than in other countries, 'know-how' is much valued more highly than 'know-that'; for example, the phrase 'nursing science', which is used commonly in other countries, is used rarely by nurses in the UK. The two kinds of knowledge are sometimes perceived as competing alternatives, and the difference between them is described as 'the theory–practice gap'. In reality, nursing, like all professional practice, requires both: although compassionate care is important, compassionate but ill-informed care may be harmful.

A third perspective, which derives from the theories of Habermas (1965), uses the term 'praxis' to describe the kind of knowledge that is linked to purpose and is necessary for practice disciplines such as nursing. Schön (1983) showed how reflection could be used to understand and thereby improve professional practice, and Johns (1995) and others have developed tools to facilitate reflective practice.

'Theory' is simply a way of organising knowledge. A theory is a statement that describes, or explains, or predicts something. The truth of the theory can be tested by the rigorous logical method that we call 'scientific method'. Theory development as a means of understanding nursing began with Florence Nightingale, but it was almost a century later before nurses began to develop theory that would describe, explain and predict nursing in a systematic way. In her book *Theoretical Nursing: Development and Progress*, Meleis (1997) traces the history of theory development in nursing from the 1950s to the present day; and Nicholl (1997) provides an excellent compilation of the most widely read and frequently cited articles that show the development of ideas about knowledge development, theory and research in nursing.

The terms 'theory' and 'theoretical' are often used pejoratively to refer to something that is idealised, or not real, or not practically useful. The phrase 'theory–practice divide' is sometimes used to argue that practising nurses do not need theory. Nothing could be further from the truth.

It has been said that 'there is nothing so practical as a good theory' because theory can explain and guide behaviour. Leonardo da Vinci is reputed to have said: 'Practice without theory is like a man who goes to sea without a map in a boat without a rudder'.

A particular focus

The focus of nursing is the whole person and the human response rather than a particular aspect of the person or a particular pathological condition.

Nurses continually stress that they care for 'the whole person'. Holism is a deeply held nursing value, and nurses sometimes claim that this is what distinguishes nursing from other health care professions. Although it is true that the nursing focus on 'human responses', which 'may be physiological, social, cultural or spiritual, and are often a combination of all of these' (RCN, 2003) is more comprehensive than the doctor's focus on the disease or the physiotherapist's focus on physical function, it would be arrogant to suggest that the value of holism is not also held by other health professionals. Moreover, the commitment to holism is not supported by the organisation of nursing education into four branches that separate, for example, mental health and learning disability from the physical care of adults. Like the other characteristics identified in the RCN definition, holism in nursing supports an extensive literature, including at least two specialist journals, and, in the USA, a recognised nursing specialty and a specialist nursing organisation.

A particular value base

Nursing is based on ethical values which respect the dignity, autonomy and uniqueness of human beings, the privileged nurse-patient relationship, and the acceptance of personal accountability for decisions and actions. These values are expressed in written codes of ethics, and supported by a system of professional regulation.

Values are enduring beliefs, attributes or ideals that establish moral boundaries of what is right or wrong in thought, judgement, character, attitude and behaviour and that form a foundation for decision-making throughout our lives (Johnson and Webber, 2001). Everybody has personal and private values, but the values that are corporately agreed and shared by a professional group are often expressed in a written code of conduct or code of ethics, to which all members of the profession are expected to conform. In the UK, the Nursing and Midwifery Council (NMC), whose purpose is to protect the public by registering qualified nurses and regulating the practice of nursing to ensure the highest possible standards, publishes the NMC Code (2008)(Appendix 1). The values expressed within it underpin all good nursing practice.

A commitment to partnership

Nurses work in partnership with patients, their relatives and other carers, and in collaboration with others as members of a multi-disciplinary team. Where appropriate they will lead the team, prescribing, delegating and supervising the work of others; at other times they will participate under the leadership of others. At all times, however, they remain personally accountable for their own decisions and actions.

This characteristic incorporates three kinds of partnership:

- partnership with patients and their informal carers;
- partnership within the nursing team;
- partnership with other health professionals in a multiprofessional team.

The first kind of partnership has already been referred to as part of nursing's mode of intervention: nurses are committed to doing things *with* rather than *to* patients. The importance of this kind of partnership has been growing in recent years and is now expressed strongly and explicitly in UK government health policy. Current terminology uses the term 'patient-centred care'; Chapter 11 discusses how access to information is strengthening the patient's role towards 'patient-controlled care'.

The second kind of partnership recognises that, as was noted at the beginning of this chapter, not all nursing is undertaken by registered nurses. Increasingly, the registered nurse leads a team that includes health care assistants, nursing students and other staff (e.g. nursery nurses) who, although they may not be managed directly by the registered nurse, are making an important contribution to nursing care. In these circumstances, the registered nurse is the leader of the team and is responsible and accountable for delegating the work and ensuring that the person to whom they delegate is competent to undertake it.

The third kind of partnership recognises that people's health needs, and the care that is necessary to meet them, are far too complex to be satisfied by any one person, however knowledgeable and skilled. The composition of the team will vary in different fields of practice but may include nurses, doctors, physiotherapists, occupational therapists, dieticians, social workers and others. As specialisation increases, it is important not only that all the available expertise is made available to patients but also that all the pieces are coordinated so that the care that the patient experiences is seamless and not fragmented. This coordination of the programme of care for an individual patient is one of the most important aspects of the nurse's role; it is often said that nursing provides the glue that holds it all together.

There is a considerable literature about multiprofessional teamwork in health care – what makes it work well and what prevents it from working well. Teamwork in primary health care in particular has been studied extensively (e.g. Poulton, 1993), but teamwork is equally important in almost every field of health care. Perhaps the best summary is the third part of Henderson's definition of nursing, which was given above:

> *As a member of the medical team, the nurse helps other members, as they in turn help the nurse to plan and carry out the total programme whether it be for the improvement of health, or the recovery from illness or support in death. No one of the team should make such heavy demands on another member that any one of them is unable to perform his or her unique function. Nor should any member of the medical team be diverted by non-medical activities, such as cleaning, clerking, and filing, as long as his or her special task must be neglected. All members of the team should consider the person (patient) served as the central figure, and should realise that primarily they are all 'assisting' the patient.*
>
> (Henderson, 1960)

Putting it all together

The RCN definition of nursing is very detailed, not least because its development included wide consultation with RCN members from many fields of practice – hospital and community, acute and long-term care, mental health and learning disability nursing, children and old people, public health and policy-making, management, education and research – each one of whom wanted to be sure that their particular focus and field of practice was included. We wanted to ensure, as far as possible, that the definition covered the whole field of nursing, recognising that one of the characteristics of modern nursing – perhaps one of its problems as a profession – is the degree of specialisation within it (Welsh Nursing Academy, 2006).

The definition does, however, show the common features of nursing, wherever and however it is performed. The four characteristics first identified by Nightingale (see above) are clearly recognisable, and the definition encompasses all of the different perspectives and emphases described in Chapter 12. It also shows the futility of arguments about whether nursing is an art or a science, or, if it is both, which is the more important. Nursing is of course both. What is clear is that the core of nursing practice is not the ability to measure vital signs, administer medication, dress wounds or manage complicated machines. It does not lie in our technical skills, many of which will be as obsolete in 5 years' time as some of the skills I learnt as a student nurse 40 years ago. It does not lie solely in our empathy or caring approach to people, for there are many others who can equal that claim. It lies in our ability to diagnose and deal with human responses to illness, frailty, disability, life transitions, and other actual or potential threats to health, and to do so within a relationship of trust and care that promotes health and healing.

Developing your own personal concept of nursing

It was suggested at the beginning of this chapter that it was important for each nurse to develop their own personal concept of nursing and that the purpose of this chapter was to help them to do so. This is in the tradition of Nightingale:

> *I do not pretend to teach her how, I ask her to teach herself, and for this purpose I venture to give her some hints*

> (Nightingale, 1859)

and of Henderson:

> *I would like to emphasise that I am not presenting my point of view as one with which I expect you to agree. Rather I would urge every nurse to develop her own concept, otherwise she is merely imitating others or acting under authority.*

> (Henderson, 1996)

This section describes how the author built up her own concept of nursing through studying the practice of a group of health visitors and developing a model to describe and explain it (Clark, 1986). Although the model was derived from health visiting practice, it may equally describe and explain other kinds of nursing, especially those where, as in health visiting, the goal is promoting rather than restoring health, and the main activities are teaching and counselling rather than physical care and technical procedures. It is also useful for analysing nursing as a 'collective', for example a nursing team or a nursing service.

Health visiting has often been seen as different from 'ordinary' nursing, and the nursing models that were popular at the time (see Chapter 12) certainly didn't fit my practice as a health visitor, for several reasons:

- They assumed that the focus of care was an individual, whereas the focus of care for a health visitor is the family as a unit.
- They assumed that nursing is concerned with people's 'problems', whereas health visitors work with normal healthy families to promote health.

- The existence of a problem that is to be resolved by nursing intervention assumes a need for change, whereas the goal for health visiting may be to maintain health – that is, not change but stability.
- They assumed a discrete 'episode' of care that begins at the point of referral or admission to hospital and ends at the point of discharge, whereas health visiting is often a serial activity that takes place over several years, in which each contact is not a new episode but builds on and is determined by where the last one left off.

I needed a model that could focus on the family or group as the 'patient'; needs rather than problems; stability rather than change; and continuity over time. I needed a new perspective on the key concepts that constitute the paradigm of nursing – the person, the environment, health and nursing (Fawcett, 1995) – and those that health visitors said directed their practice – health, prevention, needs and coping. My search for a unifying framework that would bring these elements together led me to systems theory (von Bertalanffy, 1968), which had already been used widely as a means of understanding the dynamics both of nursing and of families, as well as in fields as diverse as engineering and organisational sociology. I also drew on the work of other nursing theorists to incorporate theories about nurse–patient interaction and human development, and on Antonovski's theories about stress and coping (Antonovski, 1979).

In systems theory, the focus of concern (which may be an individual, a group or a organisation) is seen as a system – that is, a whole that functions as a unit by virtue of the interdependence of its parts; the system affects and is affected by its environment, with which it must maintain a state of balance or equilibrium if it is to survive. Within this framework I defined the key concepts as follows:

- *Health* is a dynamic equilibrium, a state of balance between the person and their environment, in which the balance is held at the level that enables the person to function physiologically, psychologically and socially at their optimum level.
- *Needs* are 'those items which the person must have in order to attain and maintain the physical and psychological balance that we call health' (Johnson and Davis, 1975).
- *Problems* occur when a person's needs are overfulfilled or underfulfilled so that the balance is disturbed; the disturbance is referred to as a patient problem.
- *Coping* is the activity by means of which the system (the individual, family or community) strives to maintain its equilibrium.

The nurse and the patient (individual, family or community) are shown as two separate systems interacting with each other in a physical and social environment (Figure 3.3).

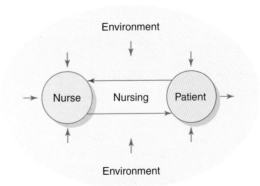

Figure 3.3 The nurse and the patient as two interacting systems in the environment.

The environment contains many elements that impinge both positively and negatively on these systems, strengthening or threatening their integrity. Nursing is shown as an interactive activity in which the goal of nursing is to maintain, and if possible improve, the patient's equilibrium or health status by helping the person to avoid or cope with actual or potential threats to health. Figure 3.4 shows how nurses achieve this goal.

This description of nursing intervention employs the widely used distinction between primary, secondary and tertiary prevention (Caplan, 1961). There are four modes of nursing intervention: primary prevention consists of heading off health-threatening stressors before they impinge on the system (e.g. helping a family living in poor housing conditions to get rehoused) or building up their coping ability (e.g. by health education). Secondary prevention includes health surveillance and screening procedures so that potential breaches of the system's boundary can be treated at an early stage. If primary and secondary prevention fail, then the system's integrity breaks down (i.e. the person becomes ill or injured) and crisis intervention is required. After the crisis has been resolved, tertiary prevention involves rehabilitation and helping the patient to maintain equilibrium (health) in a new form.

This analysis leads to what has become my personal definition of nursing: 'Helping and enabling people to cope with actual or potential threats to health.'

Of course, few nurses have the desire or the opportunity to spend 6 years on obtaining a PhD to develop their personal concept of nursing, and nor is this necessary. Each of us can build on the ideas of those who have gone before, from Nightingale onwards. But what every nurse needs is a clear understanding of the key concepts that are used in nursing, and to be able to describe, both to themselves and to others, the goal or purpose of their nursing and what they do to achieve it.

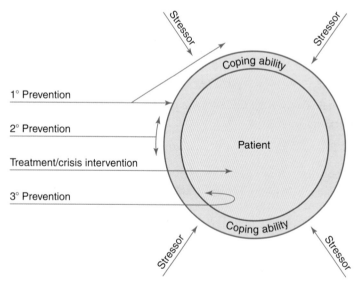

Figure 3.4 Achieving the goal of nursing.

Reflection point 3.3
Take some time to go back over this chapter and your intended learning outcomes and write down some points about your own personal concept of nursing.

There is no right or wrong answer here – but do keep your reflections and go back over them from time to time and see how your ideas might change as you gain in experience.

CONCLUSION

This chapter has tried to show how complex and rich an activity nursing is. It is not just a matter of a collection of tasks that anyone with a little training can perform at an acceptable level of competence. Of course nursing requires technical competence, a gentle touch, and care and compassion. But it is much, much more.

The constant in nursing is people's needs for nursing, and our commitment to meeting those needs. Our ability to respond to this constant within the rapidly shifting environment of health care will depend on four things:

- the way in which nursing work is organised in health care delivery systems;
- the way in which practice is regulated and the quality of care is assured;
- the way in which practitioners are prepared;
- and, fundamentally, the way nurses see their role.

References

American Nurses Association (ANA) (1973). *Standards for Nursing Practice*. Kansas City, MO: American Nurses Association.

American Nurses Association (ANA) (1980). *Nursing: A Social Policy Statement*. Kansas City, MO: American Nurses Association.

Antonovski A (1979). *Stress, Health and Coping*. New York: Jossey Bass.

Benner P (1984). *From Novice to Expert: Excellence and Power in Clinical Nursing Practice*. Menlo Park, CA: Addison-Wesley.

Bridges JM (1990). Literature review on the images of the nurse and nursing in the media. *Journal of Advanced Nursing*, **15**, 850–54.

Caplan G (1961). *An Approach to Community Mental Health*. London: Tavistock.

Carnevali D, Mitchell P, Woods N and Tanner C (1984). *Diagnostic Reasoning in Nursing*. Philadelphia, PA: Lippincott.

Carper BA (1978). Fundamental patterns of knowing in nursing. *Advances in Nursing Science*, **1**, 13–23.

Clark J (1986). A model for health visiting. In Kershaw B and Salvage J (eds). *Models for Nursing*. London: John Wiley & Sons.

Clark J and Lang N (1992). Nursing's next advance: an international classification for nursing practice. *International Nursing Review*, **39**, 109–12.

Darbyshire P and Gordon S (2005). Exploring popular images and representations of nurses and nursing. In Daly J, Speedy S, Jackson D, Lambert V and Lambert C (eds). *Professional Nursing: Concepts, Issues, and Challenges*. New York: Springer.

Evers G, Viane A, Sermeus W, Simoens-De Smet A and Delesie L (2000). Frequency of and indications for wholly compensatory nursing care related to enteral food intake: a secondary analysis of the Belgian Minimum Data Set. *Journal of Advanced Nursing*, **32**, 194–201.

Fawcett J (1995). *Analysis and Evaluation of Conceptual Models of Nursing*, 2nd edn. Philadelphia, PA: F.A. Davis.

Gordon M (1976). Nursing diagnosis and the diagnostic process. *American Journal of Nursing*, **76**, 1276–300.

Habermas J (1965). *Knowledge and Human Interests*. Cambridge: Polity Press.

Henderson V (1960). *Basic Principles of Nursing Care*. Geneva: International Council of Nurses.

Henderson V (1978). The concept of nursing. *Journal of Advanced Nursing*, **3**, 113–30. (Reprinted in *Journal of Advanced Nursing*, **53**, 21–34.)

Henderson VA (1991). *The Nature of Nursing: Reflections after 25 Years*. New York: National League for Nursing.

Hurst K (1993). *Problem-Solving in Nursing Practice*. London: Scutari Press.

Jinks A and Bradley E (2003). Angel, handmaiden, battle axe or whore? *Nurse Education Today*, **24**, 121–7.

Johns C (1995). The value of reflective practice for nursing. *Journal of Clinical Nursing*, **4**, 23–30.

Johnson M and Davis M (1975). *Problem Solving in Nursing Practice*. Dubuque, IA: W.C. Brown Co. Publishers.

Johnson PM and Webber PB (2001). *An Introduction to Theory and Reasoning in Nursing*. Philadelphia, PA: Lippincott.

Kalish B and Kalish P (1987). *The Changing Image of the Nurse*. Menlo Park, CA: Addison-Wesley.

King I (1971). *A Theory for Nursing*. New York: John Wiley & Sons.

McCloskey-Dochterman J and Bulechek G (2004). *Nursing Interventions Classification (NIC)*, 4th edn. St Louis, MO: Mosby.

Meleis AI (1997). *Theoretical Nursing: Development and Progress*, 3rd edn. Philadelphia, PA: Lippincott.

NANDA International (2007). *Nursing Diagnoses: Definitions and Classification 2007–2008*. Philadelphia, PA: NANDA International.

Newell A and Simon HA (1972). *Human Problem-Solving*. Englewood Cliffs, NJ: Prentice-Hall.

Nicholl LH (1997). *Perspectives on Nursing Theory*, 3rd edn. Philadelphia, PA: Lippincott.

Nightingale F (1859). *Notes on Nursing: What It Is and What It Is Not*. London: Harrison.

Nursing and Midwifery Council (NMC) (2008). *The Code: Standards of Conduct, Performance and Ethics for Nurses and Midwives.* London: Nursing and Midwifery Council.

Orem D (1971). *Nursing: Concepts of Practice*. New York: McGraw-Hill.

Orlando J (1972). *The Discipline and Teaching of Nursing Process*. New York: Putnam.

Peplau HE (1987). Interpersonal constructs for nursing practice. *Nurse Education Today*, **7**, 201–8.

Pesut D and Herman T (1999). *Clinical Reasoning: The Art and Science of Critical and Creative Thinking*. Albany, NY: Delmar Publications.

Polanyi M (1962). *Personal knowledge*. Chicago, IL: University of Chicago Press.

Poulton B (1993). Effective multidisciplinary teamwork in primary health care. *Journal of Advanced Nursing*, **18**, 918–25.

Rogers ME (1970). *An Introduction to the Theoretical Basis of Nursing*. Philadelphia, PA: F.A. Davis.

Roper N, Tierney A and Logan W (1985). *The Elements of Nursing: Based on a Model of Living*. Edinburgh: Churchill Livingstone.

Roy C (1970). Adaptation: a conceptual framework for nursing. *Nursing Outlook*, **18**, 42–5.

Royal College of Nursing (RCN) (2003). *Defining Nursing*. London: Royal College of Nursing.

Salvage J (1993). Nursing in action: strengthening nursing and midwifery to support health for all. *WHO Regional Publications. European Series*, **48**, 1–123.

Schön DA (1983). *The Reflective Practitioner: How Professionals Think in Action*. New York: Basic Books.

Stead C (1997). *The Letters and Journals of Katherine Mansfield: A Selection*. Harmondsworth: Penguin.

Thompson C and Dowding D (eds) (2002). *Clinical Decision Making and Judgement in Nursing*. Edinburgh: Churchill Livingstone.

Travelbee J (1966). *Interpersonal Aspects of Nursing*. Philadelphia, PA: F.A. Davis.

Von Bertalanffy L (1968). *General Systems Theory*. New York: Braziller.

Von Essen L and Sjoden PO (2003). The importance of nurse caring behaviours as perceived by Swedish hospital patients and nursing staff. *International Journal of Nursing Studies*, **40**, 487–97.

Warfield C and Manley K (1990). Developing a new philosophy in the NDU. *Nursing Standard*, **4**, 27–30.

Welsh Nursing Academy (2006) Specialisation in nursing. www.wna.org.uk.

World Health Organization (1946). *Constitution of the World Health Organization*. Geneva: World Health Organization.

Further reading

American Nurses Association (2003). *Nursing's Social Policy Statement*, 2nd edn. Washington, DC: American Nurses Association.

American Nurses Association (2004). *Nursing: Scope and Standards for Practice*. Washington, DC: American Nurses Association.

Gordon M (1994). *Nursing Diagnosis: Process and Application*, 3rd edn. St Louis, MO: Mosby.

Halloran J (ed.) (1995). *A Virginia Henderson Reader: Excellence in Nursing*. New York: Springer.

Henderson V (1997). *Basic Principles of Nursing Care*, rev. edn. Geneva: International Council of Nurses.

Meleis AI (1997). *Theoretical Nursing*, 3rd edn. Philadelphia, PA: Lippincott.

Nicholl LH (1997). *Perspectives on Nursing Theory*, 3rd edn. Philadelphia, PA: Lippincott.

Nightingale F (1992). *Notes on Nursing: What It Is and What It Is Not*, commemorative edn. Philadelphia, PA: Lippincott.

Royal College of Nursing (2003) Defining nursing. www.rcn.org.uk/publications.

PART 2

Learning nursing

4 Learning nursing

Penny Tremayne

Introduction
The aim of this chapter is to enhance the knowledge and understanding of key concepts that you will experience when learning nursing. The learning of nursing is complex and multidimensional. It cannot be compared to many other higher education courses, which can be solely academia-focused. The nurse who is learning needs not only to achieve academically according to the higher education institution (HEI) regulations but also to demonstrate competency in professional outcomes outlined by the Nursing and Midwifery Council (NMC).

Learning objectives
After studying this chapter you should be able to:
- consider the evolution of nurse education so that you can contextualise contemporary nurse education;
- identify and differentiate between the various placements settings in which you will gain clinical practice experience;
- explore the interrelationship between theory and practice and how this shapes learning nursing;
- identify the contribution of other members of the multiprofessional team towards effective patient care;
- have a raised awareness of accountability and its implications.

The historical perspective

To understand about how nursing is learnt, it is necessary, albeit briefly, to revisit the recent history of nurse training and education. Before 1979, student nurse training adopted the guise of an apprenticeship system, which, according to Bradshaw (2001), was controlled through a statutory syllabus (specified by the then General Nursing Council) and informed by nursing textbooks. It was only in 1979 that nursing as a profession became self-regulating and therefore had a very real influence on the organisation of nurse training. It was inevitable that those members of the United Kingdom Central Council for Nursing, Midwifery and Health Visiting (UKCC) (the new self-regulating body) would ultimately influence the direction of nurse training and education now that the nursing profession was set free from the previous constraints of governmental control, vocational values and medical relationships (Bradshaw, 2001). The late 1970s and early 1980s focused on the nurse developing clinical skills. However, it was beginning to be recognised that although nurses could 'do', they might not necessarily be able to explain why they were doing what they were doing. This underpinned the advent of Project 2000, which was introduced in the mid-1980s and aimed to produce a new type of nurse: a 'knowledgeable doer', a nurse who was educated and ultimately a graduate. It was not until the 1990s, though, that nursing became fully integrated within HEIs and this, in turn, influenced the manner of teaching and learning nursing.

Learning the theory and practice of nursing

Nursing draws upon theory and practice and, as such, all pre-registration programmes within the UK are made up of 4600 hours of study, of which theory comprises 2300 hours and practice comprises 2300 hours. This 50/50 attribution was identified in the UKCC (2001) report *Fitness for Practice and Purpose* and subsequently by the newly restructured self-regulating body, the NMC (2004), in *Standards of Proficiency for Pre-Registration Nursing Education*. Both documents placed emphasis on equipping nurses through education to be fit for the purpose of being a registered nurse in their chosen branch of nursing. Development of such documents is inevitably driven by governmental policy, and both of these documents were influenced by the Department of Health (1999) in *Making a Difference*. It could be argued that the introduction and subsequent implementation of Project 2000 had lost focus and the nurses qualifying in the 1990s were inadequately prepared for practice. The NMC (2004, pp. 13–16) identifies some guiding principles relating to professional standards of proficiency and fitness for practice and that should be reflected in educational programmes; these principles include the following:

- *Fitness for practice*:
  - patient-centred learning;
  - theory and practice integration;
  - evidence-based practice and learning.
- *Fitness for purpose*:
  - provision of care;
  - management of care;
  - a health-for-all orientation;
  - lifelong learning;
  - quality and excellence.
- *Fitness for award*:
  - level of learning;
  - nature of learning;
  - access and credit;
  - flexibility, integrity and progression;
  - educational quality.
- *Fitness for professional standing*:
  - adherence to the NMC Code (2008) (Appendix 1);
  - making the care of people your first concern, treating them as individuals and respecting their dignity;
  - working with others to protect and promote the health and well-being of those in your care, their families and carers, and the wider community; providing a high standard of practice and care at all times;
  - being open and honest, act with integrity and uphold the reputation of your profession.

Many of these concepts will be considered throughout this chapter.

Programmes can vary in length from 2 years and 3 months to 7 years and can be full-time or part-time. The route of entry can be either as a postgraduate or pre-registration. A full-time programme needs to be completed in no more than 5 years and a part-time programme in no more than 7 years (both inclusive of interruptions). Various pre-registration programmes are offered: diploma in higher education, advanced diploma and honours degree (BSc or BA). This means that students attain credit accumulation transfer system (CATS) ratings at a level of award. Levels of award (Table 4.1) relate to the level of accreditation influenced by the HEI's regulations that govern academic awards. CATS allows for an increase in flexibility for students. Accreditation of prior (experiential) learning (APEL) may mean that you can undertake a shorter programme, be transferred to another HEI, and receive admission with advanced standing to study for a second registration undertaking a shortened programme (NMC, 2004).

Nursing programmes include a common foundation programme (CFP) and a branch programme.

Common foundation programme

The CFP is normally a 12-month programme (or equivalent) that can embrace a number of areas, but the intention is that you get a taste and flavour of the different branches of nursing, namely adult nursing, mental health nursing, learning disabilities nursing and children's nursing. To progress to the branch programme of your choice, the NMC (2004) outcomes in relation to professional and ethical practice, care delivery, care management, and personal and professional development have to be achieved (see Appendix 2). The CFP also facilitates flexibility: should you want to transfer branches, then there is a possibility to do so, usually after discussion with your personal tutor.

Branch programme

The branch programme is a 2-year programme that focuses on one of the four branches of nursing identified previously. To enter the chosen register, you must successfully complete the standards of proficiency in relation to professional and ethical practice, care delivery, care management, and personal and professional development (NMC, 2004) (see Appendix 2).

Table 4.1 Levels of study

Level of study	Descriptor
1	Often a diagnostic level of study but may also include supportive aspects – assisting the student to make the transition to study as well as compensatory – and allowing the student to remedy deficiencies at admission
2	This level allows for exploration and development of interests/specialisms. Can also challenge; this is especially the case at level 3 study
3	At this level of academic study, the style of writing is more discursive and embraces critical analysis alongside elements of dissemination of findings. Although research may have been considered at previous levels, the student usually engages actively in the research process

Integrating theory and practice

Nursing cannot be learnt only in the classroom. Educators can replicate real-life scenarios through simulation, but nothing can replace working in the clinical practice setting. Learning from experience provides a reality and is a rich resource to the underpinning theory that provides the foundation for all clinical practice. One such method of integrating theory and practice successfully is through the development of a portfolio.

Portfolio

> **Reflection point 4.1**
>
> 1 Identify other professions that maintain a portfolio.
> 2 Discuss the strengths of maintaining a portfolio.
> 3 List what you think is included in a student portfolio.
> 4 Consider why nurses have to maintain a portfolio.

A portfolio can be defined as 'a collection of individual material that provides proof of personal growth, continuing professional development (CPD), lifelong learning and competence' (Pearce, 2003). Sometimes the term 'portfolio' is used interchangeably with 'profile'; this is a summary or 'public version' of a portfolio (Pearce, 2003). All nurses, midwives and health visitors have to maintain a portfolio so that they can fulfil the post-registration education and practice (PREP) CPD standard (NMC, 2005a). Hull *et al.* (2005) consider a portfolio to have a number of benefits from an adult and higher education perspective, including an approach to assessment, to aid a claim for prior learning and CATS points, the use of learning contracts and essentially having a student-centred approach. A common theme within many portfolios is that of reflection.

Reflection

Day in, day out, we all reflect. For example, when we are cooking a meal, on tasting it we may identify that it lacks flavour; or when we are driving, on encountering congestion at a particular place we may discover an alternative route. Reflection is often an informal, natural occurrence that centres around everyday life events.

Nursing has embraced and developed the concept of reflection with its ability to enable learning through practice (Price, 2004). Reflection, therefore, can be defined as 'a generic term for those intellectual and affective activities in which individuals engage to explore their experiences in order to lead to new understandings and appreciations' (Boud *et al.*, 1985, p. 19). Such learning not only develops nursing knowledge, skills and behaviour but ultimately enhances patient-centred care. To aid reflection, a number of acknowledged models have emerged, which provide a framework for the reflective practitioner to ensure that a systematic, logical approach is adopted. Sometimes nurses keep a reflective journal, as this can act as an aide-memoire. However, the NMC Code and the *Guidelines for Records and Record Keeping* (NMC, 2005b) should not be compromised.

> **Reflection point 4.2**
>
> There are a number of reflective models, including those of Borton (1970), Boud *et al.* (1985), Gibbs (cited in Palmer *et al.*, 1994), Kim (1999), Holm and Stephenson (1994), Marks-Maran and Rose (1997) and Johns (2000).
>
> Obtain a copy of one or two of these reflective models, as well as the reflective model that you are currently using, and attempt the following:
>
> 1 Compare and contrast the key concepts embraced within the model.
> 2 Apply a reflective model (different from the one that you are currently using) to an event from everyday life or clinical practice on which you want to reflect.
> 3 Which reflective model do think you will use in the future, and why?

Ultimately, reflection is about development, movement and change, whether personally, academically or professionally. It embraces theoretical principles to change practice. Scenario 4.1 is

SCENARIO 4.1 Example of reflection

As a student nurse I was working on a medical ward, nursing an 82-year-old lady whom I will call Alice for the purposes of confidentiality. Alice was in the end stages of lung cancer. Consequently she was often tired and frequently looked exhausted. One morning, I was undertaking her observations of temperature, pulse, respiration and blood pressure. Alice's observations were being taken four times a day.

This morning, Alice was sound asleep, but I thought that the observations were just as important. The staff nurse had asked me to record the observations of all the patients in the ward, and I wanted to do what she had asked me, and so I woke Alice up. Alice grumbled, complaining that I had disturbed her from the only bit of sleep that she had had in days. Alice told me to go away because she was getting some much-needed sleep.

I felt dreadful for depriving Alice of her precious sleep. I felt guilty and very much on the 'back foot'. Alice was clearly angry and annoyed with me. I felt that I could not go back to Alice. I felt that she thought I was stupid and incompetent and that she would always remember me for this.

In retrospect, I recognise that I was trying to please the staff nurse who was my mentor. I thought that if I got everything done, then that would go well towards me achieving my outcomes. So I did the observations, not thinking of the implications for patients such as Alice. If the observations were due, then I did them, irrespective of what the patient was doing at the time.

What went particularly well is that I did complete all the observations for the ward. I highlighted to my mentor an increase in one patient's blood pressure, and an increase in temperature for two other patients. My confidence in recording and reporting observations also improved. However, Alice's observations were entirely within normal limits, as they had been for the past week, and I had woken her needlessly.

I should have realised that any sleep that Alice got was very important to her. Despite her apparent tiredness, she was constantly interrupted by other nurses, doctors and various members of the multi-professional team. According to Rodéhn Fox (1999), sleep provides physiological and psychological restoration, and yet as a nurse I did not promote such a therapeutic intervention. Atkinson and Virdee (2001) go on to highlight that patients such as Alice have difficulty in resting because of their poor health state, which can cause anxiety and worry and numerous other symptoms. This is compounded further by the analgesic medication that Alice was receiving, namely morphine sulphate tablets 20 mg twice daily and a morphine elixir for breakthrough pain. I was unaware of the side effects of these powerful drugs. According to the *British National Formulary* (BNF), some of the side effects include drowsiness, which would explain Alice's sleepiness throughout the day. I could have left Alice and taken her observations when she was awake. I have since read literature by Carroll (2000), who highlights that the temperature is influenced by circadian rhythm and that it is at its most sensitive between 5 p.m. and 7 p.m.; therefore 6 p.m. would be the optimum time to record a temperature. I could have used my visual skills to have noted signs of a below-normal or above-normal temperature and respirations. I could have also reported the ineffectiveness of the pain relief she was receiving.

Philpin (2002) considers the 'ritualisation of undertaking nursing', and it could be said that recording observations is one such example. Nursing care, according to Walsh (1998), should be more rational and individualised, an example of which lies in the assessment and reassessment of needs and problems, as this informs all other stages of the nursing process, namely planning, implementation and evaluation. Therefore, I question the need for Alice's observations to be recorded four times daily. It would seem that once daily, at approximately 6 p.m., if Alice is awake, would be suitable, unless her clinical signs indicate otherwise.

I have learnt that, in future, I need to ensure that I individualise care and to centre care around the patient rather than the convenience to myself. Should I encounter a patient similar to Alice, I would attempt to negotiate with them so that care is delivered as and when they are able and awake and so that the patient is centrally involved in the assessment, reassessment, planning and implementation of their care.

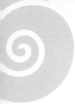

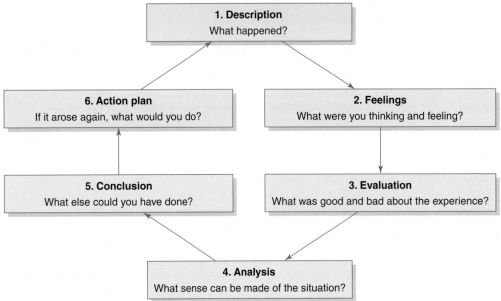

Figure 4.1 Gibb's reflective practice cycle.

an example of a reflection from a student nurse's perspective that applies the Gibbs' cycle of reflection (cited in Palmer *et al.*, 1994) (Figure 4.1).

Learning through theory

Reflection can facilitate learning from practice and can also bridge theory and practice. Although nursing is essentially a practice-based profession, it is essential that practice is informed by contemporary knowledge and underpinned by a sound evidence base. As a student nurse, while you are on placement you will learn theory in clinical practice but in a more informal manner than during your university studies. Within the CFP, you get an overview of the fundamental aspects of nursing. A range of subject areas is usually introduced within the CFP, including anatomy and physiology, psychology, sociology, communication and interpersonal skills, conceptual frameworks, models and theories of nursing, and clinical skills.

Within the branch programme, learning becomes more focused, and the knowledge and skills taught ensure that you are equipped to work effectively within your chosen branch setting. A range of subject areas is taught; these are generally related to your current placements, enabling you to apply theory to practice more readily.

Teaching embraces a number of strategies, including workshops, debates, guided study, seminars, poster presentations, formal lectures, simulations, e-learning and problem-based learning.

Learning through practice

Clinical practice contributes 50 per cent of a pre-registration nursing programme. The length of time spent in a particular practice setting varies, but learning should always be related to the theory being taught at that particular time. Within the CFP, you are exposed to the different branches of nursing. Such experience is invaluable, because as a nurse you will encounter a diversity of patients in a range of clinical practice settings (Table 4.2). Within the branch programme, clinical practice, like theory, becomes more specific to the skills that need to be acquired in order for you to become a competent practitioner. Supervised clinical practice adds richness to your learning and, because students are actively involved in the delivery of care, it is often the time when things

Table 4.2 Examples of practice placements available within the four branches of nursing

Adult	Child	Learning disability	Mental health
Accident and emergency	Adolescent unit	Young disabled unit	Acute wards
Medical	Nursery	NHS units	Elderly wards
Surgical	Special care baby unit	Challenging behaviour	Rehabilitation
Intensive care/treatment unit (ICU/ITU)	Oncology	Dual diagnosis	Community mental health
Coronary care unit (CCU)	Outpatients	Multiple complex needs	Forensic
Oncology	Community	Community	Prisons
Ophthalmology	Oncology	Social services	Crisis resolution
Outpatients	Medical	Educational sector	Assertive outreach
Community	Surgical		Common mental health problem service
Rehabilitation	Accident and emergency		Child and adolescent psychiatry
Day hospital	Theatres		
Walk-in centres	Paediatric intensive care unit		
Clinics, e.g. family planning	Schools		
Minor injury units	Young offenders' institutions		
Community hospitals	Mental health care		

'click into place'. The NMC (2004) expects the practice part of the programme to provide opportunities for you to experience 24-hour, 7-day care in order 'to enable students to develop understanding of users' experiences of health care' (NMC, 2004, p. 17).

Clinical practice can be undertaken in a variety of different settings, including primary, secondary and integrated care settings, in both the public and private sectors. Participating in aspects of nursing within these areas should expose you to differing approaches to health care and enable better contextualisation of the services offered.

Primary care refers to those health services that play a central role in the health of the local community, including family doctors (general practitioners, GPs), pharmacists, dentists and district nurses (DH, 2008). In *Our Health, Our Care, Our Say* (DH, 2006) the shift from health services within an acute setting to community services is outlined. Therefore, as a student nurse you may be placed in community hospitals and intermediate care teams. Also, more specialist teams are developing to either prevent the compromised ill individual from being admitted to the acute service and rather supported in the community and those that are admitted may be discharged more quickly and require nursing approaches to enable them for a period of time.

Secondary care comprises National Health Service (NHS) hospitals that provide acute and specialist services, treating patients with conditions that normally cannot be dealt with by primary care specialists or who are brought in as an emergency. Secondary care covers medical treatment and surgery that patients receive in hospital following referral from a GP. It is made up of foundation hospitals, ambulance services and mental health trusts.

Integrated care refers to both health and social care services working together to ensure that individuals get the treatment and care that they need in order remain in control and to live independent lives. This includes services such as cross-organisational services for drug users who have a range of difficulties, for example health, housing and education.

Clinical practice involves learning through applying knowledge to the experience being undertaken while demonstrating the standards of conduct, performance and ethics (NMC, 2008). Placements are usually coordinated by an allocations officer within the HEI, who may work collaboratively alongside clinical practice facilitators who plot your journey and ensure that repetition of a placement is avoided and therefore a breadth of experience is facilitated.

What will I be doing?

As a student nurse, you will be directly exposed to, and participate in, the assessment, planning, implementation and evaluation of individualised patient/client care. When in clinical practice, you are supervised by a mentor, who is usually a registered nurse and has attended the relevant preparation or update to support student nurses within the clinical practice setting (NMC, 2006a).

Who will I be nursing?

As a nurse, you will have the privilege of meeting, working with and caring for a wide variety of individuals, including patients, clients, residents, service users and families. The nature of the client group that you encounter depends on the branch that you follow.

It has been noted that the UK population is ageing (Population Ageing Associates, 2006), and the number of adults over the age of 50 years is projected to rise. By 2020, half the adult population will be aged over 50 years, and the number of people aged 65 years and over is projected to reach 12.5 million. This is compounded further by the number of 'older old' (people over 75 years of age) doubling from 4.5 million today to over 9 million in 2050. In contrast, there is a static and declining younger age group. Therefore, today and in the future, it is likely that you will encounter older individuals having to cope with chronic conditions and those physical, psychological and social issues that arise as a consequence of this. Nurses are faced with the unusual and difficult position of potentially caring for those who are very young (babies) and caring for patients who are dying. Therefore, they will encounter an array of emotions and behaviours from both patients and relatives, including elation, happiness, relief, worry, anxiety, fear, grief, anger, disbelief and occasional violence.

What do nurses do?

The role of the nurse is multifaceted and complex and may be influenced by the nature of the clinical practice setting in which the nurse is working. A definition of nursing therefore is to inform the role of the nurse. Nursing is an evolving profession and is in the process of achieving a unique knowledge base. Many nurse theorists have offered definitions of nursing; one of the more recent is that of the Royal College of Nursing (RCN), which states that

> . . . *nursing is the use of clinical judgement and the provision of care to enable people to promote, improve, maintain, or recover health or, when death is inevitable, to die peacefully.*
>
> (RCN, 2002)

From this definition a number of roles are derived, as Figure 4.2 shows. Further to this, the four branches of nursing offer more specific characteristics:

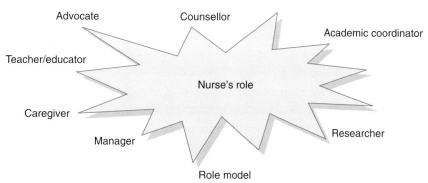

Figure 4.2 Roles of the nurse.

- *Adult nursing*: nurses in this branch assess, plan, implement and evaluate holistic nursing care for patients usually aged 18 years or older in both primary and secondary care. Sometimes the group includes adolescent patients who have reached physical maturity and who are placed within the adult clinical practice setting.
- *Mental health nursing*: this branch of nursing is 'the practice of caring for people who have mental illness, potentiating their independence and restoring their dignity' (Dexter and Wash, 1997, p. 3).
- *Learning disability*: this branch of nursing focuses on meeting the needs of individuals who have 'a significant impairment of intelligence as well as a significant impairment of social functioning and that both of these impairments were acquired before adulthood' (Carnaby, 2002, p. 8). In caring for clients with learning disability, nurses are encouraged to embrace normalisation – that is, to encourage a positive image for people with learning disabilities in order to decrease stigmatisation and to increase their acceptance into wider society (Carnaby, 2002).
- *Children's nursing*: this varied branch of nursing involves caring for both sick and well children and young people. The age range is from newborn to adolescence, and therefore a key aspect of children's nursing is the understanding of the development of the child, with the nurse being involved in partnerships with the child's parents or guardians while ensuring that the rights and uniqueness of the child are respected (Power, 2006).

Who will I be working with?

Throughout your nursing career you will work with a range of people who contribute individualised holistic patient care. The following are some of the many roles undertaken within health care (NHS Careers, 2008):

- *Art therapist*: helps clients to communicate by expressing their feelings and exploring their lives and problems through artwork.
- *Dietician*: promotes nutritional well-being and prevents and treats food-related problems.
- *Health care assistant*: works within the hospital or community setting under the guidance of a qualified health care professional, usually assisting in the delivery of care.
- *Health visitor*: a qualified nurse who has undertaken specialist education about the promotion of health and prevention of illness.
- *Midwife*: offers individual care to women and their families and helps them to take part in their own planning throughout all stages of pregnancy.
- *Occupational therapist*: helps people to overcome physical, psychological or social problems arising from illness or disability by focusing on what they can achieve.
- *Pharmacist*: has expertise relating to drugs and medicines and can be involved in all aspects of their use, including preparation, discovery, development and monitoring of effects.

- *Physiotherapist*: treats physical problems caused by accidents, illness and ageing, particularly those that affect the muscles, bones, heart, circulation and lungs.
- *Psychologist*: applies psychological theory and practice to solving problems or bringing about improvements for individuals, groups or organisations.
- *Social worker*: assesses and helps people to support their social needs, for example in relation to social care, housing, benefits and support mechanisms.
- *Speech and language therapist*: works with people who have problems with communication (usually speech defects), chewing or swallowing.

The role of the nurse when working with others is often to coordinate a multiprofessional team approach so that care can be tailored and individualised, ensuring the patient, family and carers are central in the process of collaboration.

> **Reflection point 4.3**
> Identify and briefly describe five other health care professionals that a student nurse may work alongside within the clinical practice setting. Consider what specific expertise each of these professionals offers.

Assessment of theory and practice

To ensure competency, all student nurses are assessed on both theory and practice. Assessment enables an objective measurement of learning to be made. There are a range of assessments that you may be exposed to or participate in during your nursing course (Table 4.3).

Assessment can be either formative or summative. Formative assessment enables progress to be reviewed continuously. Formative assessment still means that work, either theory or practice, will have to be submitted or undertaken. It can confirm whether learning has taken place and is useful to identify any weaknesses that may require further development. Summative assessment, on the other hand, is often undertaken at the end of a given period of time; for example, theoretical summative assessment usually occurs at the end of a period of learning such as a module or course. Clinical practice assessment, although more often continuous, has a summative element to it, as specific clinical outcomes have to be achieved. Because of their importance, some clinical skills may be assessed annually, for example basic life support.

A judgement on the effectiveness of learning is made in the form of a percentage or a descriptor such as pass, fail, satisfactory, unsatisfactory, merit, distinction or classification of degree. The results given ultimately determine progression in or completion of the programme being undertaken.

Table 4.3 Methods of assessment

Theory	Practice
Written essay	Clinical skills – continuous
Seen exam	Objective structured clinical examination
Unseen exam	
Viva	
Workbooks	
Guided study	
Poster	
Seminar	

Assessment often causes anxiety in students. First and foremost, you should never be assessed on something that you have not been taught or experienced. Assessment dates are often published well in advance, and so planning and revision around assessment should be possible. In the unfortunate instance that the assessment is unsuccessful, then the assessment can be retaken. If a number of failures are accrued (usually more than two at a particular level of study), however, this may lead to an issue with regard to progression in accordance with the assessment regulations of the HEI. It is important to ensure that any special learning needs that you have are recognised formally through the established procedures of the HEI in order that the support that can be offered is maximised; for example, a student certified with dyslexia is able to have extra time in a written exam or reader. It is also essential that nurses are aware of the support mechanisms available to them.

Supporting learning in theory and practice

Facilitation and supervision of learning in both theory and practice are available via a wide range of sources. The majority of schools of nursing and midwifery within a HEI adopt a personal tutor strategy, whereby you are allocated a named lecturer to support them throughout the course. The main aspects of the personal tutor are, according to Gidman (2001):

- *Clinical*: the personal tutor monitors your attendance and progression in clinical practice.
- *Pastoral*: the personal tutor provides assistance by identifying the services available to you should personal problems or other issues (e.g. financial, accommodation-related) arise during the course.
- *Academic*: the personal tutor may mark your academic work, monitor your academic progress, and facilitate the linking of theory to practice through reflection.

In addition, course lecturers can offer specific advice regarding issues relating to content and assessment support. The integration of theory with practice is integral; therefore, while you are in clinical placement, a visit from a lecturer may occur. The aim of such a visit is to ensure that you are being given every opportunity to achieve the clinical outcomes as stated in the practice assessment appropriate to that area and that adequate support is being offered by the clinical mentor. The visit is an opportunity for you, the clinical mentor and the academic lecturer to review your progress to date in the achievement of outcomes and proficiencies and to formulate an action plan for future professional development.

Other valuable support is available within the HEI. It is important that you become familiar with the resources offered, including counselling, occupational health, library and academic advisory services.

On each practice placement, you are allocated a named mentor (NMC, 2006a). The mentor should have appropriate education and preparation to undertake this important role and supervise you for a minimum of 40 per cent your allocated time (NMC, 2006a). In the final placement, there is an additional protected 1 hour per week to be spent with a sign-off mentor (NMC, 2006a). A sign-off mentor is an NMC registrant (on the same part or sub-part of the register as that which you are intending to enter) who makes a judgement about whether you have achieved the required standards of proficiency for safe and effective practice (NMC, 2006a). The mentor is responsible for assessing outcomes and proficiencies; other members of the nursing team, known as associate mentors, may also contribute towards the assessment of practice. Support comes also from sources other than mentors, including clinical practice facilitators and other members of the nursing and health care team, for example health care assistants, ward receptionists, members of the multiprofessional team and other students.

Learning now and in the future

Interprofessional education

The NHS is a dynamic organisation subject to continuing change in many areas, such as treatment, care and roles. Consequently the NHS continually has to develop and adapt. One such development is the increasing recognition that professionals do not work in isolation but rather work together and alongside one another in order to manage and deliver effective care. Nurse education has adapted to this and, to a varying extent, embraced the concept of interprofessional education. The Centre for the Advancement of Interprofessional Education (CAIPE) (1997) defines this 'as occasions when two or more professions learn with, from and about each other to improve collaboration and the quality of [service]'. Carlisle *et al.* (2005) consider that the term 'interprofessional education' tends to be used interchangeably with 'shared learning' and 'multi-professional learning'. Some knowledge and understanding can be shared, and this may be achieved by interprofessional learning. This is defined as 'the process through which two or more professions learn with, from and about each other to improve collaboration and the quality of service' (CAIPE, 1997). Therefore, as a nurse, throughout your career, you will be working alongside and learning with other professionals.

E-learning

Education is ever evolving, and teaching strategies are becoming increasingly diverse. One such evolution that education continues to embrace is that of information and communication technology (ICT) (Clarke, 2004). Such an approach enables a more flexible approach to be adopted. Traditional classroom teaching is being supplemented by more humanistic teaching strategies whereby learning can occur at a distance from lecturers and from the HEI. This can be disconcerting for students who prefer the immediacy of face-to-face teaching, but there are a number of benefits, including the freedom to study at any location and the flexibility of the pace, which can be set by the lecturers and other students in the group and adjusted and adapted to the individual's own learning pace (Clarke, 2004). Before students embark on any such approach to learning, it is usual to ensure adequate preparation so that learning can be maximised.

Clinical practice and nurse education are also evolving, and will continue to do so, as a response to social and health policy and initiatives from the regulatory body. As a nurse, therefore, you always have to be open, flexible and adaptable to change, while also embracing the integral concepts of accountability and responsibility.

Evidence-based practice

Although not new, the concept of evidence-based practice is emerging as being central to the standards of contemporary clinical practice. Evidence-based practice can be defined as

> *finding, appraising and applying scientific evidence to the treatment and management of health-care. Its ultimate goal is to support practitioners in their decision making in order to eliminate the use of ineffective, inappropriate, too expensive and potentially dangerous practices.*
>
> (Hamer, 2005, p. 6)

A nurse's decision or judgement should be informed because this facilitates the most effective care to be delivered. It can also enable care to come under greater scrutiny.

Accountability

Caulfield (2005) considers that the accountable nurse has confidence that allows them to take pride in being transparent about the way they carry out their practice. Decisions that nurses make are not only informed but also engage the patient or client to agree on a joint approach.

Accountability is very important, but there can be an ambiguity with nurses sometimes providing their own interpretation (Savage and Moore, 2004). To guide NMC registrants in their professional practice, there are principles within the NMC Code. For student nurses, the NMC (2006b) (Appendix 3) has provided some basic information with guidance for clinical experience, although it is highlighted that this guidance must be supplemented by information provided by the HEI.

The concept of accountability essentially means that nurses can be held to account – that is, they must be able to explain and justify their acts, omissions and decisions.

> **Reflection point 4.4**
> Read the NMC Code (see Appendix 1) and briefly summarise your interpretation of the following in relation to *An NMC Guide for Students of Nursing and Midwifery* (NMC, 2006b):
> In caring for patients and clients you must:
>
> - respect the patient or client as an individual;
> - obtain consent before you give any treatment or care;
> - protect confidential information;
> - cooperate with others in the team;
> - maintain your professional knowledge and competence;
> - be trustworthy;
> - act to identify and minimise risks to patients and clients.

Professional nurses are accountable to four pillars, namely professional, ethical, legal and employment accountability.

Professional accountability

Professional accountability means that the qualified practitioner can be called to account for their actions or omissions by the NMC. As a student nurse, you cannot be called to account professionally; this is why the NMC states that student nurses must always work under the direct supervision of a registered nurse. However, a student nurse is responsible for their actions and, if a nurse delegates a job that you feel is beyond your competence, then you should recognise this and inform the registered nurse. The delegating nurse is accountable for the decision to delegate work to others, but not the actual actions of others, and therefore the registrant should be able to justify their decision.

Scenario 4.2 describes a case study of professional accountability.

Ethical accountability

This pillar of accountability refers to morals and values that influence health care. Influences include the constraints of society, for example that nurses are expected not to torture individuals (Caulfield, 2005), and individual moral values. If a nurse has a conscientious objection, for example in relation to abortion or technological procedures used to achieve conception and pregnancy, then this can be raised.

Scenario 4.3 describes a case study of ethical accountability.

SCENARIO 4.2 Case study of professional accountability

A frail elderly woman is admitted as an inpatient to a medical ward. As part of the admission, the nurse undertakes a pressure ulcer risk assessment to identify whether the woman is at risk of developing pressure ulcers. On completion of the various categories of the assessment, the woman is not identified as being at risk. However, the nurse still thinks that the patient is at risk of developing a pressure ulcer. After explaining this to the patient, it is agreed that some pressure-relieving methods should be introduced within her care delivery.

In this instance the assessment tool acted as an aide-memoire, but the nurse had the confidence and engaged with the patient to exercise their clinical judgment and make an informed decision.

But what if . . .

. . . the nurse completed a pressure ulcer risk assessment of the elderly woman, identified that she was at high risk of developing pressure ulcers and yet did nothing about it and the patient went on to develop a grade 4 pressure ulcer, which affected her physical, social and psychological well-being?

In this instance there is an omission in the care of the patient, and the nurse has failed in their duty of care to the patient, who is entitled to receive safe and competent care.

SCENARIO 4.3 Case study of ethical accountability

A patient is admitted to the accident and emergency department after sustaining cuts to the wrist. The cuts are superficial, but while the nurse is dressing the wounds the patient informs the nurse that last night he consumed a large amount of alcohol and a quantity of illegal drugs but that he does not want anyone to know as he wants 'to end it all because life isn't worth living, as it is all so unfair'.

In this instance, the nurse would have to inform someone (a doctor), as there is a risk to the patient's physical and psychological well-being. The nurse may choose to tell the patient that she will inform a doctor, as Caulfield (2005) identifies trust is fundamental to the basis of the nurse–patient relationship. Ordinarily, nurses have a moral duty not to lie; however, the nurse has to weigh up each individual situation and decide whether telling the truth would cause the patient harm.

Legal accountability

Law, and the purpose of it, according to Watson and Tilley (2004), is to provide deterrence and compensation when things go wrong and is not a tool to punish. Nurses should be aware of the four areas of law: civil law, criminal law, public law and European law. Key concepts in relation to the law include negligence, consent, confidentiality (see Scenario 4.4 for an example), conscientious objection and palliative care.

Employment accountability

All nurses, including student nurses, are accountable to their employer by virtue of their contract of employment (Tingle, 2004). Nurses are expected to fulfil their contract and job description, and the employer expects that duties and responsibilities are undertaken safely. In turn, employers are expected to provide an appropriate environment and sufficient resources in order for nurses to fulfil their contractual arrangements; this may include training and the provision of policies and protocols (Caulfield, 2005).

Scenario 4.5 describes a case study of employment accountability.

SCENARIO 4.4 Case study of legal accountability

A nurse is in a lift full of people. She is talking with a colleague and pointing to a set of notes that she is holding, which is labelled with the patient's name, address and date of birth on the front, back and spine. The nurse says: 'Nasty cancer – starting chemo next week – the parents are really upset.' Another person in the lift recognises the patient's name and address and sends a card in the post to the child and his parents. The parents report this incident to the ward sister and enquire how someone came to know about the diagnosis: they had withheld the information from family so they could adjust to the diagnosis and protect another member of the wider family who is a full-time carer for someone with Alzheimer's disease.

In this instance the nurse has not adhered to the NMC Code and has breached confidentiality. Information has not been protected and has been used improperly and without permission. Disclosure is not in the public interest and therefore there is a legal duty under common law to keep information confidential.

SCENARIO 4.5 Case study of employment accountability

A registered nurse passes a fine-bore nasogastric tube on a young adult client with long-standing cerebral palsy who requires supplementary night-time feeding. The nurse aspirates the tube using old litmus paper, despite recently reading the updated policy that has been based upon the National Institute for Health and Clinical Excellence (NICE, 2006) guidelines. These guidelines confirm that the correct insertion of a nasogastric tube should be checked using pH indicator strips. The reading should show a pH of 5.5 or less before commencing.

The nasogastric feed commences and the client starts to cough and become breathless. The doctor is contacted immediately about the client's apparent change in condition. The nurse helps the client to sit up and offers every comfort. A chest X-ray identifies that the nasogastric tube is not in the stomach but in the lungs and that the supplementary feed has entered the lung. The client develops aspirational pneumonia and discharge is delayed.

In this instance the nurse is in breach of contract, as the policy that was circulated to all staff was not adhered to.

Other pillars of accountability are embraced within this case study, but in relation to employment accountability it would be at the discretion of the employer to apply a disciplinary measure; this could be either a warning leading to retraining or a dismissal.

Clearly accountability is a very complex concept. Each of the case studies described here demonstrates just one pillar of accountability, but other pillars would also apply. Student nurses, although not on the NMC Register during their pre-registration training, learn to work towards accountability for their own actions so that they can act as self-regulating practitioners.

Learning: it never ends

Nurse education, especially pre-registration education, is a springboard to lifelong learning. Many newly qualified nurses describe the transition from student to registered nurse as being when 'real learning' takes place. This relates inevitably to the practicalities of being a registered nurse within a clinical practice setting and becoming professionally accountable. Although the NMC (2006b) advises that there is a formal period of support called 'preceptorship' for newly registered nurses, it is worthwhile to ensure that a focus is retained regarding individual development. Personal development planning (PDP) can facilitate this. PDP is a structured process that reflects the individual's own learning, performance and achievement and enables them to plan for personal, educational and career development. This may facilitate individual performance review (IPR), sometimes known as 'appraisal', which as is undertaken on an annual basis for trained nurses.

PDP and IPR may identify training and learning needs that are required for the organisation within which you are working. This may include extending skills to provide good patient care, for example the administration of intravenous medicines, phlebotomy and venepuncture. Nurses have to be updated annually to ensure the correctness of important techniques and skills, such as moving and handling; this is called 'mandatory training'. Registered nurses must always be mindful of the PREP requirements to maintain registration and provide ongoing evidence of continuing professional development by maintaining a professional portfolio (NMC, 2005a) (see also Chapter 23).

Post-registration learning may result in the registrant returning to an HEI to undertake further study at the same or different level. This may come from a personal need to develop further or for development in a more specialist area where a more specific knowledge and understanding is required. Previously accumulated CAT points may be able to be used as part of the APEL process (e.g. advanced diploma). Post-registration education is often flexible, and part-time study is usually the preferred option. This study option may be supported by the clinical employer practice area, especially if it links directly to the practice area and the benefit will be not solely to the nurse but ultimately to the patient.

CONCLUSION

Learning to nurse should always embrace the components of theory and practice, each underpinning the other. As discussed in this chapter, in order to be competent practitioners, nurses need to have not only the requisite knowledge and understanding but also the necessary skills. Learning nursing, therefore, can be considered to be multifaceted and ever developing, as it involves caring for people often at their most vulnerable and in an environment that is subject to continuous change and challenges. To learn to become a nurse requires dedication, motivation, enthusiasm, occasional sacrifice, and commitment to the theory and practice of nursing and the challenges that this presents. To nurse a patient embraces so many roles; ultimately, though, in learning nursing, the practitioner is prepared to care and subsequently make a difference. Therefore, it is essential that we all care about learning and continuing to learn about nursing. Welcome to the lifelong journey that is nursing.

References

Atkinson J and Virdee A (2001). Promoting comfort for patients with symptoms other than pain. In Kinghorn S and Gamlin R (eds). *Palliative Nursing: Bringing Comfort and Hope*. Edinburgh: Baillière Tindall.

Borton T (1970). *Read, Touch and Teach*. London: McGraw-Hill.

Boud D, Keogh R and Walker D (1985). Promoting reflection in learning: a model. In Boud D, Keogh R and Walker D (eds). *Reflection: Turning Experience into Learning*. London: Kogan Page.

Bradshaw A (2001). *The Project 2000 Nurse*. London: Whurr.

Carlisle C, Donovan T and Mercer D (2005). Towards a shared definition of interprofessional education. In Carlisle C, Donovan T and Mercer D (eds). *Interprofessional Education: An Agenda for Healthcare Professionals*. Dinton: MA Healthcare Limited.

Carnaby S (2002). The bigger picture: understanding approaches to learning disability. In Carnaby S (ed.). *Learning Disability Today*. Brighton: Pavilion.

Carroll M (2000). An evaluation of temperature measurement. *Nursing Standard*, **14**, 39–43.

Caulfield H (2005). *Vital Notes for Nurses: Accountability*. Oxford: Blackwell.

Centre for the Advancement of Interprofessional Education (CAIPE) (1997). Definitions. www.caipe.org.uk.

Clarke A (2004). *e-Learning Skills*. Basingstoke: Palgrave Macmillan.

Department of Health (1999). *Making a Difference*. London: HMSO.

Department of Health (DH) (2006). *Our Health, Our Care, Our Say: A New Direction for Community Services*. London: Department of Health.

Department of Health (DH) (2008). Primary care. www.dh.gov.uk/en/Healthcare/Primarycare/index.htm.

Dexter G and Wash M (1997). *Psychiatric Nursing Skills: A Patient-Centred Approach*, 2nd edn. Cheltenham: Stanley Thornes.

Gidman J (2001). The role of the personal tutor: a literature review. *Nurse Education Today*, **21**, 359–65.

Hamer S (2005). Evidence-based practice. In Hamer S and Collinson G (eds). *Achieving Evidence-Based Practice: A Handbook for Practitioners*, 2nd edn. Edinburgh: Baillière Tindall Elsevier.

Holm D and Stephenson S (1994). Reflection: a student's perspective. In Palmer A, Burns S and Bulman C (eds). *Reflective Practice in Nursing*. Oxford: Blackwell Scientific.

Hull C, Redfern L and Shuttleworth A (2005). *Profiles and Portfolios: A Guide for Health and Social Care*, 2nd edn. Basingstoke: Palgrave Macmillan.

Johns C (2000). Revealing the nature of reflection. In Johns C (ed.). *Guided Reflection: Advancing Practice*. Oxford: Blackwell Science.

Kim HS (1999). Critical reflective inquiry for knowledge development in nursing practice. *Journal of Advanced Nursing*, **29**, 1205–12.

Marks-Maran D and Rose P (1997). Thinking and caring: new perspectives on reflection. In Marks-Maran D. and Rose P (eds). *Reconstructing Nursing: Beyond Art and Science*. London: Baillière Tindall.

National Institute for Health and Clinical Excellence (NICE) (2006). *Nutrition Support in Adults: Oral Nutrition Support, Enteral Tube Feeding and Parenteral Nutrition*. London: National Institute for Health and Clinical Excellence.

NHS Careers (2008). Careers A–Z. www.nhscareers.nhs.uk/atoz.shtml.

Nursing and Midwifery Council (NMC) (2004). *Standards of Proficiency for Pre-Registration Nursing Education*. London: Nursing and Midwifery Council.

Nursing and Midwifery Council (NMC) (2005a). *The PREP Handbook*. London: Nursing and Midwifery Council.

Nursing and Midwifery Council (NMC) (2005b). *Guidelines for Records and Record Keeping*. London: Nursing and Midwifery Council.

Nursing and Midwifery Council (NMC) (2006a). *Standards to Support Learning and Assessment in Practice: NMC Standards for Mentors, Practice Teachers and Teachers*. London: Nursing and Midwifery Council.

Nursing and Midwifery Council (NMC) (2006b). *An NMC Guide for Students of Nursing and Midwifery*. London: Nursing and Midwifery Council.

Nursing and Midwifery Council (NMC) (2008). *The Code Standards of Conduct, Performance and Ethics for Nurses and Midwives*. London: Nursing and Midwifery Council.

Palmer I, Burns S and Bulmer C (1994). *Reflective Practice in Nursing: The Growth of the Professional Practitioner*. Oxford: Blackwell Scientific.

Pearce R (2003). *Profiles and Portfolios of Evidence: Foundations in Nursing and Health Care*. Cheltenham: Nelson Thornes.

Philpin S (2002). Rituals and nursing: a critical commentary. *Journal of Advanced Nursing*, **38**, 144–51.

Population Ageing Associates (2006). Our population is ageing. www.populationageing.co.uk/demographics.htm. Accessed 12 January 2007.

Power K (2006). Perspectives on children's nursing. In Schober J and Ash C (eds). *Student Nurses' Guide to Professional Practice and Development*. London: Arnold.

Price A (2004). Encouraging reflection and critical thinking in practice. *Nursing Standard*, **18**, 46–53.

Rodéhn Fox M (1999). The importance of sleep. *Nursing Standard*, **13**, 44–7.

Royal College of Nursing (RCN) (2002). *Defining Nursing*. London: Royal College of Nursing.

Savage J and Moore L (2004). *Interpreting Accountability: An Ethnographic Study of Practice Nurses, Accountability and Multidisciplinary Team Decision-Making in the Context of Clinical Governance*. London: Royal College of Nursing.

Tingle J (2004). The legal accountability of the nurse. In Tilley S and Watson R (eds). *Accountability in Nursing and Midwifery*, 2nd edn. Oxford: Blackwell.

United Kingdom Central Council for Nursing, Midwifery and Health Visiting (UKCC) (2001). *Fitness for Practice and Purpose*. London: United Kingdom Central Council for Nursing, Midwifery and Health Visiting.

Walsh M (1998). *Models and Critical Pathways in Clinical Nursing: Conceptual Frameworks for Care Planning*, 2nd edn. London: Baillière Tindall.

Watson R and Tilley S (2004). Introduction: accountability and the law. In Tilley S and Watson R (eds). *Accountability in Nursing and Midwifery*, 2nd edn. Oxford: Blackwell.

Further reading

Alexander M, Fawcett JN and Runciman PJ (eds) (2006). *Nursing Practice: Hospital and Home*, 3rd edn. Edinburgh: Elsevier/Churchill Livingstone.
This comprehensive text is a one-stop shop for increasing knowledge and understanding of anatomy and physiology, applied pathophysiology and considers the nursing care required for a multitude of conditions over a number of specialties.

Barrett G, Sellman D and Thomas J (2005). *Interprofessional Working in Health and Social Care: Professional Perspectives*. Basingstoke: Palgrave Macmillan.

Coyler H, Helme M and Jones I (2006). *The Theory–Practice Relationship in Interprofessional Education*. London: Higher Education Academy Health Sciences and Practice Network.

Davis S and O'Connor S (eds) (1999). *Rehabilitation Nursing: Foundations for Practice*. Edinburgh: Baillière Tindall.

This book focuses on the concept of rehabilitation and is useful as a resource, especially as the patient group that adult student nurses encounter is mostly older and requires elements of the rehabilitation process.

Fatchett A (1998). *Nursing in the New NHS: Modern, Dependable?* Edinburgh: Baillière Tindall.

Gidman J, Humphreys A and Andrews M (2000). The role of the personal tutor in the academic context. *Nurse Education Today*, **20**, 401–7.

Hart C (2004). *Nurses and Politics: The Impact of Power and Practice*. Basingstoke: Palgrave Macmillan.

Hinchliff S (ed.) (2004). *The Practitioner as Teacher*, 3rd edn. Edinburgh: Baillière Tindall.

Rolfe G, Freshwater D and Jasper M (2001). *Critical Reflection for Nursing and the Helping Professions: A User Guide*. Basingstoke, Palgrave.

Schober J and Ash C (eds) (2006). *Student Nurses' Guide to Professional Practice and Development*. London: Arnold.
This book provides a thorough grounding in what it means to be a nurse both in theory and in clinical practice.

Stockwell F (1972). *The Unpopular Patient*. London: *Royal College of Nursing*.
A groundbreaking book at the time it was published, this provoking text sometimes makes uncomfortable reading but is still relevant to nursing today.

Walsh M (1998). *Models and Critical Pathways in Clinical Nursing: Conceptual Frameworks for Care Planning*, 2nd edn. London: Baillière Tindall.
This text provides an overview of theoretical concepts that underpin nursing practice in a convivial yet informative manner.

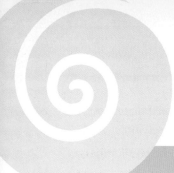

Support networks for students

5

Nick Salter

Introduction

This chapter aims to enlighten you about personal challenges that you may face before and during a programme of study. Support can offer you the chance to cope better with those challenges. The nature of support is explained, and the importance and possible benefits of support systems are discussed. Advice is given as to where information and further help can be obtained. It is hoped that, armed with this information, you will feel more able to solve problems and will look forward to the changes and challenges that lie ahead.

Learning objectives

After studying this chapter you should be able to:

- consider the challenges ahead in order to prepare for the possible changes that need to be made;
- understand where further advice can be obtained;
- have improved awareness of personal support networks;
- recognise the benefits of obtaining help and support.

Overview

This chapter discusses the nature of support and the advantages of seeking support during a programme of study. Many professional staff members give support in different situations, both formal and informal. Various types of support are needed at different times, but sometimes support does not happen. This may be due to a feeling of weakness or failure or simply to not knowing what help is on offer and from whom it can be sought. A range of support systems is available, and they form an essential part of the student experience. Additional support is available if other problems occur, for example homesickness, debt or accommodation issues.

When contemplating a university-based programme of study, there are many choices and decisions to make: Which programme? Which university? What about leaving home and living independently? What will the accommodation be like? Will it be affordable? Will paid employment be essential to supplement a bursary? There are many more questions and decisions to be made and it is hoped that this chapter will help.

Reflection point 5.1

These first questions are aimed at encouraging personal thought about some important changes that may occur and plans that need to be made. Under the following headings, make a list of ideas about these new situations that you will have to get used to when the programme starts.

How will you:

- get to know your way around the campus?
- adjust to working in practice placements?
- fit into new groups or teams?
- manage your study time?
- manage your finances?

Perceptions of student support

Perceptions of the benefits of support at university may have developed from experiences at school or the experiences that peers have shared, recently or in the distant past. Positive experiences with, for example, school teachers could induce a belief that future relationships with lecturers will be beneficial. Previous negative experiences, however, could work against a possible successful student–lecturer relationship. When at school, a summons to 'the office' created doubt and fear. Thoughts may have developed such as 'Why me?' or 'What does he want me for?' Lecturers, though, like teachers, are well able to dispense praise. They like nothing more: they enjoy helping students solve problems, guiding them and rewarding good work.

As a lecturer, it is easy to become enthusiastic about the outcome of support. The whole object of support is to help students. Support should ease your development and passage through the educational experience. A lecturer might help simply by listening or being there as a 'sounding board'. Advice could take the form of a direction or a course of action that should be taken. A lecturer might support a decision or behaviour as being acceptable, give praise for achievements and give reassurance in order to help maintain effort.

Outcomes of support

You can achieve a certain level of reassurance (as an outcome) (Teasdale, 1989) simply by knowing that support is available and that there is someone or something to turn to. Feelings of success are very positive motivators, and these can come from feedback from assignments, placement reports, tutorials and exam successes. Motivation is a great driving force. Sometimes students need encouragement to seek feedback and advice from lecturers; this can also come from peers. Often students learn together from shared experiences; the feeling of partnership can strengthen the desire to do well for each other, and learning that takes place together can seem more valuable.

Personal support can help to maintain positive behaviour and therefore learning. It can encourage the development of both personal and professional skills. So often, support attempts to enthuse students into action or decision-making. At times, when a student becomes unhappy or depressed, clarity of vision is lost. Support attempts to reorient you to reality. This process can be a difficult one, and you may need many sources of support. You may be seeking some sort of consolation or comfort during times of trouble. Symptoms of suffering are often difficult to alleviate and are often easier to spot in someone else rather than oneself.

Supporters also help by enlivening the mind and creating a sense of cheer – feelings that create hope and purpose in the mind. These positive states can help when, for example, study behaviour may need adapting to meet new situations, a change in the level of assessment, a new placement for practical experiences, or when reactions to events require new preparations for the future. Plans and arrangements for future experiences may need careful consideration, and timely effective support may make some positive difference.

One outcome of support is the creation of independence. There would be nothing gained by supporters who wish to make students dependent upon their advice. It should be obvious, then, that a significant amount of responsibility for self-determination depends on willpower. As the NMC Code (2008) (Appendix 1) indicates, nurses should:

Use the best available evidence

- *You must deliver care based on the best available evidence or best practice*
- *You must ensure any advice you give is evidence based if you are suggesting healthcare products or services*

- *You must ensure that the use of complementary or alternative therapies is safe and in the best interests of those in your care*

Keep your skills and knowledge up to date

- *You must have the knowledge and skills for safe and effective practice when working without direct supervision*
- *You must recognise and work within the limits of your competence*
- *You must keep your knowledge and skills up to date throughout your working life*
- *You must take part in appropriate learning and practice activities that maintain and develop your competence and performance.*

It can be seen that registered nurses are responsible for their own development, and so during a pre-registration programme you need to develop your own ability to be responsible for your own actions. Students work under the supervision of registered nurses; however, the aim to practise safely and effectively without direct supervision and while maintaining knowledge and skills is a requirement during training.

 SUMMARY

This discussion has described support in a general sense, with the aim of enthusing you to view support in a positive manner. The following sections discuss some of the common reasons why you might seek support or, to put it another way, some of the many needs you may experience during training. A further section discusses possible sources of support.

Possible challenges to consider

Changes to accommodation

Leaving home, especially leaving a familiar environment, routine, family members and friends, can be an upheaval. The need to learn how to perform domestic activities might be a major new set of experiences that could seem daunting. On the other hand, changes might be preferable to present arrangements, and new experiences may be those that have been looked forward to for some time. Many students, especially mature students, choose to stay at home. This can produce savings on expenses and reduce the need for change. As the need to study changes and the time spent at home changes, some allowances need to be made both by you and by the people with whom you live. Often, students describe their families and friends going through the programme with them, and so even families and friends could be making some sacrifices.

Arranging accommodation itself might be a new experience. Private accommodation is usually available, and the local advice centre, accommodation officer and students' union are all available to advise. Finding secure, safe and comfortable housing is essential, and some universities guarantee accommodation for the first year of study, especially if you are from overseas. Accommodation usually comprises premises that are owned by the university or a private landlord. University accommodation is often in halls of residence and can be situated on campus. There are many advantages to this: students value the reduced cost of travel, and often see the sense of camaraderie shared with flatmates as like having a second family. Students in shared accommodation are usually studying on different programmes, which has both advantages and disadvantages. Nursing students work during placement time, but very few other students do this. Shift patterns may create specific problems if students on other programmes do not under-stand the special needs for quietness and the fact that study time might take priority over social time. Many student nurses enjoy living with other student nurses because they gain a lot of peer support regarding programme issues, even if they are living with students in another year group or nursing branch specialty. The challenge of time management is often different for student nurses, and this can be an added stress when sharing accommodation. The way to cope is to share information, to be open and honest about expectations, and to set some universally accept-able ground rules.

Living in university halls of residence is an experience that some students relish, but others prefer to avoid it. Living in halls is a matter of taste, and no two halls are the same. Try to visit prospective halls and talk to resident students for their views before making a decision. The qual-ity of accommodation worries many students and their parents when, for example, there has been no prior viewing. There is a tendency to make friendship groups quickly in halls, and often small groups move halls in order to be with each other. Some students leave halls and rent accommodation together in order to give them a greater sense of independence.

A form P76 accompanies the final offer from the chosen university; this is the accommodation preference form. The form must be returned within 7 days for UK students.

Universities vet the private rented accommodation that they recommend through their accom-modation office or agency. The rent might be cheaper in these premises than the generally avail-able flats and houses. It is recommended that time is taken to visit areas and rental agencies as well as the university office so that comparisons can be made. Cost is not the only priority to consider. The term of the contract is an important consideration: some private landlords charge for the whole of the summer term, even though the accommodation might not be required for all the term. It is also worth finding whether belongings need to be removed during the summer.

The website www.merlinhelpsstudents.com has advice about accommodation, advice on rent-ing in the private sector, safety issues, contracts, types of tenancy, deposits, university lodgings and the benefits of staying at home. It may be worth approaching an accommodation agency. Local papers and their websites are also worth considering. Looking at the student housing on offer is often an option during university open days. Another helpful website is www.connexions-direct.com: this site displays advice about housing, including student accommoda-tion, housing benefits, and moving out/leaving home.

Inventories of contents should always be checked upon entering the accommodation for the first time. This should include an inspection of any damage already present; although accommo-dation should be in an acceptable condition, what constitutes 'acceptable' is open to debate. If it is necessary to make a complaint, try to be objective and fair and be prepared to compromise at least until after the initial settling-in period is over. With time, alternatives will be discovered and other avenues to making changes will be found.

One of the fears for some students, especially those who have not lived away from home before, is homelessness. Occasionally accommodation is arranged too late for the agency or accommodation officer to give any advance notice of location. It is important to keep a wary eye on the location and type of accommodation on offer at the interview stage and to enquire about its availability if information does not arrive when it is expected.

Managing finances

Spending money wisely will always be a difficulty for the majority of students. A lack of money might occur due to poor budgeting. You may not have had much previous experience with handling money for food, clothing, accommodation and study expenses, paying bills and fees, and living on a limited budget. Bank managers, student services departments, student loan departments, parents and partners are there to give help if necessary. Financial problems are best managed as soon as they become apparent rather than when debt has become uncontrolled. The Aim Higher website (www.aimhigher.ac.uk) has a simple cost-of-living calculator, gives good advice for hassle-free budgeting and personal banking, and has links to other useful websites. Further advice can be found from the network of Citizens Advice Bureaux (www.citizensa dvice.org.uk). These provide free and independent advice on a range of problems, including benefits, housing, immigration, debt and legal issues. The website has the contact details of the 850 local bureaux across the UK.

Students under the age of 19 years are automatically entitled to help with health care costs. Claims are made using a HC1 claim form, which can be obtained from a Jobcentre Plus office or National Health Service (NHS) hospital, and some general practitioners (GPs), dentists and opticians. The form can also be obtained by telephoning 0845 850 1166 or from the website www.ppa.org.uk/ppa/HC1_form.htm. The HC1 form can be used to claim help with NHS prescriptions; NHS dental treatment; NHS wigs and fabric supports; sight tests, glasses and contact lenses; and travel to hospital for NHS treatment.

Students from the UK or European Union (EU) qualifying for 'home student status' have their tuition fees paid and are eligible for a non-means-tested NHS bursary. For 2007–08, the amount granted is set at a basic rate of £6372 for students with additional support for parents and their children. There are no top-up tuition fees for pre-registration nursing programmes. Normally the NHS pays the tuition fees for the duration of the training. The NHS normally provides students on a diploma programme with a non-means-tested bursary. The NHS bursary website (www.nhsstudentgrants.co.uk) gives detailed information including eligibility and additional allowances for dependants. You may be eligible for the following:

- Childcare Allowance if there are children in registered childcare;
- Access to Learning fund;
- supplementary allowances for mature students, single parents, people with dependants and students incurring clinical placement costs;
- Disabled Students' Allowance;
- a grant from the Elizabeth Nuffield Educational Fund (women only).

Check the website www.nhspa.gov.uk/sgu/Allowances for further information.

Students on diploma programmes are not eligible for student loans.

For students on degree programmes, the NHS bursary is means tested (income assessed). Eligible student nurses qualify for 75 per cent of the maximum loan, regardless of income, and the rest is income-assessed. These loans accrue interest at the rate of inflation, which means that the amount repaid has the same value as the amount borrowed. The loan is unlike any other loan or credit agreement. It becomes repayable only when earnings are over £15 000 per annum. These loans are probably the lowest interest-bearing loans available. Repayments depend on earnings; a person earning over £20 000 a year repays £8.70 a week. If a nurse stops earning, they stop paying and the payment schedule does not need to be renegotiated. The starting wage for a band 5 nurse is a minimum of £19 683.

To apply for a bursary, or to obtain further information, contact:

NHS Student Grants Unit
Hesketh House
200–220 Broadway
Fleetwood
Lancashire FY7 8LG
Tel: 0845 358 6655
Fax: 01253 774490
Email: enquiries@nhspa.gov.uk
www.nhsstudentgrants.co.uk

The latest edition of *Financial Help for Health Care Students* can be downloaded from www.nhspa.gov.uk/sgu/forms/booklets/students_financial_help.pdf.

The money gained from your bursary is easily spent. Many students are in debt to banks or building societies, and many feel indebted to their parents or supporters, which can produce intense feelings of guilt. However, increasingly, students are accepting that debt is just another consequence of being at university. Many students seek employment to supplement their income (see 'Working as a student' below), whether to fund loan repayments, to help pay for basic requirements such as food and accommodation expenses, or to cover childcare fees.

ChildcareLink (www.childcarelink.gov.uk/index.asp) is a UK government-sponsored website with comprehensive information about national and local childcare and early years. It gives advice on childminders, preschool and after-school groups. The website pulls together childcare information from local authorities and facilitates searches for appropriate local care.

Christmas and other holiday times produce special demands on finances, especially for students who are parents or carers, and for mature students with family-related commitments that younger students do not experience, such as a partner's employment or business-related expenses. If hardship is experienced during the programme, you might be entitled to help from your university's Access to Learning Fund. Some students are classed as a priority, especially those with children (in particular, lone parents), those in their final year of study and those with low-income parents (see www.aimhigher.ac.uk/student_finance/other_help/access_to_learning_fund.cfm).

Scholarships are available for some students to help with costs. The Hot Courses website (www.scholarship-search.org.uk) has a database of undergraduate scholarships. The university might have a student hardship fund and there would be a specific process to follow to access this fund. Many websites offer advice on bursary issues, finance and counselling services; see www.nmc-uk.org.

New students might not fully appreciate the important issue of travelling expenses. While at school or college, your institution, parents or friends often arrange and subsidise transport. At university, bearing the cost of transport for the first time can produce worries. The burden of responsibility may also be an unknown quantity, and the expense, time and frustration of car breakdowns and missed buses and trains may add to the mounting stressors. It might be important to become aware of the process for claiming previous travel costs. Have a look at websites for cheaper travel offers.

Being in control of personal finances reduces the deleterious effects of financial hardship. This facilitates a greater focus on study and the positive effects of employment and personal management that can help improve a sense of self-esteem.

Working as a student

Learning takes place as much from experiences gained in practice as from that gained from reading, thinking and writing. The pre-registration programme is unlike many other university programmes because professional registration depends on the practical work performed. Although other university students use their non-contact time (i.e. away from lecturers) to study and socialise, much of a student nurse's non-contact time is spent practising in care establishments, studying, socialising, and perhaps running a household and family. This means that the amount of free personal time is limited and needs to be managed differently from the way it was managed before the programme started.

Working to earn money so that you can afford to stay on the programme produces its own set of stressors. Taking time away from social activities, study and sleep can have effects on wakefulness, concentration and morale. Holding down a job that helps fund studies might be relatively easy at the beginning of a programme, but some students find that the need to concentrate on studies when the academic level increases puts a strain on their ability to work in the latter part of the programme. Paid or unpaid employment reduces the time available for study, resulting in tension between the need to earn money and the need to study; the outcome is often further stress. Disappointment can occur because assessment results are lower than anticipated; alternatively, financial hardship may follow. The amount of time devoted to reading, and reflection on and assimilation of that reading, is often related to academic results, and so this is another issue that is related to work time, leisure time and time off for illness.

Some students enjoy the experience of work outside their programme and gain positive well-being from it. Working as a health care assistant or in similar role can help you gain practical experience and interactional skills. Furthermore, the experiences help to nurture a caring attitude and approach to others. However, a word of warning is necessary here: some students feel compromised when they work as bank health care assistants. They may do such work on a ward where they have worked previously in the role of student nurse; student nurses in this situation possess skills gained and practised as a student, but there is a tension when they are not able to use these skills as health care assistants. In both roles, you are responsible to the same manager, but different tasks and interactions are expected in the different roles. Students often feel restricted within the assistant role and should remember the boundaries to the role and the expectations made of them.

Many students continue the work that they enjoyed before starting university. Regardless of the job, transferable skills are learned, and these are very valuable to a student of nursing. Such skills include interpersonal skills, responsibility, autonomy, independence and teamworking. However, some jobs are low paid, and this leads to some students taking on several different jobs.

A reverse situation also exists because some students leave paid employment in order to join a programme. They may then lose status and other benefits of employment. The change in role, control and perceived competence can be an initial worry.

Other non-paid work may involve you using your time away from study and placement experiences to help others, for example in a caring role or to support their partner's employment. Some universities do not encourage their students to work outside their programme. Other universities impose a limit on the number of hours they recommend that students work per week; for example, the limit at my university is 15 hours per week. Limits, however, are usually applied loosely, and each student has a responsibility to themselves as to how much work is manageable. To put it simply, a balance of time for work and for life needs to be struck.

Managing learning

The start of any programme or module of study produces a plethora of new information to be understood and integrated into new routines. Most peers are in a similar position, and so you should talk with other students to see what sense others make of it all and to facilitate the awareness that you are not alone in your feelings and thoughts.

Using initiative for organising time might be a novel experience. An important point here is that you are responsible for your own learning. Lecturers have a responsibility to teach, but they cannot learn for their students. In practice, this means that you need to prepare for lectures, gain insights and motivation from the lecturers, and read around the subject and gain further information in order to help form opinions and alter your thinking about what you have heard and seen.

There are some potential difficulties in relation to learning resources. Obtaining books and journal articles can take a long time and cost money. There are insufficient books in most libraries for all students to be able to borrow copies of the same book at the same time. Libraries do not expect or have funds to hold sufficient copies of key texts for all students. The short loan and recall systems should be used. Library staff members are keen to help and often run introductory sessions to help you understand how best to access literature and use literature-searching facilities.

Photocopying costs money, and this expense needs to be anticipated. Again, planning will help, especially around the times when there is likely to be heavy demand on certain key texts. Book tokens for birthday presents are useful. Books should be bought only after you have looked through them and deemed them essential; a dictionary, an anatomy and physiology textbook, and key psychology and sociology texts might be recommended. The sharing of information and resources with peers is very useful, as this can save time and money and nurtures symbiotic relationships.

Meeting deadlines, handing in assignments and getting behind with work often causes stress. Time management can be a skill that takes years of practice. Setting goals by working back from assessment deadlines is essential. Lecturers, peers and more experienced students can offer advice and encouragement, and so discussion of difficulties can be very beneficial. If all else fails, lecturers may agree to extend assignment deadlines when there have been difficulties, for example illness, that prevent proper completion of work. You should not be reluctant to negotiate an extension – they are the university's way of being flexible when unpredictable events occur.

Reflection point 5.2

This is a good place to encourage thought about commitment to others. Have a look at the following questions. While thinking of the possible answers, significant others could be included in the discussion to arrive at an action plan so that changes that may have to be made can be controlled.

1 If in current employment, will the nature of the employment change as a result of the programme?
2 Will a job be essential in order to finance the programme?
3 If there are any dependent individuals, what will have to change when the programme is started?
4 Will it be possible to alter any volunteer work while on the programme?
5 If there are any regular sporting interests, will there need to be any changes to routines?

Well-being is a critical factor for success

The effects on the time available for study and recreation and on well-being are critical issues. However, the physical manifestations of tiredness and frustration can affect behaviour, and friends and associates might be the first people to recognise the results of getting the balance wrong. For this reason, helping friends to realise what is happening may be a new experience. The student who gets the balance wrong may not be the first to realise it.

Any physical or psychological work takes energy. A study day can be as draining, if not more so, than physical work. Routine academic study may lead to understimulation during the day, which may hinder sleep. Physical work can produce more deep sleep, which can create the sense of recuperation the following day. An interesting day's activities filled with variety and novelty helps to induce sleep more rapidly and provides deeper sleep. However, extra work of any kind produces a sense of weariness after an extended time. If insomnia occurs, it can lead to ill health, reduced work performance, absenteeism and accidents. If this happens, then an increase in exercise and interest during the waking hours may help. A good book to read about sleep is Morgan and Closs (1999).

You should not expect absence from work or study to be condoned. Absences can attract responses from placements or the university that prove stressful. Each university programme has different regulations regarding minimum attendance, and some relate differently to practice and theory. These regulations are usually reinforced during induction. The message is to talk to lecturers about the need to work outside the programme. Student welfare officers and occupational health departments can offer advice about health, counselling, finance and employment issues. Genuine sickness is usually not a cause for debate, but absence levels are cause for concern during professional programmes, and lecturers are there to help during times of difficulty. Absence that occurs because of the need to follow religious beliefs should also be discussed with personal tutors before events occur, so that the absence can be understood in context.

Considering all these factors, there appears to be a vicious circle that could operate (Figure 5.1).

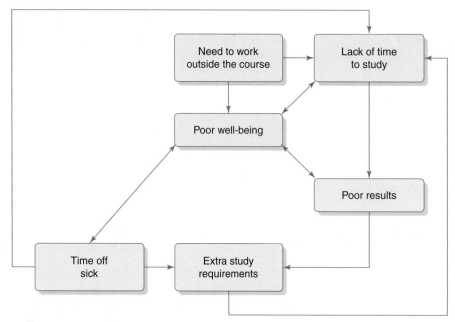

Figure 5.1 The cause and effect of poor well-being.

It is clear that students may need support at any stage of this cycle of events in order to protect their well-being. Coping strategies develop over time. McInnes (1999) comments that, although these strategies might have helped in the past, that might not be the case in a new situation. Nursing programmes help students to be more assertive, and this is one skill that should help you to challenge stressful encounters. The following is a possible stress-relieving process (after McInnes, 1999):

1 Look at what is causing the stress and try to alter it. Try to tackle bits of the problem at a time by breaking it down into manageable chunks.
2 If that cannot be done, try to change how it is perceived. Try to see it as if someone else has the problem and consider what they might do about it.
3 Try not to worry about stress. Some stress is positive and can be a motivational force for positive change. Don't strive to erase all the stress that exists in life, as this is impossible.

Physical and emotional changes will occur during the programme. One guarantee is that, at the end of the programme, every student will be a different person, not least because of their experiences but also because maturity adds insight and a changed self-awareness. The knowledge that adults can be vulnerable, wrong, unskilled and unappreciated can come as a surprise. Support is often required to help to explain and accept personal and attitudinal changes. Disenchantment with placements, colleagues, lecturers and assessment results can lead to apathy and lack of motivation and occasionally leads to students withdrawing from programmes. Problems are much better aired before they have serious effects.

Illness can happen at any time, a fact that all nurses learn quickly to appreciate. Having just a little knowledge may make the student nurse worry about many potential illnesses that are not really a problem. Furthermore, nursing ill people can make you think that patients' symptoms are similar to your own, leading to needless worry or even hypochondriasis. Personal illness must be taken seriously, as you need to be fit and well in order to be able to nurse patients.

Struggling into work when ill may lead others to question your professionalism and motives. Colds and flu, for example, may be debilitating and are contagious; as such, they are best isolated from staff and patients, and you should stay at home. Occasionally programmes have to be customised or interrupted because of illness. This is unfortunate but not a sign of personal weakness or failure. Further advice may need to be sought regarding maximum allowable sick leave from the programme. It is vital to follow any health and safety advice, policies and procedures relating to working while ill or recovering from illness.

Reflection point 5.3
The following exercise refers to questions that will help you to focus further on your need for support and relate to some of the issues discussed above.
If the programme has not yet started:

1 What changes will occur for which adjustments will have to be made? They may be the same or similar to those identified above.
2 What support might be used when at university?
3 How might any needs for support change during the programme?
4 Make a list of topics mentioned in this chapter that might need attention in the near future.

How relationships might be affected

Starting a programme might involve an element of sacrifice, a trade of a comfortable existence for an uncertain future, as born out by Earwaker (1992). The programme can produce reassurance that decisions were justified. The question of whether or not the curriculum satisfies your needs will prob-ably be a continuous affair of challenge for you, other students and lecturers. During the programme, checking progress will help to reaffirm commitment to the programme and desire to succeed.

Leaving family and friends to join a programme can be stressful, although this separation for most students is temporary. For students who travel from overseas, however, this separation might be for many months or years. It is important to maintain contact, whether by telephone, email, text or writing; family and friends can be a source of strong support at times when motiv-ation decreases, and they will want to know about your progress, especially your successes and excitements. Remaining in contact is also important for emotional well-being.

Travelling home can incur great cost, and it is sensible to budget wisely for such trips. As students set-tle down into shift patterns and blocks of study, they tend to reduce their trips home. However, it should be borne in mind that homesickness can become a serious issue. Friends may need to help each other to adjust to being away from those on whom they have significant dependence, and talking to tutors and welfare officers can also help. If homesickness is a worry, the websites www.uwec.edu/coun-sel/pubs/homesick.htm and www.counselling.cam.ac.uk/hsick.html offer useful tips.

Family problems and home life might not be disrupted and may in fact provide substantial support (Earwaker, 1992). Some problems might even be solved by changes that the programme produces. However, occasionally changes cause problems, such as separation, financial hardship, loneliness, changes to roles, or an uncooperative partner. If you are a lone parent and your children require care, this can produce enormous difficulties. Childminding, escorting to and from school, and planning and providing meals can all be stressful, especially when shift work is involved.

Most universities offer some form of childcare provision, such as crèches, out-of-school clubs, toy libraries and holiday play schemes. Information about these facilities can be discovered at university open days. There is usually a great demand for these services, so it is important to dis-cuss your needs with the university as soon as possible. The Aim Higher website (www.aimhigher.ac.uk) mentions the Daycare Trust, a charity promoting childcare facilities within higher and fur-ther education colleges across the UK, and offers information on benefits and grants available to students with children.

A lot of discipline may be required when trying to study at home surrounded by dependent chil-dren and other family members. Good timing and time management are essential. It is also import-ant to give some quality time to the family as a reward for the allowances they make. Problems regarding time and discipline are surmountable, and sometimes help from others is the key.

If you experience difficulties or problems with relationships, you might like to try some of the suggestions below that are based on the work of Counselling Services (2004):

- Admit that there is a problem.
- Talk about the problem with a family member or friend. Peer groups do work very well if there is a willingness to share feelings and emotions. Strength can come simply from having shared feelings.
- Make new friends.
- Think about what is to be gained or how change might make a difference.
- Write about your thoughts. When you see your ideas on paper, they can look different, as if they were someone else's thoughts. Imagine a friend has the problem – how would you advise them? Then try taking the same advice.
- Don't just complain. Instead, think about what change might be useful, but make your expect-ations achievable and realistic.

- Importantly, do something! Buried problems rear their ugly heads later when your ability to deal with them might be less effective.

Relationships with peers are dynamic. Meeting fellow students for the first time and making and breaking ties with peers brings a different set of uncertainties, doubts and pressures. In addition, peer pressure exists within groups of student nurses, for example pressure to take up or stop smoking. Some students are enticed to join or leave groups. Some are encouraged to lead groups, for example as an official group representative. These activities might not be an obvious first choice for many students, but peer pressure might bring positive rewards. Remember, however, that individuals have a right to express their personal thoughts and to make up their own mind (Townend, 1991).

Many students discover new interests at university. There are usually sports activities and interest groups on and around the campus. The students' union will have lots of information about their activities, which are often the centre of university life. Most student unions run social activities, such as student societies, sports clubs, nightclubs (on campus or at local venues), pubs and restaurants. All university students are entitled to become members of the union. Meeting students from other programmes is part of the university experience and is a great way of making new friends from different walks of life. Membership of the union also entitles students to discounts in certain shops, clubs and cinemas. The website of the National Union of Students (www.nusonline.co.uk) is focused on the welfare of students and contains a wealth of health-related pages.

Most students at university have more free time than students of nursing. Other students may seem to be 'getting off lightly' and may seem to be out all the time or enjoying more freedom by choosing whether to attend lectures. This can be a cause of frustration for some student nurses. Sharing accommodation with other university students can bring a unique set of pressures. However, while others are out clubbing, student nurses may have to work in placements, including during the night. Other students do not always appreciate the student nurse's need for quiet or understand that mid-week days off replace weekends, and so some mixing with others might be constrained.

Challenges for mature students

Balancing domestic responsibilities with study can be a new venture. Remember that, previously, at school or college, time had to be shared between responsibilities. Increasing age brings with it different and often more significant responsibilities and occasionally a reduced desire to change. However, change is something that students need to commit to for at least the 3 years of the programme, and coping with unforeseen difficulties will probably depend on you planning now to cope with the known difficulties. Good preparation is the key to feeling in control, which itself is the key to coping; therefore, if you have any doubts, ask questions, find sources of information, listen to advice and be prepared to make difficult decisions. When difficulties are shared, they can seem to be easier to deal with. Making new friends can help in this process. Remember: strangers might be simply friends who have not yet been met.

Some students need to continue to support their partner, for example financially, emotionally, in a health care capacity or in business. This takes time, effort and commitment. It also requires understanding and tolerance from the partner. Compromises may have to be made on both sides, and this might happen only after lengthy debate and heart searching. Understanding, compromise and assertiveness on both sides are key to overall success. In addition, the likelihood that changes are not necessarily lifelong, and may ultimately occur again, needs to be understood.

Mature students may have to adapt their lifestyle or living arrangements in order to meet their need to study effectively, for example moving furniture or bringing a desk into the house. This may affect how the house or a particular room is used – for example, the dining room may become a temporary office. Your family will also experience the changes and may not enjoy the encroachment into their space, and so the way in which changes are made and rationalised may be more important than the physical alterations themselves.

For many mature students, the challenge of re-entering education after time out causes unease. Some mature students have not studied for many years. They may have raised a family or for other reasons now have reduced demands from dependants. When they start a study programme, mature students often feel that they are in some way disadvantaged. However, mature students bring with them life experiences that others do not possess, and younger students are often grateful for the learning that they achieve by mixing with mature students. The lack of recent study can be seen as a disadvantage, but study skills such as time management can be learned easily, and the commitment to learning that mature students possess may be stronger than that in students who have just left school or college. Effective learning is often borne from commitment and motivation, and these should be seen as gifts in the mature student that should not be underestimated.

Information and communication technology (ICT) is a part of efficient learning, and the ability to use a computer is an advantage. For example, notes and references that have been recorded on a computer can be transformed into a presentable assignment, saving you time. Connection to the Internet aids communication with the university, friends and colleagues. The ability to access literature on the World Wide Web, in university libraries and in electronic journals is an advantage for study that should be a major consideration. Universities have computerised study facilities, and programmes include the use and teaching of ICT – therefore, a lack of experience or a perceived lack of skill will be overcome with practice.

Coping as a student from overseas

Adapting to a new place of study, new accommodation or new town can be stressful in itself, but what about a new country and culture? You may be fearful of encountering hostility or alienation from fellow students or neighbours because of where you come from, how you speak or what you look like. If English is your second language, it may be difficult for you to cope with translations and the speed of delivery of lectures. If in doubt, you should seek advice to find out whether the university runs any English language programmes. Some English language courses commence before official programme start dates to give students a head start. Universities usually help students from overseas through a support group, student support services or a dedicated overseas student office, some of which arrange seminars, visits and meetings.

One of the inherent difficulties faced by overseas students is the physical separation from known and trusted friends and family. The people who used to surround you are no longer near, and the isolation felt can be enormous. This can be minimised by telephone conversations, which are not always expensive, using email facilities and writing letters.

Visits home might be few but will be greatly valued. Planned annual leave and possibilities for travelling home should be checked well in advance, as it may be very difficult to rearrange placements and taught classes, which are usually planned before the start of the programme.

Most universities have student societies dedicated to certain cultures. These societies often organise social events that take place before the start of the university programme. It is worth asking at open days or during interviews when such events take place so that the valuable experience of mixing with people from different cultures is not missed. Many student unions have international welfare officers who can provide support if problems are experienced while living in Britain.

SUMMARY

This section has discussed some of the common reasons why support during training might be accessed. The reasons are numerous, and the list in this chapter is by no means exhaustive. It is hoped that it will now be clear that the challenges of change can be met through the meeting of new friends and staff and accessing new information. Knowing what to do about a problem is only half the battle; the other half is doing something to improve the ability to cope. Coping alone can work, but it might be advantageous to share experiences: coping together with others can lead to unexpected ideas for enhancing the ability to tackle present and future challenges.

Systems of support during the programme

As Phillips (1994) suggests, the main thrust of support is probably of an academic nature, but pastoral care is also an essential element. Most contacts initiated because of an academic need include some discussion related to the student's feelings about themselves or others. Interactions on placements and in university, and conflicting demands on students' time, are common discussion topics. One aim of study is to prepare you to accept responsibility for your own actions and your own learning. Learning through lectures and group sessions will not achieve this, but personal tutorials can, through individualised advice, direction, problem-solving and reflection when aimed at your own needs. You will optimise your level of self-awareness if you avail yourself of this facility.

The role of the personal tutor

It is not the sole province of one supporter, but the effective combination of all the support systems available to students, that will optimise the educational experience. A lecturer who has responsibility for coordinating the support of students may be termed a 'personal tutor'.

Individual students have different needs when entering university compared with their needs when leaving university, and the dynamics of the student–tutor relationship reflect this. At first, there will be a sense of dependence on the support structures in general. New relationships can be fraught with doubt and anxiety. However, students should try not to delay or put off meeting with a tutor. Generally, all students have an equal right to gain help from lecturers, and you should try to maintain regular meetings in order to improve rapport. Students gain more knowledge in this way, especially about their abilities, strengths and weaknesses. Self-awareness is a lifelong process of development, and it is often not possible to become aware of what others think unless they are asked or they volunteer their observations.

Writing in a diary can help you to record your thoughts, feelings and experiences. In some programmes, this can be a formal part of the curriculum. 'Reflection . . . is a generic term for those intellectual and affective activities in which individuals engage to explore their experiences in order to lead to new understandings and appreciations' (Boud *et al.*, 1985, p. 19). Reflection involves thinking about all that you do, feel and think about situations or events. Learning from reflection is helped in part by keeping a reflective diary or portfolio that you then use to recall items for discussion during tutorials; the diary can be a very powerful tool to reflect on changes in your knowledge base and, importantly, attitudinal changes (Heath, 1998). Reflection on action (see Schön, 1983) can contribute to growth of professional attitudes, and writing about your experiences, thoughts and feelings will lead to improved self-awareness. Read also Palmer *et al.* (1994) to discover more about how reflection can help your professional development.

Some tutor–student relationships will be formalised. This means that the tutor initiates the interactions and sets the intervals of meetings. Another approach is the very informal management of the scheme, whereby students initiate meetings as and when required. This informal system often occurs alongside a more official system. The reason for this is that although students and tutors are assigned to each other, students may also have so much incidental contact with another lecturer that they decide to interact for all other support requirements with that lecturer. This should not present many problems to the organisation, but students may need to inform tutors about how they are operating. Although all concerned may not find difficulties, this could lead to some students finding their tutors unavailable due to them being in demand. Line managers may as a result rationalise the support structure and formalise the system in order to produce a more equitable workload among all lecturers. Phillips (1994) advocated a formally planned framework of support to be included in curricula for this reason.

Some tutors are able to organise their time to see students in a very flexible manner. When students make a request, tutors may simply make an appointment in a diary to their mutual benefit. Alternatively, some tutors have so many demands on their time that they set certain times within their working week as 'surgery times' when they are available for students to drop in when they can. Of course, these two contrasting arrangements will not benefit all people at all times, and ad hoc arrangements will always operate. Suffice to say that although it is accepted that students have a right to see their tutors, the process is dissimilar to feeling thirsty, going to a vending machine and obtaining a drink on demand. Tutors have needs, demands on their time, and the right to coffee and lunch breaks. This should be borne in mind when knocking on a door and expecting to be seen there and then.

The variety of qualifications held by students, and their individual life experiences, indicate that students will experience differing levels of satisfaction from lectures and seminars. Further explanation and advice can be gained from the lecturing staff after or even before sessions if they are concurrent. This, of course, may not occur directly after all sessions: staff may not be available, or students may be moving on to another session. For this reason, note down any questions. The next meeting might be some time away, but reading lists and references can be followed up in the library. In addition, the answers to questions might also be gained by asking friends. The power of belief is very strong, so try to believe in the question and do not feel reluctant to ask just because it might be the wrong thing to ask. Being a student means that mistakes are allowed; often, that is how learning takes place.

Bramley (1977) advocated a model of friendship for the student–tutor relationship. You should be able to expect your personal tutor to be friendly but not your best friend. If the lecturer is required to discuss poor progress, academic failure or misdemeanours with students, then a personal relationship may make the exchange difficult and hard for students to accept. Therefore, although it should be expected that a lecturer is friendly, lecturers should attempt to protect both parties from overfamiliarity.

Friendship is not essential to the central role of support, and the personal tutor may in fact not actually teach the student. Some personal tutors may have a relationship with students for the whole of the programme or for only part of it. Different institutions will have produced their list of role responsibilities from different origins. This will be demonstrated through the operation of the role.

Personal development

Development of a plan of action for the method by which knowledge and skills will be gained in the future is important. The process of planning learning ('action planning') is very useful, as it can show clearly that learning takes place even when times are difficult to cope with. Personal development planning is an integral part of future career progression planning, which is part of the knowledge and skills framework (KSF). The KSF was introduced across the NHS in the UK on 1 December 2004 as part of the Agenda for Change (RCN, 2005). This was the biggest over-haul of NHS-wide pay, terms and conditions in over 50 years. The KSF is linked to annual devel-opmental reviews and personal development planning. Producing one or more action plans per semester is relatively easy and gives experience of a process that will be required when qualified. Practice now, because it will help you in the future. Personal tutors will be able to help you to gain the most from your personal development planning during your relationship. They will discuss your development during the programme, giving you praise and encouragement and challenging you to confront your learning needs through reflection on your action plans.

Support by placement mentors

A network of qualified nurses and experienced staff provides support for students in placements. These nurses should be appropriately qualified and experienced in their specialty and will have attended training sessions in order to familiarise themselves with curricula content and assess-ment strategies relevant to their practice setting and programme requirements. Students often say that the quality of the placement experience hinges on the quality of the relationship between them and their placement mentors. The role of the placement mentor is therefore a crucial one. Some mentors will be junior staff members who have been in their role for less than a year. Relatively new mentors can be very useful to students because their training is recent and fresh in their mind. The stressors present for students might be identifiable by the mentor, and so there is a possibility of a useful empathic relationship developing.

Mentors are good people to look to for careers advice. Mentors have experienced the prepara-tion required for getting through interviews. Student nurses are not guaranteed employment upon qualification. Previously, in many areas of the UK, there was relatively little competition for nursing jobs. Now, however, across the UK, it has become an employers' market. This means that student nurses are more likely to have to compete with their friends. The message to students now is that they must make themselves as employable as possible because potential employers have fewer vacancies to fill.

Mentors who have many years' experience in the specialty and of supporting students are often seen as oracles of knowledge. Their confidence in approaching students and knowing how to facilitate learning through contemplation and encouraging new experiences is acknowledged by students as being invaluable and is often a reason for requests to revisit a placement at a later date.

Support in placements by lecturers

Lecturers who undertake key aspects of preparation also support students in placements. Visits afford you the chance to discuss academic and practical developments together with the theoret-ical underpinnings of practice. The morale of staff in placements has an effect on students' attitude and motivation. The visiting lecturer will be able to highlight issues that students may not be aware of and possibly influence the support from other people or resources during the experience. Discussions in class also provide opportunities to explore experiences. Especially important is the need to debrief after experiences that were emotionally significant or incidents that were of a critical nature. Occasionally, explanations are not given soon after events, and worries and questions that are left unanswered can affect morale and taint beliefs that otherwise would not be a problem. Lecturers might refer you back to practice staff, but it is still important to alert lecturers to what is being experienced, either verbally or through a diary or portfolio.

Peer support

Students are a great support to each other, and some believe that they survive on a programme only because of their friends. Even during the preparation of assignments, it is important to share and perhaps review each other's work. Several students who share regularly will be helping each other, which reinforces their team spirit and thus enhances their confidence and group strength. This will help in the future when new challenges occur. Sometimes competition is healthy, as it can produce new insights and risk-taking. A group identity provides security and camaraderie; for example, if you need to relocate accommodation, friends may help with the arrangements.

Help with language was mentioned earlier. Mixing with peers can be valuable as a safe situation to practise speaking and reviewing their writing skills. This helps towards success in studies and practice. Some skills can be developed with the help of peers; these might include computer skills and the use of mathematics, which will prove useful for both studies and practice. Knowledge about practice is also shared, together with advice about how to react in certain practice situations.

Students from different groups often mix in practice areas, such as nursing students and students from medicine, pharmacy, speech and language therapy, physiotherapy, audiology and social work. There is the possibility of learning practice-related skills from these other students. Many practice skills are transferable, such as interpersonal skills and teamworking. Familiarity between junior and more senior students often results in learning that would not take place otherwise. Assertiveness and confidence, together with learning how to become part of the multiprofessional team, are all valuable developments that take place.

The buddy system

In some universities, there is a formal 'buddy' arrangement between senior and junior students, which might be maintained for the length of the programme. New students might want to discuss issues related to leaving home, or moving to a new area or country. Their senior buddy might have experienced something similar and might be able to share experiences and help in that way. As the programme progresses, advice about curriculum content, assignments and academic style might be welcomed. In the final year, advice on job applications, interviews, and the culture shock and attendant responsibility associated with becoming a new staff nurse might be useful, as the buddy has already experienced this transition.

There are several benefits to this approach to student support:

- Lecturers and personal tutors do not have to be aware of communications between the students, and so they can be the subjects of discussion outwith the official university support structure.
- The senior student will have experienced similar feelings and experiences to the junior student, thus facilitating an empathic relationship.
- Students relating with each other do so with similar perceptions; lecturers may not have a similar view of the education experience.

Many students feel a sense of security and camaraderie with their buddies. Friendships that exist between group members can produce a sense of identity within the faculty. The development of group support between year groups is an added bonus of an individualised support system of this kind and demonstrates clearly the notion that, just as nurses care for patients, so too can students care for each other. Thus, the care ethic begins before life as a nurse begins, which ultimately transfers to behaviour after qualification.

Supporting students with special needs

Special needs are usually catered for well within universities. Dyslexia, for example, presents itself in a variety of ways and occasionally is not even assessed properly until a student presents with difficulties when preparing work for assessment. Many lecturers are skilled at assessing dyslexic difficulties and routinely refer students to appropriate sources of help that can result in extra time for examinations and possibly several thousands of pounds towards computer equipment and supplemented tutorial support. Disabled Students' Allowance (DSA) does not have to be repaid, unlike a student loan. Further financial assistance can be used for specialist equipment for the whole of the programme and can be kept following the programme. Further information is available from www.dfes.gov.uk/studentsupport. The local education authority will be able to give advice before an application for a DSA is made.

Students with dyslexia have access to a free educational psychologist assessment so their needs can be assessed properly, leading to access to financial support and their studies becoming easier. Fear of being 'labelled' should be reduced in the future. Indeed, it is hoped that the positive aspects of dyslexia will be heralded, and the lessons learnt through helping dyslexic student nurses should be used to help other students.

An important point is that people with learning difficulties have previously often been labelled as 'slow learners' and therefore have been disadvantaged. Students who have special needs often do not know that specific help can be targeted effectively if proper assessments are carried out.

The Special Educational Needs and Disability Act (2001) places responsibility on institutions in respect of providing support, irrespective of funding arrangements. The Act removed education's previous exemption from the Disability Discrimination Act (1995). This meant that it became unlawful for educational establishments to discriminate against students with dyslexia; for example, it is unlawful to turn away a student from a programme simply because they have dyslexia. However, there are levels of dyslexia that would prevent a person from working as a nurse, and so it is unlikely that a university would accept a student on to a programme if their dyslexia were so profound as to preclude them from such work. This professional exception would be lawful.

Students with hearing or sight difficulties can be catered for, so long as staff are aware of the student's difficulty.

Coping with the unexpected

Planning how to tackle your workload, social life and essentials such as shopping and eating is difficult, especially when starting a new programme, but a sense of well-being exists when coping is taking place (Palmer and Puri, 2006). However, disasters do happen, and not always to other people. What might happen if your finances become exhausted, your computer breaks down, or illness prevents your attendance at placement or university? Universities have systems in place to help, such as the system of extensions for academic assessments. Extensions are normally awarded if you experience severe and unexpected difficulties that mean that your academic work might not be submitted to your usual standard. This is not a standard statement and may differ from university to university, so it is important to check with your university. Extensions might also be granted for practical assessed work. There may be a normal amount of time attached to an extension, and 1–2 weeks might be considered normal practice; however, this must be confirmed by the programme documents or lecturers. Students often regard extensions as a mark of failure, but they exist as a means to introduce some flexibility to what would otherwise be very rigid assessment timetables that could disadvantage you if, through no fault of your own, you had trouble at a late stage of your preparation for submission of assessed work.

> **Reflection point 5.4**
> The following exercise will help you to start to identify possible emergency support, some of which is mentioned in this chapter.
> Try to identify a support strategy for the following situations:
>
> 1 Your computer crashes and your hard disk will not work.
> 2 You become ill and you are advised not to attend university or practice for 2 weeks.
> 3 Your practice placement has been changed to one that will mean you have to leave your accommodation half an hour earlier than normal each morning.
> 4 You have 2 days to hand in your assignment but one of your parents falls ill and you need to return home for a few days.

Support from a professional union

Unions represent the views and interests of members. Annual subscription is required, but the benefits can be very advantageous. There is a certain sense of security achieved by membership. The sense of belonging to a like-minded group, and the awareness that third-hand advice and even counselling can be on tap, perhaps through the Internet, can bring about a good deal of reassurance. This is true not only if something goes wrong; importantly, the union is a resource of positive help that can enhance a sense of achievement and self-assurance.

The following are some very good reasons why students join a union:

- discount on merchandise and other offers;
- financial assistance, including insurance policies and advice about loans;
- information about news and events;
- indemnity insurance in placements;
- careers opportunities;
- access to anonymous counselling services;
- advice about accommodation;
- legal services.

Two main unions cater for the needs of nursing students: the Royal College of Nursing (RCN) and UNISON. The RCN is dedicated to the interests of nurses and students of nursing. It represents around 400 000 nurses, health care support workers and nursing students, in both the NHS and the private sector; it represents around 36 000 student nurse members. UNISON is the biggest UK trades union, with over 1.3 million members working across the public services, including 25 000 student nurse members.

> ## SUMMARY
>
> This section has discussed challenges that you might experience, although this is not an exhaustive list. The nature of support and where it can come from have been outlined.

CONCLUSION

This chapter has set out to encourage you to believe that you are not undertaking the programme alone. It is likely that you will gain support at different times and need it for different reasons compared with other students; this is perfectly normal and should be expected. The curriculum and the environment might not always be conducive to health, wealth and happiness. Staff members in the university and practice areas are there to encourage success. Gaining support from the networks discussed in this chapter will bring benefits to well-being. The way we act towards others affects the way they act towards us, and it is worth remembering that the job of a nurse is to make others feel better about their situation, feelings and thoughts. Carers care for each other, so do not be afraid to ask for help.

Previous experiences, attitudes and beliefs might have a significant influence not only on your achievement on the programme and your development as a student and a nurse but, importantly, also on your personal development. People who know you well can be the best guardians of what makes you who you are. When help is needed, it is good to know to whom you can turn. Keep in touch with friends and family, use their advice, and do not forget to be interested in what is going on in their lives.

There may be times when a member of your place of worship could help with difficulties. Your family doctor might be able to help, or parents, extended family members or neighbours might be the ones to approach for help. Keep in contact with personal supporters, and then they are more likely to be there if needed. This relates also to relationships with lecturers and your personal tutor. Relationships need to be worked on and will develop as a result of interactions. Share good times; then, if there are any bad times, they too will be easier to share. Good luck!

References

Boud D, Keogh R and Walker D (eds) (1985). *Reflection: Turning Experience into Learning*. London: Kogan Page.

Bramley W (1977). *Personal Tutoring in Higher Education*. Guildford: Society for Research into Higher Education.

Counselling Services (2004). Overcoming homesickness. www.uwec.edu/counsel/pubs/homesick.htm. Accessed 12 October 2007.

Earwaker J (1992). *Helping and Supporting Students: Rethinking the Issues*. Buckingham: Open University press.

Heath H (1998). Keeping a reflective practice diary: a practical guide. *Nurse Education Today*, **18**, 592–8.

McInnes B (1999). Stamp out stress. *Nursing Standard*, **13**, 53–5.

Morgan K and Closs SJ (1999). *Sleep Management in Nursing Practice: An Evidence-Based Guide*. Edinburgh: Churchill Livingstone.

Nursing and Midwifery Council (NMC) (2008). *The Code: Standards of Conduct Performance and Ethics for Nurses and Midwives*. London: Nursing and Midwifery Council.

Palmer AM, Burns S and Bulman C (1994). *Reflective Practice in Nursing: The Growth of the Professional Practitioner*. Oxford: Blackwell.

Palmer S and Puri A (2006). *Coping with Stress at University: A Survival Guide*. London: Sage.

Phillips R (1994). Providing student support systems in Project 2000 nurse education programmes: the personal tutor role of nurse teachers. *Nurse Education Today*, **14**, 216–22.

Royal College of Nursing (RCN) (2005). *Agenda for Change*. London: Royal College of Nursing.

Schön DA (1983). *The Reflective Practitioner: How Professionals Think in Action*. London: Basic Books.

Teasdale K (1989). The concept of reassurance in nursing. *Journal of Advanced Nursing*, **14**, 444–50.

Townend A (1991). *Developing Assertiveness*. London: Routledge.

Further reading

A lot of advice and information is available from schools, colleges, friends and family. As we are living in the so-called 'information era', it is pertinent to offer a list of useful websites that display relevant information for students contemplating a university programme. There is the usual warning, however, that the nature of these websites may change over time.

Aimhigher. www.aimhigher.ac.uk.
This is an excellent resource with links to other useful information resources that might help when deciding on a career, type of programme and career progression action planning. The organisation gives its key aims as follows:

A. *To offer an effective and extensively used entry point that enables prospective students to seek information about higher education institutions and programmes.*
B. *To offer information and assurance on financial matters to students entering higher education, specifically information about financial support and advice.*
C. *To help widen participation in UK higher education – and particularly among students from non-traditional backgrounds, minority groups and disabled persons.*

Directgov. Education and learning: university and higher education. www.direct.gov.uk/en/EducationAndLearning/UniversityAndHigherEducation/index.htm
This provides information on a wide range of topics to enable students and their parents and advisers to make effective decisions, especially with regard to applications and finance.

Nursing and Midwifery Council. www.nmc-uk.org.
This site enables you to search for work-related issues and regulations and helps to explain the responsibilities of staff nurses (e.g. a staff nurse is responsible for the actions of a student nurse under their supervision).

Office of Public Sector Information. www.opsi.gov.uk.
This site gives access to the Acts of Parliament referred to in the text. Explanations provide the rationale for the changes that have occurred, or will occur, in higher education in respect of the law.

Opendays.com. www.opendays.com.
This service facilitates a search for interesting university open days and allows you to book places online. It also gives advice about possible questions to consider asking when attending an open day. Open days are a great way to find out from lecturers and students what life might be like in a university and to ask questions about different programmes. You will need to consider some good points but also some not so good points before making your final decision.

Royal College of Nursing. www.rcn.org.uk.
The official home page for the RCN. There are links to learning and ways to get involved with the College.

Royal College of Nursing. Nursing students community. www.rcn.org.uk/students/home.
This site answers frequently asked questions and gives access to discussion forums for students. It provides quick links to news, publications and job vacancies, and members have special access to areas such as the electronic library.

Student Loans Company. www.slc.co.uk.
This gives important information about student loans from the Student Loans Company UK. It also has many useful links to other sites.

uni4me. www.aimhigher.ac.uk/uni4me/home.
This answers many questions about what it is like to be a university student, helping you to work out options and make decisions. It has a great jargon buster.

UNISON. www.unison.org.uk.
The official home page of UNISON. Follow the links to health care and then nursing.

UNISON. Nursing and midwifery students. www.unison.org.uk/healthcare/students.
The home page for nursing and midwifery student members of UNISON.

Universities and Colleges Admissions Service. www.ucas.com/students/coursesearch/index.html.
This site will help you to find university courses that might fit your requirements. There are links to other parts of the website.

PART 3

Practising nursing

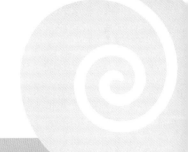

6

Principles of professional practice

Caroline Woolrich

Introduction

The first part of this chapter focuses on the key principles of what it means to be a professional. An overview of the key points in the professional evolution of nursing is provided, along with some comparisons with the growth of midwifery as a profession. The chapter explores the values and principles that surround the context of nursing as a profession and the nurse as a professional.

The second part of the chapter brings together the NMC Code (2008) (Appendix 1), which sets out the framework of professional practice for all nurses and from which all other advice and guidance is derived, and the competencies required to be fit for practice (NMC, 2004a). The two inform the public of the standard of professional conduct that they can expect of a registered nurse.

Whatever the chosen route to registration as a nurse, a key feature of registration is that it denotes membership of a recognised profession. This role and the expectations that accompany being a member of a professional group present many challenges to nurses and deserve specific attention from all those seeking to share the responsibility of such a position.

One of the key features of belonging to a profession is that it holds an acknowledged position within the society that it serves. Therefore, there are certain expectations that are required of all who seek to, and subsequently achieve, a licence to practise. An integral part of the preparation for achieving this licence is to have an understanding of what is expected from a registered nurse and how this may be nurtured during the course of any programme of education.

Programmes of education for initial registration with the Nursing and Midwifery Council (NMC) are aimed at preparing students to be able, on registration, to apply knowledge, understanding and skills when performing to the standards required in employment, to ensure that they make the care of people their first concern and to acknowledge their responsibilities and accountability for their practice. The development of nursing programmes arises from the premise that nursing is a practice-based profession, recognising the primacy of people's needs and respecting them as individuals.

An essential condition of entry to the nursing profession is the acceptance and internalisation of the NMC Code, which all nurses must uphold.

Learning objectives

After studying this chapter you should be able to understand:

- the NMC Code, its implications and how it can be used to support you in professional practice;
- professional self-regulation and how the nursing profession has developed;
- the standard of professional conduct required in professional practice;
- that accepting professional accountability for practice is fundamental to having a licence to practise and therefore being a registered nurse.

Development of nursing as a profession

The evolution of nursing as a recognised profession has been the subject of much deliberation (McGann, 1992). The early effort for recognition of the professional standing for nursing was much thwarted by its roots as an occupation carried out by women and hence of low social status (Simnett, 1986; Dingwall *et al.*, 1988). Indeed, the Registrar General's classification of social class still identifies the social status of doctors, dentists, opticians and pharmacists as being superior to that of nurses, midwives, health visitors and other health professionals allied to medicine (Davis, 1995).

To be a member of a professional group supports a general view that those who belong to the group provide some kind of personal service to clients. The traditional view of a profession, and usually a male-dominated profession such as medicine or law, is its association with certain features: professional self-governance, professional autonomy and registration of practitioners; setting and monitoring standards for practice in certain fields; education in a university; and a public ideology of service to clients (Freidson, 1970; Jackson, 1970).

All health care practitioners in contemporary practice are required to have both knowledge and understanding of the professional framework for practice and must also demonstrate this through their practice. As Fletcher and Buker (1999) explain, although the influence of the regulatory body is focused on registered practitioners, those training for the professions must recognise from the outset the commitment and responsibilities that being a professional demands and the competencies required in practice to demonstrate that accomplishment.

In order to explore the current position of nursing and the standards that symbolise its place in the world of the professional practitioner, it is important to examine how nursing has adopted some of the key features of a traditional profession.

Professional self-regulation and autonomy

Johnston (1972) asserts a commonly accepted view of a profession as an agent of occupational control of its members. The self-governing nature of a true profession is seen as critical to its success. Professions are legitimised by the state and therefore are bound by certain legal impositions on practice. As such, it was a notable point in history when the Midwives Act (1902) and the Nurses Registration Act (1919) gave statutory recognition to a regulatory framework developed through the work of the Central Midwives Board (CMB) and the General Nursing Council (GNC), respectively.

The move towards state registration did not arouse uniform acceptance from either the medical profession or some sections of the nursing and midwifery professions, which were threatened in different ways by the potential implications of self-regulation (White, 1976). The medical profession enjoyed the benefits of self-regulation, autonomy and a monopoly for practice through the establishment of the General Medical Council (GMC) in 1858 (Blane, 1988). This was not to be the experience for either nursing or midwifery; professional autonomy was a concept not validated by the 1902 and 1919 acts. Unlike doctors, nurses and midwives were to be the subject of scrutiny and control from the state and the more powerful influences of the medical profession. A number of contributory reasons have been associated with this. For many years, the legacy of Florence Nightingale's leadership style, coupled with the institutionalisation of nursing and later midwifery, did little to empower practitioners. Girvin (1998) suggests that, although Nightingale was a powerful woman and an influential figure in policy-making at the time, the dominance of the medical professions had a lasting impact on the development of nursing as a profession in its own right. Any real impact on the autonomy of the profession was yet to come.

Blane (1988) explains that the 'leading' professions, to which he assigns medicine, differ from the 'lesser' professions, to which he assigns nursing, by virtue of the position that access to clients 'is only through the instruction of the leading profession'. His examination of the major differences between the professions of nursing and medicine provides a clear reminder of the subservient role of nursing even in the latter part of the twentieth century. While the capacity to exercise self-governance evolved through the ceaseless efforts of those determined to see changes, the first major reform to the regulatory framework did not take place until the enactment of the Nurses, Midwives and Health Visitors Act (1979).

These regulatory reforms saw the demise of the CMB and GNC within the UK, with one body, the UK Central Council for Nursing, Midwifery and Health Visiting (UKCC), replacing them. This caused much dissent from some factions of the midwifery profession, concerned that the absence of a separate regulatory body for midwives would be a retrograde step to its independence from nursing.

Nonetheless, the move towards a larger and more resolute regulatory framework was proposed through the UKCC. In order for the new council to project its role and assert greater power on the professional standing of nursing and midwifery, its regulatory function and purpose needed to be more accessible to its registrants. The UKCC reviewed and presented national standards for both education and practice and, as part of its regulatory function, began to issue written advice and guidance on the expected behaviour and conduct to all its registrants. The emphasis on self-governance and autonomy of the individual registrant became an important feature, encouraging registrants to use the regulatory body as a support and guide to good practice rather than one whose main purpose was punitive.

A much clearer foundation was set from which practice could be monitored and judged. The traditional features of a profession were presented through a framework that required attention to the prevailing values and beliefs of the professional, expressed in a code of professional conduct and through a set of competencies. These not only applied through standards set for entry and initial registration but also were to reflect the requirements for sustaining a licence with a much greater focus on how the values of the profession would ensure an appropriate service to the public.

The 1992 amendment to the Nurses, Midwives and Health Visitors Act (1979) resulted in a proliferation of guidance documents from the UKCC, with a more overt quest to establish a distinct image for the professional nurse, midwife and health visitor. Public protection was at its root and was made explicit. Running parallel to the government's reforms of the NHS in the 1990s was a review of professional regulation. The Conservative government commissioned an independent review of the two sets of legislation underpinning the regulation of professions allied to medicine, and nurses, midwives and health visitors respectively. The report (JM Consulting, 1998), covering the four national boards and the UKCC, led to the most recent (at the time of writing) reforms in professional regulation and culminated in the establishment of the NMC in April 2002. The national boards, governed by the Nurses, Midwives and Health Visitors Act 1997, were present in all four countries of the UK until 2002. They were responsible for the setting of standards for courses enabling individuals to qualify for registration as nurses, midwives or health visitors, and for the framework of professional development programmes for those already registered. Changing professional regulation is part of the modernisation of the health service and continues through the initiatives of the present government (DH, 1999).

Although the focus on self-regulation and the exercise of achieving greater autonomy occupy a continued place in the professional development of nursing, exploration of the practice of nursing has followed a more complex path.

Specialist knowledge and monopoly for practice

Perhaps the most contentious aspect of the search for enhanced professional standing rests with identifying the distinctive nature of nursing and hence its monopoly for practice. Midwifery has within its statute some clearly defined boundaries from which practice is identified and governed (UKCC, 1998), but the same cannot be said for nursing. As such, the identification of a specialist field of knowledge that reflects the activity of nursing as a measure of its monopoly for practice continues to present an important challenge.

Those seeking to enhance the professional standing of nursing sought to compete with the GMC's objective that people requiring medical aid should be enabled to distinguish between qualified and unqualified practitioners (Blane, 1988). The statutory requirement that outlined the activities of a midwife demanded a concerted effort to pursue and eliminate non-bona fide mid-wives from the profession (Robinson, 1990). For nursing, the task of policing a profession, where such boundaries were more diverse, was problematic. Nonetheless, the emergence of the nurse theorist and the proliferation of the literature in both the UK and the USA saw a new approach to this challenge – one that focused on the process as much as the activity of nursing.

The development of a theory for nursing could be said to date back to Florence Nightingale's *Notes on Nursing* published in 1859 (King, 1981). Attempts to embrace the essence of nursing were to be explored later through an identification of nursing models and systems of care. In short, the concept of a model for nursing was introduced in an attempt to identify the value, belief or ideology that would underpin the practice of nursing care of individual client groups (Aggleton and Chalmers, 2000). Peplau did some of the earlier work on models in the 1950s; the dissemination of other models in the 1970s and 1980s aimed to explore the essence of nursing in a more explicit way (Peplau, 1988; Orem, 1995; Pearson, 1996; Roper, 2000).

Virginia Henderson, one of the most celebrated authors to explore the concept of nursing models as an inherent feature of a new framework for nursing practice, attempted to define the nurse's role:

> . . . to assist the individual 'sick or well' in the performance of those activities contributing to health or its recovery (or to a peaceful death) that he would perform unaided if he had the necessary strength, will or knowledge . . .

(Henderson, 1969)

Other efforts to explore the process, rather than the tasks or activities of nursing, brought a revolutionary approach to how care was managed and delivered. The 'nursing process' saw the introduction of a more systematic enquiry into how patients' needs would be assessed, planned, implemented and evaluated. It brought a new and more structured framework from which nursing could be examined (Christensen, 1995). The main purpose of this new dimension was to encourage the skills of decision-making and problem-solving in a more holistic way than had been seen in the more task-oriented approaches of the past.

Benner's work in the 1980s brought a further dimension to the discussion and provoked many debates about the differences between theoretical knowledge and its application in practice (Benner, 1984). Benner suggested that the development of skills was not always accompanied by an understanding of theory and that it was important for nurses to have the know-how as well as the 'know-what' of practice. This encouraged the shift towards nurses undertaking an increasing number of tasks normally carried out by doctors, exacerbated in part by the growing demand for a decrease in doctors' hours (Greenhalgh and Co., 1994). Over time there has been an almost inevitable expansion in the work carried out by health care assistants to fill the gap left by nurses and a significant shift in the boundaries for practice of all those involved in health care provision.

The growth and development of nursing towards an increase in activities normally carried out by doctors has perhaps failed to clarify the distinctive nature of nursing practice. However, it is towards the changes in education that this chapter now turns, to locate their impact on the professionalisation of nursing.

Education

A distinguishing feature of a profession is the nature of the education of its members, and the educational reform of nursing and midwifery has had a significant influence on the professional standing of both groups. At the end of the nineteenth century, the Nightingale training schools for nurses and midwives provided the first formal education (Woodham Smith, 1952). However, it was nearly a century before the move to university education saw any radical changes in the organisation, content and status of programmes of education.

The 1970s saw an acknowledgement for change proposed in the Briggs Report (Briggs, 1972), but this was not enacted until the review of pre-registration programmes in the 1980s (UKCC, 1986). This represented a major change in nurse education and professional nursing structures in the UK. It was anticipated that the outcomes of such programmes would see the emergence of a new 'knowledgeable doer' (Slevin, 1992).

Such reforms included the introduction of curricula based upon research, opening up new horizons for nurses on both pre- and post-registration programmes (Benner and Wrubel, 1989). The value of research as a means to underpin practice was fundamental to the growth and recognition of nursing, not only as a means of enhancing its professional status but also as means of replacing outdated practices based on custom rather than grounded in evidence.

One major theme that emerged throughout this new approach to education was the emphasis on the essence of care, described by Kirby and Slein (1992) as a 'new curriculum for care'. Other important elements of problem-solving, critical thinking and reflective practice were formalised as essential components of the competencies for the nurse of the late twentieth century. The study of ethics was introduced, where issues relating to moral responsibility were presented in a different way from the pronouncements of the past. The emphasis became that of the individual nurse being required to accept and carry the burden of judgement and decision-making (Hunt, 1992). The new reforms set out in the Project 2000 report were '. . . underpinned by the notion of a morally responsible and ethically accountable nurse, a nurse who has broken with the unthinking subservience of the past' (Hunt, 1992, p. 98).

The introduction of ethics paved the way for a more frank acknowledgement of the client's participation in the care process. Hunt explained how the new curriculum was designed to promote the concept that the nurse must learn to respect the values and desires of the individual and that students should no longer be treated as 'passive unquestioning recipients' of a limited range of practical skills. This was enhanced further by the legal sanction given through Rule 18 of the Nurses, Midwives and Health Visitors (Amendment) Act (1992), which required that practice should be measured through a set of identified nursing competencies.

In the years that followed, the drive to enhance the professional status of nursing was seen through this new approach to education (Buckenham, 1992). A new energy was released that supported an extension of the way the nurse, as a professional partner in care, should be seen. Overall, the move of nurse and midwife preparation into higher education institutions added the kudos of academic achievement to the professional qualification, with a greater emphasis on research-based practice and an acknowledgement of the shifting boundaries of practice.

However, an evaluation of the Project 2000 programmes of education demonstrated that there were concerns about nurses' fitness to practise at the point of registration (Bartlett *et al.*, 1998). As a consequence, the UKCC set up the Commission for Nursing and Midwifery Education to reassess and re-evaluate the preparation for the professional role and 'to prepare a way forward for pre-registration of nursing and midwifery education that enables fitness for practice based on health care need' (UKCC, 1999).

The resulting *Fitness for Practice* report (UKCC, 1999) identified the need for a more balanced focus on the achievement of both practice-based competencies and those that would reflect the core values of the profession. Therefore, a direct link was made between the accomplishment of competencies for registration and the professional development of the nurse, one that was seen as fundamental to the autonomy and accountability of the individual practitioner and, therefore, fundamental to the NMC Code. The requirements for pre-registration nursing programmes were revised in April 2002, following the establishment of the NMC, and again in August 2004 to bring them in line with changes to the rules brought about by the Nursing and Midwifery Order 2001. The resulting document combined the requirements for pre-registration nursing programmes and some content previously published in Statutory Instruments and Council policy to form the Standards of Proficiency for Pre-Registration Nursing Education (NMC, 2004a). These standards of proficiency define the overarching principles of being able to practise as a nurse; the context in which they are achieved defines the scope of professional practice.

The standards are underpinned by guiding principles that establish the philosophy and values of the NMC's requirements for programmes leading to entry to the register as a registered nurse. They relate directly to professional standards of proficiency and fitness for practice. As practice takes place in the real world of health care delivery, it is linked inextricably to other aspects of fitness – that is, fitness for purpose, professional academic awards and professional standing. With these beliefs and values underpinning practice, the most immutable trademark of a profession – one that seeks to identify the standard of expected conduct and behaviour as a true reflection of the ideology of the time – is strengthened.

Public ideology and standards for conduct and behaviour

As a reflection of the values and beliefs of the nursing and midwifery professions, the guidance from the regulatory body is presented in the form of statutory rules, professional codes, and competencies for practice on qualification and advisory documents. Individual accountability is the key and must be applied to people in the care of nurses, the profession, the law and, unless self-employed, the employer.

Such accountability requires nurses, on an individual basis, to engage in exploring personal values and ethics in order to participate in seeking shared outcomes with the people they care for and mutually accepted goals with other professionals. An additional dimension has been the hitherto unprecedented expectations of society, which is increasingly aware of the rights and information so often denied in the past and is more enlightened about the shortfalls and fallibility of the health service. A new culture for care has arisen, where it has become necessary to formalise an ethical framework for practice to complement those of the profession and the law. Greater consideration is given to the duty of care that underpins the nurse's role now represented within the regulatory framework, employment contract, and health care legislation, and through the requests and demands of the people in their care.

In order to examine this duty of care further, the remainder of this chapter focuses on how the NMC Code acts as a template on which all professional dimensions of practice are grounded.

SUMMARY

Membership of a professional group requires achievement and maintenance of competence and behaviour that justify the trust and confidence of the public in that profession. The development of nursing and midwifery as professions through regulation, the nature of practice, education and public expectations has been enhanced both nationally and internationally. The result is a distinct set of values and beliefs that provide a robust and unique framework for health care practice that the public needs and expects. However, maintaining the momentum of that development may mean that nursing does not have to continue to emulate all the traditional characteristics of a profession. There is a new professionalism and culture of care emerging that seeks to work with rather, than 'do to', people in the care of nurses. The practice of individual accountability within a robust framework of professional values and beliefs is the key.

The NMC Code as a framework for professional practice

The NMC Code was initially drawn up by the UKCC under the powers of the Nurses, Midwives and Health Visitors Act (1979). The NMC published a code as a reminder that this is 'the single most important document published by the regulatory body' (NMC, 2002). This code incorporated and replaced the 1992 version of the NMC Code and two other guidance documents – the UKCC Scope of Professional Practice (UKCC, 1992) and the UKCC Guidelines for Professional Practice (UKCC, 1996). In August 2004, this code was revised further, with an addendum to include indemnity insurance and renamed the Code of Professional Conduct: Standards for Conduct, Performance and Ethics, to reflect Article 21 of the Nursing and Midwifery Order 2001. Article 21 requires the council to establish and keep under review the standards of conduct, performance and ethics expected of registrants and prospective registrants and to give them such guidance on these matters as it sees fit. In 2007, to reflect changes in the professions and developments in the delivery of health care services, the NMC held UK-wide focus groups and an online consultation to seek the views of all stakeholders on how best to develop the NMC Code. The aim was to seek the broadest range of views on how the NMC Code could be developed to make the duties of nurses and midwives clear in addition to providing an effective support for professional practice. Almost 3000 people were involved in the consultation, which represents an enormous collaborative effort and resulted in a new version of the NMC Code being published in 2008 and renamed *The Code: Standards of Conduct, Performance and Ethics for Nurses and Midwives*. The NMC Code is essential for safeguarding the health and well-being of people in the care of nurses, and its principles form the basis of effective practice. The revised format of the NMC Code has been developed to reflect standards of conduct, performance and ethics that are appropriate and comprehensive, that prioritise the interests of those in the care of nurses and midwives, and that reflect up-to-date professional practice. The NMC Code is set out in six sections; the main four are detailed in Box 6.2. It continues to represent the shared values of all eight UK health care regulatory bodies. This is an important presentation of unity to people in the care of nurses and other health professionals who should have confidence that they all work within the same frame of values. A statutory overarching body, the Council for Healthcare Regulatory Excellence, governs the nine regulatory bodies:

- Nursing and Midwifery Council;
- Health Professions Council;

- General Medical Council;
- General Dental Council;
- General Optical Council;
- General Chiropractic Council;
- General Osteopathic Council;
- Royal Pharmaceutical Society of Great Britain;
- Pharmaceutical Society of Northern Ireland.

This body, separate from the government, was established in April 2003 to promote best practice and consistency in the regulation of health care professionals.

The NMC Code encompasses key principles that combine professional responsibilities with people's rights and provides an ethical dimension of accepted behaviour that would satisfy the expectations of the community. The emphasis on public protection and the accountability of each nurse to enact this cannot be overstated. This has far-reaching implications in terms of the demands it places on each individual's accountability, as it involves how people behave not only towards those for whom they care but also towards each other as professionals and towards society.

Singleton and McLaren (1995, p. 135) suggest that professional codes function as a 'framework for decision making which enshrines contemporary views of professional morality'. They add that the content of a code should be interpreted as a guide to professional conduct and moral obligation within caring relationships which are based upon trust, worth and dignity. For Hunt (1992), a professional code seeks not to resolve moral problems but to present enforceable minimum standards for practice that act as directives to be used as 'reminders' rather than 'resolutions'.

The NMC Code and proficiencies for practice

The standards set by the regulatory body are met through the successful achievement of a series of proficiencies that combine a number of different aspects of practice. These are currently expressed as 'domains' and fall into four categories (NMC, 2004a):

- professional and ethical practice;
- care delivery;
- care management;
- personal and professional development.

Entry to the profession is, therefore, seen through the development of knowledge and expertise that embrace clinical activity, interpersonal skills and a commitment to the values of the profession. In acknowledgement of this, the Council expects that an 'acceptance and internalisation of the Code' be seen as an inherent part of the process leading to registration (NMC, 2004a, Section 3, p. 16).

The regulatory body captured the essence of this as part of the new educational philosophy for the twenty-first century:

The NMC values the rights implicit in the social contract between the profession and society to participate in the health care of individuals, families and communities. Such rights also carry obligations. These include not only the responsibility to provide competent, safe and effective care but also responsibility for the highest standards of professional conduct and ethical practice.

(NMC, 2004a, Section 3, p. 16)

The standards set by the regulatory body apply from the moment a commitment is made to enter a programme of study (NMC, 2004b). It is, therefore, incumbent upon all students to grasp the link between the proficiencies for practice and the guiding principles that underpin the NMC Code, which apply to all practice interventions. The principles outlined within the NMC Code need to be examined with reference to those proficiencies – those that reflect the 'being' rather than the 'doing' element of nursing.

Reflection point 6.1
Consider how aware you were when you started your programme of the existence of the NMC Code and its connection with the proficiencies you will require on registration.

You may not be aware, but the standards set by the NMC already apply to you. The level of entry to pre-registration programmes is all part of these standards.

The NMC Code and principles for practice

The NMC Code presents an unequivocal message to reflect the personal accountability and sense of moral responsibility that an individual nurse must convey to their role (Box 6.1). Each of these requirements is expressed within the four sections of the NMC Code and reflects the personal accountability each nurse has in caring for people (Box 6.2). An expansion of these principles prompts a series of expected behaviours from which practice is judged. These principles will be considered below, with an opening reference to the proficiency for practice that relates to the principle.

BOX 6.1 Professional accountability

As a professional:

- you are personally accountable for actions and omissions in your practice and must always be able to justify your decisions;
- you must always act lawfully, whether those laws relate to your professional practice or personal life;
- the people in your care must be able to trust you with their health and well-being;
- you must act with integrity and uphold the reputation of your profession at all times.

Source: NMC Code (2008).

BOX 6.2 Principles for practice

- Make the care of people your first concern, treating them as individuals and respecting their dignity.
- Work with others to protect and promote the health and well-being of those in your care, their families and carers, and the wider community.
- Provide a high standard of practice and care at all times.
- Be open and honest, act with integrity and uphold the reputation of your profession.

Source: NMC Code (2008).

'Make the care of people your first concern, treating them as individuals and respecting their dignity'
This section of the NMC Code contains the following five principles:

- Treat people as individuals.
- Respect people's confidentiality.
- Collaborate with those in your care.
- Ensure you gain consent.
- Maintain clear professional boundaries.

'Treat people as individuals'
The related proficiencies for practice are to:

- maintain, support and acknowledge the rights of individuals or groups in the health care setting (professional and ethical practice domain);
- provide care that demonstrates sensitivity to the diversity of patients and clients (professional and ethical practice domain);
- consult with patients, clients and groups to identify their need and desire for health promotion advice (care delivery domain);
- provide relevant and current health information to patients, clients and groups in a form that facilitates their understanding and acknowledges choice/individual preference (care delivery domain);
- provide support and education in the development or maintenance of independent living skills (care delivery domain);
- establish priorities for care based on individual or group needs (care delivery domain) (NMC, 2004a).

The recognition of respect for the individual needs and preferences of people lies at the heart of the therapeutic relationship. It reflects the personal responsibility assigned to each nurse to consider the importance of the partnership with the person for whom they are caring.

Each nurse needs to recognise the rights of the individual, to accept the uniqueness and diversity of people, and to exercise respect and dignity towards others, regardless of their differences. Without doubt, this may present a major challenge at times, either when decisions made by people are in conflict with those of the professional or where opposing values may have to be addressed through compromise.

Emphasis is also placed on ensuring that nurses 'maintain clear professional boundaries' within the professional relationship, and how people in the care of nurses must be able to trust them with their health and well-being.

Reflection point 6.2
From your clinical placements so far, think back to an occasion when you or your colleagues felt that a person's rights had not been addressed sufficiently. How did you feel about this? What could have been done differently?

You may have found this situation difficult, but you must always remember that, as a registered nurse, you are personally accountable for any actions and omissions in your practice. With that in mind, consider how you would deal with these types of situations in the future.

'Respect people's confidentiality'

The related proficiency for practice (professional and ethical practice domain is to ensure the confidentiality and security of written and verbal information acquired in a professional capacity (NMC, 2004a).

Seeking the help and advice of a health care professional almost invariably involves revealing information that people usually regard as private. In addition, it often involves allowing access to a person's body and, in some cases, property. It places people in a vulnerable position and one that can be fairly described as unequal in terms of power. This inevitable imbalance places an obligation on all health care practitioners to respect the confidentiality of information that is shared. The principle of respecting people's confidentiality is a crucial commitment to the public that the trust placed in nurses will not be betrayed (Box 6.3).

BOX 6.3 Confidentiality of information

- You must respect people's right to confidentiality.
- You must ensure that people are informed about how and why information is shared by those who will be providing their care.
- You must disclose information if you believe that someone may be at risk of harm in line with the law of the country in which you are practising.

Source: NMC Code (2008).

Reflection point 6.3

Take a moment to think about the sort of information you give to your own general practitioner (GP), practice nurse or counsellor and the assumptions you make that they will not share that information with anyone else without your consent. Consider the personal implications should this information be divulged without your consent, even to family members.

You may have found yourself in situations where information has been shared, without the consent of the individual. Consider the reasons for this and the process that the multiprofessional team followed in reaching the decision to disclose. How did this make you feel? Was the disclosure justified in order to protect someone from harm? Were any legal implications considered?

The protection against disclosure of information does, nonetheless, pose some difficulties. The ethical value that underpins the need for confidentiality is one of trust. It requires honesty and an openness that respects and recognises an equal partnership between the nurse and the person for whom they are caring.

'Collaborate with those in your care'

The related proficiencies for practice are to:

- establish and maintain collaborative working relationships with members of the health and social care team and others (care management domain);
- review and evaluate care with members of the health and social care team and others (care management domain);
- consult with patients, clients and groups to identify their need and desire for health promotion advice (care delivery domain);

- collaborate with patients and clients and, when appropriate, additional carers to review and monitor the progress of individuals or groups towards planned outcomes (care delivery domain) (NMC, 2004a).

The principle makes paramount the involvement of, and respect for, people in the care of nurses and the importance of listening to them and responding appropriately to their needs. Cooperation and respect for the equally important contribution that the person in the care of a nurse can bring to the delivery of health care must remain at the forefront of the relationship. (Box 6.4). This emphasises how working with the patient is vital to a successful outcome and is now seen as a fundamental component of the current health care agenda. It presents a new pattern for practice, where the person in the care of a nurse is the central focus of the health care team's activity, which necessitates nurses sharing information with their colleagues and monitoring the quality of their work to ensure that the people for whom they are caring are safe, while remaining personally accountable for actions and omissions in their practice.

BOX 6.4 Collaborate with those in your care

- You must listen to the people in your care and respond to their concerns.
- You must support people in caring for themselves to improve and maintain their health.
- You must recognise and respect the contribution that people make to their own care and well-being.
- You must make arrangements to meet people's language and communication needs.
- You must share with people, in a way that they can understand, the information they want or need to know about their health.

Source: NMC Code (2008).

'Ensure you gain consent'

The related proficiencies for practice (professional and ethical practice domain) are to:

- act to ensure that the rights of individuals and groups are not compromised;
- respect the values, customs and beliefs of individuals and groups.

The principle relating to obtaining consent before giving any treatment or care brings with it respect for people's autonomy, while recognising the complex demands that characterise the overriding professional duty of care. On the one hand, it elevates the rights of a person to accept or decline care or treatment, while presenting, on the other hand, a duty to ensure that these rights are not violated and that the person remains at the centre of decision-making.

There are five requirements within this principle that seek to establish the current professional and legal position relating to the rights of people to receive information that should uphold these rights be shared 'in a way they can understand' (NMC Code).

It reinforces the principle of respect for autonomy for those legally competent to participate in the planning of their own care, making it clear that nurses must 'uphold peoples rights to be fully involved in decisions about their care' and that they 'must be aware of the legislation regarding mental capacity, ensuring that people who lack capacity remain at the centre of decision making and are fully safeguarded' (NMC Code).

As a reminder that working *with* people and making their care their first priority is now much more than rhetoric, nurses must be prepared for many different scenarios. For example, in demonstrating the principle of respect for a person's autonomy, they may find themselves caring for the competent person who has both the capacity and the ability to express an informed choice. Here, the nurse must demonstrate respect and support for the decisions made by that person.

Alternatively, some people have the capacity to consent but may, as Teasdale (1998) suggests, express feelings of vulnerability and powerlessness in their dealings with health professionals and require a nurse to act as an advocate to speak on their behalf. There are also people who lack the capacity to be involved in the decision-making process; this may require the nurse to exercise professional and moral judgements to ensure that they are fully safeguarded.

Reflection point 6.4

People have the right to receive information about their condition in order to make decisions on treatment. Think for a minute about a situation where you have seen a procedure or intervention explained well to a person and how they responded. Compare this with a situation where you felt that the person had been given insufficient information. How did this make you feel? Imagine yourself in this position and how you would react.

When admitted to any health care environment, people place themselves in a vulnerable position and can sometimes feel intimidated by the professionals caring for them. It is therefore every nurse's responsibility within the framework of the NMC Code to ensure that consent is always obtained before any treatment or care is given, remembering that obtaining consent is a process rather than a one-off event. The process should be rigorous and transparent and demonstrate a clear level of professional accountability. All discussions and decisions relating to obtaining consent should be recorded accurately, and the information regarding treatment or care should be given in a sensitive and understandable way. People should be given enough time to consider the information and the opportunity to ask questions if they wish to. Nurses should not assume that the person they are caring for has sufficient knowledge, even about basic treatment, for them to make a choice without an explanation.

It is essential that people are given adequate information so that they are able to make a decision. If a person feels that the information they have received is insufficient, then they could make a complaint to the NMC or take legal action. Most legal action is in the form of an allegation of negligence. In exceptional cases, for example where the person's consent was obtained by deception or where not enough information was given, this could result in an allegation of battery (or civil assault in Scotland). However, only in the most extreme cases is criminal law likely to be involved.

'Maintain clear professional boundaries'; 'Be open and honest, act with integrity and uphold the reputation of your profession'

This section contains four principles (Box 6.5). The related proficiencies for practice are to:

- practise in accordance with the NMC standards of conduct, performance and ethics for nurses and midwives (professional and ethical practice domain);
- demonstrate knowledge of contemporary ethical issues and their impact on nursing and health care (professional and ethical practice domain);
- manage the complexities arising from ethical and legal dilemmas (professional and ethical practice domain);
- act appropriately when seeking access to caring for people in their own homes (professional and ethical practice domain);

- maintain and, where appropriate, disengage from professional caring relationships that focus on meeting the patients or clients needs within professional therapeutic boundaries (care delivery domain) (NMC, 2004a).

The concept of trust, when translated into the professional relationship, is fundamental both to the individual nurse's moral standing and to that of the reputation of the profession. The NMC Code requires nurses to behave in such a way that will inspire public trust and confidence, where violation of any one of the key principles could do damage to both. The underlying maxim of any code of conduct is the principle of non-maleficence – the duty to prevent harm as a matter of professional integrity (see Chapter 9). These two parts of the NMC Code set out how this principle should be practised for the protection of the individual and of society (Box 6.6).

Avoiding inappropriate use of the registered nurse status in the promotion of products or services that are not related to health or any involvement in financial gain are examples of where the trust of the people nurses care for and the reputation of professionals need to be protected. Equally, the acceptance of gifts, favours or hospitality' that might be interpreted, as an attempt to obtain preferential treatment' are inconsistent with the behaviour expected of a registered nurse. It is also unacceptable for a nurse to 'ask for or accept loans from anyone' they care for. As Blane (1988) points out, any preoccupation with gain transgresses the notion of altruism and is not generally associated or accepted within professional practice. The important element here is, of course, to separate the gratitude that may accompany a person's discharge from their care in hospital or the community from an offer or proposal that would be dishonourable if accepted.

Abuse of the privileged relationship that a nurse has with the people they care for can take many forms and covers a wide spectrum. However, evidence from the extreme manifestations of how the professional relationship may be violated has attracted much attention in recent years, leading to criminal charges against both nurses and doctors. The actions of Beverly Allitt (DH, 1994) and

---

BOX 6.5 Be open and honest, act with integrity and uphold the reputation of your profession

- Act with integrity.
- Deal with problems.
- Be impartial.
- Uphold the reputation of your profession.

Source: NMC Code (2008).

BOX 6.6 Act with integrity and professionalism

- You must establish and actively maintain clear sexual boundaries at all times with people in your care, their families and carers.
- You must not abuse your privileged position for your own ends.
- You must uphold the reputation of your profession at all times.
- You must give a constructive and honest response to anyone who complains about the care that they have received.
- You must not allow someone's complaint to prejudice the care that you provide for them.
- Failure to comply with the NMC Code may bring your fitness to practise into question and endanger your registration.

Source: NMC Code (2008).

Harold Shipman (Baker, 2001) shocked the public and health care professions alike. Although extreme, these examples nevertheless demonstrate how individuals whose practice was way outside the boundaries of accepted moral or legal conduct managed to enter the profession and maintain their respective licences to practise unimpeded for some time. This begs painful questions about the vigilance and willingness to act in the public interest of all health care professionals.

Without doubt, such cases are exceptional, and it is within the context of avoiding harm in all situations involving people in the care of nurses that the notion of trust should be considered. The duty of care and the requirement to prevent harm have both professional and legal standing and require some personal reflection on how an individual's behaviour may be judged. The NMC Code does not identify specific examples of conduct that would be seen to be unworthy of a registered nurse. It does, however, assume an understanding that any evidence to support that the trust or confidence of the public has been damaged may lead to a judgement by the profession, the law, the employer or all three. The NMC Code now clearly stipulates that nurses must not only 'adhere to the laws of the country in which [they] are practising' but also 'inform the NMC if [they] have been cautioned, charged, or found guilty of a criminal offence'.

As part of its statutory function, the NMC deals with significant allegations of misconduct each year, where evidence supports the abuse of the therapeutic relationship between the nurse and the person for whom they are caring. Although the majority do not attract the same media attention as the examples given above, any referral to the NMC serves as a reminder of the need to preserve the privilege that a licence to practise bestows and the resultant damage and dishonour to both the individual and the profession when standards of practice and behaviour for the profession are disregarded.

Reflection point 6.5

Take a moment to think about what you expect of any nurse caring for a friend or relative or perhaps yourself. Harm can be done in many different ways of which, sometimes, we are not aware. Think about what tone of voice, facial expression and body posture convey to you. They might seem trivial, but they can be the components of persistent abuse in the unequal power relationship between the nurse and the person they are caring for.

You may have already seen or experienced behaviour from a health professional that made you feel uncomfortable. Do you know how you come across to the people for whom you care and colleagues, especially if you are stressed? It can be difficult to challenge a colleague who may be senior to you or someone who is caring for you, a friend or relative, and there is no easy answer. However, unacceptable behaviour will persist as long as it is allowed to. Safety, respect and dignity for people in the care of nurses are top priorities.

'Work with others to protect and promote the health and well-being of those in your care, their families and carers, and the wider community'

This section of the NMC Code contains the following four principles:

- Share information with your colleagues.
- Work effectively as part of a team.
- Delegate effectively.
- Manage risk.

The related proficiencies for practice are to:

- establish and maintain collaborative working relationships with members of the health and social care team and others (care management domain);

- participate with members of the health and social care team in decision-making concerning patients and clients (care management domain);
- review and evaluate care with members of the health and social care team and others (care domain);
- seek specialist or expert advice as appropriate (care management domain);
- contribute to the application of a range of interventions that support and optimise the health and well-being of patients and clients (care delivery domain);
- contribute to the learning experiences and development of others by facilitating the mutual sharing of knowledge and experience (personal and professional development domain);
- manage risk to provide care that best meets the needs and interests of patients clients and the public (care management domain);
- use appropriate risk assessment tools to identify actual and potential risks (care management domain);
- communicate safety concerns to a relevant authority (care management domain);
- apply relevant principles to ensure the safe administration of therapeutic substances (care management domain);
- identify unsafe practice and respond appropriately to ensure a safe outcome (professional and ethical practice domain);
- demonstrate the safe application of the skills required to meet the needs of patients and clients within the current sphere of practice (care delivery domain);
- take into account the role and competence of staff when delegating work (care management domain);
- maintain one's own accountability and responsibility when delegating aspects of care to others (care management domain).

This section of the NMC Code makes paramount the importance of managing risk, of involving and respecting colleagues' contribution to care delivery, and of effective communication and teamwork. Cooperation and respect for all those working within a multiprofessional team and involved in the organisation and delivery of a health care service must be paramount. Although this is not a new concept and has been seen as fundamental to the activities and role of all nurses for many years, it nevertheless presents a more overt expression of the value placed upon a respect for others working within the health care team, as a means of benefiting those for whom they care (Box 6.7).

BOX 6.7 Sharing information and working effectively as part of a team

- You must keep your colleagues informed when you are sharing the care of others.
- You must work cooperatively within teams and respect the skills, expertise and contributions of your colleagues.
- You must be willing to share your skills and experience for the benefit of your colleagues.
- You must treat your colleagues fairly and without discrimination.
- You must make a referral to another practitioner when it is in the best interest of someone in your care.
- You must make sure that everyone you are responsible for is supervised and supported.

Source: NMC Code (2008).

'Manage risk'

This part of the NMC Code affirms the key ethical principles of non-maleficence (duty to prevent harm) and beneficence (duty to promote good). It goes without saying that the basis of any caring role is the duty to ensure that an individual person is free from harm and that the care of the person is the first priority. Yet, it is in this area that 'doing nothing' and 'not being heard' led to the tragedies of Bristol, Shipman and many other less well-known examples.

The obligation placed on nurses to make appropriate professional judgements in aspects of care, driven as much by an ethical framework as by any professional or legal ruling, generates a need for a particular approach to solving problems. It is likely that the challenges that present in practice will exercise the mind of the most diligent nurse, particularly where these involve the behaviour of colleagues. Dilemmas may arise from the duty that all nurses have to make their concerns known where there is evidence to suggest that the care to a person may be compromised, whether this relates to the environment of care or the specific care of an individual (Box 6.8). 'Whistle-blowing' is never a comfortable thing to do, but using the appropriate channels and evidence with perseverance is all part of practising this principle in a person's best interest.

BOX 6.8 Managing risk

- You must act without delay if you believe that you, a colleague or anyone else may be putting someone at risk.
- You must inform someone in authority if you experience problems that prevent you working within the NMC Code or other nationally agreed standards.
- You must report your concerns in writing if problems in the environment of care are putting people at risk.
- You must act immediately to put matters right if someone in your care has suffered harm for any reason.

This clearly puts particular demands on the individual nurse who may be required to challenge the practice of a colleague or expose the shortfalls of a particular health care environment, where there may be serious implications for more than one person. At a time when the nursing profession is eager to promote the need for evidence-based knowledge to support practice and a renewed confidence to empower nurses to challenge poor practice, it is with regret that the findings from the Bristol Inquiry, the Kennedy Report (DH, 2001a), serve as a reminder of the devastating implications if poor practice goes unchallenged.

The Kennedy Report identified lessons to be learned from the inquiry into a higher death rate among children undergoing heart surgery in Bristol. Not only was it critical of those whose clinical care was substandard, but it also exposed numerous damaging aspects of the environment for care and of organisational systems; it serves as a timely warning for all nurses to revisit the demands of the principles that underlie this part of the NMC Code. Indeed, Section 46 of the Kennedy Report recommends that the relevant codes of practice for nurses and professions allied to medicine should be incorporated into their contracts of employment with hospital trusts or primary care trusts. It also suggests that 'Trusts should be able to deal as employers with breaches of the relevant code . . . independently of any action which the relevant professional body may take' (DH, 2001a).

This quote is all the more pertinent considering the public consultation undertaken by the Department of Health (DH) into the regulation of medical and non-medical health care professionals. One of the proposals in this consultation called for greater employer responsibility in their regulation.

The Bristol Inquiry described a 'club culture' within the Bristol Royal Infirmary, which could be taken as an indictment of the more traditional professional values no longer accepted in contemporary practice (Anonymous, 2001). It is hoped that a collective and professional effort will avoid such events happening again and will repair the damage done to the image of the health professions.

Other elements of this section of the NMC Code highlight the importance of reporting concerns to the appropriate person and the value of a written record to support any claims made. It also explains how a nurse's duty of care applies at all times, extending even into their off-duty hours (Box 6.9).

BOX 6.9 Duty of care

- You must be able to demonstrate that you have acted in someone's best interest if you have provided care in an emergency.
- As a professional, you are personally accountable for actions and omissions in your practice and must always be able to justify your decisions.
- You must act lawfully, whether those laws relate to your professional practice or to your personal life.

Source: NMC Code (2008).

Reflection point 6.6

You may have already become aware of practice and care environments that cause concern. During your clinical placements you might take the opportunity to discuss how situations such as these would be handled. Talking things through with others is important for future practice. It helps to shape your thinking and share the burden of a dilemma.

It is worth remembering here that your priority is to the people in your care. You must at all times ensure that their care is your first priority. You may find yourself in situations where you believe staffing levels are insufficient or the skill mix is inappropriate to meeting this requirement. Have you thought of how you would address such situations? Are you aware of systems being in place to report such concerns?

This part of the NMC Code leaves the nurse in no doubt about the professional demands that accompany a licence to practise. The licence is a privilege and a major commitment to the public that has its own reward. However, many feel that the balance of that reward is seriously undervalued in material terms, and this view will take perseverance on the part of the profession and others to change.

Within this section of the NMC Code, the Council acknowledges the right of a nurse to object to participation in certain activities that may transgress their own moral framework or religious beliefs (Box 6.10; see also Chapter 9). For some, this may appear to contradict the NMC Code, in that it suggests that the right of the nurse be protected over and above that of the person for whom they are caring.

> **BOX 6.10 Reporting concerns**
>
> • You must inform someone in authority if you experience problems that prevent you working within this NMC Code or other nationally agreed standards.
>
> *Source:* NMC Code (2008).

This part of the NMC Code seeks to preserve certain human or moral concerns that the nurse may wish to express. However, there are limitations to the application of this right based upon the current legal position that identifies only two areas where a nurse has the right conscientiously to object to take part in treatment or care. These are through the Abortion Act 1967, which gives nurses the right to refuse to take part in an abortion, and the Human Fertilisation and Embryology Act 1992, which provides rights to refuse to take part in technical procedures in assisted conception.

The expression of a person's right to choice in health care matters has, by tradition, been driven largely by the health professional. This, as noted above, was primarily the domain of the doctor, although many nurses were not without fault in their affirmation of an equally dominant position within the patient–practitioner relationship. As Girvin (1998) explains, the institutionalisation and socialisation required to survive the hierarchical styles of management seen in both public and private sector environments paved the way for a type of behaviour that was to infiltrate all professional groups.

The paternalistic values associated with that approach have, however, as a result of the growing demands and expectations of a society far more willing to express dissatisfaction with the health service, seen the emergence of a different pattern of care. Hence, we have seen a shift towards a more equitable relationship between carer and those who are cared for – one that can and should no longer tolerate a lack of respect for the autonomy of the individual.

Perhaps the strongest reinforcement of this shift has been through the Human Rights Act 1998, which came into force in the UK on 1 October 2000 and gave further effect to the rights enshrined in the European Court on Human Rights. The Act provides the legal support, within existing case law, for the courts to exercise a more forceful expression of individual rights. Those parts of the Act most likely to affect care practice are identified through a series of Articles (Box 6.11).

> **BOX 6.11 Legislation underpinning individual rights**
>
> • *Article 2*: protection of right to life.
> • *Article 3*: prohibition of torture, inhumane or degrading treatment or punishment.
> • *Article 5*: right to liberty and security.
> • *Article 8*: respect for private and family life.
> • *Article 9*: freedom of thought, conscience and religion.
> • *Article 14*: prohibition of discrimination in enjoyment of Convention rights.
>
> *Source:* Taken from the Human Rights Act 1998 (cited in DH, 2001b).

The Council expects that the appropriate emphasis is given to a person's right to make choices, reinforcing that nurses must not practise in a way that assumes that they know what is best for the person in their care.

'Provide a high standard of practice and care at all times'
This section of the NMC Code contains three principles:

- Use the best available evidence.
- Keep your skills and knowledge up to date.
- Keep clear and accurate records.

The related proficiencies for practice are to:

- use professional standards to self-assess performance (professional and ethical practice domain);
- consult other health care professionals when individual or group needs fall outside the scope of nursing practice (professional and ethical practice domain);
- consult with a registered nurse when nursing care requires expertise beyond one's own current scope of competence (professional and ethical practice domain);
- identify one's own professional development needs by engaging in activities, such as reflection in and on practice and lifelong learning (personal and professional development domain);
- develop a personal development plan that takes into account personal, professional and organisational needs (personal and professional development domain);
- share experiences with colleagues and patients and clients in order to identify the additional knowledge and skills needed to manage unfamiliar or professionally challenging situations (personal and professional development domain);
- take action to meet any identified knowledge and skills deficit likely to affect the delivery of care within the current sphere of practice (personal and professional development domain);
- ensure the confidentiality and security of written and verbal information acquired in a professional capacity (professional and ethical practice domain);
- use evidence-based knowledge from nursing and related disciplines to select and individualise nursing interventions (care delivery domain);
- demonstrate the ability to transfer skills and knowledge to a variety of circumstances and settings (care delivery domain);
- ensure that current research findings and other evidence are incorporated in practice (care delivery domain);
- engage with, and evaluate, the evidence base that underpins safe nursing practice (care delivery domain) (NMC 2004a).

The achievement and maintenance of proficiencies that led to registration and its continuance is a lifelong process and is essential to the public's confidence in the profession. This section of the NMC Code highlights the requirement to keep knowledge and skills up to date with current evidence or research and to develop any new or enhanced skills through regular learning. Also highlighted is the importance of communication through maintaining clear and accurate records on people in the care of nurses. Record-keeping is sometimes seen as being of less importance in the delivery of care and something to be fitted in if circumstances permit. It cannot be stressed enough how inaccurate this view is. Record-keeping is an integral part of nursing practice and a tool of professional practice that should help in the care process. Nurses who adhere to good record-keeping principles are helping to protect the welfare of the people for whom they care by promoting high standards of clinical care and ensuring effective communication between the wider multiprofessional health care team.

Nurses may be required to determine the individual interests of each person they are caring for in sometimes complex situations that may fall outside the scope of a particular nurse's practice. In such cases, it requires the exercise of professional judgement and skills to make a decision to recognise and work within the limits of their competence (Box 6.12).

> **BOX 6.12 Keep your skills and knowledge up to date**
> - You must have the knowledge and skills for safe and effective practice when working without direct supervision.
> - You must recognise and work within the limits of your competence.
> - You must keep your knowledge and skills up to date throughout your working life.
> - You must take part in appropriate learning and practice activities that maintain and develop your competence and performance.
>
> *Source:* NMC Code (2008).

Nurses are expected to judge the scope of their own practice and are encouraged to exercise self-determination and professional control. Although Schober (1998) suggests that this was something not widely accepted or acknowledged by nurses in the past, when new skills may have been developed in the absence of an adequate post-registration programme of learning, it has now become integral to the demands of exercising personal responsibility. With autonomy comes responsibility, as the following paragraph from the introduction to the NMC Code states: 'As a professional, you are personally accountable for actions and omissions in your practice and must always be able to justify your decisions (NMC Code 2008, p. 1).'

> **Reflection point 6.7**
> You may have been asked to do things that you do not feel sufficiently prepared for or supported to undertake, and this will almost certainly continue to happen after you are registered to practise. Take a minute to think how you would feel about such a situation and how you might handle it for the benefit of the person you are caring for.
> Perhaps you have already found yourself in such a situation. Think about how you and those around you handled it. Was it handled appropriately or did you feel that more could have been done to support you? Were you aware at the time of how you could use the NMC Code to support your practice?

As a student you are not accountable for your practice in the way you will be once registered. As a nurse you will hold a position of responsibility and other people will rely on you. By virtue of this registration with the NMC, you will have a professional accountability as well as contractual accountability to your employer. When faced with situations where nurses are asked to deliver care that they consider unsafe or harmful to the person they are caring for, they are required to carefully consider their actions. The care that nurses deliver should ultimately promote the health and well-being of the people in their care and be based on the best available evidence or best practice.

Professional indemnity insurance

The final section of the NMC Code, although not related directly to proficiencies for practice, is nevertheless just as important. This section of the NMC Code provides guidance to nurses on indemnity insurance and the importance of protecting themselves in the event that a claim for professional negligence is made against them.

The decision to include such guidance was first taken in 2003, following extensive consultation, primarily as a result of concerns surrounding nurses and midwives working in independent practice, where employers' vicarious liability would not normally be in existence. This was first published in the 2004 edition of the NMC Code, and it has been updated and incorporated into the 2008 edition of the NMC Code.

The NMC recommends that registered nurses, midwifes and specialist community public health nurses, in advising, treating and caring for patients and clients, have professional indemnity insurance. This is in the interests of clients, patients and registrants in the event of claims of professional negligence.

Although employers have vicarious liability for the negligent acts and omissions of their employees, such cover does not normally extend to activities undertaken outside the registrant's employment. Independent practice would not be covered by vicarious liability. It is the individual registrant's responsibility to establish their insurance status and to take appropriate action.

In situations where an employer does not have vicarious liability, the NMC recommends that registrants obtain adequate professional indemnity insurance. If unable to secure professional indemnity insurance, a registrant will need to demonstrate that all their clients and patients are fully informed of this fact and the implications that this might have in the event of a claim for professional negligence.

Vicarious liability is when the employer has accountability for the standard of care delivered and the responsibility when the employee is working within the sphere of competence as assessed. To remain covered by the employer's vicarious liability clause, an employee must work *only* within their abilities and sphere of assessed competence.

Reflection point 6.8

Consider the professional and financial implications of not having indemnity insurance along with finding out that you are not covered by your employer's vicarious liability insurance for any negligent acts that may occur during your practice. Remember that negligent acts are not always deliberate. Consider what factors in the work environment could contribute to or exacerbate such acts and how they could be alleviated.

There has been an increase in recent years in medical negligence claims made against not only organisations but also individual health care professionals. Possible reasons for this include the increase of health care professionals, including nurses and midwives, opting to work in independent practice, and also increased patient awareness and involvement in care. Many nurses fail to realise the importance of having adequate indemnity insurance, believing that, because they continue to be aware of and accept their professional responsibilities within the law and framework of the NMC Code, this is superfluous to requirements. However, errors are not always as a result of deliberate negligence and can be made by the most dedicated, careful and competent nurse. Factors such as poor staffing, poor skill mix and pressures of work can raise the risk of error. In this situation, as in all, nurses are required to acknowledge their accountability in ensuring that the people in their care are cared for safely. Any deficits in the environment of care that could lead to errors occurring and care being compromised must always be brought to the attention of the appropriate individuals within the organisation.

CONCLUSION

The choice to enter the nursing profession brings expectations and anticipations to be explored and owned throughout the journey towards registration. The successful achievement of professional proficiencies is the result of utilising opportunities for learning that will lead to academic, clinical and professional success. It will depend upon a number of interrelated experiences throughout the programme of learning that will be given a different priority at different stages of the process.

The traditional values of 'being a professional' are now the subject of much challenge. We have seen that the recognition of the professional element of nursing or midwifery practice is integral to the wider expression of the modern nurse or midwife practitioner. Nevertheless, it is only recently that real emphasis has been placed upon how nurses may use the regulatory framework to enhance both their personal and their professional growth in the ever-widening dimensions of health care.

With a licence to practise as a registered nurse or midwife comes the responsibility and the right to act autonomously in the interests of the people for whom they are caring. The responsibility and the right are finely balanced. For example, nurses must exercise their autonomy if they believe that they have been instructed to carry out any activity that may not be placing the needs of people in their care first. How the individual nurse demonstrates this right to autonomy is complex and the subject of much discourse. It is through a greater understanding of this right, and the coexisting duty to protect the public by exercising this right, that the principles contained within the NMC Code and the proficiencies for practice should be embraced and applied.

For students of nursing and midwifery working in contemporary practice, it is vital that the professional and ethical perspectives on practice are acknowledged as an integral part of the curriculum, with equal importance being given to those activities relating to care delivery and management. The philosophy behind the approach to learning places great emphasis on the individual student mastering the necessary proficiencies and recognising the professional accountability that registration as a nurse or midwife demands. The outcome of learning will be validated by the profession and will confirm (or not) 'fitness for award' – the assimilation of knowledge and understanding – 'fitness for purpose' – the acquisition of skills and expertise – and 'fitness for practice' – the skills and ability to practise safely and effectively without the need for direct supervision. These mark the achievement of proficiencies relating to the philosophy and values of professional practice and will confirm the final step towards registration – the licence to practise.

References

Aggleton P and Chalmers H (2000). *Nursing Models and Nursing Practice*. Basingstoke: Macmillan.

Anonymous (2001). News: Bristol report published. *Bulletin of Medical Ethics*, **169**, 3–8.

Baker R (2001). *Harold Shipman's Clinical Practice 1974–1998: A Review Commissioned by the DOH*. London: The Stationery Office.

Bartlett H, Hind P, Taylor H and Wescott EJ (1998). *An Evaluation of Pre-Registration Nursing Programmes: A Literature Review and Comparative Study of Graduate Outcomes*. Oxford: Oxford Centre for Health Care Research and Development.

Blane D (1988). Health professions. In Patrick DL and Scrambler G (eds). *Sociology as Applied to Medicine*. London: Baillière Tindall.

Benner P (1984). *From Novice to Expert: Excellence and Power in Clinical Nursing Practice*. Menlo Park, CA: Addison-Wesley.

Benner P and Wrubel J (1989). *The Primacy of Caring: Stress and Coping in Health and Illness*. Menlo Park, CA: Addison-Wesley.

Briggs A (1972). *Report of the Committee on Nursing*. London: HMSO.

Buckenham M (1992). Academic and organisational change. In Slein O and Buckenham M (eds). *Project 2000: The Teachers Speak*. Edinburgh: Campion Press.

Christensen PJ (1995). *Nursing Process: Application of Conceptual Models*. St Louis, MO: Mosby.

Davis C (1995). *Gender and the Professional Predicament in Nursing*. Oxford: Open University Press.

Department of Health (DH) (1994). *The Allitt Inquiry: Independent Inquiry Relating to Deaths and Injuries on the Children's Ward at Grantham and Kesteven General Hospital During the Period February–April 1991 (Clothier Report)*. London: HMSO.

Department of Health (DH) (1999). *Making a Difference: Strengthening the Nursing, Midwifery and Health Visiting Contribution to Health and Healthcare*. London: Department of Health.

Department of Health (DH) (2001a). *Learning form Bristol: The Report of the Public Enquiry into Children's Heart Surgery at the Bristol Royal Infirmary 1984–1995 – the Kennedy Report*. London: The Stationery Office.

Department of Health (DH) (2001b). *Reference Guide to Consent for Examination or Treatment*. London: Department of Health.

Dingwall R, Rafferty AM and Webster C (1988). *An Introduction to the Social History of Nursing*. London: Routledge.

Fletcher L and Buker P (1999). *A Legal Framework for Caring: An Introduction to Law and Ethics in Health Care*. London: Macmillan.

Freidson E (1970). *Profession of Medicine*. New York: Mead.

Girvin J (1998). *Leadership and Nursing*. London: Macmillan.

Greenhalgh and Co. (1994). *The Interface between Junior Doctors and Nurses: A Research Study for the Department of Health. Executive Summary*. Macclesfield: Greenhalgh and Co.

Henderson V (1969). *Basic Principles of Nursing Care: The Nature of Nursing – a Definition and Its Implications for Practice Research and Education*. Basel: International Council of Nurses.

Hunt G (1992). Project 2000: ethics, ambivalence and ideology. In Slein O, Singleton J and McClaren S (eds) (1995). *Ethical Foundations of Health Care*. St Louis, MO: Mosby.

Jackson JA (1970). Professions and professionalization. Cambridge: Cambridge University Press.

JM Consulting (1998). *The Regulation of Nurses, Midwives and Health Visitors*. Bristol: JM Consulting.

Johnston T (1972). *Professions and Power*. London: Macmillan.

King L (1981). *A Theory for Nursing: Systems, Concepts, Processes*. Chichester: John Wiley & Sons.

Kirby C and Slein O (1992). A new curriculum for care. In Slein O and Buckenham M (eds). *Project 2000: The Teachers Speak*. Edinburgh: Campion Press.

McGann S (1992). *The Battle of the Nurses*. London: Scutari Press.

Nursing and Midwifery Council (NMC) (2002). *Council Report*, 23. London: Nursing and Midwifery Council.

Nursing and Midwifery Council (NMC) (2004a). *Standards of Proficiency for Pre-Registration Programmes*. London: Nursing and Midwifery Council.

Nursing and Midwifery Council (NMC) (2004b). *NMC Guide for Students of Nursing and Midwifery*. London: Nursing and Midwifery Council.

Nursing and Midwifery Council (NMC) (2008). *The Code: Standards of Conduct, Performance and Ethics for Nurses and Midwives*. London: Nursing and Midwifery Council.

Orem D (1995). *Nursing Concepts of Practice*, 5th edn. St Louis, MO: Mosby.

Pearson A (1996). *Nursing Models for Practice*. Oxford: Butterworth Heinemann.

Peplau H (1988). *Interpersonal Relationships in Nursing*. New York: Putnam.

Robinson S (1990). Maintaining the independence of the midwifery profession: a continuing struggle. In Garcia J, Kilpatrick R and Richards M (eds). *The Politics of Maternity Care: Services for Childbearing Women in Twentieth Century Britain*. London: Clarendon Press.

Roper N (2000). *Models for Nursing: Based on Activities for Living*. Edinburgh: Churchill Livingstone.

Schober JE (1998). Nursing issues for effective practice. In Hinchcliff S, Norman S and Schober J (eds). *Nursing Practice and Health Care*, 3rd edn. London: Arnold.

Simnett A (1986). The pursuit of respectability: women in the nursing profession 1860–1900. In White R (ed.). *Political Issues in Nursing Past, Present and Future*. Chichester: John Wiley & Sons.

Singleton J and McClaren S (1995). *Ethical Foundations of Health Care*. St Louis, MO: Mosby.

Slevin O (1992). Knowledgeable doing: the theoretical basis for practice. In Slevin O and Buckenham M (eds). *Project 2000: The Teachers Speak*. Edinburgh: Campion Press.

Teasdale K (1998). *Advocacy in Health Care*. Oxford: Blackwell Science.

UK Central Council for Nursing, Midwifery and Health Visiting (UKCC) (1986). *Project 2000: A New Preparation for Practice*. London: UK Central Council for Nursing, Midwifery and Health Visiting.

UK Central Council for Nursing, Midwifery and Health Visiting (UKCC) (1992). *Scope of Professional Practice*. London: UK Central Council for Nursing, Midwifery and Health Visiting.

UK Central Council for Nursing, Midwifery and Health Visiting (UKCC) (1996). *Guidelines for Professional Practice*. London: UK Central Council for Nursing, Midwifery and Health Visiting.

UK Central Council for Nursing, Midwifery and Health Visiting (UKCC) (1998). *Midwives Rules and Code of Professional Practice*. London: UK Central Council for Nursing, Midwifery and Health Visiting.

UK Central Council for Nursing, Midwifery and Health Visiting (UKCC) (1999). *Fitness for Practice*. London: UK Central Council for Nursing, Midwifery and Health Visiting.

White R (1976). Some political influences surrounding the Nurses Registration Act 1919. *Journal of Advanced Nursing*, **1**, 209–17.

Woodham Smith C (1952). *Florence Nightingale*. London: Reprint Society.

Maintaining professional standards

Susan Savage

Introduction

We hear the term 'standards' used so often – standards of care, professional standards, clinical standards . . . Although we are surrounded by standards in our daily lives, we often don't stop to reflect on the standards we expect, or those expected of us. We take it for granted that we share a common understanding of standards and what is important to us. What implications does this have for standards in health care? In the past some argued that nurses placed little value on standards and did not use them in their practice (Dozier, 1998). If this is still the case, then the nursing profession is jeopardising the foundation of safe practice; at best, registered nurses are not benefiting from a useful reference and guide for their practice, and at worse they are not fulfilling their professional accountability to provide safe, good-quality care.

Standards are central to our professional practice. In order to use them effectively, it is important that we fully consider and understand such standards. Professional standards define the expected behaviour and level of competence required of registered nurses and other health professionals. Professional self-regulation provides the framework for these standards. The Nursing and Midwifery Council (NMC) acts as the regulatory body for nursing and midwifery in setting, maintaining and improving standards for our professions across the UK. Professional registration acts as an agreement with the public; in granting registered nurses and midwives the right to practise, registration places a responsibility on each practitioner to maintain professional standards. This is the essence of professional accountability.

This chapter explores professional standards that affect your practice. The topics discussed here relate to the outcomes and requirements set out in *Standards of Proficiency for Pre-Registration Nursing Education* (NMC, 2004a) as follows:

- Manage oneself, one's practice and that of others in accordance with the NMC Code (2008) (Appendix 1), recognising one's own abilities and limitations.
- Practise in accordance with an ethical and legal framework that ensures the primacy of patient and client interest and well-being and respects confidentiality.
- Practise in a fair and antidiscriminatory way, acknowledging the differences in beliefs and cultural practices of individuals or groups.
- Provide a rationale for the nursing care delivered that takes account of social, cultural, spiritual, legal, political and economic influences.
- Contribute to public protection by creating and maintaining a safe environment of care through the use of quality assurance and risk-management strategies.
- Demonstrate knowledge of effective interprofessional working practices that respect and utilise the contributions of members of the health and social care team.
- Delegate duties to others, as appropriate, ensuring that they are supervised and monitored.
- Demonstrate a commitment to the need for continuing professional development (CPD) and personal supervision activities in order to enhance knowledge, skills, values and attitudes needed for safe and effective nursing practice.
- Enhance the professional development and safe practice of others through peer support, leadership, supervision and teaching.

Learning objectives

After studying this chapter you should be able to:

- understand the meaning of standards and the types that affect practice in health care;
- recognise the role of the NMC in setting and maintaining professional standards;
- understand what it means to be professionally accountable;
- be aware of potential challenges you may face in maintaining professional standards and ways in which you can address these.

The meaning of standards

To start this chapter we will consider the meaning of standards, different perspectives and what influences standards.

What do we mean by standards?

The Concise Oxford English Dictionary definition of a standard is:

a level of quality or attainment; a required or agreed level of quality or attainment; . . . something used as a measure, norm or model in comparative evaluations; (standards) principles of honourable, decent behaviour.

Reflection point 7.1

Think of standards of health care and nursing that fit each of the definitions above.

Here are just a few examples of how the definitions of standards are used in nursing and health care:

- You would have been required to reach a set level of academic attainment before starting your nursing course.
- Waiting times for appointments are used to measure how quickly patients are seen as a way of measuring the responsiveness of services to patients needs; for example, all patients with a suspected cancer must be referred to a specialist within 2 weeks (DH, 2000a). Such standards are often used as performance measures.
- Registered nurses are bound by the NMC Code, which sets out standards of behaviour and principles of professional practice. This will be discussed in more detail later in the chapter.

Types of standard

When you considered different examples of standards that are set in health care, you may have identified some that focused on the environment of care – for example, having adequate screens to ensure patient privacy – and some that focused on nursing procedures – for example, the correct procedure to administer medicines safely (NMC, 2007a). Some standards may have described the expected outcomes of health care, such as standards for the provision of care for people living with diabetes to optimise control of blood glucose levels, blood pressure and other risk factors in order to reduce the incidence of complications and improve life expectancy (DH, 2001a).

Donabedian (2005) used such different aspects in his framework for quality, which comprised structure, process and outcome. This framework is based on the systems theory of input, throughput and output and has been used widely in the health care setting. You will often see

Donabedian's framework adapted and expanded to provide a comprehensive approach to standard setting and monitoring. For example, the Royal College of Nursing (RCN) used it, together with other health care quality approaches such as a problem-solving approach, in a quality assurance cycle to develop its standard-setting system for nursing (Morrell *et al.*, 1997). The framework continues to be used today, with the components of structure, process and outcome being used to develop indicators of quality in nursing practice (e.g. Kunaviktikul *et al.*, 2005).

These components of standards can be explored more fully using infection control as an example. Standards for infection control have been under close scrutiny in order to address the growing problem of health care-associated infections (HCAIs), such as *Clostridium difficile* and meticillin-resistant *Staphylococcus aureus* (MRSA).

The Health Protection Agency has defined HCAIs as follows:

> *Healthcare-associated infections (HCAIs or HAIs) are those that arise as a result of healthcare interventions, either in patients undergoing these interventions or in healthcare workers involved in these interventions. A wide variety of organisms can be transmitted in healthcare settings, causing in turn a wide range of different diseases.*
>
> (Health Protection Agency, 2006)

HCAIs are sometimes called 'nosocomial infections'. You can find out more about HCAIs on the Health Protection Agency's website (www.hpa.org.uk).

Standards about infection control demonstrate the importance of each of the components in Donabedian's framework, as outlined below:

- *Structure*: this includes aspects such as facilities, equipment, and the qualifications of staff and the organisation, which affect the environment of care (Donabedian, 2005). Applying this to infection control, there are standards set regarding cleaning in hospitals (DH, 2004a) and decontamination of equipment (MHRA, 2003). Although minimum staffing levels are not always explicit, Coia and colleagues (2006) report numerous research findings that show that reduced nursing staffing levels relate directly to increased infection rates.

- *Process*: Donabedian (2005) interprets aspects of process as procedures to provide care, for example patient assessment and diagnosis, and standards of competence to undertake procedures. Care pathways could also be considered as an aspect of process. Relating this to infection control, handwashing is the single most important procedure to prevent cross-infection. Standards for hand hygiene are set by national health departments, for example National Institute for Health and Clinical Excellence (NICE, 2003) guidelines in England and the Clinical Standards Board for Scotland (CSBS, 2001) (now part of NHS Quality Improvement Scotland (NHS QIS, 2005)). You can find detailed information on handwashing in the RCN document *Good Practice in Infection Prevention and Control* (RCN, 2005). Another process that is fundamental to nursing practice is aseptic technique. However, studies have shown that standards for aseptic technique are not being met, as discussed by Preston (2005), which is putting patient safety at risk. Preston (2005) describes the clinical situations in which aseptic technique should be used, the principles of aseptic technique and safe glove application. It is vital that you learn and practise this technique if you have not already done so in your clinical placements.

- *Outcome*: outcomes of health care can include recovery and survival rates, which may be relatively straightforward to measure, but other outcomes such as patient satisfaction and restoration of function may be defined less easily. Donabedian (2005, p. 694) considers outcomes to be the 'ultimate validators of the effectiveness and quality of medical care'. In relation to infection control, outcomes may be expressed in terms of prevention or the reduction of infection rates. For example, hospitals are required to reduce the rates of MRSA (DH, 2006a, 2008). For practitioners, an outcome measure could be successful wound healing without infection following surgery.

By examining the different aspects relating to infection control, we can see the importance of each aspect of Donabedian's framework in achieving good-quality care. This also reflects the complexity of achieving quality and the wide range of people involved in contributing to the quality of care.

Reflection point 7.2
Consider each of the aspects of structure, process and outcome for standards in infection control. Identify the different people who are involved in achieving these standards.

As you will have discovered, a collection of people are involved in standards, including nurses, doctors, cleaning staff, managers and those involved in maintaining equipment. What about the patient? Did you include their contribution in your reflections? Patient involvement is increasingly recognised as essential in achieving standards; such involvement ranges from sharing information – for example, giving advice to patients and their visitors regarding HCAIs (NHS QIS, 2005) – to involving patients in monitoring standards – for example, inspections of hospital cleanliness by patient environment action teams (PEATs) (DH, 2004a).

Values in standards and the importance of involving people

As we have already seen, the variety of standards and the number of people involved are likely to bring different perspectives about what the standard should be and, more fundamentally, which standards are more important. For example, a manager may view a short length of hospital stay as a success criteria, but a patient may be concerned about feeling pressurised to be discharged, which to them may indicate poor quality of care. Therefore, there is a potential for conflicting expectations of quality. Quality has a subjective dimension to which we all bring our values and beliefs. Similarly, our values and beliefs influence our behaviour in all aspects of life, including our professional behaviour. Jasper (1996) outlines six sources of our personal values:

- religious and moral upbringing;
- ethnic origins;
- educational opportunities;
- social class;
- environment in which we grew up;
- life experiences.

Reflection point 7.3
Think about Jasper's six sources of personal values and consider how your own values have developed.

- What are your own beliefs and behaviours that affect health, such as diet, smoking, alcohol and exercise? How might this affect you and influence your behaviour as a nurse?
- What values underpin your image of the professional nurse to which you aspire? Have you assumed that others share that image and those values? Take time out to discuss such values with your peers.

It follows that values and beliefs about health care and its standards are likely to be diverse. Williamson highlighted the relationship of values to standards:

> *Standards are descriptions of specific aspects of health care practices to which are attached prescriptive values . . . the values can be drawn from any field of knowledge or thought, from the highly technical to the everyday, from the scientific research to psychoanalysis, from ethics to evidence, from empirical certainties to professionals' intuitions and beliefs from their experience.*

(Williamson, 2000, p. 190)

It seems essential, then, that the values of society, patients, clients and professional groups are recognised in forming a standard. It seems obvious that the way to do this is to involve all those affected by the standard in determining what those standards should be, but this has not always been the case (Williamson, 2000).

Reflection point 7.4

Williamson (2000, p. 190) stated: 'although patients have a greater stake in standards than health professionals, health care professionals have the power to reject patients' views about what standards should be.'

- Do you agree or disagree with this statement?
- What might affect professionals' views about involving patients and clients in standards setting?
- What benefits arise from involving patients and clients in standard setting?

Here, Williamson (2000) is questioning the balance of power between the professional and the patient, which not only affects standards setting but also goes further to impact on the nature of the relationship between the professional and the patient or client. You may have considered whether some professionals find that the greater involvement of patients in making decisions about their care is challenging to their own clinical judgement. However, by involving patients and clients, such standards will be meaningful, appropriate and therefore of value to patients and clients.

The public, from a local through to a national level, rightly expects greater involvement in decisions about health care and its standards. This is reflected in health care policy across the UK. For example, in England, NICE involves patient groups in its deliberations regarding guidance and standards of clinical care. Local patient forums are involved in the implementation and monitoring of national service frameworks (NSFs), such as the management of care for people with long-term conditions (DH, 2005a).

Regulatory bodies are changing to meet public expectations, with greater public involvement in how professional standards are set. This is not only through public consultations but also in the increasing proportion of lay members (people who are not registered health professionals) on the regulatory councils themselves, such as the NMC. Further information can be found on the NMC website. However, the UK government has reviewed medical and other health professional regulation in light of the Shipman Inquiry (CMO, 2006; DH, 2006b). Following public consultation, the government proposed in its White Paper a substantially greater lay membership in all regulatory bodies so that there would be minimum parity between lay and professional membership (DH, 2007). Further information can be found on the Department of Health website (www.dh.gov.uk).

Individual patients also affect decisions about standards of care, for example through complaints, which can act as indicators of failings of standards. In responding to individual complaints organisations can rectify specific problems in the delivery of care, and by reviewing complaints received they can assess whether there are any trends – for example, quarterly figures may show an increase in complaints about waiting for appointments, or concerns about attitude, which the organisation can then address. At a national level in England, the Healthcare Commission produces reports on investigations into failing standards, so that other organisations can learn from actions taken and review their own standards. For example, the Healthcare Commission and the Commission for Social Care Inspection (CSCI) undertook a joint investigation into concerns of services for people with learning disabilities in the Cornwall Partnerships NHS Trust and made recommendations to be implemented nationally (CSCI and CHAI, 2006).

SUMMARY

- A standard is a required level of quality or attainment and can also be used to describe principles of expected behaviour.
- Standards of care need to be considered in terms of structure, process and outcomes in order to best facilitate quality of care.
- Our personal values and beliefs influence our expectations of quality and standards.
- Patients, clients and carers should be involved in determining standards of health care and those of health care professionals.

Why do we need standards?

You will be getting a picture of the variety of standards that are used in health care. Given the vast array of standards, it is helpful to pause for a moment to consider why we also need professional standards and how they can benefit your practice. You can then consider the rationale for professional standards as you explore the specific standards that you will be required to uphold or contribute to as a registered nurse.

Reflection point 7.5
What do you think is the purpose of professional standards? Discuss with your peers and with registered nurses on your clinical placement. List the drawbacks and benefits of such standards for you in practice.

The problem with standards
You probably found more positive reasons than negative for standards. However, you may have come across some negative views of professional standards. Some examples that have been stated are:

- They limit practice and are a barrier to innovation.
- They are used defensively to protect one's own position rather than to support developing roles.
- They are too general to be meaningful in contemporary practice.
- They are too prescriptive, so that individuals do not have enough freedom to practise.
- They are used as a 'stick' to make practitioners conform.

Even here you can see contradictions in people's views. This chapter challenges these views and aims to show that, when used proactively in daily practice, professional standards serve to benefit rather than hinder your practice. However, in order to achieve this, professional standards need to be understood.

Benefits of professional standards

Professional standards are the linchpin to the success of nursing; they have been described as the infrastructure beneath organisational standards, competency-based education and quality assurance programmes (Dozier, 1998). Some benefits of using professional standards described by Dozier are:

- They provide consistency across practice settings and among registered nurses.
- They provide a common understanding of the parameters in which nurses practise.
- They serve to describe the essential elements of professional practice.
- They provide the structure to integrate three key elements of professional accountability: care, quality and competence.
- They provide a benchmark and reference point on which organisations can base their care delivery.
- They support the nurse in influencing innovations in practice to be introduced safely and appropriately.
- They provide a reference point that can be used to evaluate care and professional practice.

This list is not exhaustive, and you may have identified some other benefits in your reflection.

What standards affect your practice?

Throughout your professional practice you will be expected to maintain personal standards and contribute to standards of teams and organisations. Standards in the health care setting can be broadly classified in terms of professional, clinical and organisational standards. You will also come across other terms used that relate to standards and quality of care, for example benchmarks and criteria.

Professional standards

These define the standards of professional practice and focus on the individual's conduct, education and competence to practise. It is the responsibility of the regulatory bodies such as the NMC, the Health Professions Council (HPC) and the General Medical Council (GMC) to set these standards. The duties and powers of regulatory bodies are set by legislation; for example, the Nursing and Midwifery Order (2001) sets out the responsibilities of the NMC. Professional standards are discussed in detail later in this chapter.

Clinical standards

Clinical standards relate to specific aspects of health care and treatment. Many of these are empirical standards, as they are determined by research-based evidence for the optimum treatment of disease or injury and the measurement of outcomes such as improvement of symptoms. National service frameworks describe the expected standards of clinical care for certain groups of people, for example older people (DH, 2001b), or for certain conditions, for example coronary heart disease (DH, 2000b). One of the standards in the NSF for coronary heart disease is that people with a suspected heart attack should commence thrombolysis within 60 minutes of calling for professional help (DH, 2000b).

Clinical standards also encompass the health care user's expectations and experience, which are rightly gaining more prominence in the way in which the environment and delivery of services in the NHS are developed and measured. This is discussed further under organisational standards in the next section. Five key areas have been identified by patients as areas that are most important to them in the patient experience (DH, 2005b). These are listed in Box 7.1.

BOX 7.1 The five dimensions of the patient experience

- access and waiting;
- safe, high-quality, coordinated care;
- better information, more choice;
- building closer relationships;
- clean, comfortable, friendly environment.

Source: Crown copyright material, reproduced with permission from DH (2005b, p. 11).

Reflection point 7.6

Take some time to talk to friends and relatives about their experiences of being a patient. Then talk to the team you are working with about the patient experience and seek their views about what helps and impairs this. Consider the views of your colleagues and those who have been patients in relation to the five dimensions in Box 7.1. Then read the patients' accounts in *'Now I Feel Tall': What a Patient-Led NHS Feels Like* (DH, 2005b) and compare their views with those of your colleagues. Find out what schemes or initiatives are happening where you are working to improve the patient experience. What is your contribution, as a nurse, to improving the patient experience? Which of the five dimensions can you influence the most?

You may have considered that nursing can play a part in improving all five dimensions of the patient experience listed in Box 7.1, in particular your role in ensuring safe, high-quality care, permitting more choice and improving relationships. The ways in which these can be achieved vary, depending on the different client needs or care setting.

Nursing has a fundamental role in maintaining standards to promote a positive patient experience while providing clinical care in all settings and disciplines. Schmidt (2003) highlighted that studies have shown that satisfaction with nursing care has been a primary indicator of overall satisfaction with health care provision and health outcomes. This, Schmidt argues, when set in the context of Donabedian's declaration that patient satisfaction is the ultimate outcome of care and an element of health, shows nursing to be the linchpin of quality of care.

So how does nursing measure quality of care? One way has been to benchmark standards of practice in key areas of fundamental and essential aspects of care. In 2001, the Department of Health launched the Essence of Care initiative (DH, 2001c), which provided a toolkit to measure standards of care, to learn and share good practice, and to identify areas that needed to be improved.

Benchmarking has been defined as a process of comparing, sharing and developing practice in order to achieve and sustain best practice (Modernisation Agency, 2003).

Initially, standards were developed with patients, professionals and patient representatives in eight aspects of care; a further three standards were added later (Box 7.2).

It is not solely nursing that has a significant contribution in improving standards of care in these aspects; all members of the health care team play a part. Consider who would have a key role in, for example, food and nutrition. In the hospital setting, the availability of the right diet for

---

.

> **BOX 7.2 Essence of Care benchmarks**
>
> - principles of self-care;
> - food and nutrition;
> - personal and oral hygiene;
> - continence and bladder and bowel care;
> - pressure ulcers;
> - record-keeping;
> - safety of clients with mental health needs in acute mental health and general hospital settings;
> - privacy and dignity;
> - communication (added 2003);
> - promoting health (added 2006);
> - care environment (added 2007).
>
> *Source*: Crown copyright material, reproduced with permission from Modernisation Agency (2003).

each patient is reliant on the catering services. Some patients need additional nutritional needs and need the expertise of the dietician. In the community, patients may rely on a voluntary service or social care to support them with shopping or meals service, such as meals on wheels.

The benchmarking process is set out in six stages, but it is in fact an ongoing cycle of improvement (Figure 7.1).

Benchmarking is increasingly being used across the health care setting to improve clinical performance, for example in the management of long-term conditions, maternity care and the

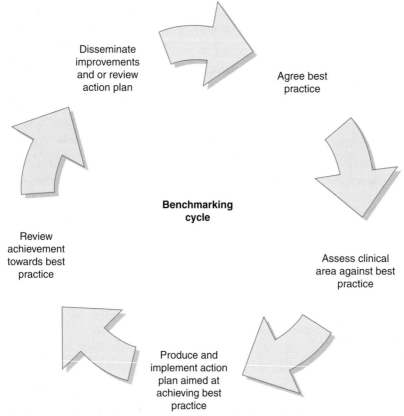

Figure 7.1 Cycle of improvement for benchmarking (Adapted from Crown copyright material, reproduced by permission of Modernisation Agency, 2003).

patient experience (Productive Time Delivery Board and the NHS Benchmarking Club, 2006). More information can be found at www.nhsbenchmarking.nhs.uk.

Organisational standards

These refer to the performance measures that indicate how the organisation ensures that professional clinical standards are facilitated and upheld. In England the standards are set by the Department of Health in *Standards for Better Health* (DH, 2006a). Standards are set in seven areas (domains) to cover the wide range of factors that affect the delivery of health care. These domains are:

- Safety
- Clinical and cost-effectiveness
- Governance
- Patient focus
- Accessible and responsive care
- Care environment and amenities
- Public health.

For each domain there are core standards that describe the minimum standard acceptable to which every organisation must comply. In addition, there are developmental standards that are used to promote ongoing improvement in standards of care, reflecting increasing patient and public expectations. Organisations are required to demonstrate ongoing progress towards the developmental standards each year.

Across the UK there are slightly different arrangements in each of the four countries. The Healthcare Commission (also known as the Commission for Healthcare Audit and Inspection – CHAI) is responsible for monitoring these standards in England and also monitors standards for organisations providing health care in the independent sector. Care homes and nursing agencies, however, are required to meet the standards set by the CSCI. In the future, the functions of the CHAI and the CSCI will be brought together under one regulatory organisation – the Care Quality Commission. In Scotland, standards are set and monitored by NHS QIS. In Northern Ireland, quality standards in health and social care are set by the Department of Health, Social Services and Public Safety (DHSSPS) and are monitored by the Regulation and Quality Improvement Authority (RQIA) (DHSSPS, 2006). In Wales, health care standards are set by the Welsh Assembly Government (Welsh Assembly Government, 2005) and are monitored by the Healthcare Inspectorate Wales (HIW).

In addition to these standards, all health care organisations are required to maintain other legal standards, such as health and safety, and employment practice.

Professional, clinical and organisational standards are inextricably linked in the framework for quality of health care. Further discussion about clinical and organisational standards can be found in Chapter 8 in relation to clinical governance.

The remainder of this chapter focuses on professional standards.

◎ SUMMARY

- In health there are three key types of standard that affect our practice: professional, clinical and organisational standards.
- Standards have benefits such as providing consistency across care settings, a common understanding of care expectations, and a reference point by which to evaluate the quality of care.
- Nursing has a key role in promoting standards and improving the patient experience.

Your professional standards

Your professional practice is determined by standards as set out by the NMC. The NMC is given powers to set these standards through legislation. The statutory framework for nursing and midwifery professional regulation is set out in the Nursing and Midwifery Order (2001), which stipulates the responsibilities and powers of the NMC. The Order specifies the key areas in which the NMC must set standards. It states that the NMC will 'establish from time to time standards of education, training, conduct and performance for nurses and midwives and to ensure the maintenance of those standards' (Part II 3(2)).

The fundamental standards for nurses and midwives are published in the NMC Code (2008) (see Appendix 1). It would be helpful to familiarise yourself with the NMC Code at this point, as these standards are discussed in detail in the next section. The importance of the NMC Code is highlighted by Jasper, who states:

> This is not a document for bedside reading, to be cast aside and filed away as yet another of the documents issued by the professional body as interesting but not really relevant to everyday practice. The code leaves one in no doubt about where responsibilities and accountability for practice lie, and therefore there is no excuse for any practitioner to claim misunderstanding or ignorance of the standards expected of them.

(Jasper, 2002, p. 189)

This may sound dramatic, but the NMC Code really is the linchpin of professional practice. However, some authors have questioned the relevance of the NMC Code to today's practice (e.g. Tschudin, 2006), and Jasper (2002) suggests that its standards may be unrealistically high, particularly when considered with constraints placed on practitioners in practice. The NCM Code is not intended, however, to act as a book of rules or procedures; the very nature of the ethical principles on which the NMC Code is based means that practice cannot be either straightforward or simplified in order to avoid difficult dilemmas in providing care.

Describing the standards as 'a code' may be the wrong terminology for contemporary nursing practice. The language stems from the introduction of the first codes of practice in nursing from the 1950s, set by the American Nurses Association (ANA) and the International Council of Nurses (ICN), at a time when some still viewed nursing as subservient to the medical profession (Esterhuizen, 2006). You can look back further into the history of nursing to the writings of Florence Nightingale about nursing the sick in 1882 to find expected behaviours and qualities of a nurse to include trustworthiness, cleanliness, neatness, and being sober and chaste (defined in terms of modesty and humility, with religious reference), which reflected the prominence of religious values and the number of nurses drawn from religious orders at that time (van de Peet, 1995).

Some standards have remained constant, albeit with their interpretation and practical application being redefined over time; for example, honesty, truthfulness and trustworthiness are still regarded as expected behaviours today within the NMC Code. These behaviours form the clauses that relate to one's professional conduct and underpin the ethical dimensions of the code.

The original language of codes, then, reflected the nature of practice, the relationship of nursing to medicine, and also the societal values of the time. Despite revisions and updates to bring the content of codes of practice and conduct up to date and relevant to modern-day practice, the continued use of the term 'code' perpetuates the image of a rule book.

Instead, the NMC Code should be used as a guide to be referred to for daily practice. (It might be interesting to ask practitioners if they have a copy to hand, to see whether it is indeed being used in this way.) Esterhuizen states:

> *. . . knowledge of a code of practice can supply the practitioner with an instrument with which to clarify values, a base upon which to build meaningful and equal dialogue with other professional disciplines (who in their turn base arguments on their ethical codes), and a set of concrete criteria for defending patient advocacy.*

> (Esterhuizen, 2006, p. 107)

Esterhuizen, then, presents the NMC Code as a tool to be used in practice, as a mechanism so that ethical principles underpin decisions to ensure that the patient's or client's best interests are upheld. However, he suggests that nurses do not apply codes to daily practice or use them in supporting decision-making for moral dilemmas, making practice dependent on the social and personal values of individual nurses. This, he argues, undermines the professionalism of nursing, because it ultimately dismantles the accountability of a practitioner as society would no longer have an agreed set of principles to which the practitioner would be expected to practise.

It is important at this stage to consider how professional regulation in maintaining standards works. Although the regulatory body sets and monitors standards, the implementation of such standards is dependent on each registered practitioner upholding the set standards. As a registered nurse you will be accountable to the regulatory body to observe the NMC standards in your own practice and in the practice of colleagues. In day-to-day practice, then, registered practitioners regulate themselves and their colleagues – that is, practise professional self-regulation. This is discussed in more detail in Chapter 6.

Reflection point 7.7
Choose a clause of the NMC Code and consider any challenges you might face in applying it in practice. What choices would you have? What would you do if faced with your scenario?

The NMC Code refers to your accountability to work collaboratively and to take account of guidance from colleagues; there may be occasions where someone who is viewed as having more expertise than you may tell you to do something that you are not happy about. What if their instruction is not best practice or you know it is against the patient's wishes? You would need to consider how you would address this potential conflict and how you would seek support to do so. This is discussed further in the section Maintaining professional standards in practice (p.134).

Professional standards for conduct

Earlier in this chapter we considered the influence of personal values on attitudes to professional standards. In particular, such values affect our views on behaviours or conduct. The NMC Code describes the required standards of behaviour that characterise the expected attitude of registered practitioners, including respect, trust, confidentiality and cooperation with others in the health care team. We have already considered how these expectations have persisted through the centuries of nursing practice. However, these standards are not exclusive to nursing and midwifery but are based on values shared across the health regulatory bodies in the UK.

Standards of professional conduct relate in particular to normative standards – that is, the definition of standards regarding expected behaviour or the norm. Such expectations reflect societal values of the time. This is exemplified in the changing nature of complaints brought to the regulatory body in relation to conduct. Cases cited in the early days of nursing regulation, after its introduction in the Nurses Registration Act 1919, included removal from the register for bearing illegitimate children, for committing adultery, and for being drunk and disorderly in a public place (Pyne, 1998). Although unrelated to nursing practice, at that time society viewed such personal behaviour as unacceptable. As societal values change, so do the expectations of registered nurses by the public. The NMC Code today demands that we uphold the good reputation of the professions. However, non-practice-related complaints account only for 3.4 per cent of cases heard by the NMC. The nature of these complaints is highlighted in the NMC's annual report about fitness to practise:

> *A registrant can be called to account for behaviour not related to practice if it is considered that public trust and confidence in the professions might be undermined, or if such behaviour constitutes a risk to the public. Most non-practice-related matters concern dishonesty, violent crime, and sexual offences (including downloading pornography).*
>
> (NMC, 2005a, p. 6)

These standards tend to be put to the test when they have not been met – for example, through complaints – rather than exemplifying when such standards have been met. Our challenge as a profession is to demonstrate standards of behaviour in positive terms and so ensure against the demise of a consistent and agreed professional standard of behaviour, as warned by Esterhuizen (2006).

Reflection point 7.8
Earlier we discussed the use of Essence of Care benchmarking to determine standards for nursing care. Now take some time to review the benchmark for privacy and dignity and identify where professional standards for conduct have been incorporated.

In reviewing standards to maintain privacy and dignity you should find that standards of professional conduct are integral to standards in clinical nursing practice.

Ethical principles in the NMC Code
Ethics are discussed in full in Chapter 9 and are not repeated here. It is worth reviewing the ethical theories and principles outlined in Chapter 9 and then considering how these are articulated in the NMC Code.

SUMMARY
- Our professional standards are set by the NMC and are primarily standards of education, conduct and performance.
- The NMC Code describes the standards of professional behaviour and practice expected of registered nurses and midwives and is underpinned by ethical principles and legal requirements.

Professional standards for education

The NMC sets standards for education that affect you throughout your professional career. These relate to:

- preparation for entry to the register;
- requirements to maintain registration;
- specific requirements for post-registration qualifications.

You will see as you look at this section that standards for education are inextricably linked with standards for practice, so that knowledge is relevant and applied to improve skills and contribute to clinical competence.

Meeting standards for entry to the NMC register

As you prepare to become a qualified nurse you will be following an educational programme through a university, through which you will be required to demonstrate an academic level of attainment and competence of clinical skills. The structured programme is designed to provide you with formal teaching and self-directed learning, linked closely with practical experience to develop your nursing skills and competence in a clinical setting. The standards against which you are assessed are set out in *Standards of Proficiency for Pre-Registration Nursing Education* (NMC, 2004a), some of which are noted at the beginning of this chapter. To be eligible for entry to the NMC register you will be required to achieve these standards of proficiency in the practice of your chosen area of nursing, namely adult nursing, children's nursing, mental health nursing or learning disabilities nursing. There are similar standards specific to the midwifery profession (NMC, 2004b).

Individuals who are registered nurses or midwives in countries outside of the UK and European Economic Area can also apply for registration to practise in the UK. The NMC considers whether the preparation and experience of each applicant in their home country meets the standards for registration with the NMC; if so, the applicant must successfully complete an Overseas Nursing Programme (NMC, 2005b). This ensures that nurses trained outside the UK are also assessed against the same standards of proficiency (NMC, 2004a).

Meeting educational standards to maintain registration

The need for education does not stop once you have become a registered nurse. With increasingly available knowledge from research and about health needs, health care continues to develop at a fast pace. Also, as your career develops, you will need to acquire new skills in new areas of practice. The expectation to maintain up-to-date knowledge is articulated in the standards stated in the NMC Code. Maintaining knowledge, then, is clearly seen as a tool for maintaining safe clinical practice. The requirements for continuing professional development (CPD) are specified in more detail in the NMC standards for post-registration education and practice (NMC, 2006a), which are outlined in Box 7.3. You may have heard these abbreviated to 'PREP standards'.

Reflection point 7.9
Take the opportunity to discuss CPD with registered nurses you have worked with.

- How do they identify their learning needs?
- What types of learning activity have they undertaken?
- How do they keep a record of their learning activity?
- Do they feel that the standards for CPD and practice that are required to renew registration are sufficient in order to maintain competence?
- What minimum standards do you think that the public would expect?

It is likely that you identified a variety of learning activities, ranging from formal courses to observing another practitioner's practice. Some examples of learning activities can be seen in Box 7.4. More information can be found in the *PREP Handbook* (NMC, 2006a). Learning activities are also discussed in more detail in Chapters 22 and 23.

BOX 7.3 Nursing and Midwifery Council PREP standards for maintaining registration

The PREP continuing professional development standard requires that you:

- undertake at least 35 hours of learning activity relevant to your practice during the 3 years before your renewal of registration;
- maintain a personal professional profile (PPP) of your learning activity;
- comply with any request from the NMC to audit how you have met these requirements.

The PREP practice standard requires the following:

- You must undertake a minimum of 450 hours of practice that uses your nursing qualification during the 3 years before renewal of registration. (Those practitioners who are also midwives must undertake 450 hours of practice for each part of the register in order to maintain each registration; e.g. a registered nurse and midwife would need to undertake 450 hours of nursing practice and 450 hours of midwifery practice, making a total of 900 hours, in order to remain registered as both a nurse and a midwife.)
- If you have not undertaken the minimum hours of practice, you are required to successfully complete an approved return-to-practice course before you can renew your registration. (Additionally, midwives need to give notice of their intention to practise, in accordance with rule 36 of the Midwives rules (NMC, 2004c).)

Source: NMC (2006a), reproduced with permission from the Nursing and Midwifery Council.

BOX 7.4 Examples of learning activity

- university courses leading to academic credits;
- distance-learning packs;
- seminars, conferences and workshops;
- reading professional journals;
- reading and analysing research articles;
- observing and practising clinical skills;
- 'shadowing' another health professional to better understand their role and work;
- analysing critical incidents or events in practice;
- reflecting on own practice;
- clinical supervision.

Learning activity

Given the breadth of self-directed learning that can be used to fulfil the requirement of 35 hours of learning activity, it is not an onerous task; nor need it incur costs for individual nurses. However, due to the demands of professional practice, it is unlikely that the minimum hours alone will equip you adequately to maintain up-to-date knowledge and skills. Is this view shared by the registered nurses with whom you have discussed CPD?

The standards for maintaining registration have been under increasing scrutiny across the health professions, particularly in relation to competence (CMO, 2006; DH, 2006b). It is likely that these standards will change in the future so that there is consistency of standards across the professions and that processes are strengthened to ensure that all registered practitioners meet these standards. One aspect of this is an expectation that employers will play a bigger role in supporting and monitoring CPD and practice.

Therefore there is increasing emphasis on CPD by employers, particularly in relation to ensuring that employees have the appropriate skills for the roles that they are asked to perform. One of the main tools used by the NHS in England is the Knowledge and Skills Framework (NHS KSF) (DH, 2004b). The NHS KSF sets out a comprehensive range of functions (dimensions) and accompanying skills and competences required to fulfil these functions. There are six core dimensions, which are relevant to all jobs in the NHS, such as communication, quality, service improvement, and personal and people development. A further 24 specific dimensions are used for specific jobs; for example, financial management is relevant for people working in finance, whereas dimensions for health and well-being, such as assessment and care planning, apply to nursing roles. The dimensions are listed in Table 7.1.

For every job in the NHS (with the exception of doctors, dentists, and some directors and senior managers) the required functions and level of skill has been determined and set out in an

Table 7.1 Core and specific dimensions of the NHS Knowledge and Skills Framework (Crown copyright material, reproduced with permission from DH, 2004b)

Core dimensions

Communication
Quality
Service improvement
Personal and people development
Health, safety and security
Equality and diversity

Specific dimensions

Health and well-being	Promotion of health and well-being and prevention of adverse effects on health and well-being
	Assessment and care-planning to meet health and well-being needs
	Protection of health and well-being
	Enablement to address health and well-being needs
	Provision of care to meet health and well-being needs
	Assessment and treatment planning
	Interventions and treatments
	Biomedical investigation and intervention
	Equipment and devices to meet health and well-being needs
	Products to meet health and well-being needs
Estates and facilities	Systems, vehicles and equipment
	Environments and buildings
	Transport and logistics
Information and knowledge	Information-processing
	Information collection and analysis
	Knowledge and information resources
General	Learning and development
	Development and innovation
	Procurement and commissioning
	Financial management
	Services and project management
	People management
	Capacity and capability
	Public relations and marketing

NHS KSF post outline. The post outline is then used to review the individual's progress and to identify learning needs. In this way, learning needs are linked closely to the competence required for the role. You may find it useful to ask the human resources department at your next clinical placement for a copy of a KSF post outline for a registered nurse.

Keeping a record of your learning activity

It is important to keep a record of your learning activity, as this is also a requirement of the NMC CPD standards. There are no hard and fast rules on how this should be done. A number of formats are presented in the professional literature, and commercially produced folders and software are widely available (Driscoll and Teh, 2001). However, you do not have to incur extra cost, as you can make your own profile simply in a notebook or electronically in a computer file. The NMC (2006a) presents a sample template in its *PREP Handbook*, which can be copied easily. Whatever format you choose, there are some key questions that can help you structure your notes (Box 7.5). This will help you to demonstrate how the learning activity has developed your practice.

> **BOX 7.5 Questions to structure your record of learning activity**
> - Where were you working when the learning activity took place?
> - What was the learning activity, when was it undertaken and how long did it take?
> - How has the learning activity informed and influenced your practice?
>
> *Source*: NMC (2006a), reproduced with permission from the Nursing and Midwifery Council.

It is also worth thinking ahead to when you qualify and start your first post as to how you will show where your learning activity supports your development in the NHS KSF. You will need to indicate how your learning is relevant to the core and specific domains in your post outline.

Reflective practice

One learning activity listed is reflective practice; however, this is part of all learning activity and central to professional practice. Reflecting on one's practice is a skill that develops with experience; in the same way that clinical skills need to be learned, practised and honed, reflective practice needs equal attention. Reflective practice will be explored a little further here, but you will find more information in Chapter 22. There are also some suggested texts about reflective practice in the further reading section in this chapter.

What is reflection?

Much has been written about reflection. Johns (2000, p. 34) stated:

> *Reflection is a window through which the practitioner can view and focus self within the context of her own lived experience in ways that help her to confront, understand and work towards resolving the contradictions within her practice between what is desirable and actual practice.*

Reflection, then, is looking at your own practice, considering how you acted in a certain event, and evaluating your own performance against what the ideal or model practice would be. Sometimes you will identify where your practice was good and, in doing so, identify what made your practice in that circumstance successful so that you can use it in order to maintain your performance in future practice. On other occasions you will identify where you felt you could have practised differently and where you may need to develop a skill or knowledge further. You can then act on this so that you can improve your practice in the future. This means that you self-monitor your own standards of practice. This should be a constructive process, so that you can critically review your own practice without castigating yourself for not getting things quite right – after all, you will never be in the perfect practice setting or circumstance in order to be able to perform 'textbook' practice. It is likely that you are already becoming familiar with this learning technique during your clinical placements in discussions with your mentors and tutors.

In order to develop reflection as a constructive activity, it needs to be structured so that a process of reflection is followed. In time this process can become internalised, so that, as in the expert practitioner, it becomes an intuitive process. There are several models of guided or structured reflection in the professional literature (e.g. Gibbs, 1988; Johns, 2000; Taylor, 2000). All assist the process by asking the practitioner key questions about their experience in clinical practice. Driscoll (2006) provides a straightforward approach to guided reflection in his What? model. This comprises three stages:

- *What?* A description of the event, including what happened, how you reacted and who else was involved.
- *So what?* An analysis of the event, how you felt about your actions, how you feel now, and what the effects of your actions were.
- *Now what?* The actions (if any) that need to be taken, what help you may need, and identifying the priorities and consideration of how you will recognise any differences to your practice.

Reflection point 7.10
Select a reflective model from the literature and apply it to an event in your recent practice. Consider which parts you found comfortable and which were more challenging in reflecting on your practice. Why do you think some aspects were more difficult than others? Consider how else you could approach reflection to help you with the process.

One of the challenges of reflection that you may have identified is that sometimes it is difficult to analyse an event objectively, being the subject of your analysis, and therefore you would benefit from another view or another's expertise. Clinical supervision provides a mechanism for practitioners to reflect on practice with the support and guidance of a colleague. This is more than reflection; Driscoll (2006) reinforces this by highlighting that clinical supervision gives the opportunity to reflect and be proactive about practice, but with the support of others to stimulate new ideas and thinking, rather than in isolation.

Clinical supervision is described briefly here, but you will find more detailed information in Chapter 8 and in the Further reading section.

Clinical supervision

There can be misconceptions about clinical supervision, ranging from views that it is just chatting with colleagues to believing it is just another term for managerial supervision. This is not the case. Clinical supervision can be defined as 'a designated interaction between two or more practitioners, within a safe/supportive environment, which enables a continuum of reflective, critical analysis of care, to ensure quality patient services' (Bishop, 1998, p. 8).

It is characterised, then, by a formal meeting to discuss and explore issues of practice. This may be between two people or between a group of practitioners. Clinical supervision does not 'just happen'; it needs to be prepared for and be given devoted time. It would be useful to ask how your colleagues in your clinical placements engage in clinical supervision in order to get a perspective on how models, guidelines and policies for clinical supervision work in practice.

SUMMARY

- CPD is essential in maintaining professional standards.
- Reflective practice and clinical supervision are essential mechanisms to support you and help you improve your practice throughout your professional career.

Professional standards for performance

We need to have standards of performance so that our practice is safe and of therapeutic value for patients and clients. Nursing is fundamentally a practice profession; knowledge alone does not ensure safe or best practice, but it is its application and demonstration through skills that matter. This is why the standards for education, as discussed earlier, are integrated closely with those for practice or performance.

In order to meet the requirements for registration, you will be developing competences in practice, which you will need to demonstrate to meet the standards of proficiency, for example undertaking nursing assessments and demonstrating sound clinical judgement across a range of differing professional and care delivery contexts (NMC, 2004a). Standards for maintaining registration include the requirement to maintain a minimum amount of practice, as seen earlier in Box 7.3. This reinforces the importance of maintaining skills in addition to knowledge.

Performance or competence?

The terms 'competence' and 'performance' are both used in relation to standards of professional practice. Although they are linked closely, they have slightly different interpretations. The Scottish OPRS Committee defines competence as the 'consistent integration of skills, knowledge, attitudes, values and abilities that underpin safe and effective performance in a professional or occupational role' (cited in DH, 2006b). Again, we see how knowledge, skills, values and abilities are inseparable in determining standards for practice. Also, this definition shows that competence is required in order to meet a standard of performance. Competence, then, such as the requirements of you to be eligible for registration, is demonstrated through your performance. Performance is used to describe consistent competence; a practitioner who performs adequately is one who always works in a safe way and so meets performance standards (DH, 2006b). This reflects how performance standards are viewed to consider practice over period of time, rather than one's competence at a single point in time.

The NMC Code links the term competence with the requirement to 'have the knowledge and skills for safe and effective professional practice without direct supervision.'

As you develop your practice skills you will be working towards demonstrating your ability to do so without the need for direct supervision. This will require you to show that you are consistently competent – that is, to show adequate performance.

Reflection point 7.11

One example of the standards of proficiency required to be eligible for registration (NMC, 2004a, p. 5) is 'Undertake and document a comprehensive, systematic and accurate nursing assessment of the physical, psychological, social and spiritual needs of patients, clients and communities.'

Think about how you would demonstrate your competence for this standard. What evidence would you use? You may wish to repeat this exercise for other standards of proficiency.

It is likely that you could identify evidence for selecting a valid assessment tool and demonstrate the assessment by documenting it, which a registered nurse confirmed was accurate and appropriate. Satisfaction expressed by the patient or client in the way in which you did the assessment could provide another indicator. Equally important in achieving competence is how you undertook the assessment, with the appropriate use of interpersonal skills, observation and listening, which may be assessed by a registered nurse observing your practice. In this one exercise you can see how theoretical knowledge, skills and their application to meet the unique needs of an individual are interwoven in standards of competence.

Standards for performance in daily practice can be seen in the NMC Code by indicating that a high standard of practice is expected at all times. It refers to recognising the limits of your competence and ensuring that you have the skills and knowledge to practise without supervision. Again, the term 'competence' is used to describe expectations of registered nurses.

Levels of competence and the law

There is very little in nursing practice that is prevented by law; professional registration and its accompanying accountability give each practitioner freedom to develop their practice in order to meet the needs of patients and clients. The development of such practice is seen across nursing and other health professions; for example, prescribing was once the domain of medicine, but independent and supplementary non-medical prescribing is increasingly seen across care. This required a change of legislation to the Medicines Act and the requirement of individuals to successfully complete accredited prescribing courses.

Most developments in professional practice do not need legislative change but remain bound by legislation to ensure appropriate competence to carry out new roles. The legal standard of what is a 'reasonable' level of competence has been defined through cases of negligence, specifically the case of Bolam v Friern Hospital Management Committee in 1957 is cited (Dimond, 1994; Walsh, 2000). This judgement defined the expected standard of a skill as 'the standard of the ordinary skilled man exercising and professing to have that special skill'.

You may hear this referred to as 'the Bolam test'. In law, then, you are required to ensure a minimum standard of care throughout your practice that would be expected of anyone qualified to provide such care and accepting responsibility to do so. This means that, although we would strive to provide the highest possible standard of care, we are judged on standards that are commonly agreed as an acceptable level. This would be founded on evidence, guidelines and protocols for practice of the time, which highlights the importance of keeping your skills and knowledge up to date.

Clearly standards for competence need to be related directly to the role that you undertake. As we discussed earlier, the NHS KSF is used to determine the level of competence required for each role. In addition, competency frameworks are also used to describe the skills and knowledge required to undertake certain roles. Many of these are taken from the work of the Skills for Health, which lists over 2000 competences and National Occupational Standards. These competences are linked closely with your professional clinical standards. For example, one of the competences relevant to nursing is supporting individuals to manage continence (HSC219) (Skills for Health, 2004). This describes the skills, knowledge and values that are required and the performance criteria to be used to demonstrate that the standard of care has been achieved in relation to assisting the management of continence.

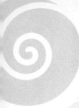

Obtain a copy of the competence for supporting individuals in managing continence from the Skills for Health website (www.skillsforhealth.org.uk) and review its performance criteria. Thinking of Donabedian's framework, consider which criteria would be associated with structure, process or outcome. Are there any gaps? Think about how you would set a performance criterion for any gaps you have identified.

You may have found that the performance criteria are predominantly about process – that is, how you carry out care – but elements of structure, for example the provision and disposal of appropriate equipment, and outcomes such as maximising privacy and preventing infection are incorporated. The most obvious outcomes of maintaining continence and patient satisfaction are not stated explicitly; you may have identified some possible ways of demonstrating these.

In the next section we will explore your standards in practice in more detail.

SUMMARY

- You are required to maintain standards of competence in your daily practice.
- You will be required to meet the NMC standards for CPD and practice in order to maintain your registration – that is, to allow you to continue to practise.
- Frameworks used by employers such as the NHS KSF and the Skills for Health competency frameworks are linked closely to our professional standards.

Maintaining professional standards in practice

So far in this chapter we have explored what is expected in relation to our professional standards and what is needed in order to fulfil such standards. In an ideal world we should be able to achieve this. We know, however, that there can be obstacles and challenges to nurses in maintaining standards in practice. This section looks at applying standards in practice.

Developing and maintaining your own standards

Throughout your professional career you will continue to develop your skills and knowledge in order to ensure standards of your practice. Here we will focus on ways to deal with developing new competences to meet changing patient need and expectations.

Dealing with new competences

When you qualify as a registered nurse you will have achieved a standard of competence with which comes an expectation of your level of skills. However, this does not mean that you can be fully competent for all aspects of practice that you will face. Indeed, all nurses at some point in their professional practice face an aspect of practice for which they feel unprepared, either because they have not undertaken a particular skill before or because they have not used a skill for some time and therefore no longer feel competent. It is important to be proactive in anticipating skills in relation to your area of work or the nature of needs within the client group you are working with. For example, consider Scenario 7.1.

SCENARIO 7.1

You are successful in getting a job as a staff nurse working with a district nursing team. Your placement in the community was at the beginning of your pre-registration programme and so you are nervous about being ready for the job.

1 Identify what skills you would want to learn or refresh.
2 Identify what knowledge and information you need.
3 Think about how you would address these gaps in your skills and knowledge, who you would approach and where you would seek information.

In Scenario 7.1, you may have identified a range of skills, such as applying aseptic technique in the patient's home, and skills in addressing wider issues in ill health such as social isolation, low income and poor housing (NHS Employers, 2006a), and identified certain people to help you, such as the district nursing team leader. In practice, it has been found that the process of developing professional competence is influenced by factors such as experience, opportunities available to nurses, personal characteristics and the environment in which nurses work (Khomeiran *et al.*, 2006). It would be worth considering what factors you think affect you in how you learn and what motivates you, in order to help you optimise these in your practice.

You will not always be able to be proactive about identifying areas of competence that you need to develop, and you may be faced with a situation where your patients or clients have an urgent care need for which you do not have, or do not feel confident in, the required skill. Although you may know that you need to seek assistance, sometimes, particularly when everyone else is very busy, nurses find this hard to actually do. Some feel they are putting more pressure on colleagues and fear being viewed as unable to do the job. This leads to the temptation to just muddle through in the hope that everything will be all right. However, it is important to take a moment in such circumstances to think about what could be the outcome of undertaking skills for which you feel inadequately prepared. In doing so, you increase the risk of making mistakes and causing injury to the patient or client and, in some circumstances, to yourself. Errors do happen in practice, but where a nurse could have prevented them by acknowledging their own limitations rather than hiding them, then their accountability is brought into question. It is much better, however difficult you feel it will be, to raise your concern with a colleague or manager in order to ensure the patient or client receives safe care and you receive support and supervision to develop the appropriate skill. In this way, you can turn your dilemma into an opportunity to develop your practice. Some nurses have described this positively as 'golden chances' that occur suddenly and are transient, to be grabbed as invaluable opportunities when they arise (Khomeiran *et al.*, 2006). Consider Scenario 7.2.

SCENARIO 7.2

Jane qualified as a registered mental health nurse 2 months ago. She works on a ward for people with acute mental health problems. Jane is caring for a patient, Jack, who experiences hallucinations, has insulin dependent diabetes and unstable glucose levels, and has been an inpatient for 4 days. Jane learned about caring for people living with diabetes in the common foundation programme, but she has not checked blood glucose levels or administered insulin since then. There is only one other registered nurse on the ward, who is with a distressed patient. Jack requires his insulin in 10 minutes and Jane has to decide what to do.

1 What would you do in Jane's situation?
2 What steps could Jane have taken in order to avoid the urgency of the situation?

In Scenario 7.2, you should have identified ways for Jane to seek help immediately from her colleague in order to ensure that her patient received the appropriate care at the right time. In addition, you should have identified future learning needs so that Jane would be prepared and skilled to provide for such care needs in the future. To do this, though, you need to have self-assertiveness and confidence in the support of the team. As a student you should receive support and guidance from mentors, and in your first employment as a registered nurse you should undergo a period of preceptorship.

Preceptorship is a formal period of support for newly registered nurses and midwives from an experienced professional colleague. It is recommended that this period is at least 4 months. The preceptor is a named individual who works in the same setting and provides help, advice and support. This individual is available when the newly registered nurse or midwife needs help with a procedure with which they are unfamiliar or a situation not encountered before, and is also able to offer guidance or help with any other aspect of practice (NMC, 2006b).

These relationships can equip you with the confidence to seek help. Chapters 5 and 22 discuss ways in which you can be supported both as a student and throughout your career. Unfortunately, occasionally nurses find themselves working in an unsupportive environment to the extent that it undermines their self-esteem, so that they feel unable to expose their own concerns about their practice for fear of the repercussions from team members. Some student nurses have described 'feeling like a waste of time', being ignored and being spoken about in front of them, to the extent that they have been unable to speak out about this and similar bullying behaviour observed towards patients (Randle, 2003). Not only is this damaging to the patient and individual nurse, but it also jeopardises safe standards of care and clearly is not acceptable. If this strikes a chord with you, it is important that you seek help immediately. NHS organisations should operate zero tolerance of bullying (NHS Employers, 2006b), but this can work only if individuals speak out if they see or experience bullying. Again, Chapters 5 and 22 will guide you to some avenues of support to do this.

Developing and maintaining standards in a team

Throughout your professional career it is unlikely that you will be working alone; rather, you will work as a member of a health care team.

Different ways of working

Increasingly nurses find roles in teams and settings that have not been typical ways of working. For example, nurses working with children are likely to be part of a team comprising education, social care and the voluntary sector. They may or may not be employed by the local NHS organisation, but they will be brought under the umbrella of a children's trust. Bringing people together in teams that focus on their shared client group facilitates more integrated working but also raises challenges about potentially different professional cultures and expectations of standards.

It is essential that there is shared understanding of different roles and responsibilities within the team, and there is agreement about shared standards of care. Ways of working in different care settings are explored further in Chapter 10.

Delegation

In all teams there will be a mix of staff in order to provide a breadth of skills required to meet the patients' needs in a cost-effective way. As a registered nurse you will have a professional responsibility for the delegation of duties as stated in the NMC Code. Primarily delegation will be to staff in assistant roles such as support workers, health care assistants and nursery nurses.

The allocation of duties to another registered nurse or midwife is not delegation, as they already have the professional authority and accompanying accountability to undertake assigned nursing functions. With the increasing blurring of professional boundaries, this could equally apply in some circumstances to other registered health professionals who are not nurses or midwives, as they may also have the authority to undertake some of the care functions and they are professionally accountable for their practice to their own regulatory bodies. Where this is not the case, then the principles of delegation can be applied equally to other registered professionals when working in a multiprofessional team, but the focus of your accountability is for delegation to assistant practitioner roles.

In order to ensure that standards are maintained, you must be assured that assistant practitioners have the skills and competence to undertake any function delegated to them. As a newly registered nurse yourself, this responsibility can seem onerous at a time when you are establishing your own practice. However, your employer also has a responsibility to ensure that assistant practitioners are competent through training and assessment for roles that are within their job requirements, for which the employer has vicarious liability (NMC, 2006b).

Having 'vicarious liability' means that the employer is accountable for the standard of care delivered and is responsible for employees working within areas of competence appropriate to their abilities. To remain covered by an employer's vicarious liability clause, an employee must work only within their abilities and sphere of assessed competence (NMC, 2006c).

With this definition, it is reasonable for you to assume, provided you are satisfied that the assistant practitioner has had such training and assessment, that they are competent to do so. If, however, you have any reservations about an individuals' competence in a particular situation, then you are responsible for raising your concerns so that their skills can be reviewed where necessary.

In delegating any aspect of care, there are principles that can safeguard the appropriateness of the delegation. In the USA, these have been described as the 'five rights of delegation' (National Council of State Boards of Nursing, 1995), which are used to facilitate the nurse's decision-making about delegation. These state that the nurse should consider whether the delegation is:

- the right task;
- in the right circumstances;
- from and to the right person;
- with the right communication;
- with the right supervision.

These factors are also reflected in the advice from the NMC (2007b) regarding delegation and so give you a useful checklist for your decision-making. Again, delegation is a skill that you will develop over time with the help of your preceptor and manager.

Contributing to standards of care development

As part of the team you will be involved in developing standards of care in the area where you work. This might be through clinical audits, benchmarking and reviews of aspects of care, for example the Essence of Care benchmarking programme (Modernisation Agency, 2003). These and other measures are discussed in detail in Chapter 8.

> ### ⊚ SUMMARY
>
> - You are responsible for identifying gaps in your competence and seeking help. Preceptorship is a mechanism to assist you in doing this.
> - As health care develops, nurses and midwives are increasingly working in new teams and organisations. It is important that there is a common understanding of standards and roles in order to maximise patient care.
> - You will have responsibility for the safe and appropriate delegation of duties to assistant practitioners. There are five key principles to use in delegating in order to ensure that standards of care are maintained.

When practice falls below acceptable standards

Sadly, we have seen cases where standards have not been maintained. This is not the sole concern of nursing and midwifery but is a concern of all health and social care professions. A fall in standards may be as an outcome of incidents or mistakes, the practice or conduct of individual practitioners, or failure at an organisational level. In all circumstances you have a professional responsibility to intervene. Some approaches in each of these circumstances are discussed below.

Dealing with errors or incidents

Mistakes happen, but it is important that factors contributing to errors or incidents are identified and addressed so that learning and action from incidents and errors minimise the opportunity for recurrence. This can happen only if there is an openness and willingness to report errors and incidents, including communicating this with patients and carers (NPSA, 2005). Organisations have incident-reporting procedures so that incidents are addressed in a consistent and comprehensive manner from which it can be determined whether there are trends of certain incidents. Such systems also include the reporting of near-misses, so that potential safety risks are identified and addressed before they escalate to actual incidents or errors. This is done at a local and national level. For example, the National Patient Safety Agency (NPSA) issued a safer practice notice in response to reports of death and patient harm due to high doses of morphine and diamorphine being given in error (NPSA, 2006).

Reflection point 7.13

Speak to the risk manager in the organisation of your next clinical placement to learn about incident-reporting mechanisms and how they are used to address standards of practice. Then discuss incident reporting with the team with which you are working. Ask whether they have reported incidents and, if so, the nature of the incident. Do they see any benefits or disadvantages to reporting errors and incidents?

It is important that you know the local systems for reporting incidents and near-misses. Although seeing the benefits in reporting incident, your colleagues may have expressed some concerns about the personal consequences in admitting an error or incident. Barriers to reporting have been identified, including feeling a sense of failure, fear of blame, fear of legal action, lack of time, and difficulty with reporting systems with perceptions that staff should be caring for patients rather than completing forms (Wilson and Sheikh, 2002). However, organisations should be working to ensure open and fair culture so that staff feel comfortable to report without fear of reprimand in their seven steps to patient safety; reporting systems should also be clear and uncomplicated (NPSA, 2004).

Chapter 8 incorporates some aspects of risk management. Further information on your contribution to patient safety, including an e-learning programme on patient safety, can be found on the NPSA website (www.npsa.nhs.uk).

Dealing with concerns about an individual practitioner

During your practice you may observe actions or behaviours of another practitioner that give you concern. There are different avenues you may need to pursue, depending on the nature and seriousness of your concern. In the first instance, you may feel confident to raise the concern yourself. This might be appropriate where your concern is minor or not an immediate risk to patients. For example, you may have observed out-of-date practice. You can introduce evidence on updating practice with the whole team, following discussion with the manager, so that it can be a learning process to review existing guidelines. A training need could be proposed to the manager or clinical leader, from which the whole team could benefit.

Alternatively, you may feel confident in speaking to the practitioner directly, particularly if you work in an open supportive team where this approach is generally accepted. However, even in a supportive environment, a practitioner may not recognise their limitations and may be reluctant to change. In such circumstances, you need to raise your concerns with the practitioner's manager. The employer is expected to take appropriate action to address this (DH and NPSA, 2006), with possible measure such as retraining, supervision and reassessment of an individual's competence.

Although you are fully aware of your primary responsibility to your patients and clients, the prospect of raising concerns can be daunting, with fears of being seen as telling tales or being disloyal to colleagues. This is particularly difficult if the work culture focuses on blaming individuals rather than addressing the standards of care in question. It is important that you seek support, whether from a trusted colleague or from a representative from a professional body.

If your concern about a practitioner relates to an immediate risk to patient or staff safety that cannot be addressed directly with the practitioner, it should be reported to the manager without delay. There are some circumstances in which a manager will intervene by requiring the practitioner to stop work in order not only to protect the patient's interest but also to protect the practitioner until the concern has been investigated. This may be where there is a serious health concern affecting the ability to practise, such as alcohol or substance misuse, or where conduct is brought into question, for example suspected verbal, physical or financial abuse.

Where an organisation takes action about serious concerns of a practitioner's competence or conduct, it has to decide whether it is also a matter for the professional regulatory body, such as the NMC. This is likely if any remedial action to address competence is persistently unsuccessful, such that the individual is unsafe to practise, or where their conduct poses a risk to patients and the public. The NMC should be informed where a practitioner's contract is terminated as a result of the action taken or the practitioner leaves before investigations into serious concerns are completed (DH and NPSA, 2006).

When the NMC receives an allegation, it investigates the matter to see whether it is an issue for the regulatory body, and if, after considering the preliminary evidence (including the practitioner's response to the allegations), it believes that there is a case to answer. If so, it will proceed to a public hearing of the case by the Conduct and Competence Committee (unless it is a matter of ill health, in which case proceedings are held in private by the Health Committee). The proceedings are a legal process set out in the Nursing and Midwifery Order (2001) and therefore are similar to a magistrate's court: a panel hears the case, people are sworn in to give evidence, and legal advisors and solicitors are involved. It is worth attending a hearing if you have the opportunity.

If the allegations are proven, the NMC has a range of sanctions that it can instigate (NMC Order, 2001: Part V, 29(5a–d)):

- *Striking off order*: the person is removed from the register.
- *Suspension order*: registration is suspended (for up to 1 year).
- *Conditions of practice order*: conditions are imposed with which the person must comply (for up to 3 years).
- *Caution order*: the person is cautioned and this is noted on the register (for not less than 1 year and not more than 5 years).

These sanctions and the processes by which the NMC deals with reported concerns are described in detail in *Reporting Unfitness to Practise: A Guide for Employers and Managers* (NMC, 2004d) and *Reporting Lack of Competence: A Guide for Employers and Managers* (NMC, 2004e). The NMC annual report on fitness to practise for 2004–05 is also of interest as it gives examples of cases heard by the NMC and their outcomes (NMC, 2005a). Further summaries of cases can be found on the NMC website (www.nmc-uk.org) under Fitness to Practise.

Dealing with other concerns about unacceptable standards in practice

There may be occasions where you have concerns about other standards in practice, for example health and safety where you work or standards of cleanliness. All organisations have mechanisms to support individuals who raise concerns, including specific policies that outline the process and to whom concerns should be raised. The first port of call is usually your manager or team leader, but policies should also include alternatives to this. Such procedures are commonly called 'whistle-blowing'. All workers, whether in the NHS or the independent sector, are afforded protection in reporting organisational concerns by the Public Disclosure Act (1998) (England, Scotland and Wales); the equivalent legislation in Northern Ireland is the Public Interest Disclosure Order (1998). Public Concern at Work (www.pcaw.co.uk) is an organisation that gives advice on whistle-blowing to organisations and supports individuals to raise concerns. It may be of interest to look at their website and their case studies of people who have reported concerns.

There are other organisations that also play a role in addressing concerns of practice and health care, so the onus does not fall solely on the shoulders of the registered professional. These include:

- Patient organisations – for example, health councils in Scotland and their equivalent in Wales and Northern Ireland; patient advice and liaison services in England; organisations such as Action for Victims of Medical Accidents (AVMA) and WITNESS (which supports victims of abuse by health professionals).
- Coroners: aspects of a case or a number of cases may trigger alarm.
- National Patient Safety Agency: established in England in 2001 to improve the safety and quality of care through reporting, analysing and learning from patient safety incidents and near-misses involving NHS patients. Their role was discussed earlier in this chapter.
- Healthcare Commission (CHAI) and its equivalent organisations in Scotland and Northern Ireland, as discussed earlier in this chapter.

SUMMARY

- Errors and incidents should be reported in order to address risks to patients and reduce the chance of recurrence. Organisations should have policies and procedures in place to encourage reporting without fear of reprisal.
- You have a responsibility to identify and minimise risks to patients by taking appropriate action where there is unacceptable practice.
- Anyone can report concerns to a regulatory body regarding the practice or conduct of a registered health professional, although this is usually done by the employer.
- Patient organisations and other agencies have an important role to play in identifying problems and risks to standards in professional practice and health care services.

CONCLUSION

It would be wrong to leave this chapter without putting into perspective the incidence of failure to meet professional standards. Of some 686 000 nurses and midwives registered with the NMC, only a small minority, considered unsafe to practise, is removed from the register. In 2006–07, 144 individuals were removed from the register (NMC, 2007c). In contrast, the overall body of the nursing and midwifery professions is continually maintaining and improving professional standards.

This chapter has explored how you can use your professional accountability to improve standards: in understanding what standards are and how they are implemented, you can fully appreciate your potential in providing optimum care. Our professional standards are the bedrock of our practice; by using the standards set by the NMC, you can develop your practice as an accountable practitioner. In this way you will not only be prepared for the challenges of professional practice but also be able to enjoy exercising your freedom to practise innovatively in the best interests of your clients and patients. Ultimately, it is they who are the true focus of any professional standard. Standards are important to patients: standards provide the mechanism by which patients can seek assurance that they are benefiting from the optimum quality of care. We must continue to work with patients and clients at individual, local and national levels to ensure that all professional standards truly reflect their perspective.

References

Bishop V (1998). Clinical supervision: what is it? In Bishop V (ed.). *Clinical Supervision in Practice*. London: Macmillan.

Chief Medical Officer (CMO) (2006). *Good Doctors, Safer Patients*. London: Department of Health.

Coia JE, Duckworth GJ, Edwards DI, *et al.* (2006). Guidelines for the control and prevention of methicillin-resistant *Staphylococcus aureus* (MRSA) in healthcare facilities. *Journal of Hospital Infection*, **63S**, S1–44.

Clinical Standards Board for Scotland (CSBS) (2001). *Standards: Healthcare Associated Infection (HAI) Infection Control*. Edinburgh: Clinical Standards Board for Scotland.

Commission for Social Care Inspection (CSCI) and Commission for Healthcare Audit and Inspection (CHAI) (2006). *Joint Investigation into the Provision of Services for People with Learning Disabilities at Cornwall Partnership NHS Trust*. London: Commission for Healthcare Audit and Inspection.

Department of Health (DH) (2000a). *The NHS Cancer Plan*. London: Department of Health.

Department of Health (DH) (2000b). *Coronary Heart Disease: National Service Framework for Coronary Heart Disease – Modern Standards and Service Models*. London: Department of Health.

Department of Health (DH) (2001a). *National Service Framework for Diabetes: Standards*. London: Department of Health.

Department of Health (DH) (2001b). *National Service Framework for Older People*. London: Department of Health.

Department of Health (DH) (2001c). *Essence of Care*. London: Department of Health.

Department of Health (DH) (2004a). *Towards Cleaner Hospitals and Lower Rates of Infection*. London: Department of Health.

Department of Health (DH) (2004b). *The NHS Knowledge and Skills Framework*. London: Department of Health.

Department of Health (DH) (2005a). *Supporting People with Long Term Conditions: An NHS and Social Care Model to Support Local Innovation and Integration*. London: Department of Health.

Department of Health (DH) (2005b). *'Now I Feel Tall': What a Patient-Led NHS Feels Like*. London: Department of Health.

Department of Health (DH) (2006a). *Standards for Better Health*. London: Department of Health.

Department of Health (DH) (2006b). *The Regulation of the Non-Medical Healthcare Professions: A Review by the Department of Health*. London: Department of Health.

Department of Health (DH) (2007). *Trust, Assurance and Safety: The Regulation of Health Professionals in the 21st Century*. London: The Stationery Office.

Department of Health (DH) (2008). *The Health Act 2006: Code of Practice for the Prevention and Control of Healthcare Associated Infections*. London: Department of Health.

Department of Health (DH) and National Patient Safety Agency (NPSA) (2006). *Handling Concerns about the Performance of Healthcare Professionals: Principles of Good Practice*. London: Department of Health and National Clinical Assessment Service.

Department of Health, Social Services and Public Safety (DHSSPS) (2006). *The Quality Standards for Health and Social Care*. Belfast: Department of Health, Social Services and Public Safety.

Dimond B (1994). Legal aspects of role expansion. In Hunt G and Wainwright P (eds). *Expanding the Role of the Nurse: The Scope of Professional Practice*. Oxford: Blackwell Science.

Donabedian A (2005). Evaluating the quality of medical care. *Milbank Quarterly*, **83**, 691–729.

Dozier AM (1998). Professional standards: linking care, competence and quality. *Journal of Nursing Care Quality*, **12**, 22–9.

Driscoll J (2006). *Practising Clinical Supervision: A Reflective Approach for Healthcare Professionals*, 2nd edn. London: Baillière Tindall.

Driscoll J and Teh B (2001). The contributions of portfolios and profiles to continuing professional development. *Journal of Orthopaedic Nursing*, **5**, 151–6.

Esterhuizen P (2006). Is the professional code still the cornerstone of clinical nursing practice? *Journal of Advanced Nursing*, **53**, 104–13.

Gibbs G (1988). *Learning by Doing: A Guide to Teaching and Learning Methods*. Oxford: Further Education Unit, Oxford Polytechnic.

Health Protection Agency (2006). Healthcare associated infections. www.hpa.org.uk/infections/topics_az/hai/default.htm.

Jasper M (1996). *Evaluating Care and Effecting Change*. Unit study guide. London: Distance Learning Centre, South Bank University.

Jasper M (2002). A plethora of standards for individual practitioners, but where does the buck stop? *Journal of Nursing Management*, **10**, 189–90.

Johns C (2000). *Becoming a Reflective Practitioner: A Reflective and Holistic Approach to Clinical Nursing, Practice Development and Clinical Supervision*. Oxford: Blackwell Science.

Khomeiran RT, Yekta ZP, Kiger AM and Ahmadi F (2006). Professional competence: factors described by nurses as influencing their development. *International Nursing Review*, **53**, 66–72.

Kunaviktikul W, Anders RL, Chontawan R, *et al.* (2005). Development of indicators to assess the quality of nursing care in Thailand. *Nursing and Health Sciences*, **7**, 273–80.

Medicines and Healthcare Products Regulatory Agency (MHRA) (2003). *Community Equipment Loan Stores: Guidance on Decontamination*. London: Medicines and Healthcare Products Regulatory Agency.

Modernisation Agency (2003). *Essence of Care: Patient-Focused Benchmarks for Clinical Governance*. London: Department of Health.

Morrell C, Harvey G and Kitson A (1997). Practitioner based quality improvement: a review of the Royal College of Nursing's dynamic standard setting system. *Quality in Health Care*, **6**, 29–34.

National Council of State Boards of Nursing (1995). *Delegation: Concepts and Decision Making Process*. Chicago, IL: National Council of State Boards of Nursing.

NHS Employers (2006a). *From Hospital to Home: Supporting Nurses to Move from Hospital to the Community*. Briefing issue 26, November 2006. London: NHS Employers.

NHS Employers (2006b). Stop bullying: it's in your hands – staff guidance. www.nhsemployers.org.

NHS Quality Improvement Scotland (NHS QIS) (2005). *Healthcare Associated Infection*. Edinburgh: NHS Quality Improvement Scotland.

National Institute for Health and Clinical Excellence (NICE) (2003). *Infection Control: Prevention of Healthcare-Associated Infections in Primary and Community Care*. Clinical guideline 2. London: National Institute for Health and Clinical Excellence.

National Patient Safety Agency (NPSA) (2004). *Seven Steps to Patient Safety: An Overview Guide for NHS Staff*. London: National Patient Safety Agency.

National Patient Safety Agency (NPSA) (2005). *Being Open When Patients Are Harmed*. Safer practice notice 10. London: National Patient Safety Agency.

National Patient Safety Agency (NPSA) (2006). *Ensuring Safer Practice with High Dose Ampoules of Diamorphine and Morphine*. Safer practice notice 12. London: National Patient Safety Agency.

Nursing and Midwifery Council (NMC) (2004a). *Standards of Proficiency for Pre-Registration Nursing Education*. London: Nursing and Midwifery Council.

Nursing and Midwifery Council (NMC) (2004b). *Standards of Proficiency for Pre-Registration Midwifery Education*. London: Nursing and Midwifery Council.

Nursing and Midwifery Council (NMC) (2004c). *Midwives Rules and Standards*. London: Nursing and Midwifery Council.

Nursing and Midwifery Council (NMC) (2004d). *Reporting Unfitness to Practise: A Guide for Employers and Managers*. London: Nursing and Midwifery Council.

Nursing and Midwifery Council (NMC) (2004e). *Reporting Lack of Competence: A Guide for Employers and Managers*. London: Nursing and Midwifery Council.

Nursing and Midwifery Council (NMC) (2005a). *Fitness to Practise Annual Report 2004–2005*. London: Nursing and Midwifery Council.

Nursing and Midwifery Council (NMC) (2005b). *Registering as a Nurse or Midwife in the United Kingdom: Information for Applicants from Outside the European Economic Area*. London: Nursing and Midwifery Council.

Nursing and Midwifery Council (NMC) (2006a).*The PREP Handbook*. London: Nursing and Midwifery Council.

Nursing and Midwifery Council (NMC) (2006b). *Preceptorship: A–Z Advice Sheet*. London: Nursing and Midwifery Council.

Nursing and Midwifery Council (NMC) (2006c). *Accountability: A–Z Advice Sheet*. London: Nursing and Midwifery Council.

Nursing and Midwifery Council (NMC) (2007a). *Standards for Medicines Management*. London: Nursing and Midwifery Council.

Nursing and Midwifery Council (NMC) (2007b). *Advice on Delegation for NMC Registrants: A–Z Advice Sheet*. London: Nursing and Midwifery Council.

Nursing and Midwifery Council (NMC) (2007c). *Fitness to Practise Annual Report: 1 April 2006 to 31 March 2007*. London: Nursing and Midwifery Council.

Nursing and Midwifery Council (NMC) (2008). *The Code: Standards of Conduct Performance and Ethics for Nurses and Midwives*. London: Nursing and Midwifery Council.

Preston RM (2005). Aseptic technique: evidence-based approach for patient safety. *British Journal of Nursing*, **14**, 540–46.

Productive Time Delivery Board and the NHS Benchmarking Club (2006). *Delivering Quality and Value: Focus on Benchmarking*. London: Productive Time Delivery Board and the NHS Benchmarking Club.

Pyne R (1998). *Professional Discipline in Nursing, Midwifery and Health Visiting*, 3rd edn. Oxford: Blackwell Science.

Randle J (2003). Bullying in the nursing profession. *Journal of Advanced Nursing*, **43**, 395–401.

Royal College of Nursing (RCN) (2005). *Good Practice in Infection Prevention and Control: Guidance for Nursing Staff*. London: Royal College of Nursing.

Schmidt LA (2003). Patients' perceptions of nursing care in the hospital setting. *Journal of Advanced Nursing*, **44**, 393–9.

Skills for Health (2004). HSC219 Support Individuals to Manage Continence. Health and Social Care suite of National Occupational Standards. www.skillsforhealth.org.uk/tools/view_ framework.php?id=39.

Taylor B (2000). *Reflective Practice: A Guide for Nurses and Midwives*. Buckingham: Open University Press.

Tschudin V (2006). How nursing ethics as a subject changes: an analysis of the first 11 years of publication of the journal *Nursing Ethics*. *Nursing Ethics*, **13**, 65–85.

Van de Peet R (1995). *The Nightingale Model of Nursing: An Analysis of Florence Nightingale's Concepts of Nursing, and their Impact on Present Day Practice*. Edinburgh: Campion Press.

Walsh M (2000). *Nursing Frontiers: Accountability and Boundaries of Care*. Oxford: Butterworth-Heinemann.

Welsh Assembly Government (2005). *Health Care Standards for Wales: Making the Connections Designed for Life*. Cardiff: Welsh Assembly Government.

Williamson C (2000). Consumer and professional standards: working towards consensus. *Quality Health Care*, **9**, 190–94.

Wilson T and Sheikh A (2002). Enhancing public safety in primary care. *British Medical Journal*, **324**, 584–7.

Further reading

Department of Health (2005). *'Now I Feel Tall': What a Patient-Led NHS Feels Like*. London: Department of Health.
An easy-to-read document telling the patient experience, with examples of how improvements have been made.

Driscoll J (2006). *Practising Clinical Supervision: A reflective Approach for Healthcare Professionals*, 2nd edn. London: Baillière Tindall.
A practical and easy-to-read guide about clinical supervision. Demystifies some of the theory surrounding reflection and supervision and explains how to get started.

Randle J (2003). Bullying in the nursing profession. *Journal of Advanced Nursing*, **43**, 395–401.
A disturbing but essential read of a study highlighting the detrimental effects of bullying on students and standards of care.

Benchmarking

NHS Benchmarking Network. Raising standards through sharing excellence. www.nhsbenchmarking.nhs.uk.
Provides information and toolkits for benchmarking in clinical areas, and gives examples of where benchmarking has been used successfully to improve patient outcomes.

Competence frameworks

Skills for Care. www.skillsforcare.org.uk.

Skills for Health. www.skillsforhealth.org.uk.

Provide information on competence development and career frameworks.

Patient safety

National Patient Safety Agency. Improving patient safety. www.npsa.nhs.uk/patientsafety/improvingpatientsafety.
Provides an introduction to patient safety, reporting and safety campaigns. There is also a learning tool (aimed at junior doctors and clinicians) called 'Safe foundations' comprising four modules covering the principles of human error, risk assessment, safer systems and when things go wrong.

Infection control

Epic. Evidence based practice in infection control. www.epic.tvu.ac.uk.
Provides research evidence-based guidelines and information in relation to infection control.

Health Protection Agency. www.hpa.org.uk.
Provides information about infectious disease and health care-associated infections.

NHS Core Learning Unit. Infection control training. www.infectioncontrol.nhs.uk.
An e-learning programme that covers the key aspects of infection control. Easy to register online and get started.

Health regulatory and governmental bodies

Department of Health, Social Services and Public Safety for Northern Ireland. www.dhsspsni.gov.uk.
Provides information about the Department's role and has links to health organisations and health councils representing patients' interests.

Healthcare Commission. www.healthcarecommission.org.uk.
Provides information about the Healthcare Commission's role as the health watchdog in England, and information about its role in Wales. You can download reports of investigations into failing organisations and find the performance ratings of health organisations.

Healthcare Inspectorate Wales. www.hiw.org.uk.
Access to the Inspectorate's standards and publications.

NHS Quality Improvement Scotland. www.nhshealthquality.org.
Provides information about performance monitoring and improvement in Scotland. There are useful links to other Scottish agencies, such as the Scottish Health Council.

Nursing and Midwifery Council. www.nmc-uk.org.
Provides information on all the work of the NMC, including downloads of its standards and guidance. There are useful case studies about fitness for practice and details of how the NMC administers professional self-regulation. The site also has useful links to other regulatory bodies.

Patient organisations

Action against Medical Accidents. www.avma.org.uk.
Provides information on the work of Action against Medical Accidents (AvMA), a charity that promotes better safety and justice for people affected by medical accidents.

Patients Association. www.patients-association.org.uk.
Lists publications that give a patient's perspectives on standards of care, and explains the Patients Association's role in raising patients' concerns.

WITNESS. www.popan.org.uk.
Information on WITNESS, which provides support to patients and campaigns for the prevention of abuse by health care professionals.

Employment matters

Ban Bullying at Work. www.banbullyingatwork.com.
Campaigns to stop bullying in the workplace and has specific guidance for people who are experiencing bullying.

NHS Employers. www.nhsemployers.org.

Provides advice for NHS employers. Has information about whistle-blowing and employment practice.

Public Concern at Work. www.pcaw.co.uk.

Supports individuals to raise concerns about standards and safety in their organisations. Describes some case studies highlighting the experience of whistle-blowing in real life.

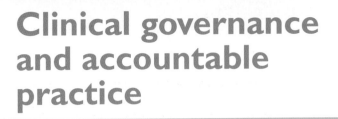

Clinical governance and accountable practice

Jacqueline McKenna

Introduction

Whatever setting nurses work in, they have a vital role in patient care and health promotion. Nurses are held accountable for their actions and omissions and should work within a clinical governance system that supports the development of their abilities. This chapter introduces clinical governance, discusses how it developed, and explains how its constituent parts support effective nursing practice. By using the different aspects of clinical governance, nurses can demonstrate accountability to themselves, their patients, peers and managers, and their professional body, in your case the Nursing and Midwifery Council (NMC). Clinical governance is a framework that allows health care workers to assure different people, and different groups of people, that care is delivered to a certain standard. It is a concept that brings true accountability into health care.

Putting it a different way, imagine you are a patient. Whether you are going to your general practitioner (GP) or into hospital for an operation, having something wrong with your health, particularly if you have not received a diagnosis, can be one of the most anxiety-provoking and vulnerable times of your life. This may be your first time in hospital or with your GP. You may not have met the nurses and doctors before, and you may not remember what they say or what you wanted to ask them. At times such as these, you need to be able to trust the staff and the systems within which they work. In other words, you need to know that there is strong clinical governance in the organisation. Although you would not necessarily know that it is called clinical governance, you would expect that the nurses:

- have been trained properly;
- have standards to work to;
- will keep you safe;
- will involve you in decisions about your care;
- will keep up to date through continued study once they are registered;
- will adhere to relevant national guidance.

The NMC Code (2008) (Appendix 1) sets out the standards of behaviour expected of nurses by their governing body and states clearly what a registered nurse is accountable for. As clinical governance reduces the risk to which the public is exposed in health care organisations, aspects of clinical governance feature in the NMC Code and are introduced in the relevant parts of this chapter.

Many books and articles have been written about clinical governance in the past decade. The Royal College of Nursing (RCN, 2003) has developed a clinical governance online resource. This has a foreword for each of the four countries in the UK, emphasising the importance of good clinical governance to twenty-first-century health care. This resource divides clinical governance into five main components in relation to nursing:

- *Placing patients' experience at the heart of health care*, and focusing on the environment of care.
- *Making information work for you*, focusing on data relating to the patient's experience.
- *Quality improvement in action*, focusing on risk management.
- *Supporting nurses in the workplace*, focusing on education and training.
- *Building blocks of clinical governance*, focusing on leadership and performance review.

This chapter describes the inception of clinical governance and its subsequent development to be a key aspect of service delivery in the NHS. It then discusses these five components of clinical governance in relation to you as an accountable practitioner. Being personally accountable for your practice means that you are answerable for both your actions and your omissions, and this is central to the NMC Code. Clinical governance and accountability are inextricably linked and therefore the two issues are discussed side by side throughout this chapter. The chapter also explains two complementary systems in which nurses may work that highlight nurses' accountability. These are: the Medway Nursing and Midwifery Accountability System (MNMAS) and shared governance. Where these systems are in place, they can demonstrate to the boards of organisations and the public they serve that decisions about patient care are made in an open way and that staff are held accountable for their clinical performance.

Learning objectives

After studying this chapter you should be able to:

- describe how a nurse can use clinical governance as a framework for accountable practice;
- explain what is meant by accountability;
- explain what accountability means to the public;
- describe different ways of being accountable to the public;
- explain how relevant parts of the NMC Code relate to accountability and clinical governance.

Development of clinical governance

Clinical governance was introduced into British health care by the Labour government in 1997. The development of clinical governance in England and Wales is described below; the other UK countries have made their own arrangements reflecting those in England.

Soon after coming to power in 1997, the Labour government published *The New NHS: Modern, Dependable* (DH, 1997). This White Paper set out the government's vision of the health service using a 10-year programme of reform based not only on finance and activity but also, for the first time, on quality of care. The White Paper was the first of many documents informing the health service and the public about the changes that were to happen in relation to delivering and monitoring the quality of care on a national basis.

A year later, *A First Class Service: Quality in the New NHS* (DH, 1998) was published as a consultation paper. The paper described the government's strategy for a modern health service; once again, it not only discussed the funding of health care but also introduced the concept of clinical governance and made clear that clinical governance would be a key aspect of performance for all health care organisations, not only hospitals. The consultation paper stated:

> . . . *clinical governance can be defined as a framework through which organisations are accountable for continuously improving the quality of their services and safeguarding high standards of care by creating an environment in which excellence in clinical care can flourish.*
>
> (DH, 1998)

This is now often used as the classic definition of clinical governance.

Following the consultation on *A First Class Service*, the government produced a health service circular, *Clinical Governance in the New NHS* (DH, 1999a). This gave detailed guidance on the action required to implement clinical governance, with time deadlines. In June of the same year,

The Health Act (DH, 1999b) was passed, which made quality a statutory duty for the first time and is a milestone in the history of clinical governance in the UK. The Act states:

> *It is the duty of each Health Authority, Primary Care Trust and NHS Trust to put and keep in place arrangements for the purpose of monitoring and improving the quality of health care which it provides to individuals.*
>
> (DH, 1999b)

As clinical governance was so important and also so new to the health service, a national organisation called the Clinical Governance Support Team was formed to support the implementation of clinical governance. The organisation continues to function and facilitate clinical governance development in health care organisations.

Clinical governance is about reducing the risk and improving the quality of care for patients. The result is improved patient safety, and this has been central to the further development of clinical governance. In 2000, *An Organisation with a Memory* (DH, 2000a) was published. The document described the scale of health care errors and found that reporting and learning from these errors was not developed enough across the country. It put forward the need to have unified systems for reporting and analysis of errors, and a more open culture, and stated that lessons learned should be put into practice. This was followed a year later with the document *Building a Safer NHS for Patients: Implementing an Organisation with a Memory* (DH, 2001a). This gave NHS organisations guidance on the actions that were expected of them and set patient safety at the centre of the government's clinical governance agenda.

The NHS Plan (DH, 2000c) was a culmination of many documents that set a 10-year plan for investment in the NHS. It was, however, made clear that with investment came reform. These reforms focused on patient care, choice and access. Clinical governance was central to this strategy, but it also emphasised the patient and public involvement aspect of clinical governance, introducing, among other things, the national patient survey (see later in this chapter).

The National Audit Office (NAO) is an organisation that audits the financial statements of all government departments and reports to Parliament on the value for money with which public bodies spend money. The NAO reported in 2003 on its review of clinical governance in *Achieving Improvements through Clinical Governance: A Progress Report on Implementation by NHS Trusts*. In summary the NAO found that:

- the safety culture within trusts is improving;
- all trusts have established effective reporting systems at a local level, although underreporting remains a problem;
- most trusts pointed to specific improvements derived from lessons learnt from their local incident reporting systems (NAO, 2003).

The report was broadly favourable and demonstrated the commitment of the NHS in grasping and implementing the concept of clinical governance.

The NHS Plan is a living document that continues to guide development of national services. To support it, the Department of Health has published reports summarising progress to date and also the next steps required to achieve the plan. One such report is *The NHS Improvement Plan* (DH, Health 2004b), which sets the priorities for the service up to 2008; clinical governance is, once again, central to the drive to improve the quality and safety of patient care. In the same year, *Standards for Better Health* (DH, 2004a) was published; this moved clinical governance one step further and integrated it into the wider governance agenda. *Standards for Better Health* proposed assessment of organisations across seven domains:

* safety;
* clinical and cost-effectiveness;
* governance;
* patient focus;
* accessible and responsive care;
* care environment and amenities;
* public health.

Standards for Better Health signalled the move away from a system where performance was measured by achievement of national access and finance targets to a system based on a new performance framework. The first measurement of health care organisations under the new performance framework took place in 2006, and *Standards for Better Health* was one aspect of this framework. For the first time, the performance of these organisations was measured not only in relation to finance and access targets but also based on patient feedback and aspects of clinical governance such as implementation of National Institute for Health and Clinical Excellence (NICE) guidance. This evaluation of performance is called the Annual Health Check (Healthcare Commission, 2005a).

Since its inception in 1997, clinical governance has become a key aspect of how health services are planned, delivered and measured. It is a statutory duty for health care organisations, and accountability is with the chief executive. As stated in *A First Class Service*, 'Effective clinical governance will make it clear that quality is everybody's business' (DH, 1998).

SUMMARY

* Clinical governance was first implemented in the UK by the 1997 government.
* Clinical governance made quality a statutory duty for all NHS organisations for the first time.
* NICE, the Commission for Health Improvement and the Clinical Governance Support Team were formed to give organisations guidance on best practice, to monitor the quality of care, and to help develop clinical governance.

Placing patients' experience at the heart of health care

Clinical governance is about making each patient's experience the best it can possibly be. This is now high on the government's agenda and has become part of the success criteria against which health care providers will be judged (DH 2008). Nurses should be totally focused on the needs of the patients and should use all the different components of clinical governance in order to improve patient care. To ensure consistency in different parts of an organisation or within different parts of the country, standards are used to guide nursing practice. Standards can be at the national or local level. The accountable nurse understands the standards and how they support their practice.

Standards

The organisation, standards and environment of care are key elements in ensuring an excellent patient experience. The person in the role of team leader, ward manager or department manager holds 24-hour responsibility for everything that happens in that environment. This does not mean that the manager should be available at the end of the phone 24 hours a day, but it does mean that they should set standards of care and behaviour that are achieved, regardless of whether they are on duty or not. At times, the nurse will find herself in the position of being responsible for the care of a group of patients or for managing a shift. At such instances, the nurse should work within the standards already set but also clearly articulate her expectations of her colleagues for that shift. It should be clear to each nurse what they are able to do competently at their level of training or at the level of their registered nurse post. A registered nurse can delegate the care of a number of patients to a student nurse, although the registered nurse remains accountable for the care, having given you adequate support.

On occasion, nurses may come under pressure from other members of the team or may want to undertake a procedure or action for which they do not have the required knowledge or skills. Proceeding in this way means practising outside of the NMC Code, which states: 'You must recognise and work within the limits of your competence'. It should be clear in the local standards what different levels of staff can do. However, if someone asks you to do something for which you are not trained, you should make it clear that you cannot do it and let your manager know that someone else who has those skills is needed. Acknowledging the limits of your competence is essential to safe and accountable practice and is not something to be afraid or ashamed of.

Organising care

Organising care is a skill and can make the difference between a good or poor patient experience, including whether risk is managed appropriately. For example, following the handover session at the beginning of a shift, the plan for the shift should be agreed between all staff. If there is no plan, then the shift will be disorganised and lack leadership, which will adversely affect standards and the patient experience. It should be remembered that a plan may be changed to incorporate the unexpected, but all staff should know what they are expected to achieve by the end of the shift. Staff breaks are important and should be part of the plan for the day. The shift leader should monitor how the staff are managing throughout the day and whether they require help. All care and changes in the patients' condition should be recorded throughout the shift and an accurate handover made to the next shift.

If you are working within a team and the shift leader has not made their expectations clear, then it is up to you to ask for clear guidance on what needs to be achieved throughout the shift and when you should plan your breaks. During the shift, you also have a responsibility to keep either your team leader or the person in charge of the shift up to date with changes in your patients' condition and changes to treatment or care due to a doctor's review or a registered nurse's evaluation or assessment. You must always record any assessment and evaluation you have done. This should be recorded in line with the NMC (2004) and the organisation's guidance on record-keeping, and should also be discussed with the patient. Good record-keeping is essential for accountable practice. As you may be recording things after an event, you should note both the time of the entry as you write and the time of the event; if you do not do this, then it will appear that the time of the entry is also when the event happened. To summarise, the NMC Code states that:

- *You must keep clear and accurate records of the discussions you have, the assessments you have made, the treatment and medicines you give and how effective they have been*
- *You must complete records as soon as possible after an event has occurred*
- *You must ensure any entries you make in someone's paper records are clearly and legibly signed, dated and times.*

Reflection point 8.1

Thinking about the last time you were at work, read the following statements and assign a rating out of 6 to each, using 1 for total disagreement and 6 for total agreement:

- I knew the patients I was responsible for.
- I knew exactly what had to be done, and I planned the shift well.
- I involved the patients in their care.
- I recorded everything that was relevant to the care of the patients.
- I had adequate breaks.
- I updated my manager on significant issues.
- I was updated on changes as the shift progressed.
- I left on time, having done everything that was expected of me.

What could have been done differently to make your patients' experience better?

Did the nurses you were working with make it clear which patients were under your care?

Did the nurses give you enough information about the care that the patients needed during that shift and, if you knew, this did you plan your time well, including when you had your breaks?

Did you explain to the patients what care was needed and negotiate with them when they wanted this to take place?

Did you record everything that you did and how the patient responded to this?

National standards

It is important to have local standards; however, in a national health service, treatment and care should be supported by national standards to aid professionals and patients with a consistent approach. Patients have the right not to be disadvantaged by where they live and should be offered the most effective procedures, treatment and care (Kennedy, 2001). To help ensure this, an accountable nurse will care for patients using as much evidence-based care as possible. There are a number of sources that will help you to do this. *The Royal Marsden Hospital Manual of Clinical Nursing Procedures* (Dougherty and Lister, 2008) is recognised as a national reference book for supporting nursing care in acute and primary care settings. There are also online reference points, such as the Cochrane Database of Systematic Reviews, a resource from the Cochrane Collaboration dedicated to making up-to-date, accurate information about the effects of health care available and the *Bandolier*, an independent journal about evidence-based health care. Both of these can be used to ensure that the care you are giving patients is based on evidence.

Integral to the government's reforms that introduced clinical governance in 1997 was the formation of the independent organisation National Institute for Health and Clinical Excellence (NICE). The purpose of NICE is to support evidence-based practice development and implementation (NICE, 2005). Health care organisations in England and Wales and, more recently, Northern Ireland (DHSSPS, 2006) implement NICE guidance, thereby ensuring that patient care is based on national guidance. In Scotland, NHS Quality Improvement Scotland (NHS QIS) has a similar remit for health care organisations.

NICE guidance is divided into the following five categories:

- *Clinical guidelines*: recommendations based on the best available evidence on the treatment and care of people by health care professionals.
- *Interventional procedures*: evaluation of the safety and efficacy of procedures used for diagnosis or treatment.
- *Technology appraisals*: recommendations on the use of new and existing medicines and treatments.

- *Public health interventions*: guidance on good health and prevention of ill health.
- *Public health programme guidance*: guidance on good health and prevention of ill health.

The majority of the guidance relates to medical treatment; however, the clinical guidelines that nurses should know about and use are listed in Box 8.1.

BOX 8.1 NICE clinical guidelines that nurses should be aware of

- Diabetes
- Falls
- Head injury
- Infection control
- Preoperative tests
- Pressure-relieving devices
- Pressure ulcer management
- Pressure ulcers

Reflection point 8.2

Access the NICE website (www.nice.org.uk) and look at a clinical guideline that relates to your current clinical placement.

1 Having read it, to what extent is the team adhering to this guidance?
2 If there is something that the team is not doing, is there a valid reason for it?
3 How does this clinical guideline benefit patient care?

NICE provides health care professionals with up-to-date guidance for their practice. There are organisations in each of the UK countries that monitor the quality of care against national standards:

- *England*: Healthcare Commission.
- *Wales*: Healthcare Inspectorate Wales.
- *Scotland*: NHS Quality Improvement Scotland.
- *Northern Ireland*: Regulation and Quality Improvement Authority.

These four organisations report on health care compliance with national standards. The public can access these reports to see how good hospitals and primary care trusts (PCTs) are in terms of clinical governance. With patient choice, this will be one source of information for patients to use to decide where they want to be treated.

Adhering to national and local standards is good clinical governance, and nurses should be aware of the policies and guidelines that are in use to support their professional practice. In some health care organisations, clinical nurses are involved in setting standards; an example of this is shared governance.

Shared governance

Although shared governance does not exist routinely in the UK, it is an excellent system for account-able practitioners to work within. In shared governance, the senior nurses work with clinical nurses to make the necessary decisions about different aspects of nursing practice, such as nurse education, standards, risk management and policies, therefore sharing the accountability for major decisions rather than it being vested solely in senior nurses' responsibility (Geoghegan and Farrington, 1995).

For some nurses, this is a difficult model to work within because it requires active participation. Often it is easier to work passively within a system where responsibility is passed from one level to another. In shared governance, this cannot happen as clinical nurses accept accountability by working in a shared framework with senior nurses. Once shared governance is implemented, however, most nurses thrive in the environment, motivated by seeing how their contribution influences practice in their organisation.

The shared governance model works by deciding what issues are important for nursing and patient care. Groups are developed to lead on these issues; for example, there may be three groups, one each looking at the aspects of education, risk management standards and policies. The members of these groups consist of nurses and midwives at all levels of the hierarchy from band 8 to band 2. There should also be members of the public and user groups, where appropriate, plus colleagues co-opted for expertise in different disciplines, such as dieticians and physiotherapists. It is best if the chair of the group is a nurse of band 7 or lower, so that senior nurses are not seen to be controlling the group. The group will have a work schedule and will be expected to deliver on the objectives within agreed timescales. As this is a different way of working, nurses in these groups should be given training to fulfil their role, such as being able to chair meetings if they have not done this before. All of these groups feed into a coordinating group, which has senior and clinical nurses as members (Figure 8.1).

There are many benefits to such a system, including clinical and managerial nurses working together on a common agenda, professional and personal development for clinical nurses, networking across different specialties, and having clinical input into policy decisions. This can result in more realistic planning and delivery of policy, and nurses working in an accountable framework to improve the patient and staff experience.

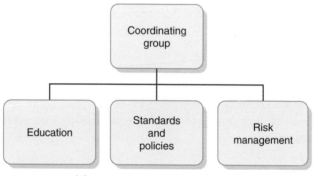

Figure 8.1 Shared governance model.

SUMMARY

- Standards of care should be set by the team leader and upheld by the staff.
- Standards of care help to ensure consistently good-quality nursing practice.
- Nurses must work within their level of competence.
- Good organisation of care improves the patient's experience.
- Care must be recorded in line with NMC guidelines for record-keeping.
- Health care organisations are monitored to assess the effectiveness of their clinical governance structures.
- Systems such as shared governance improve staff involvement and accountability.

Making information work for you

Health care organisations understand how well they are performing by using a wide range of metrics, including financial income and expenditure, theatre utilisation, bed occupancy and nurse staffing levels. The important and more challenging task is to transform these data into information that will help progress the business of the organisation, working towards an excellent patient experience. One way of obtaining information about the patient experience is by asking patients and the public. Compliments, suggestions and complaints should all be used to paint a picture of the public's experience of health care.

Patient feedback: complaints

All NHS organisations should have a formal complaints system reflecting national guidance (DH, 2006b). Complaints, no matter how trivial they may seem, should be treated seriously and with respect. Complaints offer the patient's or carer's perception of the health care experience at a point in time. Used in a positive way, complaints can be very helpful in improving patient care in one area and changing practice across an organisation.

Complaints take a lot of time to address properly, and an accountable practitioner will understand their role in making the patient experience as good as possible so that there is no need to make a complaint. Patients should be asked routinely if there is anything that would improve their stay in hospital or their care at home. If the nurse cannot meet the patient's or carer's requirements, then, rather than ignore their requests, the nurse should make the person in charge of the shift, or the line manager, aware of the patient's needs. Being accountable means acting within your remit and communicating to someone else if you are unable, for what ever reason, to carry out an action or procedure. In acute and community hospitals, the modern matron role, which is discussed later, has a clear remit in allaying patients' concerns, and therefore modern matrons should be a good resource to turn to in such a situation.

> **Reflection point 8.3**
> On your next shift, ask the patients you care for whether there is anything that could be done differently that would make their experience in the clinic, home or ward better. Feed this information back to your manager. It will be particularly interesting if a number of patients say the same thing.

Most patients enjoy talking to staff and will give information readily. It may be daunting asking the first patient, but it gets easier and most patients are likely to say that their experience has been good. If a patient says, for example, that the food is always cold because he is always served last, then the manager should be informed so that the routine can be changed.

It is important to note in relation to the activity of any health care organisation that only a very small number of people complain formally. If you are involved in a complaint, then it is likely that you will be asked to write a statement. Formal complaints are not common, but they deserve serious attention and as prompt a response as possible.

Patient feedback: surveys

At the ward and department level, examples of how patients and the public have developed the service, and how patients are involved in monitoring the standard of care in the ward or in the community, should be made known. Involvement may happen in different ways; questionnaires are a simple example. Acute trusts and PCTs in England have to participate in annual national patient surveys, the results of which are published nationally (Healthcare Commission, 2005c). There are many benefits to these surveys. Organisations receive a high-level summary of how patients feel about many aspects of their health care experience, including communication, dignity, cleanliness and treatment. Organisations are also able to benchmark their results against that of their peers across the country, giving clinicians and managers a measure of how they compare with their neighbours and competitors.

The national survey can give the organisation a steer on the issues that are important to patients, such as what is good about the patient experience and what needs to be improved. This is a good basis on which to develop local surveys. For example, if a nurse considers the issues where patients gave a lower score than the national average, then a local survey could be used to focus in more depth on these issues and to find out why patients think improvement is needed. Once the results are collated, a team of nurses can identify what is important to patients and then work out how to make the improvements. Some improvements will be simple and will not require funding, but others may require financial support, for which a convincing case will have to be made and negotiated with managers. When different initiatives have been put in place, improvements in the patient experience can be evaluated, either by obtaining continuous feedback or by undertaking another survey. The process and outcomes can be shared across the organisation and with other organisations to help improve the service to, and health care experience of, patients.

Medway Nursing and Midwifery Accountability System (MNMAS)

Traditionally it has been very difficult to measure a nurse's performance as a contribution to a patient's experience, and there is very little information in the literature about how to do so. Performance management in the health service has been implemented relatively recently and in many ways is a result of having to make the health service more cost-effective and to ensure achievement of government targets. There are many examples to support the view that, if you measure something, then it gets managed. For example, access targets set for the NHS since 2000 have resulted in reduced waiting times for treatment for patients (DH, 2003). Chief executives are held to account for their organisation's achievement against these and other targets, which is one way to measure and manage performance. Other public services, such as the police force, have managed their performance in this way since the 1990s and have proved in many ways that, if you measure performance, then it usually improves.

The MNMAS was inspired by the way Mayor Rudolf Giuliani led improved police performance in the 1990s and made New York a much safer city. A performance management tool called Compstat (Giuliani, 2003) was used, with the characteristics being:

- a set of agreed performance indicators;
- weekly data collection on each indicator;
- weekly meetings;
- staff held to account for their performance.

The MNMAS (Geoghegan, 2006) uses a similar tool to measure nurses' performance and makes them accountable for their performance. A set of performance indicators (Box 8.2) were agreed by senior nurses, matrons and ward managers. Nurses and midwives have a direct impact on all of these indicators and can therefore be held to account for them. For instance, in this system, the nurses are responsible for identifying the numbers of patients with methicillin-resistant

> **BOX 8.2 Medway Nursing and Midwifery Accountability System performance indicators**
>
> Number of patients with MRSA   a Admitted
>   b Acquired
>
> Number of patients with *Clostridium difficile*   a Admitted
>   b Acquired
>
> Bed days lost due to closure
>
> Hours lost due to short-term sickness <7 days
>
> Results of weekly documentation audit
>
> Nurses not wearing uniform properly
>
> Hours of agency staff used
>
> Hours of bank staff used
>
> Number of people with pressure sores   a Admitted
>   b Acquired
>
> Number of complaints about nurses and nursing care

Staphylococcus aureus (MRSA) and the number who were already MRSA-positive when admitted. Nurses cannot be held to account for those patients who were admitted with MRSA, but their practice will impact on whether patients acquire MRSA during their stay. If patients do acquire MRSA, then the nurses are required to explain why this might be so and what measures have been taken in order to minimise risk to the infected and other patients.

Critical to making this accountability system work is the weekly collection of data based on each of the modern matron's areas of responsibility. This may be all the wards in the medical directorate or just one department, such as the neonatal intensive care unit. Modern matrons' posts were created in response to the public wanting a visible accountable presence for standards of nursing care in hospitals (DH, 2001b). Their key remit is to be visible to the public, to allay patient concerns, to reduce infections, and to ensure a clean and tidy environment.

The weekly data collection is collated for discussion and agreed action at the weekly MNMAS meeting chaired by the director of nursing. All the modern matrons attend this meeting. The meeting focuses on two modern matrons' performance every week, and they share good practice and are held to account when their performance is not improving. As the director of nursing is at these meetings, patient care issues are ensured to be included on the trust board agenda and nursing performance is accounted for right up to board level. Increasingly, boards must pay as much attention to patient care matters as to financial matters. Taking their eye off patient care can lead to disastrous patient care situations, such as those revealed at Stoke Mandeville Hospital (Healthcare Commission, 2006) and the Maidstone and Tunbridge Wells NHS Trust (Healthcare Commission, 2007).

In MNMAS meetings, two matrons present their performance in relation to the key performance indicators over the previous 8 weeks. It is important to note that matrons are not compared with each other, because they have such different areas; however, there is a constant comparison of their previous performance and current performance. When the matrons are accounting for what has happened in their area over the past 2 months, they are praised when things have improved. They are invited to share why the improvement has happened and what interventions they have made, thus enabling other matrons to learn what has worked in other areas and whether this has the same positive effect in their own. If, however, performance has deteriorated, then the matron will be held to account and invited to explain what has happened and the actions they intend to put in place in order to improve the situation.

By measuring performance on a weekly basis, the nurses have an up-to-date picture of performance in their area. They cannot criticise the information by saying it is old and that practice has changed, which could be the case if quarterly data were used. At these meetings, the matrons should be accompanied by the band 7 nurses and staff nurses. Student nurses may also attend if they wish. This is a powerful way to hold practitioners to account; in the majority of cases, simply by measuring the performance and understanding accountability to the organisation and patients, performance will improve steadily. Although the MNMAS is based in the acute setting, it can be transferred easily to the primary care and mental health settings by agreeing the performance indicators that demonstrate how nursing adds value to the organisation in question and for what nurses can be held accountable.

Reflection point 8.4

Review the performance indicators in Box 8.2 used in MNMAS that are relevant to the area in which you are currently working. Write an account of how you have contributed to your team's performance for each of the indicators.

You may have thought of your practice in relation to the number of patients who have infections or pressure ulcers or in relation to the number of hours of sickness on the ward. Is there anything you could have done differently to improve the performance of your area?

SUMMARY

- A lot of data exist about the patient experience. These data need to be analysed in order to become useful information.
- Patients should be asked routinely how they believe their health care experience could be improved.
- Patient feedback offers a different and essential perspective on the standard of health care.
- Feedback can be gained through surveys, complaints and compliments.
- Information about the patient experience should be discussed at board level.
- Performance management systems such as MNMAS can improve patient care and inform the board about the patient experience.
- Nurses should be held to account for their performance.

Quality improvement in action

Health care professionals should always look for ways to improve the care of their patients. This chapter highlights a number of approaches, such as finding out what patients want from the service and working to agreed standards. Reducing risk is an essential approach to improving the quality of care. Once you reduce any risk to a patient, for instance by using correct pressure-relieving devices, then you immediately improve the quality of care.

Risk

Clinical governance is all about improving the quality of patient care and reducing risk to patients; therefore, managing risk is an important activity for an accountable nurse. The NMC Code states that 'you must act without delay if you believe that you, a colleague or anyone else may be putting someone at risk'. A risk is defined by the Health and Safety Executive (2006) as 'the likelihood that a hazard (anything with potential to cause harm) will cause a specified harm to someone or something'. We manage the risks in our life almost automatically. For example, if rain is forecast and there is a risk of getting wet, then you may carry an umbrella to minimise the risk. Similarly, if you are driving to a place that you have not been to before and you need to arrive on time, then you may plan the route on a map, use an Internet route planner or install a satellite navigation device in your car; all of these reduce the risk of you getting lost and being late – or, put another way, increase the likelihood of you taking the right route and arriving on time. Likewise, to improve the quality of care for patients, it is important that nurses manage the risk to patients. The NMC Code highlights that nurses must identify and minimise risks to patients.

Risks have to be managed for patients in hospital. Patients are unfamiliar with the environment and routine. Equally, they may not feel sufficiently in control to be able to manage the risks around them at home or in a clinic or hospital. Clear identification of the risks, and effective procedures or controls to minimise or eradicate them, are part of accountable practice.

Examples of risk include the following:

- *Clinical*: patients taking the wrong medicine, falling or developing pressure sores.
- *Environmental*: staff working with unsafe equipment; unsafe or trailing wiring; poor cleaning; obstacles such as furniture.
- *Financial*: not managing within the given budget due to having more patients than planned, using agency staff, or staff not being aware of the financial limits and thus wasting resources.
- *Human*: staff working outside of agreed policies and protocols or making poor decisions.
- *Equipment*: staff using equipment that they are not trained to use; equipment not being maintained correctly and therefore not working consistently.
- *Perception/reputation*: patients being unhappy with the care they receive and contacting the media – poses a risk to the reputation of your area of work and the organisation.
- *Information*: breach of confidentiality or not keeping accurate patient records – you should work within the Data Protection Act at all times.

Reflection point 8.5

Choose three of the categories above and think about your past week at work. Write down a risk or potential risk that you experienced that falls into each of the three categories. What was your participation in managing these risks? Did you identify, measure and manage any of these? Did you see other members of the team managing the risk, or was the risk left unmanaged?

This exercise should make you more aware of the risks that are inherent in health care. Take, for example, an equipment risk: you may have had to use a piece of equipment with which you are not familiar. This poses a potential risk to you and the patient. What actions would you take? Would you tell a nurse and ask them to do the task? Or would you ask them to teach you how to use the equipment so you would know in the future?

Managing risk

Risk can be managed in four ways:

- terminate;
- treat;
- transfer;
- tolerate.

For example, you have done an assessment on a newly admitted patient and you identify that they have a nutritional risk. It is difficult to *terminate* or *transfer* this risk. However, there are a number of ways in which the risk could be *treated*, such as referring the patient to a dietician, ordering nutritional supplements, using a food chart, and ensuring that the patient has adequate assistance with eating. It would be unacceptable practice to *tolerate* such a risk. Clearly, the best way to manage this risk to the patient is to *treat* it as described above, to document it on the care plan, and to evaluate it to see how successful the interventions were.

Taking another example, consider a patient's relative being abusive to a member of staff. The risk could be *terminated* by calling security and getting the relative removed from the organisation. *Treating* the risk would be taking the relative into a quiet place on the ward and explaining that their behaviour is threatening, that it is not acceptable and that, if they continue, security staff will be called. *Transferring* the risk is difficult, other than by moving the patient to another ward. Once again, it is not acceptable to *tolerate* the risk, as the relative may be a potential threat to the safety of patients and staff. However, a compromise may be reached whereby future visits are tolerated on the understanding that staff would take action if any abusive behaviour reoccurs. The choice in this instance has been to *treat* the risk.

Community nurses will face similar risks, but these can be more difficult to manage because in many instances these nurses work in smaller teams without easy access to support such as health and safety officers. An example of a risk specific to a community practitioner is the personal risk when visiting people alone. This risk can be *tolerated* by continuing to make lone visits but being aware of and prepared for the risk. The risk can be *transferred* so that a different member of staff visits the patient. Or the risk can be *terminated*, by moving to another post in which the nurse does not have to put themselves at risk. *Treating* this risk is the safest option for the nurse and the organisation. Most organisations now have lone worker policies to which nurses should adhere by ensuring that their work-base knows where they are planning to go and checks are made as to their safety at the end of the day.

The accountable practitioner must be aware that risks are everywhere and that, in order to ensure no harm comes to the patient, these must be identified and managed. This is good clinical governance.

Clinical risk

Assessment forms the critical foundation of good care for any patient for whom you are responsible. A patient should have a general assessment of their health status and the extent to which they are able to care for themselves. This assessment should be done in conjunction with the patient or their relatives and is usually accompanied by more detailed assessments of their nutritional state, tissue viability and risk of falling. There are numerous stand-alone assessments that allow the practitioner to carry out an initial general assessment and then a more detailed assessment of the risks that the patient faces. Examples include the Waterlow score (Waterlow, 1996) for pressure ulcers, the malnutrition universal screening tool (MUST) for nutrition status (Malnutrition Advisory Group, 2008) and the obesity assessment (DH, 2006a). All of these assessment tools give the practitioner a comprehensive picture of the patient, enabling them to identify what risks there are to patients and their care.

The clinical risk cycle is as follows: the assessment and the risks are recorded in the care plan as potential problems. The way to treat (reduce) or terminate the risks is recorded under the plan of care, the care is implemented, and the accountable practitioner evaluates the effect of the implemented care on the risks and therefore the patient. If the risk reduces or increases, then the care planned needs to change to reflect this, and so the cycle continues. Good care-planning is good clinical governance.

The assessment and plan of care are inextricably linked. If both are done effectively, then they will reduce the risk and improve the quality of care. Look at the assessment: have you assessed something, for example eating, where the patient is not self-caring? Is there a link to the care plan that reflects this need? Are appropriate actions planned in the care plan, for example referring the patient to a dietician?

Non-clinical risk

All other risks, such as financial and environmental risks, should also be identified, usually by the ward manager or the team leader who has responsibility for managing risk across their whole area. This is important, as knowledge and management of the risks will have an effect on how well the team can do their work. Identified risks should feed into an organisational risk register so that the senior management team knows what risks exist, how they are being managed, and whether corporate resources need to be used in order to reduce or terminate them to make the organisation safer. If you identify risks that you are unable to manage, then you must report these to someone more senior who can influence how the risks are addressed. It is recognised that you will not be able to manage every risk and that you are part of a team, where other members will be able to act on the information that you give them.

Recording risk

As part of the importance of maintaining clear, accurate records of patient care, recording of risk to the patient in any of the examples described above, such as clinical or environmental, is essential. Doing so demonstrates that risks have been identified and measured and actions put in place to manage them. As mentioned previously, clinical risk that has the potential to slow patient recovery should be recorded on the care plan. If, however, the risk is in one of the other categories, then it should still be recorded on a risk register, which then feeds into an assurance framework for the ward, department or community team.

Documentation of a risk and how it was managed is necessary so that if it did cause harm to the patient and you were called to account for your actions, then your records could show what and why you did what you did. Remember that if it is not written down, then it is very difficult to remember the rationale for your actions and even more difficult to prove that you actually took the appropriate actions. Without a written record, it could be construed that you tolerated the risk and took no action to minimise it. Good record-keeping helps demonstrate good clinical governance.

Risk register and assurance framework

Clinical risks to patients are identified by assessment and recorded and managed through their care plans. All other risks are identified by assessment but are recorded on risk registers and managed using assurance frameworks. Each ward, department or community team should have a risk register; this is the initial way to identify and record the risks, which then feed into a departmental assurance framework. Examples of a risk register and an assurance framework are given in Tables 8.1 and 8.2.

Table 8.1 Risk register

Risk	Likelihood	Consequence	Total risk score
Staff sickness	4	5	20

Table 8.2 Assurance framework

Objective	Risk	Measure	Internal control	External control
To use no bank or agency staff	Sickness	20	Monthly establishments	Acute hospital portfolio ward staffing report
	Maternity leave	16	Human resource statistics	
	Staff leaving	10	Appraisals	

All departments and the staff within them should work to objectives. In the example in Tables 8.1 and 8.2, the objective for the nursing team is to not use any bank or agency staff. The risks are then measured by calculating the likelihood out of 5 and the consequence out of 5, with 1 being the least and 5 being the most likely (NPSA, 2002). The likelihood measures the probability of the risk happening and the consequence measures the effect the risk would have if it happened. These two scores are then multiplied to calculate the total risk out of 25. The risk register states the risk and the risk score as seen in Table 8.1. In this example, the likelihood of a member of staff being sick is 4 and the consequence of staff sickness is 5, as the nursing team would need bank or agency staff to ensure staffing numbers. You can see that, in this instance, 4×5 gives a score of 20, which is a high risk.

The risk register (Table 8.1) feeds into the assurance framework, which is like the care plan in that it shows how the risk is to be managed. The assurance framework (Table 8.2) relates to the original objective and then adds two elements – the internal and external controls. The control part of the assurance framework is what the nurses will use to show that they are not using bank or agency nurses. Internal control is evidence from within the organisation – for example, budget statements – and external control is evidence from outside – for example, national reports. Controls are important so that everyone can see that, having identified and measured risks, there are actions or other measures that demonstrate how well the risk is being managed.

In this case, the internal control comes from the team manager's staffing figures, appraisals and the organisation's human resource statistics. The external control comes from the national acute hospital portfolio (Healthcare Commission, 2005b), which is a collection of acute care reviews measuring NHS trusts' performance and regularly examining and benchmarking nurse staffing levels.

Reflection point 8.7

Look at the risks you identified in Exercise 8.3. Now measure the risks using the 5×5 matrix. What is the likelihood (out of 5) of the risk occurring in the future? What would be the consequence (out of 5) of the risk happening in the future? Multiply these scores. What is the highest risk you experienced last week?

If the previous example of using a piece of equipment for the first time is used, then the risk is calculated like this: the likelihood of having to use a new piece of equipment is high (4), and the consequence of not knowing how to use the piece of equipment correctly is also high (4). Multiplying these figures shows that the risk is 16. Now think of your examples of risk: multiply the likelihood and consequence to find how large a risk they are.

The risks that were identified in the ward/department/team risk register then feed into a directorate risk register. The highest risks here will then transfer to the organisation's risk register. The top risks to the organisation can then be identified from the whole organisation risk register, which should be reviewed at board level so that the directors understand the risks to the organisation and the actions being taken to improve the quality of care and reduce the risk to the business of the organisation. Nurses have a role to play in ensuring that serious risks are identified and escalated via established systems to board level. This is good clinical governance.

Consider Scenario 8.1.

SCENARIO 8.1

You have identified that a nursing colleague is not competent in a certain skill. You have discussed this with her, but she does not agree with you. Using your organisation's risk management policy, work through what you should do to ensure that the risk your colleague poses is identified and managed.

Ask the nurse in charge or your mentor where you can find a copy of the organisation's risk management policy. Then read it. What options does it give you to manage the scenario above? Does it encourage you to tell your manager, to report it formally or to talk to your colleague?

Reporting when things go wrong

The risk management scenarios discussed above show how clinical and non-clinical risk can be managed proactively. However, despite everyone's best efforts, there are always going to be times when a risk goes unmanaged and results in a near-miss or actual harm to a patient, employee or visitor. At these times, it is essential that accountable practitioners manage the situation in an open and honest way. All organisations should have policies that support such situations. When a near-miss or actual harm happens, the first thing that should be done is to ensure that the person is examined and, if appropriate, receives the treatment they require. Following this, the line manager should be involved, and an incident report form should be completed clearly and fully and sent to the relevant manager.

If the incident is serious, then a full investigation should take place. If you were involved in any way, you should write a clear statement of your actions before, during and after the incident. This statement should state your name, your role, and the date and time of the statement. You should include what you did, why and how you did it, where you were at the time, and who you were interacting with. It helps to write a statement as soon after the incident as possible so that the facts are clear and you remember as much as you can. Remember that the NMC Code states that 'you must cooperate with internal and external investigations'. In most instances, this information will be used to see how the risk of such an incident can be minimised in the future, although in some cases employer or professional (NMC) disciplinary action may be taken.

In-depth investigation may not be necessary for the majority of reported incidents. Nevertheless, it is still important to collect the information, as it can be used to identify trends across the organisation or in individual clinical areas. Once again, when trends are found, actions can be taken either to reduce the likelihood of incidents recurring or to add them as an identified risk on the team, directorate or organisational risk register. Hiding incidents is not helpful to patients, staff or the organisation. If incidents are not reported, then measures cannot be taken to manage the risk, to make the care safer for patients to create a better patient experience. The consequence of not reporting incidents is, in many cases, worse than reporting them, whatever the anxiety you may feel about doing so. An accountable practitioner knows that reporting such situations will result in care being improved through safer practices – and that is good clinical governance.

> ## SUMMARY
>
> - Risks are everywhere, at work and in our home life.
> - There are a number of different categories of risk.
> - Risks can be managed in four ways: treated, tolerated, transferred or terminated.
> - Clinical risks to patients are identified by assessment and managed and evaluated via care plans.
> - Risk can be measured by multiplying the likelihood and the consequence of the risk happening.
> - Once identified and measured on a risk register, risks are managed and monitored via an assurance framework.
> - Accurate recording is critical to risk management and improved patient care.
> - Managing risk is part of the NMC Code.

Supporting nurses in the workplace

An organisation's staff is its main and most important resource. It costs an organisation a lot in terms not only of money but also of time to recruit new people. Therefore, most organisations have in place strategies to support and retain their nursing staff. *The Improving Working Lives Standard* (DH, 2000b) encourages employers to develop flexible working practices, to offer access to childcare and generally to improve the working environment. In relation to clinical governance, the organisation has a responsibility to support nurses so they are equipped with up-to-date knowledge and skills to care for patients competently; it is this aspect that we discuss here.

Gaining feedback on your practice

Once registered, a nurse or midwife has a duty to maintain their knowledge and skills, which means being a lifelong learner. Becoming registered is the start, not the end, of learning and development. This is set out clearly in the NMC Code: 'you must keep your knowledge and skills up to date throughout your working life'.

As a student, you should take part regularly in learning activities that develop your competence and performance. Ensuring that your skills and knowledge are appropriate for your job must be a priority and provides a foundation for being an accountable practitioner. Feedback is one of the most productive ways of finding out what your performance is like. Feedback can be obtained in many ways, for example informally during your working day from patients and others, formally at appraisal, and by auditing your practice through self-assessment.

Informal feedback can be given by anyone you come into contact with. It is useful to ask rather than wait for feedback. Most people will be pleased to help you; they may give you both positive feedback and constructive thoughts about areas you may need to develop further. As a student, you will gain feedback throughout your course, especially during clinical assessments and assignments.

Feedback from patients is important, as they are the recipients of your care. Their view offers an alternative perspective to your performance. Patients can give feedback on a personal basis;

alternatively, if the *Essence of Care Standards* (DH, 2001c) are being used, patients can offer feedback more generally about the care on a ward or department or at home. However, it should be remembered that patients tend to give a more positive view when asked for feedback, as they are dependent on nurses while being cared for.

Appraisal

Once registered, it is expected that you will participate in a formal appraisal system when you are working for any health care organisation. If not, you should ask that you have appraisals at least every 6 months. Formal appraisals give you and your manager a good opportunity to reflect on your performance and to agree objectives for the future. In preparing for an appraisal, think about what aspects of your work are going well and what aspects you have found more difficult and need to improve. The appraisal should be a positive experience where your own and your manager's perceptions of your performance can be discussed constructively. If your manager has a concern over some aspect of your practice, they should discuss this with you at the time and not store it up for your appraisal. There should be no surprises at this important feedback session. It is advisable to think about your objectives before the meeting, as this will demonstrate that you have reflected on your practice and will guide your manager towards agreed objectives. These can be personal objectives or, as you may well work in a team, team objectives.

Reflection point 8.8
Take some time to prepare for your next meeting to discuss your progress in your current clinical placement. Use the points raised above so that the discussion is positive and useful.
  Think about what you have been involved in and experienced during this placement. What three things have gone well? Do you feel part of the team? What have you learnt? What has not gone so well? Is anything worrying you?

Knowledge and skills framework

Another component of the appraisal is based on the *Knowledge and Skills Framework* (KSF) (DH, 2004c). The KSF states the level of knowledge and skills required to perform different roles. The knowledge and skill is described at a number of levels to reflect the desired level of competence for each role. The KSF forms part of the appraisal process and helps to ensure that staff have identified appropriate development and are supported to perform their jobs effectively. A framework exists for the whole of the NHS, and every post except those for doctors, dentists and directors has an associated KSF. Using the KSF as a registered nurse will offer you some very specific feedback regarding your clinical performance in relation to what is the expected standard for your particular post. It also gives you a benchmark as to whether you are ready for promotion. You must be aware of the level of each knowledge and skill that relates to your post. If you are worried that you will not be able to meet a certain standard, then you should discuss this with your manager and ask for development in this area. A way in which you can obtain the standard will be agreed and form part of your personal development plan (PDP). This is a dynamic document and is an aspect of lifelong learning. You must keep your annual PDPs as they demonstrate how you have developed over the years.

Audit

Auditing the care you give is an excellent way to gain feedback on how well you are doing. This can be done on a personal level or as a team. The process involves comparing what you actually do with the required standard of how it should be done. The standard that is to be audited should be clear and understandable. The actual care given is then observed and compared with the criteria in the standard. By comparing the actual practice with the standard, nurses can measure and articulate the quality of care. If the actual care falls short of the standard, then you will know that you need to learn more or practise this aspect of care and then re-audit your practice. Clearly, practice changes from time to time and therefore standards and audit criteria need to change to reflect this.

Take, for example, giving a subcutaneous insulin injection. There should be a standard for this procedure, as shown in Table 8.3.

Table 8.3 Standards for administration of subcutaneous insulin injection

Action	First audit (yes or no)	Re-audit (yes or no)
Explain and discuss the procedure with the patient (to ensure that the patient understands the procedure and gives consent to receive the injection from the nurse)		
Wash your hands (to minimise risk of infection)		
Consult the patient's prescription sheet in relation to the following points: drug, dose, date and time of administration, route and method of administration, validity of the prescription, signature of prescriber; prepare injection		
Assist the patient into the required position to expose site for injection		
Choose the site – arm, abdomen, thigh or buttock; ensure rotation of site is carried out for each injection (for rotation, move approximately one finger's breadth from last injection point and alternate between right and left side of any site)		
Ensure correct needle length is chosen (in general 8 mm, or 5 mm for underweight people) (to minimise the risk of missing the subcutaneous tissue)		
Insert 8-mm needle into lifted skin fold at 90-degree angle (5-mm needle needs no skin fold technique) (to raise subcutaneous tissue away from underlying muscle and further maximise subcutaneous tissue injection); inject insulin		
Withdraw needle and drop skin fold; ensure skin site left clean and undamaged		
Dispose of sharps safely in accordance with organisation's policy		
Wash your hands (to reduce risk of cross-infection)		

Reproduced with permission from the Medway NHS Foundation Trust, based on The Royal Marsden Hospital Manual of Clinical Nursing Procedures, 6th edition, Dougherty and Lister, 2006, p. 208–9. Reproduced with permission from Wiley-Blackwell Publishing.

Reflection point 8.9
You are going to audit your insulin subcutaneous injection procedure. To audit your care, you should compare how you gave your last subcutaneous injection with the audit criteria on the standard of how to give an injection shown in Table 8.3. Write 'yes' or 'no' next to each point of the standard, depending on whether you met the criteria or not.

By doing this, you will be able to see the extent to which your care met the standard. You will also find out the aspects of the standard with which you did not comply, enabling you to alter your practice to meet the standard. After a time, you should re-audit your injection administration technique to see whether it has improved. Even when the work of a team is being audited, you can identify your contribution and how your own improvement can help the team's results to improve.

Training and development

Feedback is essential in order for an accountable practitioner to gain a picture of how they are developing and where their strengths and weaknesses lie. Formal feedback is the foundation of a nurse's professional development plan, a dynamic document that changes as the nurse's knowledge, skills or post change. Once a development need has been identified, it should be highlighted on the professional development plan, including the way in which it is going to be met and the timescale. Post-registration education and practice (PREP) is the NMC's framework for lifelong learning (NMC, 2006). Registered nurses have to renew their registration with the NMC every 3 years, although from 2006 registered nurses are required to pay for the 3-year registration on an annual basis. In order to renew registration, a nurse has to undertake at least 35 hours of learning activity relevant to their practice during the 3 years before renewing registration, has to maintain a professional profile and has to comply with any request from the NMC to audit how they have met the requirements. The following gives some ideas of how you can meet the requirement for 35 hours of study and support your development.

A post-registration course is sometimes seen as the most ideal way to meet a development need, but it is by no means the only way; the most appropriate way depends on your development need. However, to gain promotion later in your career, and to specialise, a post-registration course may be a prerequisite. There is a whole range of post-registration courses to choose from; to help you make an informed choice, seek advice within your organisation or from your local higher education provider.

Other ways to develop skills and knowledge include visiting a different department of your organisation or visiting another organisation. This can be organised quite easily and can be highly motivating for both the visitor and those hosting the visit.

If you are thinking about moving to another type of post or seeking promotion, your development need may be to know more about the new post. A shadowing visit could be arranged for a few days with someone already undertaking the role. Again, this is easy to arrange and gives you a clearer view of what is entailed in the different post and what skills, knowledge and experience you need to be successful in the post.

An important way to keep up to date is to read the professional journals and the national and local press – something you will have done for assignments as a student. There are a number of national nursing journals that give current news stories and offer clinical and research articles. If you decide to specialise, then there are specialist nursing journals that will enable you to keep up to date with new initiatives within your chosen field. The national press often prints news stories about the health service due to its profile on the political agenda, and some newspapers have a heath supplement on a certain day of the week. The local press will carry news stories that involve your organisation and neighbouring organisations.

SUMMARY

- Nurses should ask for, listen to and act on feedback from their manager, peers and patients.
- Every nurse should have a professional development plan to reflect their learning needs and KSF.
- Nurses should be lifelong learners and use their development plan and profile to guide this.
- PREP is a requirement for continuing registration and your licence to practise.

Building blocks of clinical governance

Health care organisations' boards, and chief executives in particular, have a statutory duty for the quality of care in their organisation (DH, 1997). An effective system of clinical governance and clear lines of accountability will be in place only when the leaders at board level and throughout the organisation commit to:

- placing the patients' experience at the centre of the business;
- using information intelligently;
- promoting continuous quality improvement;
- supporting their staff.

By having effective leadership, information about the patient's experience and practitioner's performance will inform the board about what is being achieved and what needs to improve. Acting on this will lead to a better patient experience.

Patient involvement

Standards can no longer be set and monitored by professionals alone. Patient and public involvement in setting and monitoring standards of care is integral to good clinical governance and accountable practice. There should be a system in place to encourage public and patient involvement at all levels of the organisation, from the boardroom to the bedside. This is a central part of the government's health care reforms in England. Indeed, all four UK countries have documented patient and public involvement policies in health care. All English NHS trusts are encouraged to become foundation trusts, which have built in to their constitution greater accountability to the community that they serve.

A good way to involve the patients and public is to invite them to participate in meetings to discuss issues, for example developing staff handover at the patient's bedside. Understanding this from the patient's perspective is necessary, as patients are the main beneficiaries of such an approach and it would be wrong to proceed without their input.

In terms of clinical governance, patients and the public should be members of any group that is making decisions about patient care and services. Openness and transparency about how an organisation or profession governs clinical standards and patient care are the required norm – decisions cannot be made behind closed doors.

Getting members of the public to join groups can be relatively easy. Hospitals and GPs' practices in many places are a vital part of the community, and a proportion of the public will want to be involved in helping them to be as good as they can possibly be. The public can be invited by advertisements in the local press, GPs' practices and health centres. Patients and their relatives can be asked whether they would like to become involved when they are inpatients. Another source is patient members of local support and voluntary groups. Any developmental initiative should try to reach and invite members of the public who reflect the whole community. Where this might be difficult, the organisation should meet the community's leaders in order to overcome actual or perceived barriers to working together for the development of services that will benefit them.

Having said that, it can be quite daunting for members of the public to be in the same meetings as professional health care workers, and it is always a good idea to have relevant induction meetings for the public. They need to know how the organisation works, what is expected of them, what they can expect in return, information about the project or group, and the desired outcomes of the group. The group leader should ensure that patient and public members are made to feel welcome and are kept well informed and that their contributions are valued and respected. Working with the public in this way is extremely helpful, as the public brings a different perspective to the issues under discussion. However, it can also be challenging for both parties and complicated by the different levels of knowledge and expectations as to what can be achieved. Diplomatic compromises may have to be made in order to achieve an agreed outcome. Being able to demonstrate these processes to the public and regulators, such as the Healthcare Commission, is all part of good clinical governance.

Consider Scenario 8.2.

SCENARIO 8.2

Mary is a 62-year-old retired teacher. She is due to join a group at her local GP practice to help the practice improve communication with its patients. What information would Mary need about the practice and its community to help her contribute to the group?

It is both exciting and challenging for members of the public to join groups in any health care organisation. It helps the members if they have some background information. You may think about the objectives of the practice and how it currently communicates with patients, but are there other things that would help?

SUMMARY

- Patient and public involvement is a key policy for all four UK governments' health administrations and NHS boards.
- Members of the public should be proactively involved in committees and groups that make decisions on issues that affect patient care.

CONCLUSION

Since its inception in 1997, clinical governance has become a major driver in health care provision. It influences not only the way health care is planned and commissioned but also every health care professional's approach to patient care. The RCN states that there are five components to clinical governance:

- placing patients' experience at the heart of health care;
- making information work for you;
- quality improvement in action;
- supporting nurses in the workplace;
- building blocks of clinical governance.

Each one of these is a fundamental part of the nurse's role. By being conscious of all the components of clinical governance and using it as a framework for practice, the nurse can demonstrate accountability.

Placing the patient's experience at the heart of health care and as the key focus for nursing is both an organisational and a professional responsibility. The purpose is to ensure every aspect of a patient's experience is as good as possible and is the reason why evidence-based guidelines and nationally and locally set standards are developed, used and monitored. Organisations that have a shared governance ethos will develop a culture where nurse managers work alongside clinical

CONCLUSION (continued)

nurses to develop, implement and monitor standards for all aspects of patient care that have the patient's experience at its heart.

There is a vast amount of data regarding the patient's experience and the nurse's contribution to this. However, to be useful, the data need to be transformed into information and then analysed. This will help nursing teams learn how their culture, behaviour or practice should be changed in order to improve patient care. Using the information intelligently demonstrates accountability; ignoring it is a managerial and professional omission. The MNMAS is an innovative nursing performance management tool that translates data into information. The information is used on a weekly basis, and the matrons are held to account for poor performance and asked to share their interventions that result in improved performance.

Clinical governance is about improving the quality and reducing the risk to the patient. Risk management is not a paper exercise. To improve the quality of patient care, nurses have to assess the risk posed to patients and decide the best course of action to minimise the risk to patients.

To be accountable practitioners, nurses need to be lifelong learners. This is necessary not only for the nurse to renew registration, which is essential to practise, but also for the nurse to be competent and have up-to-date knowledge and skills. Patients deserve and should expect nurses who practise using current guidance and techniques.

An essential aspect of clinical governance is patient involvement. Involving patients not only in their care but also in developing and monitoring services offers nurses benefits and challenges. Working in collaboration with patients allows nurses to be truly accountable to the people they serve and should be encouraged at all times.

References

Department of Health (DH) (1997). *The New NHS: Modern, Dependable*. London: Department of Health.

Department of Health (DH) (1998). *A First Class Service: Quality in the New NHS*. London: Department of Health.

Department of Health (DH) (1999a). *Clinical Governance in the New NHS*. London: Department of Health.

Department of Health (DH) (1999b). *The Health Act 1999*. London: The Stationery Office.

Department of Health (DH) (2000a). *An Organisation with a Memory*. London: Department of Health.

Department of Health (DH) (2000b). *Improving Working Lives Standard*. London: Department of Health.

Department of Health (DH) (2000c). *The NHS Plan*. London: Department of Health.

Department of Health (DH) (2001a). *Building a Safer NHS for Patients: Implementing an Organisation with a Memory*. London: Department of Health.

Department of Health (DH) (2001b). *Implementing the NHS Plan: Modern Matrons – Strengthening the Role of Ward Sisters and Introducing Senior Sisters*. London: Department of Health.

Department of Health (DH) (2001c). *The Essence of Care: Patient-Focused Benchmarking for Health Care Practitioners*. London: Department of Health.

Department of Health (DH) (2003). *The NHS Plan: A Progress Report*. London: Department of Health.

Department of Health (DH) (2004a). *Standards for Better Health*. London: Department of Health.

Department of Health (DH) (2004b). *The NHS Improvement Plan*. London: Department of Health.

Department of Health (DH) (2004c). *The NHS Knowledge and Skills Framework (NHS KSF) and the Development Review Process*. London: Department of Health.

Department of Health (DH) (2006a). *Raising the Issue of Weight*. London: Department of Health.

Department of Health (DH) (2006b). *The National Health Service (Complaints) Amendment Regulations*. Statutory Instrument no 2084. London: The Stationery Office.

Department of Health (DH) (2008). *High Quality Care for All: NHS Next Stage Review Final Report*. London: Department of Health.

Department of Health, Social Services and Public Safety (DHSSPS) (2006). *Implementation of National Institute for Health and Clinical Excellence Guidance in the HPSS*. Belfast: Department of Health, Social Services and Public Safety.

Dougherty L and Lister S (eds) (2008). *The Royal Marsden Hospital Manual of Clinical Nursing Procedures*, 6th edition. Oxford: Blackwell.

Geoghegan J (2006). Managing modern matrons. *Nursing Management*, **13**, 26–9.

Geoghegan J and Farrington A (1995). Shared governance: developing a British model. *British Journal of Nursing*, **4**, 780–83.

Giuliani R (2003). *Leadership*. New York: Time Warner.

Health and Safety Executive (2006). Five steps to risk assessment. www.hse.gov.uk/risk/fivesteps.htm.

Healthcare Commission (2005a). *Assessment for Improvement: The Annual Health Check*. London: Healthcare Commission.

Healthcare Commission (2005b). *Acute Hospital Portfolio: Reviews of Findings*. London: Healthcare Commission.

Healthcare Commission (2005c). *Variations in the Experiences of Patients in England*. London: Healthcare Commission.

Healthcare Commission (2006). *Investigation into Outbreaks of* Clostridium difficile *at Stoke Mandeville Hospital, Buckinghamshire Hospitals NHS Trust*. London: Healthcare Commission.

Healthcare Commission (2007). *Report of the Healthcare Commission's Visit to the Maidstone and Tunbridge Wells NHS Trust*. London: Healthcare Commission.

Kennedy I (2001). *The Report of the Public Inquiry into Children's Heart Surgery at the Bristol Royal Infirmary 1984–1995: Learning from Bristol*. London: The Stationery Office.

Malnutrition Advisory Group (2008). Malnutrition Universal Screening Tool. Redditch: British Association for Parenteral and Enteral Nutrition.

National Audit Office (2003). *Achieving Improvements through Clinical Governance: A Progress Report on Implementation by NHS Trusts*. London: National Audit Office.

National Institute for Health and Clinical Excellence (NICE) (2005). *A Guide to NICE*. London: National Institute for Health and Clinical Excellence.

National Patient Safety Agency (NPSA) (2002). *A Risk Assessment Tool for Assessing the Level of Incident Investigation Required*. London: National Patient Safety Agency.

Nursing and Midwifery Council (NMC) (2004). *Guidelines for Records and Record Keeping*. London: Nursing and Midwifery Council.

Nursing and Midwifery Council (NMC) (2006). *The PREP Handbook*. London: Nursing and Midwifery Council.

Nursing and Midwifery Council (NMC) (2008). *The Code: Standards of Conduct, Performance and Ethics for Nurses and Midwives*. London: Nursing and Midwifery Council.

Royal College of Nursing (RCN) (2003). *Clinical Governance: An RCN Resource Guide*. London: Royal College of Nursing.

Waterlow J (1996). *Pressure Sore Prevention Manual*. Taunton: Waterlow.

Further reading

Bandolier. www.ebandolier.com.

Cochrane Collaboration. www.cochrane.org.

Department of Health (2002). *Supporting the Implementation of Patient Advice and Liaison Services (PALS): A Resource Pack*. London: Department of Health.

Department of Health (2003). *Building an Assurance Framework: A Practical Guide for NHS Boards*. London: Department of Health.

Department of Health (2003). *Strengthening Accountability: Involving Patients and the Public*. London: Department of Health.

Department of Health (2004). *A Matron's Charter: An Action Plan for Cleaner Hospitals*. London: Department of Health.

Department of Health (2004). *How to Make a Complaint about the NHS*. London: Department of Health.

Department of Health (2005). *A Short Guide to NHS Foundation Trusts*. London: Department of Health.

Department of Health (2006). *The Regulation of Non-Medical Healthcare Professions*. London: Department of Health.

Department of Health, Social Services and Public Safety of Northern Ireland (2003). *Local Health and Social Care Groups: Community and Service User Involvement*. Belfast: Department of Health, Social Services and Public Safety of Northern Ireland.

Harrison S, Milewa T and Dowswell G (2002). Public and user 'involvement' in the National Health Service. *Health and Social Care in the Community*, **10**, 63–6.

Healthcare Commission. www.healthcarecommission.org.uk.

Healthcare Inspectorate Wales. www.hiw.org.uk.

National Assembly for Wales (2001). *Sign Posts: A Practical Guide to Public and Patient Involvement in Wales*. Cardiff: National Assembly for Wales.

National Institute for Health and Clinical Excellence. www.nice.org.uk.

National Patient Safety Agency. www.npsa.nhs.uk.

NHS Quality Improvement Scotland. www.nhshealthquality.org.

Nursing and Midwifery Council. www.nmc-uk.org.

Nursing and Midwifery Council (2006). *The Preceptorship Handbook*. London: Nursing and Midwifery Council.

Regulation and Quality Improvement Authority. www.rqia.org.uk.

Royal College of Nursing. www.rcn.org.uk.

Scottish Executive (2003). *Sustainable Patient Focus and Patient Involvement*. Edinburgh: Scottish Executive.

Waterlow J. Pressure ulcer risk assessment and prevention: understanding the causes. www.judy-waterlow.co.uk.

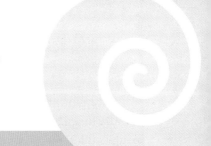

9

Ethical dimensions of practice

Paul Gibbons

Introduction

The purpose of this chapter is to introduce the ethical dimension of professional nursing practice and to consider what this means for both patients and nurses. A working definition of ethics is established and three major ethical theories discussed briefly. From this theoretical basis, principles that can guide the practitioner in identifying and addressing difficult situations are outlined and then applied to a range of everyday situations around aspects of day-to-day care, the beginning and end of life, and the implications for the population of research, resource allocation and health promotion.

The chapter aims to promote understanding of the competencies for ethical and professional practice specified by the Nursing and Midwifery Council (NMC) for those completing pre-registration nursing programmes. What follows should also assist in interpreting the NMC Code (2008) (Appendix 1).

Learning objectives

After studying this chapter you should be able to:
- understand the importance of ethics in the practice of nursing;
- begin to understand three ethical theories and their underpinning principles;
- understand the importance of the nurse–patient relationship and describe its boundaries;
- apply these first three outcomes to areas of clinical practice affecting the individual patient and the population;
- understand consent and confidentiality as key areas of professional practice;
- apply this learning to meeting the requirements of the NMC Code.

What is ethics?

The New Oxford Dictionary of English defines ethics as 'moral principles which govern a person's behaviour or the conduct of an activity'. At a more philosophical level, ethics is defined as 'the branch of knowledge that deals with moral principles'. Therefore, in the context of nursing practice, ethics can be summarised as a systematic approach based on moral principles that can underpin practice and assist the practitioner to act in a manner that fulfils the obligation to the public of being a member of a regulated profession.

Ethics are important in self-regulated professions, including nursing, medicine, allied health professions and the law, in order that both those who practise the professions and those whom they seek to serve have no doubt about what represents proper practice and where the boundaries between proper and improper behaviour in respect of their patients or clients and themselves lie. Most regulated professions in the sphere of health have codes of conduct or similar ethically based publications, which they make widely available to both practitioners and the public to provide information and advice on standards expected. For nurses, midwives and specialist community public health nurses, the core document is the NMC Code.

Ethical theories

In order to apply ethics to practice, it is necessary to have a basic understanding of three fundamental ethical theories:

- *Virtue-based ethics* (as typified by Aristotle), which hold that the virtues – including honesty, justice, charity, kindness, compassion and generosity – provide a basis that enables individuals to fulfil their duty to society and contribute to the overall good of that society. In return, society rewards its virtuous members. For instance, individuals who act from compassion and charity to relieve hunger or poverty in the developing world act ethically according to a virtue-based code and in return can expect the approbation of society for their actions.
- *Duty-based ethics* (as typified in 1781 by Immanuel Kant in his work 'Critique of pure reason') are based on the rightness or wrongness of an act and hold that rational human beings have an obligation to act in the correct way and fulfil their duties to society by so doing. Here, the individual who sees it as a duty to give money to relieve hunger or poverty in the developing world acts ethically according to a duty-based code. Acting from compassion would be less acceptable to a person who believes in duty-based ethics, as it allows for equivocation as to what is duty. For these individuals, their recognition would come from knowing and being seen to have done their duty.
- *Consequence-based ethics* (as typified Jeremy Bentham in his 1789 treatise 'Introduction to morals and legislation' and modified by JS Mill in 1863 when he published 'Utilitarianism'.) This ethical theory, which has continued to be called 'utilitarianism', holds that the right act in any given circumstance is the one that maximises the benefit and minimises the harm to society and individuals within that society. In this instance, the individual who acts ethically is the one who gives money to relieve hunger in the developing world because humanity as a whole benefits as fewer people die of starvation.

Seldom, if ever, do individuals or societies consciously categorise their professional and personal relationships or ethical decisions in this way. Rather, their actions are aimed at differentiating between right and wrong or between good and bad. Actions and decisions are influenced extrinsically by cultural and religious influences and acquired values. Intrinsic influences include conscience, personal development, education, inherent values and conditioning in society. Ethical principles, distilled from these theoretical frameworks, can provide a useful guide for individual actions.

Nurse–patient relationships

Before considering these ethical principles in depth, it is opportune to consider their interface with the relationship between nurses and patients. There are many facets of the nurse–patient relationship that impact on ethical considerations. Here, three of them are considered.

The first aspect to consider is the balance of power between practitioners and those they serve. This balance is skewed heavily towards the practitioner. This is the person with the knowledge, skills and experience to directly influence the outcome of the episode of care; this is the person on whom the patient depends for varying components of physical and emotional welfare, often including the most intimate aspects of care; this is the person whom the patient entrusts with the most sensitive information about themselves, their families and others who are close to them.

In each of these areas, the potential exists for intentional or accidental abuse. Take, for example, the case of a person who has had a stroke and who is dependent on their carers for meeting all their care needs, including feeding; the nurse has total power over the patient and could intentionally deny them food for whatever reason, for example as punishment; equally, accidental abuse of power could occur if the nurse fails to feed the patient in a dignified manner or waits until the food is cold.

Reflection point 9.1
Review the care plan of a patient whom your team have cared for recently. Note down the potential opportunities for accidental or intentional abuse of power in the nurse–patient relationship.

In your reflection you may have considered the following:

* meeting the care needs of the patient;
* failure to administer required medication on time;
* consideration of the patient's views when planning care;
* failure to provide appropriate information to the patient;
* accuracy in recording information relating to the patient.

The second aspect of the nurse–patient relationship meriting attention is trust. Patients should always be able to trust implicitly those charged with caring for them. This trust must be demonstrated in terms both of acting always in the best interests of the patient and in handling patient information and their belongings.

Third, the issue of respect is important. It is essential that there is mutual respect between the patient and the nurse. Much of what follows in this chapter relates to respect by the nurse for the patient in all aspects of the episode of care. Equally, it is vital that the patient shows respect for the nurse; failure to do so can only weaken the nurse–patient relationship and open up the potential for accusations of discrimination or other difficulties in the interaction.

Finally, it is important that the nurse–patient relationship is non-judgemental. Those providing care for patients must ensure that they are not seen by action or omission to be treating patients judgementally because of their lifestyle or personal habits.

Reflection point 9.2
Consider the range of lifestyles and habits that may lead to the nurse appearing to be judgemental if care is not taken to avoid this.

In your reflection you may have considered issues relating to:

* sexuality;
* personal hygiene;
* use of addictive substances, including tobacco and alcohol;
* status, for example prisoner or professional;
* social circumstances, for example homelessness;
* race and faith.

The boundaries of the nurse–patient relationship must also be considered. The nurse, the patient and society all have their individual perceptions of where the boundaries of the relationship lie. Clearly, all would regard the intentional killing of the patient by the nurse, or vice versa, as outwith the boundaries of the professional relationship; assault, rape or a sexual relationship (given the issue of power raised above, this includes even consensual relationships) would also be regarded as inappropriate by most people.

To ensure that the boundaries of the professional relationship are maintained, it is important that the nurse recognises the responsibility to put the needs of the patient at the core of the relationship and that the relationship is targeted to meet the needs of the patient alone. The nurse must also accept responsibility for defining the point at which the professional relationship ends. In acute episodes of care, the end point will normally be clear to everyone involved – the discharge of the patient from hospital. Where the patient has complex needs for emotional or physical care, the professional relationship may continue for many months or even years. Here, the potential for the boundaries between practitioner and patient to become blurred increases with the length of the relationship, and the vigilance with which the nurse guards against crossing the boundaries must increase. Clinical leaders and those providing supervision also have a role to play in monitoring the caseloads of those such as community staff (who tend to provide care for the same client group over long periods) and in ensuring that individuals are supported and given opportunities to share concerns and to 'disconnect' from patients where they believe they are in danger of being put in a position where the boundaries of the relationship may be transgressed.

Consider Scenario 9.1 in discussion with your peers.

SCENARIO 9.1

You are the team leader of a community mental health team and are covering the visits of John Philips, a registered nurse on the team, during his absence on holiday. All is well in the course of these visits, until you visit Helen, a 22-year-old woman with bipolar disorder. During the visit, Helen tells you that she is missing John but is pleased because she has received a postcard from him. Helen shows you the postcard. You note that John has written that he wishes Helen were on holiday with him and that he is missing her company; he promises to call on her as soon as he gets home, 3 days before he returns to work.

Make brief notes of what you would do.

In considering this scenario you may have thought about how you would approach the issue with John on his return. There would be a handover session, which would present an opportunity for discussion. If clinical supervision operates within the team, then this would present another chance to reflect with John on those of his patients you have seen during his holiday and to give him the opportunity to raise any issues in his professional relationship with Helen. Ultimately, as the team leader, it is your professional responsibility to safeguard Helen's position and you must therefore raise what you have seen with John and take appropriate action, including devising an exit strategy to remove him from being Helen's primary nurse in a way that ensures that she remains supported and that her distress at the change will be limited. You also have to consider whether John has acted outwith any local policy or has breached the NMC Code.

Breaches of the boundaries of professional relationships will not always be clear-cut. For example, many patients wish to show their gratitude for the care they have been given and will sometimes seek to give gifts to individual members of staff or teams. This is acceptable where the gift is small, for example chocolates, flowers or cosmetics. Where money is offered or where the gift proposed is more significant, then care must be taken in accepting the gift. In some organisations, there are policies to cover these situations.

Ethical principles

Having looked at some of the founding principles of the nurse–patient relationship, the ethical principles that underpin all aspects of practice can now be considered. The first ethical principle for the nurse is to always act in the best interests of the patient. This principle underpins all the others and is central to the nurse fulfilling their obligation to the patient. In essence, what is being required here is that the practitioner puts the best interests of the patient or client before all others in the course of any interaction with them.

Flowing from the principle of acting in the patient's best interests are two sub-principles. The first is the absolute principle of never harming the patient or client; the ethical name for this notion is 'non-maleficence'. The second sub-principle is the principle of doing good for the patient or client wherever possible; ethically, this is known as 'beneficence'.

Alongside best interests and its two sub-principles are two other ethical principles that inform and guide nursing practice. The first of these is the principle of recognition of the autonomy of the individual. Autonomy is the ability of the individual to exercise self-determination and to plan their own actions and act on those plans without interference from others. In recognising the autonomy of another person, it is also necessary to respect the autonomous decisions that they make. Clearly, autonomy can never be an absolute right. The autonomy of the individual has to be tempered with the best interests of the wider society, especially respect for other people; for instance, no one would support the autonomous actions of a driver who made a decision to ignore a red traffic light at a busy crossroads and who consequently collided with a school bus. This is a simple example of where the law regulates autonomy in the interests of the safety of society. A point that will be considered further when discussing the ethical implications of resources and decision-making is that respect for the autonomy of individuals does not grant them the right to have their own needs, demands and aspirations met at the expense of other autonomous individuals.

As will be seen later, the principle of autonomy, especially with regard to the capacity of individuals to make decisions, is of the utmost importance when dealing with certain types of patient in relation to consent to treatment. Respect for autonomy, especially when the decision of the patient is different from the decision that the nurse would have made, is an essential dimension of the nurse–patient relationship.

The final principle is justice. Patients and clients have a right to expect that those who nurse them will treat them justly and in accordance with their needs. Justice demands that patients and clients receive the care they require, free from any discrimination. The principle of justice is also important when considering matters of resource allocation.

As mentioned above, religious beliefs are important in helping the individual to construct their individual moral and ethical compass. By its nature, nursing practice in twenty-first-century Britain is pluralistic and multi-cultural; however, none of the world's major religions would appear to find difficulty in embracing these ethical principles when delivered to or by its adherents.

SUMMARY

In the first section of this chapter, the nurse–patient relationship and three ethical codes have been examined and from them a number of ethical principles identified that can underpin nursing practice and guide the nurse in the general approach to providing care. The next section builds on these themes.

Ethics in practice

In this section the ethical principles are considered further and applied to a number of situations that nurses will encounter in their daily practice.

Rights and responsibilities are fundamental to ethical professional practice. The rights of one person or group of people are normally matched by the responsibility of another person, group or agency. The NMC Code places a responsibility on registered nurses to act always in the best interests of their patients or clients and to ensure, as far as they can, that those in their care suffer no discrimination; therefore, the matched right of the client is the expectation that those giving them professional care will work in this way. Although the expectation of nursing practice is that the rights of the patient are paramount, nurses, too, have rights. The responsibility for honouring these rights falls on both patients and employers. The most obvious right enjoyed by nurses is the right to respect for their own autonomy and the right to be treated with respect. The responsibility for ensuring personal safety lies both with individuals, who have a duty to safeguard themselves, and with employers, who have a duty to take all reasonable steps to provide an environment in which staff can work safely. In addition to the basic right to freedom from verbal and physical abuse, nurses also have the right not to be discriminated against or harassed by patients, peers, colleagues or managers on grounds of race, religious belief, gender, sexuality or any other reason. Most importantly, they have the right not to be asked by patients, clients or colleagues (of any discipline) to act unlawfully or contrary to best professional practice. This is an important area where matters such as being truthful about issues of diagnosis and treatment, euthanasia or assisted suicide are concerned. It is important that all those working directly with patients and their families have access to appropriate professional support to enable them to reflect upon their practice.

Reflection point 9.3
Pause and identify situations where nurses may come under pressure from (i) patients or their relatives and (ii) colleagues to act in a way that is potentially in conflict with professional rights and responsibilities.

Possible considerations here include:

- pressure from relatives to withhold information from patients;
- pressure from patients to use medication inappropriately or to supply relatives;
- pressure from colleagues to make incorrect entries in records in order to cover up an act or omission;
- pressure from managers to discharge patients early in order to meet delayed discharge targets;
- pressure from other agencies to supply personal clinical data inappropriately;

Some of these issues will be covered elsewhere in this chapter.

A contentious area of individual rights for some nurses relates to the role of personal conscience. With very limited exceptions, which are written into the law relating to abortion and assisted fertility services, nurses enjoy no more and no less legal protection for their conscience than does any other health worker. The part played in practice by conscience is recognised in the NMC Code, which supports individuals in drawing matters of conscience that cause conflict with professional practice to the attention of senior professional colleagues. This area is important in discussing the nurse–patient relationship. The nurse who has issues of conscience relating to individual aspects of care must ensure that they always behave professionally and put the requirements of the patient at the centre of all interactions. Where conscience precludes an individual from participating in delivery of some parts of care, the onus remains on the practitioner to arrange for colleagues to provide the care required. In an emergency, it is the duty of each individual to ensure that all steps to ensure the patient's well-being are taken; this requirement is in no way weakened by the limited legal recognition of conscience.

Reflection point 9.4

Think about issues where individual conscience may impact on professional practice and how these can be addressed (i) by the individual nurse and (ii) by professional leaders.

Your reflection may have led you to consider:

- how an individual practitioner, finding themselves faced with difficulty caused by a matter of conscience, can ensure that the patient receives the care needed from other members of the team;
- how those in leadership positions can best balance the need to ensure continuity of high-quality patient care, the smooth running of clinical areas and the need to support the individual member of staff;
- how those in professional education and development can ensure that those they educate and support realise that conscience cannot be used as an abdication of professional responsibility to give care to individual patients or groups whose lifestyle, personal habits or diagnosis are offensive to the practitioner;
- how all staff are made aware of where they can obtain impartial professional support, including occupational health teams, spiritual care services (chaplaincy) and employee counselling services.

The next focus is on the particular ethical and moral issues which affect professional practice at the beginning and end of life.

The beginning of life

To start, three issues related to the beginning of life – termination of pregnancy, management of infertility and sterilisation – will be examined. Each of these subjects warrants an entire chapter, and the outline nature of the present coverage must be recognised.

Termination of pregnancy

The issue of termination of pregnancy remains a significant ethical dilemma for many health care professionals. Legally, termination of pregnancy by medical or surgical means is permissible before the twenty-fourth week if two doctors form the opinion that continuing the pregnancy would involve a greater risk to the mental or physical health of the mother than would the termination of the pregnancy (Abortion Act 1967). Given that infants of 20–22 weeks' gestation now routinely survive due to advances in neonatal care, there is an ongoing debate as to whether the time limit for termination of pregnancy should be reviewed and shortened, possibly to 20 weeks.

One of the main ethical debates in this area concerns the rights of the fetus. As the right to life is universally assumed to be a good thing, then questions around the moral consequences of terminating the life of the fetus must arise. The fundamental question here is: does a fetus have a right to life? Two responses are possible to this question, each of them proving acceptable to those who advocate the individual position supported by that response. The first response, supported by those who would give a woman total control over her body, is that the fetus, being incapable of separate existence from the mother, has no right to life. The second response, supported by those of conservative views and certain religious persuasions, is that the fetus has the potential to become a person in his or her own right and therefore has an inalienable right to life. Neither of these extreme positions provides a one-size-fits-all response to this most difficult of issues.

The first position fails to recognise that, from an early point in its development, a fetus has a beating heart, developing nervous system and the presumed ability to feel pain. As the pregnancy progresses, the fetus becomes increasingly aware of its environment and able to respond to stimuli and capable of independent existence until the pregnancy reaches the twenty-fourth week, when it is assumed, at least in law, that the fetus is capable of independent existence. Against this background it must be added that, in law, the fetus has no status until it draws its first breath.

The second position fails to acknowledge that, in certain circumstances, such as following rape or an act of incest against a young person or a person vulnerable through learning disability or profound mental health problems, termination of a pregnancy may be justified. A particularly sensitive area in consideration of whether termination of pregnancy is justified relates to situations where antenatal testing has revealed that the fetus has a physical abnormality. Understandably, many people with disabilities and groups working with them are vehemently opposed to termination on these grounds.

In considering the ethics of termination of pregnancy, it is important that all nurses consider the issues carefully and non-judgementally. As stated earlier, termination of pregnancy is one of very few areas of activity where nurses have a legal right, except in emergency situations, to voice a conscientious objection to participation. It is important that this right is respected and that nurses who make such a decision are supported. Equally, it is important that those nurses who are willing to participate in termination services are also supported so that they, in turn, can support women who face what will probably be one of the most difficult decisions of their lives. Recognition must also be given to the fact that the psychological sequelae of a termination may stay with women for many years, even their whole lifetime.

Reflection point 9.5
Consider how both those who feel that conscience precludes their involvement and those who do participate can be supported effectively.

In addition to the points considered in response to Reflection point 9.3, you may also have considered:

- how effective staff rotation arrangements can ensure that those who do care for women having pregnancies terminated are supported to ensure that they do not suffer adverse consequences;
- how continuing professional development (CPD) programmes can support and refresh staff in ensuring that they are updated in techniques of offering both physical and psychological support to women undergoing termination of pregnancy.

The management of infertility
The management of infertility is another area of practice that can be riddled with ethical dilemmas. Research into treatments for infertility is among the fastest-growing areas for clinical study. Techniques currently available span the whole range of interventions, from artificial insemination of a naturally produced ovum by a woman's partner or an anonymous donor, through in vitro fertilisation using naturally occurring or donated ova and sperm, to surrogacy in which a woman carries a child and at birth passes it to another woman to raise as her own child. These techniques have significant ethical implications, and none more so than the ethical issues surrounding the use and storage of embryos created in vitro and then stored by freezing rather than implanted at the point of fertilisation. In this situation, the same question arises over the status of the embryo as arises over the status of the fetus. Given the conclusion reached relating to approaches to the

status of the fetus, it will come as no surprise to discover that identical arguments may apply to the embryo. The same responses to those arguments can also apply. However, in the case of the embryo, the arguments on the potential person from the moment of conception are weakened by the fact that, as science currently stands, without implantation there can be no development beyond a cell mass and therefore no potential person can exist. That said, it would be wrong to assume that the fertilised human embryo can be treated as an item of science. It is widely accepted that the embryo is entitled to special respect on the basis that it represents human tissue.

Genetic manipulation and embryo research

As techniques for developing and modifying embryos evolve, so too do the ethical implications of the technology. For example, the UK courts have approved the selection of embryos to maximise the potential for matching tissue to be created to allow a sibling with a degenerative disorder to be treated; the same techniques can be used to facilitate the genetic manipulation of embryos to provide 'spare parts' or stem cells capable of developing into any type of body tissue.

Reflection point 9.6
Discuss the above ruling and assess how far embryo research should allow tissues to be used for the benefit of the parents and relatives or complete strangers.

- Did you consider how you regard the embryo – collection of cells or potential human being?
- Did you consider whether the intended beneficiary – parent, relative, sibling, stranger – made any difference to your decision?
- Did you consider whether the nature of the disease to be treated by the embryo made any difference to your decision?
- Does limitation of present knowledge plays any part in your decision?
- Can you envisage any future factors that may change your view?

A similar discussion surrounds the selection of embryos for implantation on grounds of gender. This raises an interesting topic for ethical debate. The immediate response of most people to this question would probably be a firm no; however, if the question is then posed to them in terms of preventing the transmission of diseases such as haemophilia, which are transmitted through the female line but affect only males, then a different response may ensue. Further questions also arise about the benefit for society as a whole that may come from research on embryos, especially genetic manipulation to yield possible treatments and cures for previously untreatable, distressing and, in some cases, fatal diseases, such as cystic fibrosis. Many people would be prepared to allow embryos not required for implantation or storage to be used for the greater good of the human race knowing that they would derive no personal benefit (the notion of altruism), while others may raise serious and legitimate questions about research on an embryo that cannot benefit directly from the research findings. A further differentiation needs to be drawn between embryos used for research, having been created for implantation and being surplus to the number required, and those created specifically for research purposes. A more pertinent question may be: what should be the fate of stored embryos? For those who subscribe to the cell mass theory, then the answer is straightforward: disposal in the same way as any similar collection of cells. For those subscribing to the potential person theory, then a real problem exists: human life is sacred and cannot be ended by the action of another individual or body. The current legal position is that embryos cannot be allowed to develop beyond the fourteenth day following fertilisation and cannot be stored for more than 5 years after fertilisation.

Control of fertility

From the management of infertility, we now move to look at the ethical issues surrounding control of fertility. Surgical sterilisation and chemical and barrier contraception have all been accepted elements of clinical practice for many years. In most circumstances, the use of contraception and sterilisation give rise to few ethical issues. That said, there are times when nurses may find themselves caring for people in situations where contraception and sterilisation are problematic.

Current ethical issues around contraception relate to the prescription and supply of the contraceptive pill in two circumstances: to girls under the age of 16 years and as the so-called 'morning-after pill'. In relation to the first issue, the main ethical question is: as it is illegal for a man to have sexual intercourse with a girl under 16 years of age, even with her consent, can a doctor or nurse prescribe or supply the girl with contraception? This illegality does not prevent some girls under the age of 16 years from engaging in consensual sexual intercourse. Therefore, falling back on the injunctions discussed earlier never to do harm to the patient and to do good wherever possible, health professionals have to perform a difficult balancing act between denying contraception and running the risk of an unwanted and potentially psychologically devastating pregnancy or prescribing contraception in the knowledge that sexual intercourse is going to take place and a crime be committed against the girl. Like many of the other issues discussed throughout this chapter, there is no easy answer to this conundrum. In reality, the health professional has to make a judgement as to the maturity and understanding of the girl, to offer wise counsel in regard to responsible sexual behaviour, and to offer advice on the availability and use of contraceptives that have fewer potential side effects than the contraceptive pill. Given the earlier comments on the need for nurses to be non-judgemental, it is important that the judgement here is the professional's judgement of the capacity of the individual to understand the information to be imparted rather than any judgemental assessment of the habits of the individual. Ultimately, knowing that sexual intercourse will take place regardless of whether or not contraception is used, many health professionals would meet the patient's wishes. A separate and equally contentious issue is the debate as to whether or not the girl's parents should be told. We shall look further at this when examining matters of consent.

The issues associated with the morning-after pill relate to its mode of action and availability. The morning-after pill is effective because it prevents the fertilised embryo from implanting into the endometrium and leads to its spontaneous ejection. Those groups and individuals who hold that the embryo has special status, because of its 'person potential' qualities, argue that this mode of action means that the morning-after pill leads to a termination as surely as if medical or surgical means had been used. With regard to availability, those responsible have determined that, subject to training and counselling being available, the morning-after pill should be made widely available from pharmacies and in other settings, including in some instances at school, where it may be administered by a school nurse.

Reflection point 9.7
Consider the pros and cons of school nurses being empowered to prescribe and administer the morning-after pill to students in their care.

Arguments in favour that you may have considered include the following:

- The school nurse may already have a caring relationship with the student, and this can be built on to provide support and offer ongoing, confidential advice on sexual health and contraception in order to avoid recurrence of the morning-after pill being required.
- The school nurse can provide support in managing the physical consequences following the administration of the morning-after pill.

Arguments against may include the following:

- The school and local health services could be seen to be condoning under-age sexual activity.
- Prescribing and administering the morning-after pill detracts from the time the school nurse has to fulfil their main role of health promotion.

When thinking about surgical sterilisation, the ethical implications relate to the presumed permanence of the procedure, the consequences of failure, and cases where sterilisation is proposed (normally for women) in the absence of capacity to consent. Most individuals seeking sterilisation do so with the firm intention of preventing future pregnancy. There are a number of lifestyle reasons why this decision may be regretted; a change in partner, the death of a child and change of mind about family size are all good examples. Some sterilisations may be reversible, but many are not. For this reason, it is important that the patient receives adequate counselling about the nature of the procedure that they are requesting and give truly informed consent before the operation takes place. The opposite situation is also true; in a very small minority of cases, the effect of the sterilisation (especially in males) may not be permanent if the vas deferens becomes rejoined. Again, frank discussion of the possibility of rejoining and obtaining fully informed consent before surgery is essential.

The final point relating to sterilisation that has ethical implications relates to individuals who lack the capacity to consent either to sterilisation or to consensual sexual relationships. This is a matter of profound concern to the parents, other relatives and carers of women of childbearing age with learning disabilities or mental health problems who are at risk of sexual exploitation and who are also wholly incapable, through no fault of their own, of managing menstruation or pregnancy or caring for a child. Very few such cases arise, but those that do cause great angst for those who care for and about the person concerned. Ultimately, it may be necessary for the facts to be presented to the courts and a judgement obtained as to the legality and appropriateness of sterilisation taking place. The ethical considerations that both health professionals and the courts need to take into account are the same: the need to ensure that the proposed procedure is the only way of protecting the best interests of the woman, and the need to ensure that the risks of rendering her incapable of having a child are less than the risks of her being sexually exploited and finding herself pregnant and facing the distress of either having the pregnancy terminated or having a child that may have to be taken into care.

Ethics in day-to-day care

Consent to treatment

In considering the practical ethical implications of day-to-day activities of care, consent to treatment is a useful starting point. Obtaining informed consent before undertaking any activity involving an autonomous individual lies at the heart of ethical practice. Indeed, any member of the care team who treats an autonomous person without their consent not only acts unethically but also potentially breaches both criminal and civil law.

Beauchamp and Childress (2001) spell out four components, all of which must be fulfilled, in order to secure informed consent: competence, disclosure, understanding and voluntariness. Before consent can be given or withheld, the person seeking consent must be satisfied that the patient has the intellectual and mental capacity to appreciate what is proposed. The practitioner must give information in an accessible format, which is in line with the patient's or client's level of comprehension, about the planned action. This information should include details of the intervention, details about the potential or actual benefits to the patient or client, and details of any possible alternatives, complications or side effects. Once this information has been given, it is for the practitioner to satisfy themselves that the patient or client has understood the information and been given the opportunity to ask questions or seek further information, including, if appropriate, information from an independent source. The final requirement is for the consent to have been sought free from inducement or pressure. Once these tests have been met, informed consent can be said to have been given or withheld.

For most patients, explicitly giving or withholding consent is something that happens at a fixed point in time before undergoing surgery or other invasive procedure. The patient or client is seen by a health professional, discussion takes place and a document is signed.

For, nurses this explicit and documented process is the tip of the iceberg. By cooperating in their care, patients and clients give their implied but unwritten consent on a daily basis to both physical and psychological interventions.

Reflection point 9.8
Think about a patient or client you have worked with recently. Consider the interactions that took place and list ways in which the patient or client gave implied consent.

You may have listed:

- keeping an appointment for a counselling session;
- holding out their arm to allow venepuncture to take place;
- answering questions during the taking of a nursing history;
- removing clothing to allow an ultrasound examination.

There will always be areas where the ability of the individual to give consent is less clear. These situations can present those caring for such patients with real dilemmas.

Intellectual competence and consent

If the patient or client does not have sufficient intellectual competence to give or withhold consent based on understanding of the information given, then the practitioner must always act in the best interests of the individual. There should be protocols in place to guide staff involved in determining how best interests can be met when competence is lacking. This guidance should include criteria for the assessment of competence and also should highlight the importance of language and method of communication to ensure maximum comprehension. All members of the clinical team must bear in mind that, in most circumstances, no one, including the next of kin, can give consent on behalf of another adult.

Legal frameworks to protect the rights of those who cannot make decisions for themselves exist in England and Wales in the Mental Capacity Act 2005 (introduced in October 2007) and in Scotland in the Incapable Adults (Scotland) Act 2000. Each of these pieces of legislation specifies arrangements to ensure that those who lack the capacity to make decisions for themselves are safeguarded and at the same time can access services (including health care) that they need in order to maximise their quality of life. In the most difficult cases, NHS bodies can make application to the courts for permission to carry out treatments on adults who lack the capability to give informed consent in their own right.

There may be circumstances when a patient anticipates approaching incompetence and makes an advance directive (also known as a living will), specifying the circumstances under which defined treatments would be acceptable or unacceptable. Subject to certain conditions, including the statement being in writing, dated and witnessed, being met, the Mental Capacity Act gives such directives a statutory status. A further condition that the Act places on advance directives is the requirement for the document to specify that the writer wishes the directive to be followed even in life-threatening situations.

Consent to the administration of medicines is just as important as consent to any other intervention. The nurse must be able to justify administering medication covertly in the same way as any other non-emergency treatment without consent would be justified. Circumstances where patients who are confused, mentally ill or otherwise uncooperative refuse to take oral medication present real challenges to care teams. These situations require skills of persuasion and patience to achieve compliance. Where all such efforts fail, other members of the clinical team, including prescribers and pharmacists, should be involved to ensure that the treatment being attempted is the most appropriate drug and preparation. Where, after full consideration, covert administration is agreed as being in the best interests of the patient, the full details of the decision should be entered into the patient's record. Such decisions should always be kept under review by senior members of the clinical team and should remain as part of the treatment for as short a period as possible.

Reflection point 9.9
List the possible approaches that can be employed to gain compliance with medicine regimes and avoid the need for covert administration without consent.

Among others, your list may include the following:

- the provision of information regarding medication in alternative formats, for example written, audio or Braille;
- the presentation of medication in a format more acceptable to the patient, for example liquid preparations;
- ensuring that coercion is avoided, utilising the expertise of relatives or others whom the patient trusts in order to explain the benefits of taking the medication;
- where side effects, such as dryness of the mouth, are problematic, considering the prescription of alternatives.

Perhaps the most difficult area of all facing practitioners is the withholding of consent by a competent adult, where the effect is deterioration in health or even death. Providing competence has been established, no intervention (apart from exerting influence in a sensitive and professional manner, which avoids any suggestion of coercion, in order to ensure that the patient is in possession of and understands the facts) is justified in these circumstances. To intervene is to undermine the right of the competent individual to autonomous self-determination. This important principle of consent was reaffirmed in the spring of 2002 by Dame Elizabeth Butler-Sloss, then President of the Family Division of the High Court in England and Wales. The case concerned Miss B, whose respiration was maintained by a ventilator following damage to her spinal cord caused by a haemorrhage. Miss B requested the clinical team caring for her to withdraw her ventilation. Her request, which was refused, was made in the knowledge that she would probably die. On appeal to the High Court, the president decided that Miss B had the competence to understand her request and the probable outcome and thus found that Miss B's autonomy was infringed by the refusal of the clinical team to comply with her wishes. The appeal was allowed and Miss B was subsequently transferred to another hospital where the clinical team was prepared to comply with her request; her ventilation was withdrawn and she died peacefully. She was also awarded nominal damages against the first NHS trust for its failure to comply with her wishes.

Another complex area of consent relates to children and young people. For children who, because of their age and immaturity, cannot satisfy the four criteria for informed consent, consent can be given by the parents (or those with parental responsibility). In England, Wales and

Northern Ireland, a young person is normally deemed competent to give consent on their own behalf at the age of 16 years. However, since the Gillick case in 1984, if the practitioner seeking consent believes that a young person under the age of 16 years has the maturity, understanding and competence to appreciate the details of the proposed intervention, then that individual can give consent without parental involvement. In Scotland, children of 16 years have a statutory right to give consent when the practitioner is satisfied that they can understand what is planned.

There are certain circumstances where staff are unable to obtain consent, for example where a patient is in extremis or where a practitioner witnesses a sudden cardiac arrest. In these and similar emergency circumstances, nurses will normally be deemed to have acted ethically where they provide appropriate treatment within their professional skills, knowledge and experience and in the patient's best interest.

Nurses must also be aware that there will always be a small number of patients in mental health settings who do not have to give consent to treatment if, in the view of psychiatrists and the legally competent authorities, they meet the requirements of the Mental Health Act (1983) operating in England and Wales and the Mental Health (Care and Treatment Scotland) Act 2003.

Consider Scenario 9.2.

SCENARIO 9.2 Informed consent

Mrs Mary Smith is a 78-year-old woman who has fractured the neck of her left femur. She has a degree of heart failure and is mildly deaf. These physical conditions aside, she is well and is completely competent mentally.

You are Mrs Smith's named or primary nurse and accompany the junior doctor who examines her and seeks her consent before surgery to fix her hip fracture. Having listened to the doctor, Mrs Smith signs her consent form. Some hours later, you discover that Mrs Smith is in a distressed state. On questioning, you find that she is unsure what the form was that she signed – as owing to the high level of background noise in the ward, she couldn't hear the doctor clearly.

Looking at the four components of consent outlined above, what steps must you take to ensure that Mrs Smith is empowered to give her informed consent for the procedure?

Examples of issues considered in Scenario 9.2 could include the following:

- recalling the doctor and ensuring that Mrs Smith is moved to a quieter area to have a discussion regarding her consent form;
- ensuring that Mrs Smith is wearing her hearing aid (if she uses one) and that it is in working order;
- providing Mrs Smith with written materials to support her in giving informed, voluntary consent;
- if Mrs Smith can understand sign language, providing an appropriate translator;
- with her consent, asking a family member who regularly communicates with Mrs Smith to be present during her discussion in order to provide support and to help her to ask questions.

Confidentiality

Confidentiality is another area of nursing practice with a significant ethical dimension. Trust and respect lie at the heart of the ethical relationship between the nurse and the patient. Patients must have confidence that nurses will always act in their best interest in all aspects of the professional relationship. This expectation of trust extends beyond the assumption that the therapeutic interventions carried out by the practitioner will be carried out responsibly and using appropriate skills, knowledge and experience. It also embraces the assumption that any information imparted by the patient to the nurse, either formally (e.g. the clinical history) or informally (e.g. in a social chat over a cup of coffee), will not be used to the client's detriment – that is, that confidentiality will be respected. From the perspective of the nurse, the principle must be that in all but the most extraordinary circumstances, the presumption of clients that their confidentiality will be respected will prevail. The NMC Code specifically requires practitioners to 'treat information about patients and clients as confidential' and make disclosures outside the team involved in the delivery of care only with consent, by order of a court or where the practitioner can justify disclosure in the wider public interest.

Some examples of when a nurse may be justified in breaching confidentiality include the following:

- where a court orders the information to be released;
- where the practitioner believes that, by doing so, a serious crime may be avoided or the detection of a serious crime assisted; in this case, serious crime would normally mean a serious crime against the person, such as terrorism, murder, manslaughter, rape or child abuse;
- where there are grounds to believe that the patient or another person may be at risk of death or serious physical or mental injury if information is not disclosed;
- where there are grounds to believe that there is a significant risk to public health in not disclosing information.

Formally disclosing information about a patient without consent is always a matter of the utmost gravity. Nurses must also bear in mind that informal breaches of confidentiality can take place more easily than formal breaches. Consider, for instance, the impact of a patient's relative overhearing two nurses in a supermarket on their way home from work discussing that patient; this may seem improbable in a large city, but it is entirely feasible in a small town. Staff may also come under pressure from other bodies to provide informal information, for example by the police investigating crimes where they believe a suspect may have been injured. In this situation, the patient has the same right to respect for his confidentiality as any other hospital patient.

Reflection point 9.10
Consider how inadvertent breaches of confidentiality can take place and how they can be averted.

Among other inadvertent breaches, your list may include the following:

- ensuring that sensitive patient information is not left lying around, visible to visitors or non-clinical staff;
- checking the identity of telephone callers before releasing information; where there is doubt, the patient should be asked explicitly what information should be released;
- avoiding the discussion of patients in non-clinical settings, such as canteens;
- conducting sensitive conversations with patients in appropriate settings. Remember how easy it is to be overheard – screen curtains are not sound-proof!

Having considered the importance of consent and confidentiality in day-to-day nursing practice, the chapter's consideration of ethics in practice concludes with ethical issues surrounding death and dying.

Ethical issues at the end of life

Before considering ethical issues at the end of life, it is important to be clear about when life ends. The answer to this question a century ago was straightforward: life ended when the heart ceased to beat, thus ending the supply of oxygenated blood to the brain. All the other main organs of the body stopped operating as a result of the ensuing hypoxia and metabolic disturbance. The advent of intensive care, artificial ventilation, drugs that support core body systems, and mechanical assistance to support the failing heart have changed this. While these artificial aids remain in place, oxygen exchange can continue, the cells can be supplied, and one level of life, which we call physiological life, can continue. Recognition of this in the 1960s and 1970s led to brain stem death being accepted as a defining measure of death in the developed world. In the UK, the process of confirming brain stem death has three phases:

1 Identifying the cause of the patient's coma and ensuring that it is not reversible and then ensuring that the coma is not due to any drug overdose or interaction, hypothermia or metabolic disturbance.
2 Performing a standard range of physiological tests to ensure that all the centres in the brain stem that control the body's vital functions are destroyed.
3 Ensuring that the patient cannot breathe when artificial supports are withdrawn.

To establish that brain death has occurred, each phase is repeated at least twice over a period of several hours or days.

This discussion of when (brain) death occurs is highly relevant when considering the ethical implications of organ transplantation.

Organ transplantation

In the UK, most transplants are undertaken using freely donated organs from cadavers. In these situations, organs are donated, where the person, while alive, carried an organ donor card, entered their name on the organ donor register or expressed a wish to donate. New legislation introduced in 2006 (Human Tissue Act 2006) removed the right of those close to the patient (relatives, registered civil partners or recognised next of kin) to object to the donation and subsequent transplantation if the individual had registered their desire to donate or carried a donor card. Although the emphasis here is on the wishes of the individual while alive, the good practice outlined previously on informed consent can be helpful in assisting communications with those in a bereaved and distressed state. In spite of the new legislation, significant ethical problems arise when those close to the patient continue to object. In this situation, it is important that the nursing staff who have cared for the patient continue to support those close to the patient through their grief. In the absence of any expressed wishes by the patient, the views of those closest to the patient must be paramount, and coercive behaviour aimed at securing their agreement must be avoided.

Transplantation using organs from a living donor is potentially far more ethically complex than transplants using cadaver organs. Living donors, usually of kidneys but sometimes of portions of the liver, submit themselves to both long- and short-term risks. Short-term risks arise from the significant surgery required to obtain the tissue for transplantation, and long-term risks arise from the possibility of future harmful effects occasioned as a result of having only one kidney or an incomplete liver. In the UK, living donor transplants are strictly regulated. The purpose of this regulation is to ensure that any decision to make a donation is free from duress and does not involve any payment or other reward. The regulatory system also monitors that the decision to make the donation is made with full information regarding the possible consequences for the donor.

A major difficulty facing the UK lies in the inadequate numbers of organs being made available for transplant. There is little doubt that some patients who could be saved if an organ were available for transplant die while they are waiting. To address this, some people propose that, rather than carry a donor card and indicate a willingness for their organs to be used, individuals should have to register, while alive, their objection to their organs being used. The ethical implications of such a practice would require detailed consideration to ensure that an individual's autonomy over their body continues to be accorded its proper priority. The establishment of such a register could also represent the start of a slippery slope. Need to register objection to organ usage today could lead to a need to register an objection to other procedures tomorrow and eventually could bring about a need to register individual objections to life being ended prematurely.

Withdrawal of food and fluids

Another complex area related to the end of life is the withdrawal of food and fluids when it is obvious that a patient's condition has deteriorated to the point that no further treatment can bring about an improvement and death is inevitable. When faced with a patient lying in a hospital bed with eyes open but unseeing, unable to communicate in any way, unable to undertake any of the activities that were important in health, and unable to recognise those close to them, there comes a point where the members of the care team must ask themselves whether they are acting in the patient's best interests by working hard to keep them alive. In the UK the intentional killing of a person is never considered to be in their best interests; however, when curative treatment is not possible, allowing a person to die free from pain and with all possible dignity may be. In the UK the question was first addressed legally in the 1993 case of Airedale NHS Trust v Bland. Anthony Bland was one of the spectators who suffered grave injury in the Hillsborough Stadium football tragedy in 1989; he remained in a persistent vegetative state until 1992. In that year, the NHS Trust that managed the hospital in which he was receiving care sought the permission of the courts to stop life-sustaining treatment, including artificial feeding and hydration, and restrict future treatment to those measures that would allow him to die free from pain and with dignity. The English courts, including the House of Lords, upheld the argument that withdrawal of treatment could be in the person's best interests. Once treatment has ended, the patient normally dies from dehydration within a matter of days. Several aspects of the decision to end treatment may be a cause of ethical unease, including the withdrawal of artificial food and nutrition, the inevitability of death, and the manner of that death by dehydration. Ultimately, in addressing these ethical dilemmas, health professionals need to be satisfied that accepting inevitable death is in the best interests of the patient. Only on that basis can the court decide, as has happened in a number of cases since 1993, that withdrawal of treatment is lawful and that action can be taken, in accordance with the ethical principles that underpin good nursing practice.

Euthanasia

Although the withdrawal of food and fluids from people faced with the inevitability of death is an area where the ethical and legal considerations are not clear-cut, the position relating to euthanasia – the deliberate, premature ending of life – is quite clear. In UK law, the intentional ending of a person's life by act or omission is unlawful. Two forms of euthanasia are often identified, voluntary and involuntary. The latter involves a belief that the person carrying out the process knows what is best for the individual who is bearing the suffering, which the procedure is intended to relieve, and that, because of mental or physical frailty, the person's best interests are being met by bringing their life to an end. This is not a position that finds favour even with those who advocate voluntary euthanasia, which involves a person who believes their suffering is intolerable asking those caring for them to take steps to bring their life to an end. The steps sought may be active – for example, the deliberate administration of a drug or obstruction of the airway – or passive – for example, failing to do something, such as withholding antibiotic therapy in patients with pneumonia in the knowledge that life will end. It is noteworthy that opposition to euthanasia is not universal. The Dutch government recognises that a person who requests, on an ongoing basis, that their life be ended because of very severe mental or physical suffering that cannot be relieved may be assisted to die. Closer to home, a Bill was introduced into the House of Lords by Lord Joffee in 2004 (the Assisted Dying for the Terminally Ill Bill 2004), which, had it become law, would have legalised voluntary euthanasia by means of assisting those in great suffering and where there was no hope of recovery, to commit suicide. As Lord Joffee's Bill did not pass into law, assisting another person to commit suicide remains both unlawful and unethical in the UK. A voluntary body in Switzerland, named Dignitas, has arranged for a number of Britons to leave the UK and commit suicide in Switzerland. Those who lead resistance to calls for the UK to make euthanasia legal argue that euthanasia is not necessary where there is sufficient provision of high-quality hospice and palliative care.

Reflection point 9.11

If you have experience of caring for patients in the last stages of their life, think how effective palliative care interventions can help to prevent an individual coming to the point where they might seek the assistance of the care team to end their life.

You may have listed some of the following:

- effective control of pain and other distressing symptoms;
- support both for the patient and for those close to them;
- enabling the patient to spend what remains of their life in a way that best meets their needs and ambitions;
- allowing the patient to die in the setting of their choice – often at home;
- affirming death as a natural part of life and providing suitable spiritual care.

An important ethical issue that must be recognised when considering the ethics of the end of life is the doctrine of double effect. This doctrine holds that certain actions, although foreseen, are not intended. Perhaps the best example of this is the administration of powerful opiates to patients with cancer who have intractable pain. Those prescribing and administering these drugs do so with the intention of relieving the patient's pain, while at the same time recognising that the respiratory depression that the drugs cause may also hasten death. As long as the intention in giving the drug is to relieve pain and not bring about death, then the patient's best interests are served and the members of the care team are not behaving unethically.

It is important that those caring for a patient who is dying are sensitive to the spiritual care requirements of the various faith groups and are able to secure the attendance of religious and faith representatives as required. Equally, the wishes of patients such as humanists who make clear statements about the non-spiritual nature of their death must also be respected.

Those caring for patients after death in all care settings must have information available to them about the requirements of the various faith groups and be sensitive to them. These requirements may include, but are not be limited to, the care of the body (including the religious belief and gender of those giving the care), the arrangements for storage of the body, time limits within which burial or cremation are required, and views on post-mortem examinations and the dissection and storage of tissues. It is good practice for comprehensive protocols to be agreed with recognised representatives of major local faith groups and widely disseminated.

SUMMARY

This section has looked at the translation of the ethical codes and principles into the practice of nursing on a day-to-day basis, as well as at moments of ethical vulnerability – the beginning and end of life.

The professional standing of the nurse

The previous section concentrated on those aspects of the direct care of patients with an ethical dimension. In this section, the impact of professional ethics on the nurse is examined.

Professional relationships

Acting in the best interests of patients requires nurses not only to take matters such as consent, respect and confidentiality seriously, but also to use their practical skills, knowledge and experience appropriately, to recognise the limitations of their ability, and to know when to call in other members of the care team. These are all matters that require the nurse to reflect regularly on her practice to ensure that professional relationships contribute to the overall well-being of the patient. Any action or omission on the part of the nurse that abuses the privileged relationship with the patient, be it physical, sexual, emotional or financial abuse or neglect, inducement or coercion by the nurse on the patient, is always against the patient's best interests and therefore unethical and professionally unacceptable. Disciplinary action by employers and professional regulatory bodies may be taken against a nurse found to have abused the professional relationship with a patient. Where the action or omission is judged to constitute gross misconduct, removal from the professional register may ensue. This is the reality of the interface between professional ethics, employment and professional registration.

Relationships that respect ethical boundaries between professions and with other colleagues are as important as relationships between nurse and the patient. Health care relies on teamworking and interprofessional cooperation. No single profession working in isolation can meet all the care needs of a patient. Therefore, each member of the team has to recognise and respect the role of the other members. The features of relationships between professions replicate those of the relationship between nurse and patient: trust, honesty and integrity. The best interests of patients are not served by disharmony within the care team, with members not trusting each other to play their part, by interprofessional rivalry, or by demarcation disputes leading to avoidable gaps in care.

A significant factor in care in recent years has been the extent to which nurses and other professionals have taken over responsibility for roles previously restricted to doctors. Before taking on these roles, nurses must ask themselves whether doing so is in the best interests of the patient. Where this is the case, then the nurse must ensure that they have the appropriate skills, knowledge, experience and resources to undertake the role safely and effectively. The nurse must also ensure that, by taking on new roles, the nursing elements of the patient's care will not suffer. Where these criteria cannot be met, the nurse should not agree to the reallocation of responsibilities and should seek the advice of senior colleagues. The NMC has produced guidance to support the professions in the NMC Code.

Just as nurses have taken on roles previously in the remit of doctors, so staff who are not registered nurses have taken on roles previously undertaken by nurses. There is no ethical objection to this, but the nurse must be aware that he/she retains responsibility for acting in the best interests of the patient. This is best done by establishing that those delivering the care have the skills, knowledge, experience and resources to give the care, and by ensuring that delegation is appropriate and adequate supervision is afforded to the direct caregiver.

Professional communications

Clear communication is essential to effective and ethical professional relationships. In order to maintain professional integrity and act in the best interests of the patient, the nurse must communicate openly and honestly, not only with the patient but also with colleagues within the wider health care team. When communicating with patients, the nurse must ensure that what is being said is actually being understood. Developing a range of communication skills, styles and techniques that best meet the needs of the patient group must be a priority for every registered nurse. This entails reviewing both verbal and non-verbal communication methods in order to find the most effective. An important practical ethical consideration relates to translation and interpretation for patients whose first language is not English. For convenience and speed, it may seem obvious to use family members (sometimes from extended families) to provide interpretation and translation between the patient and the care team. When taking decisions around interpretation and translation, the need to maintain the patient's expectation of confidentiality must be paramount. Wherever possible, except in emergency situations, specialist interpretation and translation services should be used. The use of professional interpreters and translators who are familiar with clinical terminology also diminishes the likelihood of potentially dangerous mistranslation.

Truthfulness in communication with patients is another potentially difficult area for nurses. All practitioners will experience dilemmas over what information should be given to patients and how it should be given. These dilemmas are never more acute than in situations where bad news about a condition or prognosis has to be given. In these situations, the element of trust that forms a key part of the nurse–patient relationship is paramount, and the guiding ethical principle is the principle of non-maleficence: the nurse's first duty is always to avoid harm to the patient. The general rule must always be that the patient is given truthful answers to direct questions. The skill for the person giving the answer lies in assessing how much information the patient can cope with and having the empathy, knowledge and patience to support understanding of the answers. Where direct questions are not asked, patients should still be given sufficient truthful information to meet their needs at that point in time.

Consider Scenario 9.3.

SCENARIO 9.3 Communicating truthfully

You are the named nurse of James Worth, a 60-year-old man who has just been diagnosed with a brain tumour. The clinical team believes that Mr Worth must be told about his condition and that, as no active treatment is possible, he will live for only a matter of a few weeks, during which time he will require ongoing and increasing care.

Mr Worth's wife and some of his family insist that he must be told that he will get better and be back in his own home very shortly. Other members of the family support the view of the clinical team. The differing views lead to increasing tension at visiting times, until finally a confrontation takes place just outside the ward but within hearing of Mr Worth. Mr Worth is, understandably, upset to hear his family confronting each other, and he asks you and his wife what is happening.

Bearing in mind that the nurse's prime responsibility is to the patient, how would you handle this situation with regard to both Mr Worth and his family?

In relation to the scenario, you may have thought about the following:

- given the nature of Mr Worth's illness, his need for active sensitive reassurance from the care team;
- moving the family members into a more private area, where their argument is not going to cause distress to other patients and visitors;
- assessing the needs of the family and involving other members of the care team, including the consultant responsible for Mr Worth's care and members of the spiritual care team;
- aiming to agree with the family that there is nothing to be gained by withholding the truth from Mr Worth and then agreeing with them how the news of his prognosis should be imparted;
- once the prognosis has been explained, how both the patient and his family can be supported, including by colleagues such as Macmillan nurses.

Communication with colleagues in health care teams is perhaps one of the areas requiring the greatest attention to working in the best interests of the patient. Although each team member has individual roles to fulfil and responsibilities towards the patient, poor communication within and between teams and their members can lead to patient care being affected adversely, with patients being given confusing information and mixed messages. The more complex the patient's care needs and the longer the episode of care, the greater the need for effective and coordinated communication. The named nurse or other identified key worker is well placed to be an effective coordinator of the whole team; communication is an essential part of the coordination process.

Maintaining appropriate records relating to a patient is a key part of the effective communication that serves the patient's best interests. Effective documentation should enable a reader with the requisite professional knowledge picking up the record to:

- find out the patient's history;
- determine what problems and care needs have been identified;
- see the plans made for addressing the problems and meeting the identified needs;
- find evidence of evaluation and review sufficient to enable care-planning to be dynamic in response to changing needs;
- identify what information has been given to the patient and those close to them, including specific terms used to describe the condition, for example 'lump', 'tumour', 'cancer' or 'malignancy'.

Regardless of whether uni- or multiprofessional documentation systems are used, it is the responsibility of the registered nurse to ensure that an adequate and honest record of all aspects of the nursing care given to the patient is maintained in a comprehensive and timely fashion. In compiling records, nurses should be aware that, with very few exceptions, patients have a statutory right to read their own records. They should also be aware that patient records are key items of evidence in the handling of complaints, professional conduct proceedings, litigation, and inquests or similar enquiries into patient deaths. As nurses may find themselves involved in any of these situations as a witness under oath, the importance of accurate record-keeping cannot be overemphasised. Again, this is an area covered by the NMC Code.

Reflection point 9.12
Critically appraise the last patient record you completed before reading the above and the NMC Code and list any improvements that could enhance the quality of the documentation.

Your reflection may have led you to think about:

- legibility;
- comprehensiveness;
- whether unnecessary abbreviations are used;
- what the patient would understand if they read the record;
- whether a professional reading the record in 5 years' time would be able to follow the care delivered.

SUMMARY

This section has examined the importance of professional relationships for patient care and considered the need for effective communication and record-keeping.

Ethical issues affecting populations

There are a number of situations where the ethical implications of professional practice go beyond the individual patient and affect larger groups within the population. In this last section, three such areas are examined: research ethics, the ethical issues relating to resource decision-making, and the ethics of health promotion.

Drug trials

Research is essential in ensuring that the boundaries of health care are advanced for the benefit of the population. Without research, many of the interventions and drug treatments now taken for granted would never have come about. For example, if researchers had not examined why an extract of the bark and sap from a particular type of willow tree appeared to be able to relieve pain and reduce fever, salicylic acid would never have been discovered and the humble, yet potentially life-saving, aspirin would never have become available. Increasingly, nurses are involved in or conduct research during their careers. All research on individuals, who may be patients or healthy volunteers, is regulated by a network of local and regional research ethics committees, the role of which is to ensure that all research undertaken complies with national and international good practice, including the Declaration of Helsinki. Important considerations for ethics committees are the design of the study, in terms of ensuring that it will meet its aims and will do so with the lowest number of participants exposed to the lowest risk, the recruitment of participants to ensure that no coercion is used, and the quality of documentation relating to patient information and consent. For individual patients, the requirements for obtaining informed consent and safeguarding confidentiality are as applicable to research activity as to other interventions. By its nature, research will always throw up ethical problems. Consider, for example, a drug trial, in which one group of patients who receive the active drug, without them or their doctors knowing it, show a marked improvement in their symptoms, while another group of patients in the same trial receive a drug with no active ingredient (a placebo), again unknown to them or their doctors, and show no improvement. The dilemma here is: at what point does it become unethical to continue the trial, knowing that the active drug is beneficial and would improve the condition of the whole patient group?

Allocation of resources

Following on from research ethics, new drugs form a useful case study bridge to a consideration of the ethical issues around the allocation of scarce resources for heath care. Every week trials for new drugs are completed and the drugs are licensed for use. Invariably, these drugs (which are often targeted at diseases such as cancer or heart disease) come at a considerable cost to the NHS. The availability and cost of these new drugs can pit patients, clinicians, service planners and funders against each other. Patients are better informed than ever before, both about their conditions and about the treatments, including new drugs, available to them. Clinicians, as has been emphasised throughout this chapter, have both a moral obligation and an overwhelming desire to act in the best interests of patients, including prescribing newly available drugs where clinically indicated. Those who commission and fund services are under constant pressure to meet targets, deliver efficiency savings, and expand the range of services available, all within a constrained budget. Bodies such as the National Institute for Health and Clinical Excellence (NICE) are charged with assessing new drugs and treatments and, following public and professional consultation, advising ministers and the NHS on whether the drugs should be generally available. In cases where drugs recommended by clinicians have not been prescribed on cost grounds, a number of patients and patient groups have taken legal action against NHS bodies and, in some cases, have succeeded in gaining access to the drugs. One example of this relates to the drug trastuzumab (Herceptin®), trials of which showed it to have a marked effect on the management of breast cancer. A number of patients sought legal remedies against local NHS bodies' refusal to allow the prescription of the drug in the months before NICE approved its use.

Since the foundation of the NHS in 1948 there have always been groups arguing that the service is insufficiently funded. Now, 60 years later, it looks increasingly unlikely that there ever will be a consensus that funding is wholly adequate. Clearly, all additional funding made available is to be welcomed and will be useful, but the pace of change in technology, combined with the increasing longevity of the population, will probably always outstrip the ability or willingness of the taxpayer to contribute the level of funding required to meet every need or demand. The question of whether need or demand should be met is a further ethical challenge, with ethical principles being available to support both views. The meeting of need implies that an organisation or other body will take a view of what the individuals who make up society need and this will become what is available. The meeting of demand recognises the autonomy of the individual but also disregards the wider good. This dichotomy lies at the heart of debate on the rationing of health care. Regardless of its political persuasion, the government of the day propounds the argument that the UK has a comprehensive health care system that is free at the point of delivery. This is true to a point; however, increasing prescription, dental and optical charges give a different view to those who pay them. What central government never says is whether the system should meet need or demand. A glance at the annual report of any body that commissions health services in each of the UK countries will show that in excess of 95 per cent of the total NHS budget in any one year is taken up in the delivery of core services such as emergency ambulances, district nursing, acute medicine and surgery, mental health teams and caring for older people. Each of these areas, together with rare conditions that require very costly treatment to enable individuals to have the best quality of life, competes alongside new drugs and new techniques, such as interventional radiology and minimally invasive surgery, for a share of the small amount of the NHS cake that is left for development. In this situation, both need (for timely treatment, such as hip replacement, which can make an individual pain-free and promote independence) and demand (for cosmetic surgery or complicated fertility treatment, which would meet a psychological need) remain unmet, giving rise to very real distress to a number of individuals. The fact that individuals lie at the heart of decisions about resource allocation must never be forgotten. Where 60 patients can receive treatment for varicose ulcers for a year for the same cost as one patient can receive the latest drug to treat schizophrenia for a month, the decision appears easy; easy, that is, for the 60 people who will receive treatment, their families and their carers. But what of the schizophrenic patient, his family and his carers, and also the people who have to make the decision? It is not so easy for them.

There is, of course, no simple solution to this problem. What tends to happen is that blunt instruments, such as waiting lists, are used to regulate the service delivered within the resources available, and new developments are introduced in a piecemeal fashion as finances allow. The inevitable result of this method of resource allocation is that both those with needs and those with demands accept their lot and carry on, or become dissatisfied and complain, often involving politicians in making representations on their behalf, in the hope that this will bring the desired result. What is needed is an open and inclusive debate aimed at agreeing that the population would be prepared to pay, through taxation, sufficient monies to meet every need and demand – or, if this is not the case, then to reach agreement on what level of service can be provided with the money that taxpayers are willing to pay. On present evidence, none of the main UK political parties seems to have an appetite for such a debate; it seems, therefore, as if the present system will continue. Perhaps the best example of this debate having taken place is in the US state of Oregon, where, following wide public and professional debate, the state legislature has reached agreement on a list of interventions that are available from publicly funded providers of health care (Oregon Health Plan 1998, reported by Ham, 1998).

Reflection point 9.13
Identify treatments and procedures to which you personally would not allocate development funding, and explain why. By reference to your peer group, identify commonalities or differences.

You may have considered:

- the range of treatments that you would include or exclude based on your life and professional experience to date;
- any treatments that you consider to offer little benefit to the individual;
- your personal balance in the need-versus-demand equation;
- how you would shift the balance of treatments offered in order to free up resource for developments;
- how you would explain your decisions to the public.

Health promotion

The final area of population ethics relates to health promotion. Society increasingly recognises the benefit of encouraging people to maximise their own health and well-being by their own efforts, and the NHS devotes increasing resources and the time of health professionals, including nurses, to this end. When considering the promotion of health, it is important to consider the ethical implications of organised activities. Throughout this chapter, much emphasis has been laid on a respect for the autonomy of the individual, which can be restrained only in exceptional circumstances. Most health promotion initiatives operate by seeking to influence lifestyle and, although this does not directly interfere with individual autonomy (individuals remain free to act in whatever way they see fit, providing it is legal), critics would argue that the line between freedom of action and coercion into taking a course of action that is not the individual's free choice could easily be crossed. A good example of this is the campaign against cigarette smoking. For good reason, much health promotion and education activity is aimed at reducing the number of people who smoke or encourage people who do smoke to smoke less. The number of places where smoking is permitted is being reduced. Throughout the UK and Ireland, bans on smoking in public areas, including obvious places such as restaurants and bars but also less self-evident areas such as railway stations, are in place. This leads to those who cannot cease smoking becoming increasingly stigmatised. This could be construed as infringement of their autonomy. Conversely, the antismoking lobby could lay claim to the moral and ethical high ground by advancing the argument that their efforts to restrict smoking avoids people who make an autonomous decision not to smoke receiving passive doses of smoke.

At a macro-level, questions must be asked about the ethics of society in relation to health promotion. Staying with smoking as an example, it is well known that a large proportion of the cost of any tobacco product is government-imposed taxation. This taxation makes an important contribution to the income of the government, part of which is expended on the NHS. Most health promotion professionals would support a ban on the advertising of tobacco products. In terms of securing the greatest health benefit for the population, the ethical position would demand that all reasonable steps be taken to minimise the amount of smoking. However, against this position, governments of any political complexion must weigh the disadvantage they may suffer, both in financial losses from taxation and in political losses, by potentially damaging their electoral popularity. A moot point is the extent to which reduced demand for resources to fund NHS services, by reducing the number of smoking-related illnesses, would offset the reduction in income caused by the loss of taxation. As outlined above, given the increasing needs and demands faced by the NHS, any supportive argument along these lines is probably specious.

A final example of the ethical dilemmas posed by health promotion activities relates to the fluoridation of public water supplies to prevent tooth decay, especially in young children. The fact that tooth decay can be prevented by adding fluoride to water is well established, as is the fact that in certain parts of the UK fluoride exists naturally. On this basis, the health of children and young people could be improved by reducing their likelihood of developing dental caries. In terms of securing the greatest health benefit and minimising harm to one large cohort of the population, the addition of fluoride is ethically supportable. The other perspective is that, where fluoride does not occur naturally, it becomes yet another chemical added to water and forced on the population, who have no choice but to drink it and use it for cooking. Where the addition lacks consent, this may be seen as acting against the autonomy of a large proportion of the population, especially those with no natural teeth who cannot derive the intended benefit.

◎ SUMMARY

Moving from the individual to the population, this section has addressed ethical issues that affect the whole of society, including funding for the NHS.

⊚ CONCLUSION

This chapter has sought to give a brief overview of the importance of nurse–patient relationships and a number of important ethical principles. These principles are then applied to the beginning of life, the treatment of adults and children, and issues at the end of life. An overview of the importance of ethics on the population has also been explored. What has not been provided is an answer to every relationship and ethical problem that the reader will face in a career in nursing. Nevertheless, useful pointers will hopefully have been gained by the reader to help them seek solutions (rather than right or wrong answers) to ethical difficulties, and that the chapter has stimulated further exploration in this fascinating area.

References

Beauchamp TL and Childress JF (2001). *Principles of Biomedical Ethics*, 5th edn. New York: Oxford University Press.

Ham C (1998). Retracing the Oregon Trail: the appearance of rationing and the Oregon Health Plan. *British Medical Journal*, **316**, 1965–8.

Nursing and Midwifery Council (NMC) (2008). *The Code: Standards of Conduct, Performance and Ethics for Nurses and Midwives*. London: Nursing and Midwifery Council.

Further reading

Beauchamp TL and Childress JF (2001). *Principles of Biomedical Ethics*, 5th edn. New York: Oxford University Press.
A standard work for those seeking an in-depth grounding in the ethical basis of professional practice. Good for describing the nature of ethical theories and professional–patient relationships and also the concepts of autonomy, non-maleficence and beneficence.

British Medical Association (2004). *Medical Ethics Today*, 2nd edn. London: BMJ Books.

Hursthouse R (1987). *Beginning Lives*. Oxford: Blackwell.
Written by a philosopher, this book explores the moral status of the fetus and relates it to abortion and women's rights. Also contains a brief but useful overview of the Warnock Report.

Journal of Medical Ethics. http://jme.bmj.com/.
Authoritative source material widely respected in UK for its practical guidance on ethical and legal issues affecting health care.

Kuhse H and Singer P (eds) (2006). *Bioethics: An Anthology*, 2nd edn. Oxford: Blackwell.
A useful book for those who wish to have a deeper understanding of the key current issues in bioethics.

Mason JK and McCall Smith A (2005). *Law and Medical Ethics*, 7th edn. Oxford: Oxford University Press.
An important text that brings together the law and ethics. This book contains strong chapters on issues around the beginning and end of life as well as confidentiality, consent and negligence. Also helpful in helping the reading to understand some population issues, including research. Appendices reproduce a number of codes and declarations.

Nuffield Council on Bioethics. www.nuffieldbioethics.org.
Internationally respected centre examining ethical issues.

10

Care settings

Rosemary Cook

Introduction

This chapter looks at the wide range of settings in which people seek, obtain or undertake for themselves care related to their health. It encourages an approach that looks at health care first from the perspective of the individual rather than the NHS, the wider care system or the professionals working in the system. It also looks at the difference between people's wants, needs and choices related to health care and the setting for care.

The perspectives of the commissioners of health care are explored, together with the many political and practical influences that determine which services are commissioned and the way in which they are delivered. This chapter also looks at the professional and practice issues that arise in different care settings, and the impact on nurses' employment options of the move towards a wider range of care providers in the health care provision 'market'.

Information in this chapter will help you to achieve some of the Nursing and Midwifery Council's (NMC) required standards of proficiency in the domains of professional and ethical practice, care delivery and care management (Appendix 2).

Learning objectives

After studying this chapter you should be able to:

- describe the various influences on individuals' health and choice of health services;
- explain the role of the commissioners of health care;
- identify ways in which nursing practice differs in different settings;
- identify core principles for practice from the NMC Code (2008) (Appendix 1) that apply across all care settings.

Taking the individual's view on care settings

It is tempting to think about care settings in terms of NHS service delivery settings. Any such list is likely to start with hospitals and health centres, followed perhaps by 'the community' and general practitioners (GPs). You might also think in terms of 'primary care' (outside hospitals) and 'secondary care' or 'acute care' (hospitals). This is a 'system-centric' approach, which has two main problems: it excludes a lot of other settings in which people seek or obtain health care, and it does not reflect the way that the vast majority of people experience health care.

Reflection point 10.1

Think about your own experiences of health care (see Box 10.1 on the terminology on health care used in this chapter). List the different settings in which you have sought and/or received health care or information.

You will probably find that you have used a wide variety of sources in many different settings, even if you have never had a serious illness or disability. Notice how many of these settings and sources are outside of the mainstream NHS services.

The depiction of health care in the media – both in the news and in fiction such as television dramas – tends to be 'system-centric'. Hospitals, particularly the more acute areas such as accident and emergency departments, intensive care units and inpatient wards, feature strongly. Outside of hospitals, the media focus is generally on the professionals, such as GPs or district nurses, as 'characters'. It is not surprising, therefore, that people think of health care in terms of its major centres, buildings and professions, rather than in terms of their own needs and how they are best met.

Reviewing your list of settings in which you have received health care or information, check whether they include the following:

- where you were looked after when you were born;
- the school or clinic where you received some of your childhood immunisations;
- your home, where your parents dealt with your minor illnesses and injuries;
- the magazines in which you read health advice;
- the pharmacies and shops where you have bought medicines over the counter for self-administration;
- the occupational health department where you were screened before employment or acceptance on to a course.

Thinking of health care in these much broader terms, and seeing how it links with normal growth and development, helps to demonstrate the perspective of the 'ordinary' individual rather than that of the health care professional. These different perspectives are illustrated in Figure 10.1.

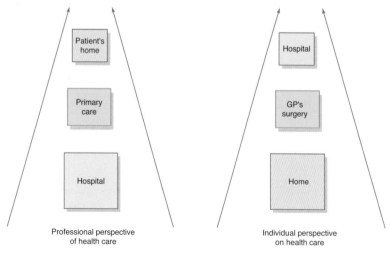

Figure 10.1 Different perspectives on health care settings.

For most individuals, their home is the setting in which they deal with most health issues and from which they access health care and information. Their GP and other community-based professionals are the first port of call for help and advice beyond that which they can obtain from informal sources such as relatives, friends, magazines or television. Hospitals are a much more distant, rarely used source of health care. In fact, 90 per cent of health care interventions are delivered outside of hospitals (DH, 2006a).

It is also important to recognise that, because health issues are part of people's ordinary, home-based lives, they are not neatly compartmentalised as 'health issues' and kept separate from other important aspects of life.

Reflection point 10.2
Write down any other areas of people's lives that you think might have an impact on their health, or make a difference to the way their health needs are expressed or met.

You will probably find that almost every aspect of a person's life has the potential to affect their health. Compare your list with the examples below.

Here are some of the key areas where health and other aspects of a person's daily life overlap:

- *Social circumstances*: for example, being in a close relationship such as marriage has been shown to be beneficial to health (Lee, 2001). Having family, friends or neighbours to talk to and consult can be an alternative to seeking professional advice on health concerns. Difficult relationships with a partner or neighbour can increase stress and the chance of ill health. Having someone prepared to provide practical care can make the difference between needing to go into hospital for treatment or to a residential home, and staying at home. There is some evidence that having a pet has a positive impact on some aspects of health, such as blood pressure and stress (McNicholas *et al.*, 2005).
- *Housing*: housing conditions can cause stress, exacerbate physical illnesses such as asthma, or force a move into residential care if, for example, the home cannot be adapted to accommodate mobility problems.
- *Employment*: some jobs may present physical dangers, exacerbate existing conditions or cause stress-related illness. Unemployment inevitably increases stress, and the reduced family income may predispose to ill health (see below).
- *Income*: lack of money may make healthy choices more difficult in relation to food, exercise and other aspects of lifestyle. A good income can widen the choices of health care. A study from the Institute of Fiscal Studies and University College London found that people are ten times more likely to die in their fifties if they come from the poorest fifth of the population than the richest fifth (Institute of Fiscal Studies, 2006).
- *Neighbourhood*: geographical isolation, lack of transport links or antisocial behaviour in the locality can increase stress and make access to some forms of health care more difficult. 'Good neighbours', involvement in the community, and a sense of 'rootedness' and belonging provide psychological and practical support that can mitigate poor health and change the nature of care needs.

Needs, wants and choices regarding health care settings

What people ask for and receive from health services is rarely a straightforward match. This is inevitable when people's expectations arise from a combination of their needs, their desires and their choices, and when what is available to them depends on a wide range of other factors, including government policy, funding, geography, infrastructure and workforce. These factors affecting the provision of health care will be explored in more detail later in this chapter, and there is more on the influences on people's needs, wants and choices in Chapter 20. For now, we consider how people's needs, wants and choices differ, and how they affect where health care is provided.

Reflection point 10.3
Think of three examples of conditions or circumstances that you would regard as an unequivocal health need. Then check with someone else whether they would agree with you.

Notice that it is difficult to agree on an unequivocal health need, even in what appears to be a very straightforward case, as need is very dependent on circumstances. For example, you might think that a cardiac arrest is a situation when the person's need (for emergency resuscitation) is absolutely undeniable; but if the person is the subject of a 'do not resuscitate' order because of their underlying condition, then this changes the care needed.

Needs, wants and choices are never straightforward to define. They are influenced by many different factors in an individual's life, including the person's:

- cultural and community background;
- access to and understanding of relevant information;
- past experiences and the experiences of others around them;
- degree of mobility and independence;
- physical, mental and emotional health;
- insight into, and ability to express, their views;
- character and personality;
- external circumstances.

An individual may believe they have a need ('I need this tattoo removed'), while a professional might consider it only a 'want'. Conversely, a professional might see a need ('this patient needs to come in for a blood transfusion') that the individual does not accept ('I just want a prescription for some iron tablets'). Different people with exactly the same condition may have different needs because of their social circumstances. Someone living unsupported in an unheated caravan may need to be admitted to hospital for treatment that someone else could have at home, in the view of the health professional assessing them – although the individual may not accept the need for admission. Care that once 'needed' to be given in hospital, such as chemotherapy, intravenous medication and mechanical ventilation, can now be managed with the patient at home. So, individual views and circumstances play a part in deciding where care will be given; there is rarely a single right answer to the question of where a person needs to receive their care; and patient and professional may not agree on what is and is not a care 'need'.

There is similar complexity behind what a person 'wants'. One individual may want to be treated in a day-care centre so that they can go home to their family at night, and another may want to be admitted to hospital because they are lonely at home. The person may want to go to a specialist centre some miles away because of its reputation, or they may reject the 'better' centre because they want to stay close to home. They may want to go farther away not for medical reasons but to escape an abusive home life. However, where health professionals or the health system are geared only to dealing with 'needs', then a person's wants are sometimes disregarded or overruled.

Choice is the area in which there has been most radical change in recent years. In the past, people might have had a view about their own needs and preferences about health care and where they received it, but they had little choice. There were few services provided outside hospitals or their GP's surgery, and their GP decided when and where they would be referred for specialist care. Outpatient and admission appointments were issued without any consultation with the individual about the suitability or convenience of the date. Over recent years, increasing diversity in the types and settings for care provision, and, in England, explicit government policies designed to enable people to choose where and when they are treated (DH, 2005a), have bolstered people's expectations about the degree of choice they should have. So, some people will choose a private hospital over an NHS one, or choose to travel further for treatment in order to avoid local waiting lists. Others will have a choice of a single room or shared bay in hospital, or of end-of-life care in their own home or in a hospice setting. There are, however, many limitations that make choice in health care illusory for some people:

- There is no choice if people are not made aware of the options available.
- Choice is not realistic if someone cannot understand the options and relative risks because of a severe learning disability or mental illness, or because the situation is too urgent for them to have time to consider options.
- Choice is not available to the patient if they are unconscious, although choice may be given instead to relatives.
- Some choices are not available to people in certain circumstances, such as those who are homeless, on low incomes, in prison or being held under provisions in the Mental Health Act.

Where care is asked for and delivered depends on the interaction of the individual's needs, wants and choices, and how the health professionals and health system dealing with them respond to these factors.

Perspectives of different groups of individuals

Although every individual will have their own perspective on health care and where it should happen, filtered through their own needs, wants and choices, there are some broad groupings of people whom we might expect to have similar approaches to the question of care settings because of their shared circumstances. These are:

- people who consider themselves well;
- people with short-term conditions (mental and physical);
- people with long-term conditions (mental and physical);

- people living with disability (mental and physical);
- people with caring responsibilities (including both adult and child carers);
- people needing palliative and terminal care.

Naturally these groups are very fluid, with people moving between them as their circumstances change. It is also important to realise that people may belong to more than one group at any one time. Someone with a long-term mental illness will also develop short-term physical illnesses, but research shows that people with long-term mental illness are less likely to receive good physical health care (Cohen and Hove, 2001). This may be because professionals have stereotyped expectations of the care needs of people with mental illness. People also define themselves as they see themselves: someone with a disability may consider themselves a 'well' person, as long as they don't have a specific physical illness. It is the individual's view, rather than the professionals' view, that should take precedence when planning health promotion, care or treatment.

People who are well may expect little from health services other than information and preventive care, such as screening. They are likely to want to have choices about these services and to receive them at convenient locations and times.

When people have short-term conditions, they usually want rapid access to diagnosis, treatment and advice, but they may not mind who provides it. Convenience and speed of access may be more important than the relationship with the care provider, and so a walk-in centre at a railway station may suit a commuter better than staying at home for an appointment with their GP.

For people with long-term conditions, the relationship with the care provider and continuity of care from someone with knowledge of their history are often more important. An individual may be prepared to travel further and wait longer to see the same professional or to receive care in the same setting.

People who live with a disability have seen, and driven, a significant change in attitudes in recent years. Now they may expect any care needs to be met where they live, with consideration for their convenience and commitments, rather than receiving a standard service based around a hospital or residential setting. They expect health and social aspects of care, and the commissioning of and payment for different aspects of care, to be integrated, not separated. Increasingly, with the advent of individual budgets for social care, some people with disabilities expect to be able to choose and commission much of their own care.

People with caring responsibilities are de facto experts in the care of the person they look after, and they should expect to be consulted about the setting in which routine health care, respite care and supportive care are delivered. They have a lot of valuable experience of health and social services that can benefit the health professionals who take time to listen to them.

When palliative or terminal care is required, people generally expect the options of being cared for at home, in hospital or in a specialist setting, such as a hospice. Continuity of relationships with carers is important, as is the availability of the necessary equipment and specialist expertise for end-of-life care, but these factors have to be balanced against the ability and willingness of the family to cope in different settings.

Reflection point 10.4
Consider each of the circumstances above in relation to you and your family. Where do you think you would expect to receive care, and what would affect your choices, in these circumstances?

In identifying things that affect your choice, have you thought about your personal mobility, the availability of transport, your family's capabilities and other commitments, and the time you have available?

SUMMARY

Individuals' views of health care start from the opposite perspective to the traditional professional or NHS service view, which focuses on hospitals and health centres. For the individual, their home — whatever form that takes — is where health needs and wants arise and are mostly met. The setting in which people receive care depends partly on their needs, wants and choices, and partly on the response of health care professionals and the provisions of the health system. People with different health circumstances will take slightly different views of the health system and what they want from it.

Service commissioners' perspectives of care settings

Commissioning is the process of 'using the available resources to achieve the best outcomes by securing the best possible health and care services for local people' (DH, 2006a). In 2005 commissioners spent £23.6 billion on out-of-hospital health services and £12 billion on adult social care (DH, 2006a). In the provision of free-at-the-point-of-delivery national health services, it is the commissioners of health services who decide in which settings services will be provided, having consulted with local communities.

Who holds responsibility for commissioning health care for patients and communities in the UK depends on the government health policy of the day in each of the four countries of the UK, which determines the structure and roles of health organisations. At the time of writing, commissioning responsibilities are devolved as follows:

- in Scotland, to 14 health boards;
- in Northern Ireland, to four area boards;
- in Wales, to 22 local health boards (LHBs) and local authorities;
- in England, multiprofessional practice-based commissioning groups are beginning to take on the commissioning role, supported by commissioners in primary care trusts (PCTs). The great majority of PCTs are now coterminous with local authorities, which is intended to make joint commissioning for health and social services simpler.

In making their decisions about the setting, nature and amount of health care services, commissioning organisations have to take account of a wide range of factors, as shown in Box 10.2. Some of these will conflict with each other. For example, local people may want a midwife-run birth centre in a small town, when a shortage of midwives means that maternity services have to be consolidated in a single site in the nearest city. Or commissioners may want to close an old community hospital building and reinvest the money in a home visiting team but be thwarted by the geographical size of the area to be covered by the teams. Balancing such considerations within a limited budget is the challenge of commissioning.

Reflection point 10.5
Take one of the factors listed in Box 10.2 and discuss it with a colleague or fellow student. In what way will this factor influence the setting for care? What could be done to change its impact?

BOX 10.2 Factors affecting commissioners' decisions on the setting for health care

- government policy;
- cost of care in each setting;
- geographical factors;
- workforce (generic and specialist) availability;
- infrastructure (existing and planned), e.g. buildings, equipment, transport;
- availability of service providers;
- local factors, e.g. bilingualism;
- local community opinion.

In your discussion, you should have considered how the factor chosen impacts on different community and age groups and come up with some practical suggestions for changing its impact.

Factors affecting the commissioning of care in different settings

Government policies

Policies on settings for care have a significant impact on commissioning decisions. In recent years, there has been a strong policy focus across the UK (DHSSPS, 2004; Scottish Executive, 2005; Welsh Assembly Government, 2005; DH, 2006b) on:

- moving care from acute (hospital) to primary care (community) settings;
- making access to health services easier and more convenient for people, and giving them a choice of services to use;
- integrating health and social care more effectively for all;
- avoiding hospital admission for vulnerable people by focusing on the management of complex care for long-term conditions at home;
- integrating health services with other services for specific groups of people, such as children and older people;
- helping people to change their lifestyle in order to avoid ill health.

In England, there is also a strong policy drive for encouraging a diversity of providers of health care, to include the independent sector and not-for-profit organisations, as well as NHS organisations (DH, 2006b).

Government departments of health expect that commissioners will reflect these policy drivers in their health care commissioning decisions.

Cost

The cost of providing services in different settings is inevitably a strong factor in decision-making. Commissioners have to balance the economies of scale provided by centralised settings against the lower infrastructure costs, but possibly higher workforce costs, of providing care closer to, or in, people's homes. Capital costs of building a new centre for care need to be judged against potential savings if the care provided will be more effective or cheaper to deliver in the new premises.

Geographical factors

Factors such as the area covered by services, distance between centres of population, and population density are taken into account when planning where to deliver care. Solutions for big cities will differ from those in rural areas. When commissioning over a large area, there is frequently a tension between the wishes of local people for a service close to their homes, and insufficient funding to have multiple centres instead of one.

Workforce

The availability of the required workforce expertise – in terms of both numbers and specialist skills – can determine which settings are viable for a service. Commissioners frequently have to weigh the desire for services in local settings with the need to concentrate scarce staff and expertise in one centre further away.

Infrastructure

The condition and suitability of existing buildings and equipment is a key factor. An old hospital building requiring expensive repair might need to be closed against the wishes of local people. Or government investment in a particular type of setting, such as GP surgeries, may mean that these can be purpose-built and other services transferred there.

Providers

The availability of service providers can also influence where care is given. For example, in England, a partnership called 'OwnHealth', between a health authority, a PCT, the telephone helpline NHS Direct and a pharmaceutical company, has been set up to provide follow-up through telephone contact at home to people with long-term conditions. In another example, the nurses and carers from the charity Marie Curie Cancer Care provide care for terminally ill people at home through the night. Areas without these non-traditional provider organisations may have to provide care in other settings.

Local factors

Local factors such as ethnic minority communities and bilingualism may affect the settings for care if some settings are more culturally appropriate, or effective, than others. For example, health promotion targeting Muslim men may be more effective in a mosque than in a traditional health centre.

Community views

When they are considering any changes, commissioners have a statutory duty to consult with local communities and to take account of their views about where services are provided. Commissioners cannot simply decide to make changes to services and to inform the local community of their decision.

Influencing the commissioners

The decisions that commissioners make about where services should be provided are open to influence both by local people and by health professionals.

Reflection point 10.6
Think of three ways in which the public can try to influence decisions about their local services.
Compare your ideas with the paragraphs below.

It is a statutory requirement for health commissioners to hold public consultations when they plan significant change to NHS services. Many such consultations are about reconfiguration of multiple hospital sites or buildings, involving a change in where specific services are provided, or a proposal to close inpatient facilities and provide community-based services instead. These consultations can spark further public action to try to influence decisions about the location of services, including:

- demonstrations at public meetings for or against change;
- letter campaigns to local newspapers or health officials;
- fundraising campaigns to 'save' a service;
- mobilisation of the media or public figures to support or oppose the change.

In more routine circumstances, the public can be involved in service decisions through membership of a foundation trust (Box 10.3), by responding to surveys in their locality or GP's surgery, by voting for local councillors or Members of Parliament who support their favoured option for local health services, or by joining a local patients' forum or action group.

Perhaps most significantly, many people – although not all, depending on their health care needs – have the option of 'voting with their feet' to influence where their services are provided.

BOX 10.3 Public membership of NHS foundation trusts

Residents and patients in areas served by an NHS foundation trust, as well as staff, can register as members of the organisation. Membership allows local communities to have social ownership of their NHS foundation trust. Membership in NHS foundation trusts is currently heading towards the half a million mark.

Members are able to stand and vote in elections for governors of the NHS foundation trust and can expect to receive regular information about the trust and be consulted on plans for its services and future development.

NHS foundation trusts have a duty to engage with local communities and encourage local people to become members and ensure that the membership is representative of the communities they serve. They need to demonstrate that the full range of potential members' interests is represented and that there is a proper balance between different groups.

Becoming a member
Membership of an NHS foundation trust is open to local residents and staff. Individual NHS foundation trusts may provide membership opportunities for people who live outside the area but have been patients or carers at one of the trust's hospitals. There is no limit to the number of people who can register as members, providing they meet the eligibility criteria.

What does being a member mean?
Members of a NHS foundation trust have a number of important roles to perform, as they are able to:

- elect representatives to the board of governors;
- stand for election to the board of governors;
- put themselves forward for appointment as chair of the trust or as non-executive directors on the board of directors.

Source: DH (2005c).

Commissioners sometimes complain that people use accident and emergency departments 'inappropriately' when they should go to their GP's surgery, a walk-in centre or a minor injuries unit; however, rather than being a 'wrong' decision, the choice of the 'inappropriate' setting may indicate that the care in these other settings is failing these people in terms of accessibility, convenience or quality of service. Rather than blaming people for making the 'wrong' choice, commissioners should review what is available in different settings and consult local people about how well it meets their needs.

Practice-based commissioning

Health professionals can also influence the commissioning of care, including where it is provided. The introduction of practice-based commissioning (PBC) (DH, 2005b) in England enables multiprofessional groups of primary care clinicians, including doctors, nurses and allied health professionals, to decide what their local population's health needs are, and where and by whom health services should be provided in order to meet these needs. The PCT commissioners undertake the contracting process and monitor the delivery of the commissioned services on behalf of all the PBC groups in their area. PBC groups can also decide whether they want to provide some services themselves, for example by providing care that is traditionally given in hospital in a home setting or a health centre.

The influences on PBC groups are very similar to those on PCT commissioners. However, as group members are local GPs, nurses or therapists working directly with patients from the local population, there are some differences:

- The professionals may have a clearer idea of the way the local community thinks, and its culture (or cultures). For example, when the primary care groups (PCGs) that preceded PCTs were first set up in England, there was a proposal in a major city to incorporate a particular area into one PCG. Local clinicians warned that this would be a problem because the area was bisected by a major road and local people were very strongly opposed to crossing the road (for cultural rather than physical reasons), preferring to travel further in the other direction. Service providers could not simply treat both sides of the road as one area when local people felt so strongly about the divide.
- Local clinicians may feel more pressure to take people's views into account and find it harder to balance them against more remote factors, such as cost or government policy, when making decisions.

Reflection point 10.7
How would you feel about explaining the pros and cons of different options for services to patients you care for? Would it present you with any ethical dilemmas as a nurse?

You should have taken account of your professional responsibilities under the NMC Code in answering this question. Ethical dilemmas might arise if you found yourself in a situation when your professional responsibility to protect the interests of patients and clients was threatened by a service change that you felt would not be in patients' best interests.

SUMMARY

The organisations that commission health services for local people can decide where these services should be provided. However, they have to take into account a wide range of factors in reaching these decisions, and they will very often have to compromise on the ideal.

Practice-based commissioning brings these decisions into the realm of practising clinicians, who often have good local knowledge of the community and its health care needs.

Different settings for care

Having considered both patients' and service commissioners' perspectives on care settings, it is worth exploring in more detail the variety of settings in which health care can be delivered.

Care at home

More and more 'hands-on' care that would once have required a stay in hospital is now provided in the home. Supported care using technology such as ventilators, parenteral feeding and continuous oxygen therapy is available to people at home. Very complex packages of care for people with multiple, serious or terminal conditions are coordinated by case managers, who may be nurses or other professionals. Health needs and social care needs often overlap, and 'joint assessments' have been introduced to ensure that all the individual's needs are identified and met appropriately. As a result, care in the home can be provided by a combination of nursing and social care staff. The care coordinator – whether the community nurse team leader, case manager or, in England, community matron – can call on other community nurses or allied health professionals, such as therapists, when they are needed, and in some places the care coordinator has the authority to admit people for inpatient care when necessary. Some case management services include the use of remote monitoring technology – which the patient uses to monitor their condition and transmit results through the telephone – in place of some routine staff visits. See Scenario 10.1.

> ### SCENARIO 10.1 Combining case management with technology
>
> Dartford, Gravesham and Swanley Primary Care Trust introduced community matrons as part of its district nurse 'renaissance' project. The community matrons case-manage around 750 local people who have been identified as having frequent hospital admissions, mostly because of long-term conditions such as diabetes and chronic obstructive airways disease. Associate matrons are being introduced to focus on the large cohort of people with cancer-related diagnoses rather than long-term conditions who are also at risk of frequent admission.
>
> Simultaneously, Kent County Council started a pilot scheme that involves more than 200 people with long-term conditions using technology in the home to enable them to monitor their own or their relative's blood pressure, blood sugar, blood oxygen levels, temperature, weight and peak flow (for people with asthma). Results are downloaded securely to the patient's general practice surgery and then reviewed by a doctor or nurse there. Abnormal results are colour-coded on the computer to highlight them, and the clinician responds by contacting the patient to change medication or take other therapeutic action, or to arrange a visit.
>
> When the system was piloted in the USA for people in nursing homes in Seattle, hospital admissions were reduced by 49 per cent, and length of stay for people admitted dropped by a third. The cost of care for these patients fell by 43 per cent.
>
> *Source*: Nolan (2006).

As well as traditional hands-on care, some care in the home is provided remotely without involving local health services. NHS Direct in England, NHS Direct Wales and NHS24 in Scotland, nurse-led telephone helplines, provide advice, information and help with minor illnesses and injuries that are suitable for self-care. Where professional care is required, the caller is referred to their GP, pharmacist, or local accident and emergency department. NHS Direct in

England receives around 6.5 million calls a year, and the related website (www.nhsdirect.nhs.uk) receives more than 1 million visits per month.

Other forms of 'telecare' that have been shown to give positive outcomes or to improve care include telephone or text reminders about appointments or medication regimes, telephone follow-up and counselling, and telephone screening (Future Healthcare Network, 2006).

People also have access to many more elements of health care at home. They can obtain information, guidance and support, and order medicines and genetic testing and diagnostic kits over the Internet. Pharmacies sell diagnostic kits, medical equipment, monitoring devices, and a very wide range of medicines, machines and devices for use at home. This is a clear example of the 'control' of health-related information and products moving away from professionals and into the domain of individuals. Although this helps to encourage a more equal relationship between the individual and their health advisors and carers, it can also increase the individual's concern about their health. There is no quality control on information provided on the Internet, and some of it may be wrong, biased, alarmist or misleading. The ability to test oneself for a condition without any counselling or awareness of the support services available can be traumatic if the result is positive. Nurses need to be aware of these possibilities when dealing with individuals who come for advice or care after using such self-help options.

Reflection point 10.8
Before reading on, identify ten other places outside hospitals where people can go for health advice, care or treatment.
Now compare your list with the settings described below.

Care close to home

Outside of the home, health care is delivered in a wide variety of local settings. As well as the familiar GP surgery and health centre, care is provided in the following:

- *Pharmacies*: increasingly offer confidential consultations and treatments for a range of minor illnesses, long-term conditions and health needs.
- *Workplaces*: offer care through occupational health services, which are often run by nurses.
- *Schools*: school nurses have a major role in health promotion and protection issues, such as immunisation, contraception, dealing with stress, child protection issues (including abuse and bullying), obesity, smoking and substance misuse (DH, 2004).
- *Walk-in centres*, e.g. in railway stations or city centres: these are nurse-led services offering treatment and advice on a drop-in basis; patients do not have to register as they do at a GP's surgery.
- *Nursing and residential homes*: where older, frail or severely disabled people both live and receive care. As many homes are run independently, they are outside the mainstream NHS, and it can be harder to maintain standards of care in line with those within the service. See Scenario 10.2.
- *Supermarkets*: with the introduction of alternative provider medical services contracts, it is now possible for non-traditional organisations to provide primary care services (Box 10.4). Several major supermarkets have expressed interest in employing GPs and nurses to work in their premises offering health care to customers.

SCENARIO 10.2 Improving care for people with diabetes in a care home

A general practice in the Wye Valley found that although 53 per cent of its patients with diabetes received an annual review and glycaemic monitoring, in residential care less than 2 per cent of people with diabetes were managed in this way. The project team developed a multiprofessional assessment tool and introduced training for care staff, new healthier diets for residents, and a programme of diabetes screening by the practice nurse.

By the end of the project, all people with diabetes in the home had had a full assessment of their condition, and all new residents are now screened routinely for the disease. A practice nurse holds a regular clinic in the home to ensure that this standard of care can be maintained.

Source: Queen's Nursing Institute (www.qni.org.uk).

BOX 10.4 Different providers of primary health services

Personal medical services (PMS) are equivalent to general medical services (GMS) – that is, services traditionally provided by general practitioners (GPs). GMS practices must have at least one GP as a partner in the practice.

PMS can be provided by any member of the NHS family, e.g. a doctor, nurse or therapist. There is no need for a GP to be a partner in a PMS practice, although the partnership will need to employ a GP to perform some of the services provided by the practice to meet the needs of the practice population.

Alternative provider personal medical services (APMS) can be provided by partners from outside the NHS family, e.g. private companies and not-for-profit and charitable organizations. Such providers also employ GPs and other professionals to perform the necessary services.

Where no other provider is in place to provide GMS/PMS, these services can be provided by a primary care trust (PCT) – these are known as primary care trust medical services (PCTMS). This is usually on a temporary basis, while the PCT advertises for and appoints a more permanent provider.

No home or temporary home

People who are homeless or living in temporary accommodation can have difficulty accessing mainstream health services. Sometimes they are prevented from registering with a GP because they do not have a permanent address. Their lifestyle, location or limited income can make it impossible for them to keep appointments at designated times or to travel to an out-of-hours centre or duty pharmacy. Homeless people often have serious physical and mental illness, however, and a higher proportion of homeless people than the general population have substance misuse problems (Box 10.5). Health care for these people is often provided in very informal settings, such as drop-in centres or hostels, or from a specially-equipped van or bus.

Health care also needs to be provided to people who are away from home for temporary reasons, such as people detained in prison or police custody suites, many of whom have acute or long-term health needs. The prison population collectively has more ill health and greater health need than the general population (Box 10.6). Since April 2006, PCTs have been fully responsible for commissioning prison health services.

Communities of people who travel as a lifestyle, using their caravan as a permanent home but in temporary locations, use mainstream health services differently from the general population as a consequence. These people are often accused of 'inappropriate' use of GP surgeries and accident and emergency departments, and, because of fear, prejudice or practical difficulties, sometimes

BOX 10.5 Health needs of homeless people

- Homeless people are 40 times more likely than the general public not to be registered with a GP (based on interviews with 100 hidden homeless people in London; Crisis, 2002a).
- 55 per cent had no contact with a GP in the previous year (Crisis, 2002a).
- Compared with the general population, people in hostels and bed-and-breakfasts are twice as likely, and rough sleepers three times as likely, to have chronic chest and breathing problems (Crisis, 2003).

Addictions

- 81 per cent of homeless people are addicted to drugs or alcohol. Heroin comes top of the league, followed by alcohol (Crisis, 2002b).
- Two-thirds of homeless people cite drug or alcohol use as a reason for becoming homeless (Crisis, 2002b).
- Four in five homeless people have started using at least one new drug while homeless (Crisis, 2002b).
- People who are dependent on drugs or alcohol are almost twice as likely as non-dependent users to be banned from homelessness services (Crisis, 2002b).

Mental health

- Women have a higher percentage of mental health problems than men (Crisis, 2003).
- Mental health problems are up to eight times more common in the homeless population (Bines, 1994).
- Nine per cent of households accepted as unintentionally homeless and in priority need by local authorities in 2004 are in priority need due to mental illness (ODPM, 2005).

Source: www.crisis.org.uk.

BOX 10.6 Health needs of prisoners

- Prisoners have a very high incidence of mental health problems (in particular, neurotic disorders), compared with the general population. By International Statistical Classification of Diseases and Related Health Problems (ICD-10) criteria, in any week, almost half of prisoners have a neurotic disorder such as anxiety or depression.
- One in ten prisoners has had a psychotic disorder in the past year.
- Suicide is about eight times more common among prisoners than in an equivalent community population.
- Incidents of deliberate self-harm are reported in 1 in 60 prisoners per year.
- Half of prisoners are heavy alcohol users, and about 1 in 20 has a serious alcohol problem.
- About half of prisoners are dependent on drugs (mainly opiates, cannabis and stimulants), and at least one-quarter of prisoners have injected drugs. A minority of prisoners continue to use drugs while in prison.
- One in four adult prisoners has engaged in activities likely to put them at risk of infection with human immunodeficiency virus (HIV), hepatitis B or hepatitis C.

Source: Marshall *et al.* (2000).

they do not receive continuity of care for medical problems, preventive health screening and education. This has a measurable impact on the health of travellers – a male traveller's average life expectancy is 10 years less, and a female traveller's 12 years less, than that of people in settled accommodation (Barry *et al.*, 1989). In some places, the health needs of this group of people are addressed by taking health care to the travellers' site (see Scenario 10.3); in others, the health

SCENARIO 10.3 Care for travellers

In a project funded by the Queen's Nursing Institute and the Burdett Trust for Nursing, a health visitor in Essex is improving the health of a large group of Irish travellers by providing an outreach clinic in a mobile police unit on the site. At the start of the project, 60 per cent of the travellers were not registered with a GP, and 70 per cent of the women had not had any ante- or postnatal care. Ninety per cent of the men had never seen a doctor or had any health screening. Many of the travellers were illiterate and unaware of the existence of preventive health care. On the first day that the clinic was held on the site, there were 44 visits from residents in 4 hours. Since then, 50–60 people have attended each clinic session, and the health visitor has started health education sessions using visual materials displayed on a laptop computer.

Following the introduction of the clinic sessions, local environmental health officers have booked sessions to work with the community on sanitation and water testing. A Catholic nun also visits the site to deliver pre-confirmation classes to the children of this largely Catholic community. One local GP practice reports that 'inappropriate' visits have fallen by 80 per cent.

Source: the Queen's Nursing Institute (www.qni.org.uk).

needs are addressed by working to ensure that travellers are accepted into mainstream services through registration with a GP surgery.

For all people with a temporary home or mobile lifestyle, who may use many different services and see many different professionals for health care, continuity of care and the care record is a key issue. The National Programme for Information Technology (NPfIT), currently being implemented in England by the Connecting for Health (CfH) agency, aims to implement new systems, including an electronic patient record that is accessible from any health care setting, which should help to mitigate the problem of continuity and sharing records (Box 10.7). The Scottish Executive also plans to introduce a single electronic health record for every patient (Scottish Executive, 2005).

BOX 10.7 National Programme for IT in England

NHS Connecting for Health (CfH) is an agency of the Department of Health set up to deliver the National Programme for IT (NPfIT) in the NHS (www.connectingforhealth.nhs.uk). The programme consists of seven key elements:

- *NHS Care Records Service (NHS CRS)*: provides 'an individual electronic NHS care record for every patient in England, securely accessible by patients and those caring for them'.
- *Choose and Book*: an electronic appointment booking service 'offering patients greater choice of hospitals or clinics and more convenience in the date and time of their appointment'.
- *Electronic Prescription Service (EPS)*: enables prescriptions to be transferred from GP to pharmacy electronically.
- *New National Network (N3)*: 'the IT infrastructure and broadband connectivity for the NHS so patient information can be shared between organisations'.
- *Contact*: a central email and directory service for the NHS, enabling the secure transfer of patient information between staff.
- *Picture archiving and communication systems (PACS)*: 'to capture, store, display and distribute static and moving digital medical images, providing clearer x-rays and scans and faster, more accurate diagnosis'.
- *IT for GPs*: including the Quality Management and Analysis System (QMAS), support for the GPs' Quality and Outcomes Framework, and a system for GP-to-GP record transfer.

Care further away

When care is required (or a person thinks it is required) beyond that available through the various services described above, the setting for care tends to move further away from the individual's home. Appointments in hospital outpatient clinics and attendances at accident and emergency departments are two examples. In these settings, care – whether diagnostic, educational or therapeutic – is delivered in a setting unfamiliar and considerably less convenient to most people. A wait for a clinic appointment is required, sometimes with a further wait on the day of the appointment or visit. Considerable travel, and associated costs may be involved, which may be particularly difficult for people with mobility problems, caring responsibilities at home, or low incomes. For some people, the hospital is an intimidating environment and may be associated with the serious illness or death of a relative. All of these factors affect the individual's demeanour and behaviour when they attend for care.

Another example of more distant care is attendance at an independent treatment centre (ITC). The first wave of ITCs was established as part of the government's drive to increase the number of people treated as day cases rather than being admitted to hospital overnight for surgery. ITCs carry out some of the more common surgical treatments, such as cataract surgery and hernia repairs, for which long waiting lists have built up. Some ITCs are run by private companies under contract to the NHS, an approach that may be unfamiliar to patients attending for surgery. Being treated and discharged on the same day may be more convenient and less intimidating to the patient than being admitted to a hospital overnight. Alternatively, it can be more stressful and frightening, as the individual has to rely on family or friends for postoperative care and support.

'Going in' for care

Community hospitals, district general hospitals, local hospices and respite centres provide the most distant care both psychologically and geographically. Although some individuals may travel many miles for an outpatient consultation at a specialist centre, this is still quite different in terms of its impact on the person's life compared with being admitted to hospital as an inpatient. If the hospital to which they are admitted is also geographically remote – for example, because it is a specialist centre with a wide catchment area – then the impact is even greater.

> **Reflection point 10.9**
> Pause and think about how it might feel to be admitted to hospital a long way from home. What practical effect would this have on the individual and their family? What would be the psychological impact? How could you as a nurse help the patient and their family when they come from another part of the country?

You should have considered issues related to visiting at long distance, such as loneliness and isolation; unfamiliar surroundings, accents and local idioms; and arranging transport home. To help, you might have considered giving information on the local area, explaining the hospital's surroundings and layout, being flexible about visiting hours and numbers of visitors, arranging for easy use of a telephone, and early discharge planning.

Within the inpatient hospital arena, there are many different settings for care, each having a different impact on the individual and requiring a different approach from nurses involved in caring for the individual. Practical, psychological, spiritual and emotional care are different in intensive care units compared with children's wards, and in maternity units compared with oncology centres. The principle of adapting care to ensure that it meets the individual's needs as fully as possible, and in the most acceptable way for the individual, applies as much in different parts of the hospital setting as in the person's home.

SUMMARY

Many conditions that would once have been treated in hospital are now treated at home. There is a wide variety of other settings in local communities where people seek and receive health information, advice and care. There are also many opportunities for people to obtain information, diagnosis, medication and equipment without consulting a health professional. Being admitted to hospital is psychologically different from receiving care in other settings, and the hospital itself provides a range of different environments, each requiring a different approach to nursing care. The familiarity or strangeness of the setting, and its distance from the individual's home or family, affects how the person reacts and behaves in receiving care. Nurses have to be prepared to adapt their care and approach for the maximum benefit of the individual in each setting.

Professional and practice issues in different care settings

The different settings for health care are more than mere geographical or organisational variations on a theme. Nursing care – in fact, the delivery of health care in general – has to adapt to each environment of care, and nurses need to be aware of, and respond to, some key issues that present differently in different settings.

Issues to be aware of include:

- variations in the physical environment and the equipment available;
- the degree of teamwork or isolation they experience in delivering care;
- maintenance of the quality of care in different circumstances;
- continuity of care and information;
- different relationships with patients in different settings;
- legal issues in different settings;
- different employers and their expectations.

The physical environment

It is clearly easier to perform a sterile or complicated procedure in a well-equipped, well-maintained hospital ward, GP surgery or independent treatment centre, with a range of equipment and other team members to hand, than alone with the patient in a living room or a caravan. However, it would be wrong to assume that informal settings are always less clean and more difficult to nurse in. People treated outside of hospitals are, of course, less likely to pick up a hospital-acquired infection, and their home environment may be at least as clean as the hospital.

Where it is difficult to carry out procedures according to the usual protocols, then it is the underlying principles, and the use of professional judgement in applying them in the context, that matter. The intention must always be to provide care to the highest standard possible in the circumstances.

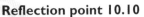

Reflection point 10.10
Look at the NMC Code and discuss the requirements of the section headed 'Provide a high
standard of practice and care at all times', in relation to your experience of providing care.

You should have considered times in your experience when you have (i) undertaken learning
activities, (ii) checked that you were competent to perform a task given, (iii) considered whether
your care was based on the best available evidence, and (iv) completed clear and accurate records.

Safeguarding the patient's confidentiality, privacy and dignity will present different challenges
in different environments. A busy ward with only screens between beds, or a crowded family
living room, can threaten confidentiality and may affect what the individual feels able to tell or
show you. On the other hand, in a quiet corner of a hostel or during a telephone call, you may
find out much more about a person than you expected to. It is important to do everything possible to provide the privacy the patient needs, while recognising that you can only negotiate with –
not give orders to – the individual and the others present. Sometimes, inventive and subtle ways
are needed to meet the individual's needs for care or information when privacy is threatened (see
Scenario 10.4).

It is important to recognise that the duty of confidentiality applies as much in informal settings
close to home as in hospital. The closeness of other family members, a long-term relationship
with a family, and the informality of the encounters can make it more difficult to resist sharing
information or answering concerned questions. Unless the individual receiving care explicitly
gives permission, however, the information should not be shared.

**SCENARIO 10.4 Ingenuity in practice: providing information on domestic
violence**

A project in Enfield provided training to more than 200 health professionals to enable them to
find effective ways of asking patients about domestic violence, and to identify and help those who
disclose abuse.

Information about emergency helplines, tips on leaving an abusive situation safely, and how and
where to find emergency support was produced for victims of violence. As simply possessing
such information can provoke further violence if it is discovered by the abuser, the information
was produced in forms that could be easily concealed, such as on bookmarks, on 'credit-cards' and
in a fold-up form designed to be hidden in a bra.

Source: Queen's Nursing Institute (www.qni.org.uk).

Supervision and isolation

Settings where individuals' care is delivered in the context of a physically adjacent team, such as
a ward, clinic or surgery, provide the opportunity to consult others if you are unsure or concerned
about something. Colleagues from nursing or other professions can be called on to advise, witness, protect or assist within a matter of minutes. This contrasts with nursing undertaken in the
home, school, hostel or workplace, when the nurse may be the only health professional present.
In these latter settings, it is important to consider both professional security – where and how you
could get help or advice if needed – and personal security. (For more on working in isolated settings, see Chapter 20.)

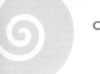
Quality of care

Although technical nursing practices may need to differ in different settings, and inventive ways of delivering care may be needed, the aim should be that the quality of care is constant across care settings. If you find it impossible to provide care of sufficient quality, then the NMC Codes states: 'you must report your concerns in writing if problems in the environment of care are putting people at risk'.

Continuity of care and information

The more settings people use for their health care, the more important it is that health professionals are aware of the treatment, advice, referrals and information that their colleagues have given to the individual. At best, conflicting practice can cause confusion and distress to the patient; at worst, the patient's health can be compromised by, for example, inappropriate multiple prescribing or lack of communication about their condition. Traditionally, information has been passed from GP to hospital and vice versa via referral letters and discharge letters. Copies in the hospital patient's record ensured that this information was available to other teams if the individual was admitted again. Copies in the GP-held record (paper and/or computer) ensured that the GP and primary care team had access to it. This information is not always shared routinely with community nursing teams, however, who may hold their own nursing records; further information may be held on disease registers, by other non-nursing professionals and by staff in walk-in centres attended by the individual. The introduction of parent-held records for babies, shared maternity records, and special records for conditions such as asthma and diabetes were all attempts to ensure continuity of the record, and so of treatment, by making the individual responsible for holding and sharing their own information.

Part of the NPfIT in England is a plan to introduce nationally an electronic patient record, already being trialled in some places, which will in future be securely accessible by both health professionals and the individual to whom it relates. The record can then be used in any setting for care, in order to ensure that the health professionals assessing or treating the individual have all the relevant information immediately available to help decision-making. A similar electronic record is to be introduced in Scotland.

Relationships with patients

More than the tangible differences in equipment, environment and processes for care, it is the nature of the relationship between nurses and those for whom they care that most differentiates the various settings for care. Writing about the difference between hospital and community settings generally, Carr (2001) describes the central issue as 'control distribution', which, she says:

> . . . is not as simple as being on one 'home-ground' or another i.e. the nurse having more control in the hospital and the patient more control in their own home. It [is] about practising to a 'real life agenda' where levels of passivity and assertiveness are dynamically negotiated in relationships. The differences between hospital and community may be explained by suggesting that the 'false' and 'temporary' environment of the hospital settings imposes a change in the normal dynamics of the relationships which is not so vigorously imposed in the community setting. Practitioners are also engaged in accommodating to the patient's life.

Reflection point 10.11

Think about the statement quoted above in relation to non-hospital settings other than the individual's home. What do you think would be different about negotiating care with someone in (i) a care home, (ii) a walk-in centre and (iii) a GP's surgery?

You should have considered, in each case, the differences in the individual's options, in the balance of power between patient and professional, in the length or brevity of the expected relationship, and in the potential consequences to the individual of non-compliance with the professional's suggestions.

Some of the elements of the real-life agenda that will influence the relationship and negotiation between you as a nurse and the individual seeking or being offered care in different settings include:

- the person's perception of themselves, especially if they consider themselves 'well' or at least 'getting by', and so have a 'take it or leave it' attitude to health information or care;
- the other demands on their life, such as children, job, family, hobbies and cultural demands;
- the balance between how much the person feels they need information or care, and how much effort is required to obtain it;
- the 'cost' of the care, both financially such as prescription charges and travel to clinics, as well as time and opportunity costs and the emotional cost of ceding some control to the professional.

These are factors which carry different weight in different care settings and vary between individuals. They are different to those that apply to the relationship between nurses and patients in hospital. To be successful in caring for people in all care settings, it is essential to be sensitive to the different dynamics and to be prepared to negotiate agreement with each individual.

Legal issues

Consent to treatment almost always has to be negotiated with an individual, whatever setting they are in, other than in very specific circumstances. However, when a person presents for treatment at recognised health premises, such as a hospital or GP surgery, then the seeking of consent starts from a mutual expectation that some form of care is both needed and desired.

The situation may not be so straightforward in other settings. In mental health care, for example, nurses need to be aware of the provisions of the Mental Health Act regarding compulsory detention and treatment. There are specific requirements for establishing the need for such treatment, and for the activation of appropriate authority to detain and treat, which are subject to regular review. If you are going to work in such services, you should be given, or seek, the most up-to-date information, together with the policies and procedures of your employing organisation, through which it is put into practice.

When caring for people in their own home, the nurse or other professional has no legal right of entry to the home, even if they believe that the individual or a member of the family needs care. This is one of the clearest examples of the importance of building effective relationships with individuals, and practising the art of negotiation, in order to successfully balance two requirements of the NMC Code: to 'work with others to protect and promote the health and wellbeing of those in your care' and to 'respect and support people's rights to accept or decline treatment and care'.

There are other situations in which legal requirements impinge on the delivery of health care in specific settings, notably when caring for people in police custody suites and prison settings. The timing, nature and extent of care, and the availability of treatments, may be limited by the setting and the legal processes involving the individual.

As always, when caring in these settings, you need to adhere to the laws of the country in which you are practising, as well as employers' policies and procedures, and, within those constraints, to protect and support the health of your patient or client.

More areas of law that affect practice in health care in community settings are discussed in Chapter 20.

Different employers

There are many different employers for whom nurses may work in order to deliver care in these different environments, including the following:

- *The NHS*: in the case of most hospitals and current community-based services, primary care services for prisons, and most walk-in centres.
- *Private companies*: for some hospitals, some walk-in centres and independent treatment centres, a few GP practices, some schools, most care homes and almost all workplaces.
- *Charities*: increasingly for specialist care provision and advice, e.g. Marie Curie Cancer Care, British Heart Foundation, Terence Higgins Trust, Turning Point.
- *Social enterprises*: in various legal forms, including mutual organisations, cooperatives and limited companies, sharing the principle of reinvestment of profit for the benefit of the enterprise, for some community nursing services, out-of-hours triage and treatment services, and primary medical care services.
- *General practitioners*: for primary care services, including 'first contact' care, care of long-term conditions, and screening and immunisation programmes that are largely delivered by nurses.
- *Local authorities*: for integrated health and social care services, some public health roles, residential care and some children's services.

Although the NMC Code always applies to registered nurses and midwives, regardless of who employs them, NHS terms and conditions of service, protocols and practices do not apply when nurses are employed by other bodies. Each employer has its own terms and conditions of service and expects nurses employed by it to work to its policies and procedures. Many nurses work very successfully for non-NHS employers, and current government policy in England is encouraging more diversity of providers in health care (DH, 2006b), which is likely to increase this proportion. For some nurses, the different nature of the employing organisation can cause concern, for example where they feel that pressure to work in the most profitable way for a private company could adversely affect the quality of patient care. The NMC Code states specifically that 'you must ensure that your professional judgement is not influenced by any commercial considerations' in its section headed 'Be open and honest, act with integrity and uphold the reputation of your profession'.

SUMMARY

Each different setting for health care generates a range of practical and professional issues that nurses must take into account when planning, offering and providing care. The requirements of the NMC Code are invariable and provide the bedrock for practice in any setting. The organisation for which the nurse works is one of the variables, and a large and increasing number of nurses work outside of the NHS. Where the expectations of employers or the environment for care jeopardises optimal patient care, the nurse has a duty to report it and try to remedy it, in line with the professional obligations of the NMC Code.

CONCLUSION

Learning to provide optimal and effective nursing care requires far more than the acquisition of theoretical knowledge and technical skills. It requires a conscious focus on the perspectives of individuals needing or seeking care in order to begin to understand the factors that influence not only their health but also their decisions and choices about asking for and receiving health care. It is important to recognise the many different sources of health information, support, advice and treatment now available that do not involve the traditional health services or professionals at all.

The settings in which health care, including nursing care, is delivered have never been so diverse. Government policies across the UK have encouraged a much greater focus on the provision of care in settings other than hospitals, and the growth of new care settings and new health care organisations provide new employment opportunities for nurses and other professionals. The most significant changes to nursing careers in recent years have been largely implied rather than acknowledged in documents about the future of nursing. Where once the majority of nurses would expect to spend their careers working in hospitals, many more will now work outside hospitals; and where they would have expected to spend their career employed by the NHS, many more will work for other health care organisations.

With regard to care settings, the principal aim for nurses in training should be twofold:

- to develop the confidence to use their skills and knowledge in a variety of settings, and with due regard for the unique circumstances of every individual requiring care;
- to base their practice on the principles of the NMC Code, and exercise those principles within their employer's policies and procedures.

References

Barry J, Herity B and Solan J (1989). *The Travellers' Health Status Study: Vital Statistics of Travelling People 1987*. Dublin: Health Research Board.

Bines W (1994). The Health of Single Homeless People. York: Centre for Housing Policy, University of York.

Carr S (2001). Community nursing: does the title fit the talents? *Journal of Community Nursing*, **15**.

Cohen A and Hove M (2001). *Physical Health of the Severe and Enduring Mentally Ill: A Training Pack for GP Educators*. London: Sainsbury Centre for Mental Health.

Crisis (2002a). *Critical Condition: Homeless People's Access to GPs*. London: Crisis.

Crisis (2002b). *Home and Dry? Homelessness and Substance Use*. London: Crisis.

Crisis (2003). *Homelessness Factfile*. London: Crisis.

Department of Health (DH) (2004). *Choosing Health: Making Healthy Choices Easier*. London: Department of Health.

Department of Health (DH) (2005a). *Creating a Patient-Led NHS: Delivering the NHS Improvement Plan*. London: Department of Health.

Department of Health (DH) (2005b). *Commissioning a Patient-Led NHS. Letter from Sir Nigel Crisp*. London: Department of Health.

Department of Health (DH) (2005c). *A Short Guide to NHS Foundation Trusts*. London: Department of Health.

Department of Health (DH) (2006a). *Health Reform in England: Update and Commissioning Framework*. London: Department of Health.

Department of Health (DH) (2006b). *Our Health, Our Care, Our Say: A New Direction for Community Services*. London: Department of Health.

Department of Health, Social Services and Public Safety (DHSSPS) (2004). *A Healthier Future: A Twenty Year Vision for Health and Wellbeing in Northern Ireland*. Belfast: Department of Health, Social Services and Public Safety.

Future Healthcare Network (2006). *Telecare and Telecaring*. London: NHS Confederation.

Institute of Fiscal Studies (2006). Longitudinal study of ageing reveals health and wealth relationship. Press release. London: Institute of Fiscal Studies.

Lee A (2001). Married to good health. *Psychology Today*, **34**, 26.

Marshall T, Simpson S and Stevens A (2000). *Health Care in Prisons: A Health Care Needs Assessment*. Birmingham: University of Birmingham.

McNicholas J, Gilbey A, Rennie A, *et al.* (2005). Pet ownership and human health: a brief review of evidence and issues. *British Medical Journal*, **331**, 1252.

Nolan A (2006). Teleaddicts. *Health Service Journal*, **116**, 10–11.

Nursing and Midwifery Council (NMC) (2008). *The Code: Standards of Conduct, Performance and Ethics for Nurses and Midwives*. London: Nursing and Midwifery Council.

Scottish Executive (2005). *Delivering for Health*. Edinburgh: Scottish Executive Health Department.

Office of the Deputy Prime Minister (ODPM) (2005). *Best Value Performance Indicators 2005/06: Guidance Document*. London: Office of the Deputy Prime Minister.

Welsh Assembly Government (2005). *Designed for Life: Creating World Class Health and Social Care for Wales in the 21st Century*. Cardiff: Welsh Assembly Government.

Further reading

Communities and Local Government. www.communities.gov.uk.
Government department set up in 2006 with responsibility for communities, including homelessness, housing, social inclusion and equality.

Department of Health. www.dh.gov.uk.

Department of Health, Social Services and Public Safety, Northern Ireland. www.dhsspsni.gov.uk.

Home Office. www.homeoffice.gov.uk.
Discusses issues relating to drugs, antisocial behaviour, prisons and victims of crime.

Kai J (2003). *Ethnicity, Health and Primary Care*. Oxford: Oxford University Press.
Gives a detailed account of the impact of ethnicity on health, and the challenges to health services to meet different needs.

Nursing and Midwifery Council. www.nmc-uk.org.

Primary Care Contracting. www.primarycarecontracting.nhs.uk.
Provides information on new forms of contracting for the delivery of primary medical services by non-traditional providers, e.g. nurse-led surgeries, and services provided, e.g. private companies.

Queen's Nursing Institute. www.qni.org.uk.
Charity providing project grants and professional information and support to nurses in primary and community care.

Scottish Executive Health Department. www.scotland.gov.uk.

Timmins N (2006). *Designing the 'new' NHS: Ideas to Make a Supplier Market in Health Care Work.* London: King's Fund.
Report of an independent working party that looks in detail at the English government's aim to bring new providers into health care, and the implications for the role of the NHS as a 'brand' rather than a service.

Wanless D (2003). *Review of Health and Social Care in Wales.* Cardiff: Welsh Assembly Government.
This report looked at the provision of health and social care in Wales and concluded that the then current position was unsustainable. The report recommended that there should be a strategic adjustment of services to focus on prevention and early intervention, and that the public health agenda should be given primacy.

Wanless D (2004). *Securing Good Health for the Whole Population: Final Report.* London: HM Treasury.
Derek Wanless' 2002 report Securing Our Future Health: Taking a Long-Term View set out an assessment of the resources required to provide high-quality health services in the future in England. This final report considers the consistency of current policy with the public health aspects of the scenario in which people are 'fully engaged' with their health, outlined in the 2002 report.

Welsh Assembly Government Health and Social Care Department. www.wales/subihealth/index.htm.

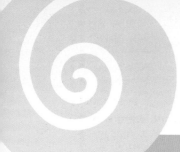

Nursing in an electronic world

June Clark

11

Introduction

Information communication technology (ICT) pervades every aspect of life in the twenty-first century. We use mobile phones to communicate by both speech and text. Every item that we buy in a supermarket carries a barcode that enables automatic stock control. We have digital radio and digital television. We have MP3s. We bank via the Internet and draw money from the 'hole in the wall'. We use the Internet for shopping, booking our holidays and finding out all kinds of information.

Learning objectives

After studying this chapter you should be able to:

- identify examples of the use of ICT in your health care practice;
- ensure that you are familiar with the terminology of ICT;
- realise the importance of nursing documentation;
- discuss the value of a single patient record;
- reflect on the pros and cons of electronic patient records;
- state the significance of nursing diagnoses.

e-Health: getting ICT into health care

Strangely, we have been slow to incorporate ICT into health care – much slower than, for example, banking or the entertainment industry. In particular, nursing has been slow to incorporate ICT into nursing practice. But all that is now changing – and fast. ICT is now seen as the key to the 'modernisation' of our health care system, and the governments of all four countries of the UK are implementing national programmes for the introduction of ICT into the NHS. The detail of the programmes and the stage of development in each country varies, but within the next few years nurses throughout the UK will be using computerised systems for:

- access to guidelines, protocols and research for evidence-based practice;
- communicating (voice and text messages) with other health professionals and with patients and carers;
- nursing documentation and patient records;
- ordering and receiving test results (including X-rays) and drugs;
- referrals and transfers of care across services (e.g. discharge from hospital);
- administrative procedures to book appointments, organise staffing and manage budgets.

Nurses working in particular areas or specialist services may also be using:

- decision support systems, such as currently used by NHS Direct and NHS24;
- video links with a doctor many miles away to diagnose or advise on the care of a patient;
- systems for monitoring a patient's physiological measurements (e.g. blood sugar, blood pressure) when the patient is in a place (e.g. their home) remote from the nurse (e.g. at the hospital);
- sensors to detect when a frail or elderly person in their own home falls or wanders into an unsafe environment (telecare).

All of these things are available and in use in some places now. They are likely to rapidly become available more widely and improve in quality, and new technologies are developing all the time. A report by the Royal Society (2006) called *Digital Healthcare: The Impact of Information and Communication Technologies on Health and Healthcare* describes developments in information technology (IT) within the next decade that, if applied in health care, will dramatically change the way we work.

Predicting the future is notoriously risky, and some predictions may turn out to be wrong – things may move even further and faster than anyone imagines. A book published in 1977 called *Science Fact: Astounding and Exciting Developments that Will Transform Your Life* stated:

> *The idea of everyone having a hand-held or wristwatch-sized transmitter and receiver to communicate with other people anywhere in the world is still in the realm of science fiction and unlikely ever to move out of it.*

(George, 1977)

Now, less than 30 years after this book was published, mobile phones that do exactly this are used by millions of people all over the world, and can record, store and transmit pictures, music and speech.

What is clear is that IT will dramatically change the way that nurses work. In particular, it will both drive and enable the following:

- *More patient-centred and patient-controlled care*: patients will have access (e.g. via the Internet) to as much information about their condition and treatment options as the health professionals who are caring for them. This will change the professional–client relationship by increasing the power of patients to challenge what professionals tell them and to negotiate their treatment.
- *More dispersed care*: there will be no need for patients to go to a hospital or for nurses to visit patients at home simply to monitor physiological measurements (e.g. blood sugar, blood pressure, heart rate) or to check on medications – the data from body sensors can be transmitted directly to the doctor or nurse, who can immediately transmit advice if needed.
- *Evidence-based care*: front-line nurses will have immediate online access to, for example, best practice guidelines and protocols, and nurse managers will use aggregated patient data to make decisions about staffing, resource management and service planning.
- *New ways of recording information*: for example, electronic patient records.

These new ways of working will require nurses to develop new skills. Information management must become a core skill for all nurses, including how to get, how to record, how to retrieve and how to use the information, how to communicate the information, and how to incorporate the use of IT as an integral part of their practice. This means not only having basic computer skills (e.g. how to use a computer, how to use a particular information system) but also understanding what information is necessary in order to support nursing practice, how this information is represented in information systems, and how to find, manipulate and use the information. In addition to information management, nurses will need other new skills, such as how to manage a consultation and the nurse–patient relationship when the nurse and the patient are not physically face to face, and completely new ways of thinking about nursing.

To younger nurses who have been brought up on computer games and mobile phones, using IT will be no problem. But for more mature entrants, and especially for older nurses who have been in practice for 20–30 years, this will involve a major cultural change and having to learn many new skills. For all of us, it requires new ways of thinking about nursing, for example in ways that were discussed in Chapter 3.

Understanding the jargon

The technological developments have required the development of new terms to describe them, and the terminology is still evolving. Some of the terms used are explained in Box 11.1.

The term 'e-health', which is currently used to refer to the whole scope of the use of ICT in health care, includes:

- methods of accessing knowledge for evidence-based practice (e.g. research, protocols, guidelines) or patients accessing knowledge about their conditions, services and treatments;
- electronic patient records;
- methods of monitoring patients' physiological measurements;
- systems for ordering and receiving test results (including X-rays) and drugs;
- systems for referrals or transfers of care across services (e.g. discharge from hospital) or among the members of a multiprofessional team;
- telephone advice services supported by decision support systems, such as NHS Direct and NHS24;

BOX 11.1 Understanding the jargon

- *Information management (IM)*: obtaining, processing and using data (the raw elements or pieces that together make up the information) to create knowledge and support decision-making. Since clinical decision-making depends on information, and nursing is defined as 'the use of clinical judgement in the provision of care' (RCN, 2003), IM is at the heart of nursing practice and is a core skill required by every nurse.
- *Information technology (IT)*: or, more correctly, information and communication technology (ICT) – the technology or set of tools that enables information to be managed – that is, to be collected, recorded, stored, processed and transmitted. IT includes hardware and software.
- *Hardware*: devices such as computers, personal digital assistants (PDAs) and mobile phones that contain data and software.
- *Software*: instructions (written in programs) held electronically inside the computer that tell the computer what to do with the data that it contains.
- *Telemedicine*: use of ICT (e.g. a video conferencing link) to enable a doctor in one place to examine a patient located in another place. The term has been widened to include *telenursing*, for example when a nurse uses a webcam link to the patient's television set at home to monitor medication or to provide advice and support.
- *Telecare (assistive technology)*: delivery of health care to individuals within their home or in the wider community, with the support of devices enabled by ICT, such as sensors to detect when a person falls.
- *Informatics*: science that underpins the use of ICT; the combination of computer science and information science that is concerned with generating, recording, classifying, processing, analysing, retrieving and transmitting information. *Health informatics* is the application of this science in health and health care. *Nursing informatics* combines computer science and information science with nursing science to do all of this in support of nursing.
- *Telehealth, e-health and digital health care*: overarching terms to refer to the whole scope of the use of ICT in health care.

- a doctor or nurse using a video link to diagnose or advise on the care of a patient while separated by distance (telemedicine, telenursing);
- the use of sensors to detect when a frail or elderly person in their own home falls or wanders into an unsafe environment (telecare);
- administrative systems to support staffing and resource management.

Data that are collected as part of any of these activities may also subsequently be retrieved and analysed and used for other purposes, such as audit, research, epidemiology, service planning and policy development.

The stories contained in Boxes 11.2 (below) and 11.3 (see p. 231) give some illustrations of nursing practice using ICT. This chapter discusses just one application of IT in nursing practice – nursing documentation using computerised patient records.

BOX 11.2 Nursing in 2020: Rachel

This story, which describes a typical morning for a Canadian nurse in 2020, was published in a Canadian nursing journal in 1995. Even at that time, all the technology required was already available and in use somewhere in the world.

The computer gently hums to life as community health specialist Rachel Muhammat logs into NurseNet. She asks a research partner, a cyberware specialist in London, England, for the results from a trial on neurological side effects of ocular biochips. Rachel, as part of a 61 member research team in 23 countries, is studying six clients with the chips. Then it's down to local business. Rachel e-mails information on air contaminant syndrome to a client down the street whose son is susceptible to the condition, and tells her about a support group in Philadelphia. She contacts a Quigong specialist to see if he can teach the boy breathing exercises, and schedules an appointment with an environmental nurse specialist. Moments before her 9.45 appointment, Rachel gets into her El-van and programs it to an address two kilometres away. Her patient, Mr. Chan, lost both legs in a subway accident and needs to be prepared for a bionic double leg transplant. Together they assess his needs and put together a team of health workers: surgeon, physiotherapist, acupuncturist, and home care helpers. She talks to him about the transplant; they hook up to his virtual reality computer to see and talk to another client who underwent the same procedure. Before leaving, Mr Chan grasps her hand and thanks her for helping him. Rachel hugs him and urges him to e-mail her if he has any more questions.

(Sibbald, 1995) Reprinted with permission from the Canadian Nurses Association.

Note in particular:

- Rachel is what we would call a 'nurse practitioner'.
- Rachel's work base could be anywhere, and not necessarily in a hospital.
- Research and the development of nursing knowledge are an integral part of Rachel's nursing practice.
- Rachel uses email to keep in touch both with patients and with colleagues all over the world.
- Rachel accesses information and puts patients in contact with a support group.
- Rachel coordinates the multiprofessional team and the programme of care.
- Rachel works in partnership with Mr Chan and uses ICT to provide the information that he needs in order to prepare him for the procedure.
- Rachel 'hugs him'. Whatever the technology, the fundamentals of nursing continue. Virginia Henderson (1985) wrote:

Nursing has never been more important than in this age when the comforting, caring presence and touch of the nurse enable the patient to tolerate invasive, often frightening and sometimes painful technology.

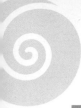
Why nursing documentation is important

In spite of constant exhortations by the Nursing and Midwifery Council (NMC) and others, inadequacies in nursing documentation continue to be the biggest category of offence identified in reports of professional conduct published by the NMC and continue to be the most frequent criticism expressed by the Health Care Ombudsman, who investigates patient complaints. Something is going badly wrong.

We noted in Chapter 3 the distinction between 'nursing as doing' and 'nursing as decision-making' and the Royal College of Nursing (RCN, 2003) definition of nursing as 'the use of clinical judgement in the provision of care'. In the 'nursing as doing' model, nursing documentation can be seen as merely a (boring) time-consuming task that takes nurses away from the more important tasks of direct patient care and that is necessitated primarily by the need to provide a defence in the event of a complaint or litigation. Seen in this light, it is perhaps not surprising that it is done badly. Guidance on good practice in record-keeping, such as that set out by the NMC (2007) and offered by lawyers, similarly focuses on exhortations about what the nurse must do (and not do) and how they must (or must not) do it, for example that patient records should:

- be factual, consistent, accurate and written in a way that the meaning is clear;
- be recorded as soon as possible after an event has occurred, providing current information on the care and condition of the patient or client;
- be recorded clearly and in such a manner that the text cannot be erased or deleted without a record of change;
- be recorded in such a manner that any justifiable alterations or additions are dated, timed and signed or clearly attributed to a named person in an identifiable role in such a way that the original entry can still be read clearly;
- be accurately dated, timed and signed, with the signature printed alongside the first entry where this is a written record, and attributed to a named person in an identifiable role for electronic records;
- not include abbreviations, jargon, meaningless phrases, irrelevant speculation, or offensive or subjective statements;
- be readable when photocopied or scanned.

Although this guidance is sound, it is inadequate. It focuses on the process of recording, but it says nothing about the most important part – the content. The 'nursing as decision-making' model described in Chapter 3 provides a completely different perspective on documentation: its purpose is to provide information for decision-making, and therefore the content is critically important.

The financier Paul Getty is reputed to have said that 'No man's decision is better than his information', and Florence Nightingale, whose contribution to information science is probably at least as great (although this is not often recognised) as her contribution to nursing, wrote:

> *In attempting to arrive at the truth, I have applied everywhere for information, but in scarcely an instance have I been able to obtain hospital records fit for any purpose of comparison. If they could be obtained, they would enable us to decide many other questions besides the one alluded to. They would show the subscribers how their money was being spent, what good was really being done with it, or whether the money was not doing mischief rather than good.*

(Nightingale, 1859)

Seen from this perspective, the important issues in thinking about documentation are:

- Who is going to read or use the information, and for what purposes?
- What type of information does the reader require in order to achieve these purposes?
- How can the information be presented so that it is accessible to the reader – that is, so that the reader can most easily find the relevant information?

Communicating information among all who are involved in the care of a patient, including the patient and their carers, is essential for patient safety and consistency and continuity of care. This information includes the patient's identification and personal details, the nature of the patient's problems (the diagnoses), the assessment data (including test results) that have led to the diagnoses, the interventions (by all disciplines) that are planned and delivered to resolve the problems, who delivered the various interventions and how, and an evaluation of the outcomes (so that interventions can be continued, stopped or changed as necessary). Unfortunately, however, most of the information that underpins nurses' decisions is exchanged orally, for example in handovers and informal conversations, and is therefore lost as soon as it is uttered. The only permanent record is the documentation in the patient's 'notes', and, as we mentioned above, the purpose of the documentation is to provide information to someone who needs to use it. It is important that the record includes all the relevant nursing data as well as medical data. A (true) story that illustrates the difficulty of making decisions about patient care without adequate documentation is given in Box 11.3.

BOX 11.3 Using telecare: Mr Thomas

This story illustrates how telecare can help us to meet the challenges of caring for frail older people in their own homes, especially at a time when changes in family structure mean that being old often also means being alone.

Telecare is the delivery of health care to individuals within the home or the wider community, with the support of devices enabled by ICT. Such devices include sensors that can detect when a person falls or wanders, or changes in the environment (e.g. because a cooker has been left on), or changes in a patient's physiological state (e.g. heart rate or blood pressure). The data are transmitted to a centre, where they can trigger a range of appropriate actions. The communication can be two-way: the patient can immediately contact the nurse, and the nurse can contact the patient.

First we tell the story of what happens without ICT; then we see how telecare can help.

Mr Thomas is an 80-year-old man who has lived alone since the death of his wife from cancer 5 years ago. One day he trips over the edge of the carpet and falls. Several hours pass before a neighbour finds him. She calls the local general practitioner (GP) surgery. The receptionist alerts the district nurse, who goes to Mr Thomas's house. The district nurse picks him up, puts him to bed but cannot find anything obviously wrong, except some confusion. To be on the safe side, she asks the GP to do a home visit. Unfortunately, the GP is a locum who does not know Mr Thomas and does not know that he is not normally confused. (Mr Thomas is alert and writes books when he is well.) Before the GP gets there, Mr Thomas tries to get out of bed and falls a second time. The GP does not make a diagnosis as to the cause of the fall, but, recognising that Mr Thomas is at risk on his own at home, he arranges for him to be admitted to a local care home for a 'period

BOX 11.3 (Continued)

of convalescence'. (Convalescence from what is yet to be determined, but the GP thinks that at least the care home will act as a place of safety.) Unfortunately, the staff at the home do not know Mr Thomas. He is miserable and soon becomes bed-bound. His regular GP, returning from annual leave 2 weeks later, goes to visit Mr Thomas in the residential home and finds him in a very sorry state. Mr Thomas has extensive pressure sores, probably created when he lay on the hard floor for several hours 2 weeks before, and worsened by the fact that he is now bed-bound. He also has bronchopneumonia. The GP admits Mr Thomas to the local hospital, where he remains for the next 3 months, just surviving the pneumonia, desperately debilitated by the pressure sores and remaining relatively immobile. The kind of medical treatment that acute hospitals provide is not, however, what Mr Thomas needs. He becomes what is pejoratively called a 'bed blocker', preventing the admission of acutely ill patients and receiving care quite inappropriate to his real needs. The hospital suggests that Mr Thomas should be discharged to a nursing home. Mr Thomas refuses to go. He says that it would kill him, and he is probably right. His daughter does not want him to be institutionalised either. He is referred and admitted to a rehabilitation unit. The rehabilitation unit does a good job, and 2 months later Mr Thomas goes home. His sacral sores have finally healed. He is gaining some stamina. Initially he walks with a frame, but he discards that a few weeks later. He is back to writing books and managing well – until the next time.

Now with ICT and telecare:

At the time of his first fall, Mr Thomas, like many thousands of elderly people, is wearing a pendant alarm. He summons help immediately, and he talks to and is reassured by the person at the call centre, who sends round an appropriate carer and alerts the GP. Even though Mr Thomas's regular GP, who knows him well, is on holiday, the locum and the district nurse are able to access Mr Thomas's health record electronically on the spot, including his last routine overview assessment. They know that he does not suffer from dementia and is not usually confused, and an infection is diagnosed and antibiotics prescribed. In response to his second fall, a fuller risk assessment by the domiciliary team is begun. This includes discussion with Mr Thomas and his family, with advice from the assistive technology department. An interim telecare package is quickly installed in Mr Thomas's home; there is no need to admit him for institutional 'convalescence', and the speedy intervention prevents the pressure sores and the bronchopneumonia, so he does not need admission to the acute hospital. Telecare and careful care-planning take account of the 'supported risks'. At the end of his rehabilitation programme (which is provided by the domiciliary team, avoiding hospital admission), his telecare package is reviewed and adjusted; the relevant devices are installed in his home and Mr Thomas learns to use them. The district nurse keeps in touch, using a planned programme of visits interspersed with telephone contact, ensuring support when it is needed. Mr Thomas remains in his own home, avoiding inappropriate admission to hospital; he treasures his independence and feels safe in the knowledge that his well-being is monitored and help would be available if ever he needed it.

If Mr Thomas had dementia, the difference between the two scenarios would have been even more dramatic. Technology can be used to improve orientation, to compensate for short-term memory loss and to minimise risk. The voice of a family member can be used in reminders to eat or take medication. Devices can monitor when an individual places himself at risk, for example wanders at night. If Mr Thomas had a chronic disease, body sensor networks would allow sensors to be placed on (or inside) the body to monitor many aspects of physiological state, including blood pressure, cardiac functioning and blood sugar. These functions can be measured continuously to give early warning of abnormalities, even if the patient is miles away from the supporting health professional. This enables both patients and health professionals to avoid the inconvenience of long journeys and means that treatment need not involve hospitalisation. It can enable fewer staff to care for more patients. It also enables more and better self-care. It also gives patients much greater control over their care, which research has shown to lead to better outcomes.

The most immediate use of documentation is to support current decision-making about a patient's care. However, once recorded, the patient record contains information that may be important for a subsequent episode of care. It will provide much of the history that is required for the assessment of the further problem; without it, there is no baseline with which to compare the present problem, the patient is forced to repeat information that they have given before (often several times before), and important items may be forgotten or missed. The individual patient record may also be needed to investigate a later complaint or to review what happened for audit, research or educational purposes.

When the anonymised data contained in multiple patient records are aggregated and analysed statistically (i.e. 'mined'), they can provide information for other decisions. For example, the database can be analysed to identify the frequency of particular items, and the relationships between items, including (if the database is big enough) cause and effect. Thus, the data can be used to answer questions such as:

- What are the most common problems experienced by a particular group of patients? (Epidemiological data to be used for service planning, resource allocation, education and knowledge development.)
- What interventions have been used for what problems?
- What were the outcomes of particular interventions? (Which worked best?)
- What was the contribution of nursing in a programme of multiprofessional care?
- What is the relationship between outcomes and staffing factors, such as who performed the intervention?

The aim is to record once, but to use many times and for different purposes. However, this can be achieved only if the record contains the appropriate information and in a form that enables it to be retrieved.

Sharing records with other health professionals and patients

Since the care of an individual patient is very rarely provided by a single health professional but usually involves several health professionals working as a multiprofessional team, it would seem sensible for them to share all their information about their shared patient, ideally in a single record to which all carers could have access and could contribute. Unfortunately, this is still rare. Separate records are maintained by different health workers in different locations, and these are almost never shared with workers in other services, such as social services or education, even though they are concerned with the same person. Even within a single hospital, nurses, physiotherapists and other clinicians usually maintain their own records separately from the main 'notes' in which medical information is recorded.

Traditionally, medical records in paper form have been 'owned' by hospitals and GPs, and only comparatively recently (since the Access to Health Records Act 1990) have patients had a legal right to see their records. In child health and maternity care, there is a longer tradition of patients not only having access to but also holding their own records. District nurses have for a long time left 'nursing notes' in the patient's home, primarily to inform the next nurse who will be providing the nursing care at the next visit.

Although the legal framework and the need to maintain patient confidentiality (see below) are very important, the idea of sharing information with the rest of the multiprofessional team, and especially with the patient and informal carers, is an issue for the approach to nursing practice discussed in Chapter 3: the commitment to partnership that is one of the defining characteristics of nursing. This is illustrated by the (true) story in Box 11.4. Things have changed considerably since 1981, but many nurses are still reluctant to expose their practice to such scrutiny in the belief that it exposes them to personal criticism. Castledine (1998) lists five questions that nurses need to clarify for themselves:

- *Self-clarification*: relates to the values that the nurse holds.
- *Professional accountability*: relates to the nurse's personal accountability for their nursing decisions and actions.
- Employer *clarification*: relates to the guidelines, directions, protocols, rules and regulations specified by the nurse's employer.
- Patient *clarification*: considers the patient's views, values and needs.
- *Public clarification*: relates to society's current views on sensitive issues such as mental health and sexual behaviour.

BOX 11.4 Sharing records with patients

I remember one visit in particular that I made with a health visitor in Finland. It was to a young mother with a baby of about 3 months. After the usual greetings, the mother undressed the baby while the health visitor got out her portable weighing scales (still unheard of in the UK) and the baby's health record – an A4 folder (we were still using A5 cards at that time), which she opened at the centile weight charts. The mother already had out the little book that was her parent-held child health record. Remember this was 1981, long before we had such things. The health visitor weighed the baby and recorded the weight both on her own chart and in the mother's book. I could see that the line of the baby's weight was below the printed curve, and I could see that the health visitor looked a bit worried. They talked for a while – of course I couldn't understand the language, but I could guess the discussion. Then the mother left us for a moment to fetch – guess what? – another little book, which was her own record from when she was a baby. They compared the two charts, they laughed, they talked a bit more, the health visitor wrote in both the records, and then the mother dressed the baby as the health visitor watched, and the visit was ended.

When we got outside I asked the health visitor to tell me about what had been going on. She said that they had talked about the baby's weight, and they had made some decisions about changing the baby's feeding, but she wasn't worried any more because the mother's own weight pattern had been exactly the same when she was a baby. I said that I had never seen records used in this way but what a great way to teach! The health visitor was surprised and asked me what we did, and I told her.

'Well', I said, 'we aren't supposed to take records out of the office, but of course if I have four visits to do in a morning I can never remember which baby has had which immunisations, so I do take the records with me. And then when I park the car (yes, I had moved on from a bicycle) I look at the records of the children I am just about to see, and then I do the visit, and then back in the car, I jot down just the most important things so that I won't forget, and then I fill in the rest when I get back to the office.'

Her eyes got wider and wider, and then she said 'You mean you write down things about people without them knowing? But that's unethical!' It was like a blow between the eyes. I had honestly never thought of it that way before.

Confidentiality and security

Maintaining the patient's confidentiality is a key requirement of the NMC Code (2008) (Appendix 1). The principle is as old as the Hippocratic Oath (fourth century BC). In recent years there has been considerable discussion and controversy about sharing information among different professionals and different services, mainly in relation to electronic records (see below) and concerned with maintaining patient confidentiality, especially sensitive information about issues such as mental health, sexual health and child protection. The patient's consent to sharing their health information, and its security, is a key issue. The RCN has published guidance for nurses as a document entitled *Competencies: An Integrated Career and Competency Framework for Information Sharing in Nursing Practice* (RCN, 2006).

From paper records to electronic records

In theory, all these issues apply equally, whether the documentation is in the form of paper records or computerised records. In practice, the ability of computers to store, sort and analyse vast amounts of information within the space of a small microchip, and to transmit the information instantaneously to multiple locations, revolutionises the usefulness of the information contained in the record and transforms the way in which it can be used. For example, all the information contained in a patient's separate paper records were previously dispersed between a GP's locked surgery and several different hospitals in different towns, but this information can now be combined and made immediately available to a doctor who needs to treat the patient in an accident and emergency department following an accident when the patient is miles from home. The move to computerised records focuses attention on issues such as security and confidentiality, which always existed but were not previously the focus of much attention; for example, we have not in the past given much attention to the reality that the transport of piles of paper records from department to department in a hospital, and their availability in an open office to anyone who wanted to steal them, is at least as great a threat to confidentiality and security as a criminal computer hacker.

Problems associated with paper records

Paper records are associated with a number of problems:

- Notes frequently get lost. Many outpatient consultations have to be cancelled or are wasted because the patient's history or test results are not available.
- The volume of paper records (many pieces of paper for millions of patients) creates storage problems and difficulties in carrying them from place to place.
- Paper records are available only in one place at one time, and important information may not be available to a person who needs it in another place.
- Paper records held in different places may contain different information, and there is no way of getting all the information together.
- Confidentiality and security are not safeguarded (see above).
- Lack of structure (which provides prompts about what to include) means that important information may not be included.

- It is difficult to find the relevant information in them quickly (Box 11.5).
- Illegible handwriting and signatures create risks to patient safety (e.g. drug errors).
- Audit is difficult and time-consuming, and it is limited to analysis of what is in the record and what can be retrieved.
- Patient data cannot easily be aggregated to provide information, for example for resource management and service planning.

Most of these problems disappear (in addition to achieving other benefits) when nurses properly use properly designed computerised information systems for documenting nursing. But the words 'properly use' and 'properly designed' are important.

BOX 11.5 The limitations of unstructured paper records

I started my new job, taking over a caseload where the previous health visitor had left about 3 months previously. On my first day, top of the pile of urgent visits, there was a request to visit an Asian family with a 4-year-old boy with learning disabilities, who should be starting school that week, but the relevant forms had still to be completed. When I visited the family at home, I found a mother who spoke no English, holding the boy on her lap while feeding him from a bottle. The 12-year-old daughter, who acted as interpreter, told me how proud they were of her little brother because he was the only boy in the family and she was the youngest of four daughters. The implications of the situation are obvious.

I went back to the office and consulted the child's records. There was a pile 6 inches high, including letters from various agencies, and one form about immunisations from the Child Health Computer System, which was then just beginning. Since they were totally unstructured, after an hour's struggle I still couldn't find who had done what when, or what the family had been told or had understood about the child's disability, or what had been planned for him. I spent a further hour on the telephone, but of course the relevant people were out or had changed jobs.

I had to visit the family several more times to collect the information I needed to even begin to work with the family. They told me that they had already told my predecessor much of what I was now asking, and repeating it was painful for both of us.

Computerised patient records

It has to be recognised that computerised records also carry risks that have to be managed and minimised, such as the following:

- Improved availability may increase risks to confidentiality and security (see above).
- Computers sometimes break down. Permanent technical support and backup systems are essential.
- Many current systems do not contain appropriate nursing data and therefore do not adequately support nursing practice. It is very important that nurses are involved fully and knowledgeably in the design and development of information systems, as well as in their implementation.
- There may be overreliance on the system at the expense of clinical judgement (see Box 3.1, p. 25).

Computerisation requires us to change the way in which we document nursing practice, including changes that we should in any case have made in using paper records. It is important to recognise that it is not enough simply to computerise documentation in its existing format. It is technically possible to do this, but it loses most of the benefits that computerised documentation offers. What is needed is a fundamental transformation of nursing documentation based on the suggestion that the purpose of documentation is to provide information for decision-making (both immediate and longer term, and both clinical and managerial) and based on the three questions that we raised earlier:

- Who is going to read or use the information, and for what purposes?
- What type of information does the reader require in order to achieve these purposes?
- How can the information be presented so that it is accessible to the reader – that is, so that the reader can most easily find the relevant information?

We also need to recognise that documentation is the outward and visible representation of our internal and invisible thinking. Restructuring documentation requires restructuring our thinking, in particular thinking about what decisions we make, and how and when we make them. Table 11.1 summarises the relationship between what happens in practice and what needs to be recorded, with some suggestions about information that can be incorporated into the system to support the nurse's decisions.

Although this kind of tabulation suggests a linear process, the ordering may vary; for example, Trigger can lead straight to Act, or Act can lead to Plan the assessment. Steps may be repeated and may take seconds or months. The practice and the record reflect the 'nursing process', but with some important differences from the format of the nursing process as it is usually used in the UK.

Rethinking the nursing process: the significance of nursing diagnosis

As we saw in Chapter 3, the 'nursing process' is in fact the same 'clinical process' as is used by all the clinical professions: what makes it 'nursing' is the nursing knowledge (as opposed to any other kind of knowledge) that is used. It is similar to the problem-solving process that most people use intuitively to manage the challenges of everyday life, but for clinical practice it is made systematic and formalised. The nursing process is simply the way that nurses structure their thinking in order to identify and solve their patients' problems.

We noted in Chapter 3, however, that since it was first formalised and introduced into nursing in the USA in the 1950s, the nursing process has been refined and developed, but UK nursing is generally still using the first-generation model – that is, the linear model consisting of the four stages of assessment, planning, implementation and evaluation. It was also noted that, since that time, better understanding derived from the research into clinical decision-making, and recognition of the significance of nursing diagnosis, has led to a third generation (Pesut and Harman, 1999), in which several more steps can be identified and the process is seen as interactive and iterative rather than linear. Other clinical professions (notably medicine) already incorporate the concept of diagnosis into their thinking, and medical diagnoses are already included in patient records.

It is a mistake to think that 'only doctors diagnose'. Each clinical profession uses its distinctive knowledge base to identify (i.e. diagnose) the 'patient problems' (diagnoses) that it knows about and is competent to treat. First-level registered nurses do not generally know enough about

Table 11.1 Using an electronic patient record to capture and support nursing practice

Practice	The record	Decision support system
Trigger (first contact with the patient), e.g. referral, admission, walk-in	Record the reason for the contact (referral, admission, walk-in); incorporate referral communication	The patient's record containing information from previous contact may be available
Plan the (nursing) assessment; decide what to assess and how; select assessment tools	Record tools used, including specific tools such as pressure sore risk	The screen format shows a particular framework (e.g. Activities of Living, Gordon's Functional Health Patterns); the system can suggest specific assessment tools (e.g. Waterlow scale)
Do the (nursing) assessment, e.g. observe, take history, examine, do tests	Record assessment data	System can include formats to plot on a chart, or calculate score; system can trigger automatic action (e.g. allergy alerts); system can suggest possible diagnoses or action
Make (nursing) diagnoses, e.g. make judgement (probable diagnoses); validate with patient	Record diagnoses	Knowledge source about various diagnoses (e.g. NANDA list); can suggest expected outcomes, pathway and actions
Agree expected outcomes (goals), e.g. using knowledge of what is possible; agree with patient what is acceptable	Record agreed expected outcomes	Can suggest possible outcomes associated with diagnoses; can offer terminology to describe outcomes (e.g. NOC, Omaha system)
Plan, e.g. decide what to do, when, when, how, by whom, including plan for review, discharge, etc.	Record planned actions	Knowledge sources; protocols; terminology to describe interventions (e.g. NIC)
Act, e.g. monitor, treat, care, refer, discharge	Record completed actions; record variance from pathway; communication re referral, discharge, etc.	Guidelines; terminology to describe interventions (e.g. NIC, SNOMED-CT)
Review, e.g. make judgement about outcome and effectiveness	Record outcomes	Terminology to describe outcomes (e.g. NOC, Omaha system); can link recorded outcomes to interventions to show effectiveness

The decision support listed is illustrative only and is not comprehensive. At any point, the user can look up knowledge sources or print the record or information for the patient.

NANDA, North American Nursing Diagnosis Association; NIC, Nursing Interventions Classification; NOC, Nursing Outcomes Classification; SNOMED-CT, Systematised Nomenclature of Medicine – Clinical Terms.

Adapted with permission from work by Ann Casey, personal communication.

specific diseases (medical diagnoses) to be able to diagnose them, and, as we saw in Chapter 3, their interventions are usually focused not on treating the disease (e.g. pneumonia) but on the patient's response to the disease (e.g. ineffective breathing pattern). Peplau (1987) has defined nursing diagnoses as simply 'the problems that nurses fix'. Since 1973, the organisation NANDA International (formerly the North American Nursing Diagnosis Association) has been identifying, naming and defining these conditions. It publishes a list of the conditions with their names and definitions, which is updated every 2 years (NANDA International, 2007).

The concept of nursing diagnosis is very important to nursing for several reasons:

- It is essential for the achievement of patient-centred, as opposed to disease-centred, care.
- The nursing diagnosis provides the focus and the rationale for selecting the appropriate nursing intervention. (If you don't know what the problem is, how do you know what to do?)
- As noted in Chapter 3, nursing diagnoses, together with their associated interventions (i.e. what nurses know about and can treat), constitute the knowledge domain of nursing.
- The nursing diagnosis provides the baseline (i.e. the condition as it existed before the intervention) for identifying the outcome and evaluating the effectiveness of the intervention.
- Data about nursing diagnoses are the building blocks that can be used to build nursing epidemiology, in the same way that data about the pattern of diseases are used to build medical epidemiology.

Nursing diagnoses are also important for patients for the following reasons:

- If the nurse has not correctly identified the problem, then they cannot identify the correct intervention and instead may use an intervention that is ineffective or even harmful.
- Nursing diagnoses do not necessarily correlate with medical diagnoses: two patients with the same medical diagnosis may have very different nursing needs, and so identifying the patient's nursing diagnoses alongside the medical diagnosis is essential for individualised care.

Diagnosis is fundamental to the clinical use of the electronic health record. The diagnosis is the data element that provides the focus for all other data elements because it is the element to which all the other elements need to be linked, especially when the data are aggregated for later use. This idea is not new: 'problem-oriented' recording has been advocated in medical care for many years (Weed, 1969). Figure 11.1 shows the relationships between diagnosis, intervention

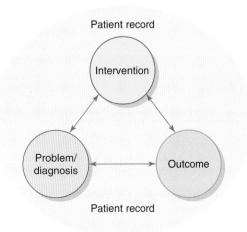

Figure 11.1 Interaction between diagnoses, interventions and outcomes.

and outcome; for example, it is impossible to understand an intervention without knowing the problem to which it is directed, or to identify an outcome without knowing the pre-existing condition that the intervention was intended to change.

The risk for nursing is that, if the nursing diagnosis is not recorded, there is no focus for understanding nursing interventions or identifying nursing outcomes, either in the care of an individual patient or more generally. In both cases, the nursing contribution to patient care remains invisible.

Requirements for computerisation

Although computers can receive, store and manipulate millions of items of data, they are much more restricted in other ways compared with human beings. For example, computers cannot see and use people's facial expressions, gestures or body language to interpret the nuances of communication (it has been estimated that up to 75 per cent of communication between human beings is non-verbal). These millions of data items, and the instructions that the computer needs about how to process them, must be expressed in a form that the computer can use. This means that the data must be standardised, structured and coded. National and international standards organisations (e.g. International Standards Organisation (ISO) and HL7) are developing standards for computerised health information systems to enable different computers and computer systems to 'talk' to one another in a 'language' that they can 'understand', in the same way as standards are developed for, for example, the labelling of food. Interoperability (the ability of computer systems to 'talk' to one another) is one of the biggest challenges in developing computer systems for the NHS, which includes hundreds of different hospitals and thousands of GP practices, most of which have, until now, used different and independent systems.

Standardising the documentation does not, of course, mean standardising practice, although it is true to say that the use of 'best practice' as specified in decision support systems, protocols, guidelines and care pathways does (and is intended to) reduce variation. Nor does it mean that what is documented will not be comprehensive or will not describe things with sufficient subtlety; that depends on the way that the computer system is configured – which is why it is so important that nurses who understand the intricacies of the care process, and how to represent these concepts in the computer system, are involved in system development.

The specific requirements for computerised documentation include:

- content (which must be coded);
- structure;
- standardised terminology.

Content

There must be an agreed common core of data elements (known as the minimum dataset), and it is important that this includes the relevant nursing data. The essential elements for any patient record include the following:

- *Patient identification*: in addition to the patient's name, address and date of birth, computerisation requires a unique identification number. Countries that have a system of national identity cards usually use the number that is issued to citizens at birth; in the UK, the NHS has developed a NHS number, which is now issued to every baby at birth and is gradually being extended to cover the whole population.

- *Patient demographic data*: this includes the patient's age, sex, ethnicity, and sometimes other elements such as language or family structure.
- *Service identification*: this includes the current service provider (e.g. the hospital that is providing the current episode of care) and information about other service providers (e.g. the patient's GP). It may also include information about agencies such as social services departments or a child's school. This heading also covers the identification of named individuals providing care (e.g. which doctor performed a particular patient's operation, or who prescribed, issued or administered a particular drug), often in the form of an electronic signature.
- *Other service data*: this includes date of current and previous hospital admissions and discharges, referrals and so on. Much of these administrative data are already collected in paper records. The paper file also often includes numerous letters, forms and other items, so that it becomes very bulky. The problem is that, because it is not usually standardised, structured or coded, it is difficult to retrieve, aggregate or compare items, for example for auditing, epidemiology or management purposes. From the patient's point of view, an additional problem is that they are asked to give this information over and over again, every time they start a new episode of care or even when they move from department to department within the same hospital. As well as wasting valuable time, this repetition encourages errors.
- *Clinical data*: these include information about the problems with which the patient presents, assessment data (including specific assessments, e.g. risk for pressure sores, results of blood tests, X-rays), allergies, current and past medications, medical diagnoses, interventions and treatments, and progress notes. In paper records, the same problems occur as in the case of administrative information, and the difficulty of linking one clinical item to another, or clinical items to administrative items, makes activities such as quality monitoring, clinical audit and performance management very difficult.

The particular problem for nursing is that, in the UK and many other countries, almost all of the clinical data currently collected are medical data. The lack of nursing information means that even if the nursing care that the patient receives is comprehensive, the record of the patient's care is incomplete and the nursing contribution to it is invisible. Moreover, nurses are vulnerable as litigation increases and courts take the view that 'if it isn't documented, then it wasn't done'.

To overcome this problem, nursing minimum datasets have been developed in several countries, and a project coordinated by the International Council of Nurses is developing and testing an international nursing minimum dataset (i-NMDS). The earliest NMDS, developed in the USA (Werley and Lang, 1988) specified four nursing elements: nursing diagnosis, nursing intervention, nursing outcome, and intensity of nursing care; these elements remain the essential core in all NMDSs. In some other countries, a more elaborate NMDS has been developed; for example, the Netherlands NMDS includes 11 nursing elements:

- nursing assessment;
- patient problem/nursing diagnoses (list of 24);
- goals;
- interventions (list of 32);
- daily (progress) reports;
- flow chart/care pathway;
- continuity of care;
- risk for pressure sore;
- vital signs;

- risk for falls;
- complexity of care (3 items) (Delaney, 2006).

Structure

The data must be structured in such a way that the user can easily find the data they are seeking. The structure is an important part of the software that is 'behind the screen' and unseen by the computer user, but the way that it is presented on the screen (the graphical user interface; GUI) is also important. The way in which the data are organised on the screen is similar to the way in which standardised forms are used in paper records. In both cases, research has shown that the data collected are more comprehensive when the person recording it has a 'picking list' that acts as a reminder. Good computerised information systems can also use decision support systems to provide a 'pop-up' or 'window' that suggests possible linkages or next steps in response to a particular input. The software must enable the elements to be linked, so that patterns and trends can be seen, errors can be identified and investigated, clinical and service outcomes can be identified, and services can be managed and costed. However, nurses traditionally write their patient records in the form of 'stories' using unstructured narrative, from which it is difficult to retrieve and impossible to analyse the relevant data.

Standardising nursing language

Another problem is that at present we have no common language for describing nursing practice. Without a language in which to express our concepts, we cannot know whether our understanding of their meaning is the same, and so we cannot communicate them to other people with any certainty. As Norma Lang has said: 'if we cannot name it, we cannot control it, finance it, teach it, research it, or put it into public policy' (Clark and Lang, 1992).

Of course, nurses do communicate with one another, and with patients, about what they are thinking and doing, but we do so (and sometimes pride ourselves on doing so) in 'ordinary' language, which, simply because it is 'ordinary', cannot convey with any precision concepts that are highly complex and specific. The words are not standardised, and so their meaning varies according to context and the private understanding of the people using them. Casey and Hoy (1997) have used the idea of a continuum to show how the informal kind of language used between people sharing the clinical care of a particular patient, and that relies heavily on context and the shared knowledge of the participants, has to become more objective and more formal as contextual information gets less. Two nurses sharing the care of a frail elderly patient understand very well what is behind phrases such as 'watch that heel' and 'needs help with ADLs', but such words are not useful, and may even be dangerous, in an audit of pressure sores or determining skill mix, and they cannot be summarised or aggregated for use in computerised information systems. Computerised records require standardised terminology.

Medicine has recognised the need for standardised language for some time. Over a century and a half ago, in his *First Annual Report of the Registrar-General of Births, Deaths and Marriages in England*, William Farr wrote: 'The nomenclature is of as much importance in this department of inquiry as weights and measures in the physical sciences, and should be settled without delay' (Farr, 1839).

Building on Farr's foundation, the World Health Organization (WHO) International Classification of Diseases (ICD) is now used to enable morbidity and mortality data from different countries around the world to be systematically collected, analysed and compared. Over the past decade, the advance of computerised health information has stimulated the development of a number of standardised terminologies for nursing. In the USA, a strong lead has been taken by the American Nurses Association (ANA), which, as far back as 1990, established its Steering Committee on Databases to Support Clinical Practice. Since then, the ANA has published several guidance documents and has established systems for 'approving' nursing languages and for evaluating the nursing documentation systems produced by commercial vendors (Warren, 2003). The best known nursing terminologies, which have been translated into several languages and are in use in various parts of the world, are:

- the NANDA classification of nursing diagnoses (NANDA International, 2007);
- the Omaha system (Martin, 2005);
- the Clinical Care Classification System (Saba, 2006);
- the Nursing Interventions Classification (NIC) (Dochterman and Bulechek, 2004);
- the Nursing Outcomes Classification (NOC) (Moorhead *et al.*, 2004).

In the UK, the government has decided that the terminology to be used for all computerised health information in the NHS will be the Systematised Nomenclature of Medicine – Clinical Terms (SNOMED-CT). This is a merging of the US-developed Systematized Nomenclature of Human and Veterinary Medicine (SNOMED) with the UK-developed Read Codes (still used by many GPs). SNOMED-CT is a comprehensive health care terminology that can be used for describing patient conditions and to support documentation of multiprofessional care. It contains over 300 000 terms describing more than 100 000 concepts. SNOMED-CT includes the ANA-recognised nursing terminologies, and so it includes coverage of nursing diagnoses, interventions and nurse-sensitive patient outcomes, and contains concepts and relationships to represent nursing clinical knowledge across the full scope of nursing practice. A nursing group (the SNOMED Convergent Terminology Group for Nursing) has been established, charged with ensuring a terminology supportive of nursing's requirement for describing patient care.

Reflection point 11.1
Some of what you have read here may not be part of your current experience. Make a note of what you are already familiar with in this field and keep your notes. It will be interesting to revisit them in 3–4 years to see where we, and you, have advanced to.

 CONCLUSION

Electronic patient records are already in use in some areas, especially in general practice, but it will be some years before the full electronic health record envisaged in this chapter is available everywhere. A summary record containing basic data has already been developed in Scotland and England and will soon be available in Wales. The need to develop and learn to use structured and standardised documentation and standardised terminology in nursing is an urgent task, and it is the business of every practising nurse.

References

Casey A (2005). Assessing and planning care in partnership. In Glasper EA and Richardson J (eds). *A Textbook of Children's Nursing*. Edinburgh: Elsevier.

Casey A and Hoy D (1997). Language for research and practice. *Journal of Interprofessional Care*, **11**, 35–42.

Clark J and Lang N (1992). Nursing's next advance: an international classification for nursing practice. *International Nursing Review*, **39**: 109–12.

Castledine G (1998). *Writing, Documentation and Communication for Nurses*. Dinton: Quay Books.

Delaney CW (2006). Nursing minimum data sets. In Saba VK and McCormick KA (eds). *Essentials of Nursing Informatics*, 4th edn. New York: McGraw-Hill.

Dochterman JM and Bulechek G (eds) (2004). *Nursing Interventions Classification (NIC)*, 4th edn. St Louis, MO: Mosby.

Farr W (1839). *First Annual Report of the Registrar-General of Births, Deaths and Marriages in England*. London: Longman.

George F (ed.) (1977). *Astounding and Exciting Developments that Will Transform Your Life*. New York: Sterling.

Henderson VA (1985). The essence of nursing in high technology. *Nursing Administration Quarterly*, **9**, 1–9.

Martin K (2005). *The Omaha System: A Key to Practice, Documentation, and Information Management*, 2nd edn. St Louis, MO: Elsevier.

Moorhead S, Johnson M and Maas M (2004). *Nursing Outcomes Classification (NOC)*, 3rd edn. St Louis, MO: Mosby.

NANDA International (2007). *Nursing Diagnoses: Definitions and Classification 2007–2008*. Philadelphia, PA: NANDA International.

Nightingale F (1859). *Notes on Nursing*. London: Harrison.

Nursing and Midwifery Council (NMC) (2007). *A–Z Advice Sheet: Record Keeping Guidance*. London. Nursing and Midwifery Council.

Nursing and Midwifery Council (NMC) (2008). *The Code: Standards of Conduct, Performance and Ethics for Nurses and Midwives*. London: Nursing and Midwifery Council.

Peplau HE (1987). Interpersonal constructs for nursing practice. *Nurse Education Today*, **7**, 201–8.

Pesut D and Harman T (1999). *Clinical Reasoning: The Art and Science of Critical and Creative Thinking*. Albany, NY: Delmar.

Royal College of Nursing (RCN) (2003). *Defining Nursing*. London: Royal College of Nursing.

Royal College of Nursing (RCN) (2006). Competencies: an integrated career and competency framework for information sharing in nursing practice. London. www.rcn.org.uk/development/publications.

Royal Society (2006). *Digital Healthcare: The Impact of Information Communication Technologies on Health and Healthcare*. London: Royal Society.

Saba V (2006). *Clinical Care Classification System Manual: A Guide to Nursing Documentation*. New York: Springer.

Sibbald B (1995). 2020 vision for nursing. *Canadian Nurse*, **91**, 30–33.

Warren JJ (2003). Preparing for the electronic health record: the USA experience. In Clark J (ed.). *Naming Nursing: Proceedings of the First ACENDIO Ireland/UK Conference.* Bern: Verlag Hans Huber.

Weed L (1969). *Medical Records, Medical Education and Patient Care: The Problem-Oriented Record as Basic Tool.* Cleveland, OH: Case Western Reserve University Press.

Werley H and Lang N (1988). *Identification of the Nursing Minimum Data Set.* New York: Springer.

Further reading

Clark J (ed.) (2003). *Naming Nursing: Proceedings of the First ACENDIO Ireland/UK Conference.* Bern: Verlag Hans Huber.

Royal Society (2006). *Digital Healthcare: The Impact of Information Communication Technologies on Health and Healthcare.* London: Royal Society.

Weaver C, Delaney C, Weber P and Carr A (eds) (2006). *Nursing and Informatics for the 21st Century.* Chicago, IL: Healthcare Information and Management Systems Society.

PART 4

Key aspects
of care

Frameworks for practice

12

Jane Schober

Introduction

The aim of this chapter is to explore factors that are important to the quality of nursing care. The nurse–patient relationship is central to this and may take many forms, require a range of skills and be a profound experience for everyone involved. People often need nurses when they are at their most vulnerable, and so the way care is conducted, organised, resourced and evaluated will impact on the quality of any outcomes. Meeting the individual needs of patients within the context of a complex health care system will always be a challenge for those with care delivery responsibilities. Effective, skilled, well-managed care relies on well-prepared practitioners. They need the abilities to meet the increasing health needs of, for example, an ageing population and for those with a long-term condition within a society that is becoming more complex as social, racial and cultural diversity increase. Nurses need to draw on a range of resources to meet these demands Frameworks for practice can contribute to this process as they inform decision-making and problem-solving, both of which are central to the effective management of care delivery.

Learning objectives

After studying this chapter you should be able to:
- consider the nature of individuality;
- explore the contribution that the nursing process makes to nursing practice and the organisation of care;
- realise the place of nursing process, nursing theory and nursing knowledge in relation to nursing care;
- explore the features of a selection of nursing models.

The nature of individuality

Being expected to respond, adapt and rise to the demands of meeting the needs of individuals in your care is one of the many reasons why nursing is such an interesting challenge. We all possess characteristics and qualities that make us who we are. These characteristics and qualities may be challenged and affected by, for example, changes in health, social circumstances, educational opportunity and our ability to cope, adapt and realise our potential. Carl Rogers (1969) recognises the complexities of being human and offers a range of propositions that help us to understand the phenomenon of individuality. Key features are summarised here and suggest that, as individuals, we

- are exposed to constant change;
- have varying insights into our own personalities and selves;
- experience our own reality;
- are influenced greatly by our educational and learning experiences;
- interact with, and are affected, by our environments;
- strive to satisfy our needs and enhance our well-being;
- react to experiences and values in a range of ways – we may adopt them as relevant, deny them or ignore them;

- live well, are open and trusting, and have confidence from experiences and relationships featuring unconditional positive regard;
- become defensive and threatened without associated learning experiences and adaptation skills.

So, as individuals, we are characterised by biological, psychological and intellectual components. These factors affect our personalities, behaviours and perceptions of ourselves. They also affect our reactions to the world around us, our relationships, and how we cope with change. We have much to motivate us, and this is a fundamental drive. We need to learn, grow and develop, but the quality and outcome of this will depend on situations and environments characterised by trust, respect and acceptance. Relationships that bear these features allow those involved to participate and share in decisions and take responsibility for their actions. These feature within a 'healthy' environment. Conversely, an environment that is threatening and stressful, or where we feel undervalued, may result in much of our energy being used to adapt, cope and indeed survive the circumstances we face. For many people requiring health care, the environment where this occurs may be new, contain a range of alien features and be managed by strangers. Nurses, therefore, have a profound role in supporting those needing care in such a way as to limit the stresses such experiences may generate.

Reflection point 12.1
Consider how an understanding of what makes us who we are may help nurses approach patients for the first time. List the factors you should bear in mind.

This exercise is about not only each patient's individuality but also the nurse's individuality. If you have recognised this in your response, then you have acknowledged part of the complexity of the nurse–patient relationship.

Therefore, from the patient's viewpoint, their experience of your approach will be influenced by:

- their previous experiences of health care;
- their ability to respond, in accordance with their current state of health;
- their understanding of the current situation;
- how threatening this situation is perceived to be;
- their ability to cope and adapt to the current situation;
- their willingness and ability to learn, cooperate and take responsibility as required;
- their willingness to trust members of the health care team;
- support from their family and friends.

Much of what nurses do relates to those who are ill. Pellegrino captures comprehensively the impact of illness and the potential power and influence of professional carers:

> *The fact of illness afflicts our humanity and diminishes it and renders us less able to function as moral agents and as human agents and as human persons. Illness wounds, diminishes, and compromises our very humanity and places us in a uniquely vulnerable situation in relation to the professional healer. The relationship of healing is inherently one of inequality, vulnerability. The obligations of those who profess to heal directly . . . are grounded in the phenomenon of illness.*
>
> (Pellegrino, 1982, p. 165)

Pellegrino challenges professional carers to recognise the overwhelming impact of illness for individuals and suggests the comprehensive potential of professional carers to heal.

The realisation that nurses need to apply their knowledge and skills to a wide range of circumstances is therefore complicated by the demands and uncertainties of individuality. In addition, the range of health and nursing needs demands that nurses draw on skills and approaches to care to make their interventions as effective and efficient as possible.

In Chapter 3 of this book, the nature of nursing is described and a range of definitions are explored. Chapter 3 also recognises the intellectual, emotional, moral and political perspectives influencing nursing today. Tracing the history of how nursing is described and defined, it appears that there is some consensus about what nursing is (RCN, 2003); but perhaps the real question is 'What do nurses do?' From the patient's point of view, this is what really matters. The RCN (2003) analysis has culminated in a definition supported by six characteristics:

[Nursing is] the use of clinical judgement in the provision of care to enable people to improve, maintain, or recover health, to cope with health problems, and to achieve the best possible quality of life, whatever their disease or disability, until death.

(RCN, 2003, p. 3)

The six defining characteristics are summarised here:

- The 'purpose of nursing is to promote health, healing, growth and development, and to prevent disease, illness, injury, and disability'.
- 'Nursing interventions are concerned with empowering people and helping them to achieve, maintain or recover independence'. Key aspects of nursing practice also include 'the identification of nursing needs; therapeutic interventions and personal care; information, education, advice and advocacy'.
- 'A particular domain: the specific domain of nursing is people's unique responses to and experience of health, illness, frailty, disability and health-related life events in whatever environment or circumstances they find themselves'.
- The 'focus of nursing is the whole person and the human response rather than a particular aspect of the person or a particular pathological condition'.
- 'A particular value base: nursing is based on ethical values which respect the dignity, autonomy and uniqueness of human beings, the privileged nurse–patient relationship, and the acceptance of personal accountability for decisions and actions'.
- 'A commitment to partnership: nurses work in partnership with patients, their relatives and other carers, and in collaboration with others as members of a multi-disciplinary team' (RCN, 2003).

The way nurses execute their interpretation of the information they have about the needs of patients determines the quality of care for patients. Therefore, their skill base, ability to prioritise, apply, relate to and communicate with patients is central to this outcome. Everyone responds differently to their state of health, be it physically, emotionally or intellectually. The complexity of this response process is also shaped by culture, ethnicity, spirituality, previous experiences and expectations. The demands on nurses are great, both to meet needs and to provide efficient, effective evidence-based care. However, care environments may not have sufficient resources to meet these demands. Thus, nurses are left with the ultimate professional challenge: to maintain the required standards of care as in the NMC Code (2008) (Appendix 1), and to combine them with the need to be able to diagnose needs in such a way as to help patients feel safe, cared for and supported in whatever state of health they find themselves in (NMC, 2004). For nurses to deliver care in such a manner, they must recognise their responsibilities within their roles and practise accordingly, which means that nurses need to be prepared and supported and care organised to this end. This chapter now considers models and frameworks for organising and planning nursing care. These are a means to educating, guiding and inspiring nurses to interpret patient information and responses effectively and to make informed, patient-centred diagnostic decisions.

Organising nursing care

Well organised nursing care relies on a range of resources, skills and educational support within the context of a multiprofessional team. This is a technological age and therefore systems for organising and recording nursing care must incorporate the required evidence-based care (see also Chapter 11).

Nursing actions are inevitably influenced by the nurse's attitudes, beliefs and values. Decisions relating to patient care and nursing practice need to be informed, systematic, and based on sound understanding and interpretation of events, as well as on a thorough knowledge of practice, theory and research. In the 1970s, the nursing process was introduced into the UK. This was implemented as a model of decision-making and problem-solving. It had its roots in the comprehensive rational model of decision-making based on the work of Simon (1950). This model makes a key assumption that the decision-maker will take into consideration all possible options and consequences, in the light of a thorough understanding of the situation. The systematic assessment, planning, implementation and evaluation of care were the core features of this process. By implication, this demands a high level of skill relating to the care demands of the associated patient group. In the main, nurses have never lost sight of the need for individualised care, the need for shared decision-making and patient involvement, as highlighted in the RCN (2003) statement. However, there remains a tension between the demands for comprehensive, accurate nursing records and the contribution that the nursing process makes to the intellectual thought processes. This is evident in the volume of paperwork produced, perhaps at the expense of time engaged in direct patient care.

Applying evidence-based outcomes to patient care is central to informed effective care management, but nurses need to be able to organise and apply these outcomes to individual patients in a systematic way. It is an NMC requirement for care delivery for entry to the professional register that student nurses assess, plan, organise, analyse and manage care plans, under the supervision of a registered nurse (Appendix 2). Critical thinking and quality decision-making when organising and managing nursing care may be supported in a number of ways, and information technology is one. However, without the ability to reason and process the range of information associated with patients needs in a personalised and sensitive manner, the care of patients may be compromised.

Alfaro-LeFevre (2006) recognises the nursing process as a means to this end. This approach to organising information gained from patients relies on systematic assessment, diagnosis, planning, implementation and evaluation.

The nursing process

Patient assessment

Patient assessment is an essential component of care. It is ongoing and complex, and it demands a range of communication, observational, technical and decision-making skills by nurses. Patient assessment goes way beyond the required collection of data, for example, when a patient is admitted to a ward environment. For patients needing care in any health care setting, ongoing assessment for the total period of care facilitates the accurate identification of information and data necessary for comprehensive individualised care-planning. (See also Chapter 14 for further information about patient assessment.)

Assessment is characterised by:

- determining the immediate health needs of the patient in order to ensure and prioritise their safety;
- promoting a caring, compassionate rapport;
- collecting information and data through interviewing and observation;
- examining the patient to determine their nursing needs;
- validating information by distinguishing objective from subjective data;
- using sources of information to contribute to this process;
- using critical thinking and judgements to determine and identify problems based on sufficient information;
- organising and recording information and establishing a plan of care.

Reflection point 12.2
The patient is usually the primary source of assessment information, but there are circumstances when this may be difficult or impossible. List the factors that may interfere with the patient being the primary source of verbal information, and list the possible alternative sources of information that could be used to improve the information about a patient.

Anything that interferes with a patient's ability to communicate clearly, rationally and comprehensively requires the nurse to explore other sources of information. Examples include patients with poor language skills, collapsed or traumatised patients, infants, patients unable to communicate coherently, and people who are frightened and stressed due to their situation. Key sources of information include the patient's next of kin, partner or carer, other health care professionals, and members of the emergency services.

Nursing diagnosis

In general, interpreting information and data gained through the assessment process informs a nursing diagnosis. Nursing diagnosis in the UK is not a commonly applied feature of nursing process, unlike in many other countries, such as the USA, where nursing diagnosis is an integral part of the nursing process, with standardised national classifications such as that of NANDA International (2007) (Carpenito-Moyet, 2006). Hogston (1997), among others, has recognised for many years the potential disadvantages to UK nurses of not having a comprehensive nursing diagnosis classification system, as it is through such a system that nurses develop consensus about the phenomena that are their concern and contribute to the development of nursing theory and science.

The main difference between nursing diagnosis and medical diagnosis is the impact of the changes in health on the individual and the resultant problems, as opposed to the diagnosis of the disease process itself. Although both recognise that health issues have the potential to impact on quality of life, lifestyle, relationships and level of dependence, nurses usually act as catalysts for managing the totality of care. This is also manifested in nurses being concerned with actual and potential problems, the psychosocial aspects of care, and the utilisation of a comprehensive plan of care to manage needs, as well as correcting and controlling problems, managing risk and preventing side effects. Thus, nursing diagnosis has three components:

- *Problems and their definition*: this describes the problem and health state and serves to direct goal-setting and possible patient outcomes.

- *Aetiology*: this relates to the possible causes of the problem and risk factors and supports the notion of individuality, as the causes may highlight experiences unique to the patient, such as an accident, a side effect of treatment or the effects of an established diagnosis, for example depression following diagnosis of Parkinson's disease.
- *Defining characteristics*: these are the signs and symptoms with which the patient presents, which in turn can be related to the NANDA International (2007) list for clarification and to the extensive list of standardised terminology in the following five categories:
  - actual diagnosis;
  - risk diagnosis;
  - possible diagnosis;
  - syndrome diagnosis;
  - wellness diagnosis.

Planning care

Nursing care plans represent essential documentation and records of decisions relating to nursing goals and interventions. Any plan suggests that there is an intended, deliberate purpose and understanding of how this is to be achieved. There are different types of care plan:

- *Initial plan*: established from the initial admission and assessment.
- *Ongoing plan*: reflects the progress, new goals and changes as care progresses.
- *Discharge plan*: ensures a smooth transition from a ward or unit to home, where care may need to be continued. Where a hospital stay is likely to be short (e.g. 24–48 hours), the discharge plan may commence alongside the initial plan.

The nursing care plan, therefore, provides a tool for:

- documenting all aspects of planned care;
- determining goals for care that reflect actual and potential problems;
- informing the patient, as appropriate, of how the care is proceeding;
- involving the patient, as appropriate, with care activities and decisions;
- identifying patient behaviours necessary to achieve goals;
- identifying targets for care, and the support and interventions required to achieve them;
- writing instructions for care delivery;
- communicating planned care between members of the nursing and multiprofessional staff;
- recording care that is evidence of nursing interventions;
- evaluating care and reassessing, modifying and updating the plan;
- recording care that can be used for legal and research purposes;
- making a permanent record of care.

Thus, care-planning is the catalyst for interventions and combines processes for professional nursing decision-making with a record of nursing actions and interventions for the benefit of individualised patient care.

Care delivery and care management are two of the four domains that make up Standard 7 of the NMC Standards of Proficiency for Pre-Registration Nursing Education (NMC, 2004; see also Appendix 2). Care-planning is an integral part of the skills required of nurses, and the skills should not be underestimated. Care-planning is more than responding to, for example, the stated problem, the reason for admission, the instruction from a senior colleague or the initial diagnosis. It is also about comprehensive assessment of the physiological, psychological and sociological impact of the health status on the individual. Nurses face a real challenge here, both to meet needs and to do so within the constraints of work patterns, the time available to be with the patient, and the reliability of the information available. Nurses, therefore, need to be taught to focus on and prioritise needs in order to alleviate suffering and stress, for example, as well as to promote safety, comfort, dignity and individuality.

Evaluating care

The quality of the nursing process and care-planning depends on the evaluative judgements nurses make about whether the patient has achieved the goals set out in the plan. To do this well, each of the following steps in the process must be evaluated with patient involvement:

- *Assessment*: to identify any changes and additional information relevant to the patient's condition.
- *Diagnosis*: to identify any new problems and risk factors that are impacting on the patient's well-being.
- *Goals*: have they been achieved? Do they need to be updated?
- *Plan of care*: to ascertain whether the planned interventions remain appropriate to the patient's care needs and priorities.

Conclusions about the progress, or otherwise, of the patient's condition are documented and help to shape the ongoing plan of care.

SUMMARY

- Nursing care is a complex integration of knowledge, skills and attitudes.
- Care-planning is a professional requirement for care delivery (NMC, 2004).
- Nursing process facilitates systematic decision-making and care-planning.

Nursing theory and nursing knowledge

So far in this chapter, the complexities of the nurse's role and the demands of systematic care-planning have been explored. Although nursing is generally regarded as a practice discipline, to practise effectively and to acquire expertise in practice implies a symbiotic relationship between what nurses do and what nurses know. Nurse education was integrated into higher education institutions in the 1990s. This was a deliberate strategy to provide a recognised academic programme of study at diploma or degree level combining equal allocation of time for theoretical input and practice experience, along with the professional requirements laid down by the NMC.

Much nursing knowledge has a theoretical and practice component. Carper (1978) recognised the range of knowledge and described patterns of knowing or theoretical knowledge. The four aspects of knowledge are as follows:

- *Empirics*: scientific knowledge, to describe, explain and predict.
- *Aesthetic*: an art – understanding and perceiving.
- *Personal*: subjective and existential.
- *Ethical*: moral.

Effective decision-making ,expert knowledge and practice, therefore, rely on nurses being able to use sources of knowledge, ranging from the scientific research-based information (e.g. relating to infection control) to the moral impact of decisions on patient care that are influenced by the NMC Code.

By implication, there appears to be more to the relationship between theory and practice than simply an understanding of what is done and why. In order to discuss the relevance of theory in nursing practice, it is necessary to understand two main relationships – first, the relationship between knowledge and nursing practice, and second, the relationship between nursing theory, its interpretation and its relevance to practice.

Knowledge and nursing practice

Knowledge is generally defined as practical or theoretical understanding. It is about having evidence and facts to work with, and it is part of expertise.

Benner (1984) considered the differences between practical and theoretical knowledge in detail and suggested that those who acquire practical skills may not always be able to account for their actions – that is, provide a rationale or research evidence. There may be many reasons for this, such as the level of nurse education and training, the nurse's experience, the value and importance placed by the nurse on these professional demands, and the nurse's commitment to keeping up to date, even though this is a professional requirement according to the NMC Code.

Here lies a paradox, recognised by nurses for decades: a significant amount of care is delivered to patients by those without professional registration and qualifications.

Applying theory to practice means that nurses are using sources of knowledge and evidence, including those from research studies, scientific enquiry and laws (Meleis, 2007). This is apparent in the development of evidence-based practice and research in nursing in recent years. However, when determining the theoretical base of nursing, it is necessary to examine a range of sources.

Nursing theory and practice

Theories about the nature and purpose of nursing provide nurses with sources of insight, experience and understanding about the range of approaches to nursing care. Theories tend to consist of concepts that are often referred to as 'conceptual models' or 'frameworks' that provide an approach or view about nursing. Many examples of nursing models may be found in the nursing literature; they contribute a great deal to the debate about how care may be approached for patients, depending on their needs.

Marriner-Tomey and Alligood (2006) suggest that the key terms used to explain nursing theories may be defined as follows:

- *Metaparadigms*: abstract concepts used to organise a theory. They are central to nursing and relate to the pattern of interaction between the *person*, *health*, the *environment* and *nursing*. These four key concepts form the basis of nursing theories. The nurse theorist usually defines each of these concepts in relation to their approach to nursing.
- *Philosophy*: many nurse theorists are influenced by beliefs, moral values, ethical principles and values from Eastern and Western philosophy. These may manifest themselves in the way a nursing theory is developed.
- *Conceptual/nursing models*: these provide views about nursing; for example, Orem (2001) suggests that the promotion of self-care is the core aim within her model.

Nursing theory and nursing models

The complexity of nursing, and the range of approaches that may be taken to execute effective care, demand that nurses draw on a range of decision-making options to fit the purpose. Models often contain the ideas and experiences of nurses. It could be said that individual nurses have their own model of nursing, which is usually demonstrated through their actions, attitudes and expertise – that is, through their practice.

Nurses who have applied themselves to a greater understanding of nursing through the formulation of a model have usually taken their ideas and their experiences about nursing, health, humankind and the environment (or society) and sought to explain the interrelationship between them. Specific models assist nurses in their understanding about the nature and complexity of nursing. It is not uncommon to find nursing documentation representing the features of such work. However, the model itself should not dictate the care for a patient but should serve to assist nurses in their decision-making and approach to the individual care requirements of patients.

The features of nursing models

Contemporary nursing models have key features in common:

- Priority is given to the integrity of the individual.
- Assessment of health needs of the individual is the foundation for all decision-making and problem-solving activities concerned with care.
- Nursing process is often an explicit feature of the systematic organisation of care-planning.
- Value is placed on the promotion of optimum health for that individual throughout the period of care.
- Each model offers a theme or approach to nursing that provides a means of focusing on the needs of the individual, for example adaptation and self-care.

Choosing a nursing model

The choice of a nursing model and approach to nursing care may follow one of two general perspectives. The choice may be influenced by the needs of patients and may be selected after a comprehensive assessment and an understanding of care priorities. Alternatively, the choice may depend on broader criteria and take into consideration not only the needs of a larger group of patients but also factors associated with the health care team, the care environment and resources.

The work of key nurse theorists

There are over 30 theories of nursing. Most originate from North America and from academic developments in nursing research and education. However, it is clear from the writings of such theorists as Callista Roy and Dorothea Orem that nursing practice and their experiences of patient care played a very influential part in theory development. In the UK, the Roper–Logan–Tierney Activities of Living model (Roper *et al.*, 2000) has influenced nursing practice and the implementation of the nursing process for more than 20 years. It remains a very influential model, and one that has shaped both the management of care and the design of nursing documentation.

It is useful to have a means of evaluating models of nursing in order to judge their potential value, application and relevance in differing care situations. Box 12.1 summarises the issues to consider.

There now follows an overview of four models of nursing. These are well recognised, universally applied and good examples of the potential contribution that models make to the understanding of nursing care. They may be applied in a variety of care settings, and they have the potential to contribute to the care of patients, regardless of age, in both acute and primary health care settings, and regardless of whether the patient's health status is acute or chronic in nature.

BOX 12.1 Evaluating a model or theory of nursing

Background of the model
Consider the origins of the model, such as when and where it was devised and developed. This should alert the reader to the context of the model, possible cultural influences, and the original intentions of the work.

Aims of the model
Examine the aims of the model. These may be expressed as aims of nursing. These will reveal the focus of the model and usually inform the reader as to whether the approach extends from the nurse–patient relationship or whether nursing aims to respond to states of health. Consider also how the author explains or defines the key concepts of nursing, health, environment and humankind, and the relationships between them, as this often reveals the overall aim of the model.

Theories associated with the model
Many authors refer to theories from, for example, the life or social sciences in order to strengthen the rationale for their approach to nursing. Roy (1997), for example, refers to theories relating to stress, in the development of her theory of adaptation.

Application of the model to clinical practice
The author may offer examples of the model's application to practice and the patients' needs that may respond positively to the proposed outcomes. The literature may also contain examples of care plans and care studies based on the model. Some authors have their own websites, so accessing these will be helpful (e.g. Orem – www.scdnt.com).

The Roper–Logan–Tierney Model of Nursing

This was the first model of nursing to be developed in the UK. The authors produced the work initially to support the education of student nurses. It has also supported developments in nursing internationally. Since its inception in 1980, the model has made a significant contribution to the understanding between the factors symbolising a person's individuality and the responses required of nurses to meet changes resulting from health care needs.

The development of the model was influenced by the work of Virginia Henderson (1966) and Maslow (1954). These works considered human needs and their importance in relation to behaviour and motivation. The identification of 12 activities of living (Box 12.2) served as the basis of identification of health needs, the emphasis being on the need to assess the biological, sociocultural, psychological, environmental and politico-economic perspective of each activity of living in relation to the patient's state of health. As well as the activities of living, Roper *et al.* (2000) emphasise the interrelationship between the activities of living, our lifespan, our level of dependence, and the need for nurses to assess and plan care accordingly.

The aim of the model is to promote the independence and individuality of each person requiring care and to assess, plan, implement and evaluate care in accordance with the activities of living. (See also Further reading.)

BOX 12.2 Activities of living

- Maintaining a safe environment
- Communicating
- Breathing
- Eating and drinking
- Eliminating
- Personal cleansing and dressing
- Controlling body temperature
- Mobilising
- Working and playing
- Expressing sexuality
- Sleeping
- Dying

Hildegard Peplau's theory of interpersonal relationships

Peplau's (1952) model is generally regarded as the first nursing model and was developed from her work with people who were mentally ill. Her major work was published in the 1950s, but readers should not be deterred by its age. Her work grew from her belief that the nurse–patient relationship is a therapeutic tool. She states:

> *Psychodynamic nursing is being able to understand one's own behaviour to help other identify felt difficulties and to apply principles of human relations to the problems that arise at all levels of experience.*

(Peplau, 1952, p. xiii)

The aim of the model is to use the nurse–patient relationship to help patients explore and understand the meaning of their feelings, to identify with what is happening, and to be involved in care.

Peplau describes four phases of the interpersonal relationship:

1 *Orientation*: the beginning of the relationship, when both parties are getting to know each other. This is the beginning of an assessment period, a time for the nurse to help the patient recognise their needs and to understand their role in care.
2 *Identification*: a time for further assessment, exploration and development within the relationship. The nurse needs to promote a trusting relationship and to promote patient confidence. Goals may begin to emerge.
3 *Exploitation*: the nurse maximises opportunities for helping the patient to take responsibilities and to identify further goals.
4 *Resolution*: new goals replace old ones and the nurse helps the patient to prepare for ending the relationship and to feel secure when separated from the support that the relationship offers.

A further strength to the model is Peplau's suggestion of six roles for the nurse engaged in a therapeutic relationship:

- *Stranger*: the first role – nurses and patients usually meet as strangers. The nurse is instrumental in extending social and professional skills in order to establish a relationship.
- *Resource*: the nurse is a source of information and encourages patient involvement and understanding.

- *Teacher*: the nurse guides and facilitates.
- *Leader*: the nurse leads the process to identify goals.
- *Surrogate*: the nurse represents people relevant to the patient and helps the patient to recall experiences.
- *Counsellor*: the nurse helps the person to reflect on, recognise and come to terms with aspects of their experiences and feelings.

Although significant changes in the care and treatment of people who are mentally ill have occurred since the 1950s, it remains that the relationship established between nurses and patients is central to aspects of the quality of care. Peplau suggests that the principles may be applied to any other setting where such interpersonal relationships exist.

Roy's Adaptation Model

Callista Roy developed her model in California in the early 1960s. Her ideas about nursing developed from observations of patients, many of them children, and how they coped with, and adapted to, their health states.

The aim of the model is to promote adaptation and the coping abilities of patients. Roy studied stress theories and ways of coping and suggested that individuals have different ways and levels of adapting to changes in health, which the nurse needs to identify and respond to (Roy, 1997).

Roy suggests four modes of adaptation:

- *Physiological*: responses to physiological and biological demands and change.
- *Self-concept*: responses to beliefs and feelings about oneself.
- *Role functions*: responses to role function in relation to one's roles.
- *Interdependence*: responses to relationships with people and other sources of comfort and support.

Roy advocates two levels of assessment. The first level of assessment is based on the four modes of adaptation that prompt the nurse to consider how changes in health have affected key aspects of the individual's life, role, relationships and physical well-being. Table 12.1 gives examples of problems affecting adaptation, causing stress, and requiring support and interventions. Each mode is interrelated and is used to guide assessment. With this model, the nurse may be prompted to explore the problems in more detail. Roy suggests that, by applying a second-level assessment, the true nature of the problem, or stressors, can be explored, understood, and used as the basis for prioritising interventions and care-planning. By exploring the stimuli underpinning each problem, care will be more individualised and targeted. These stimuli are described as follows:

- *Focal*: the main reason for the problem.
- *Contextual*: all other factors influencing the focal stimulus.
- *Residual*: associated beliefs, feelings and attitudes relating to the situation, as expressed by the patient.

This offers a detailed approach to assessment, emphasising the value of quality assessment data as outlined earlier in the chapter. It stresses the need for ongoing assessment and a relationship based on continuity. For many care environments, such as day-care wards, this is an obvious challenge. However, the principles of determining the impact of health changes on the patient's adaptive, coping behaviours through systematic assessment may lead to greater understanding of individual needs and ultimately reductions in stress.

Table 12.1 Roy's first level of assessment

	Mode of adaptation	**Example of problems**
Physiological	Physiological mode	
Exercise and rest		Insomnia
Nutrition		Nausea
Elimination		Incontinence
Fluid and electrolytes		Hypovolaemia
Oxygenation and circulation		Dyspnoea
Regulation of temperature, senses and endocrine system		Pyrexia
Self-concept	Self-concept mode	
Physical self		Poor self-image
Personal self		Guilt, loss of confidence
Role function	Role function mode	
Primary roles		Role change
Secondary roles		Role failure
Tertiary roles		Role dependency
Interdependence	Interdependence mode	
On others		Loneliness
With others		Isolation

Orem's Self-Care Model

Orem (1995) developed her model in the USA at a time when consumerism was gaining momentum and the US public was seeking value for money for their health care. This model offers an opportunity to explore the implications of self-care nursing for the patient and the nurse. Self-care is concerned with shifting responsibilities for decision-making about caring activities, appropriately, from nurses to patients. However, as Orem acknowledges, self-care activities are dependent on the patient's abilities and dependency, for example, and are about maximising opportunities for patients to be in control of, and be able to contribute to, the management of their health.

Nursing, based on this model, is seen as a system in which the promotion of self-care is therapeutic for the patient. Care-planning is dependent on the assessment of three areas of self-care requisites:

- *Universal self-care requisites*: individual needs to maintain health and well-being, e.g. nutrition, social interaction, preventing hazards.
- *Developmental self-care requisites*: these relate to the experience and maturation of the individual.
- *Health deviation self-care requisites*: these result from disease, injury, trauma or treatment.

In order to facilitate the notion that self-care may be promoted across, for example, levels of dependency, Orem describes three nursing systems:

- *Wholly compensatory nursing*: the nurse takes responsibility for the total care of patients unable to carry out any activities, e.g. unconscious patients.
- *Partly compensatory nursing*: the nurse undertakes aspects of care that the person is unable to do independently or without help.
- *Supportive–educative nursing*: the nurse supports and guides the patient to carry out self-care that the patient cannot do without knowledge, skill, practice or assistance.

Based on this model, care-planning depends on the nurse adopting one or more of these approaches to care, depending on the needs and skills of the patient, the patient's willingness to undertake self-care activities, and the the patient's ability to be self-caring. During a period of care, one or all of the systems may be applied as changes in health and dependency occur.

SUMMARY

- Nursing models, though abstract in nature, have contributed much to the understanding of approaches to nursing care and the development of nursing theory.
- Nursing process is a feature of theoretical nursing frameworks and assists the organisation of care and care plans.
- Nursing theory contributes to our understanding of the complexity of nursing and the range of needs that may need a nursing response.
- Theories have a fundamental part to play in our thinking, decision-making and ability to analyse care, all of which are essential to effective practice and care management.

CONCLUSION

In this chapter we have briefly explored the nature of individuality and how that plays into the relationship between nurse and patient – a key determinant of the quality of nursing care. Although much depends on individual interaction, this does not exist in a vacuum. The organisation of nursing care is equally important, as are the resources, skills and educational support on which it depends. Systematic patient assessment, nursing diagnosis, planning and evaluation of care are facilitated by the nursing process and underpinned by nursing theory and knowledge. Theoretical nursing frameworks offer nurses a range of approaches to promote individualised care, prioritise needs and promote effective decision-making. The nursing process is integral to the application of nursing theories and organising care systematically.

These are not academic niceties but critical components of the professional judgement that exemplifies what the care of people through nursing is all about.

References

Alfaro-LeFevre R (2006). *Applying Nursing Process: A Tool for Critical Thinking*, 6th edn. Philadelphia, PA: Lippincott Williams & Wilkins.

Benner P (1984). *From Novice to Expert: Excellence and Power in Clinical Nursing Practice*. New York: Addison-Wesley.

Carpenito-Moyet L (2006). *Nursing Diagnosis: Application to Clinical Practice*, 11th edn. Philadelphia, PA: Lippincott Williams & Wilkins.

Carper BA (1978). Fundamental patterns of knowing in nursing. *Advances in Nursing Science*, **1**, 13–23.

Henderson V (1966). *The Nature of Nursing: A Definition and its Implications for Practice, Research, and Education*. Riverside, NJ: Macmillan.

Hogston R (1997). Nursing diagnosis and classification systems: a position paper. *Journal of Advanced Nursing*, **26**, 496–500.

Marriner-Tomey A and Alligood MR (2006) *Nursing Theorists and Their Work*, 6th edn. St Louis, MO: Mosby.

Maslow A (1954). *Motivation and Personality*. New York: Harper.

Meleis AI (2007). *Theoretical Nursing*, 4th edn. Philadelphia, PA: Lippincott Williams & Wilkins.

NANDA International (2007). *Nursing Diagnoses: Definitions and Classification 2007–2008*. Philadelphia, PA: NANDA International.

Nursing and Midwifery Council (NMC) (2004). *Standards of Proficiency for Pre-Registration Nursing Education*. London: Nursing and Midwifery Council.

Nursing and Midwifery Council (NMC) (2008). *The Code: Standards of Conduct, Performance and Ethics for Nurses and Midwives*. London: Nursing and Midwifery Council.

Orem DE (1995). *Nursing: Concepts of Practice*, 5th edn. St Louis, MO: Mosby.

Orem DE (2001). *Nursing: Concepts of Practice*, 6th edn. St Louis, MO: Mosby.

Pellegrino ED (1982). Being ill and being healed: some reflections on the grounding of medical morality. In Kestenbaum V (ed.) *The Humanity of the Ill: Phenonemenological Perspectives*. Knoxville, TN: University of Tennessee Press.

Peplau HE (1952). *Interpersonal Relations in Nursing*. New York: Putnam.

Rogers C (1969). *Freedom to Learn: A View of what Education Might Become*. Columbus, OH: Merrill.

Roper N, Logan W and Tierney AJ (2000). *The Roper–Logan–Tierney Model of Nursing*. Edinburgh: Churchill Livingstone.

Roy C (1997). Future of the Roy model: challenge to redefine adaptation. *Nursing Science Quarterly*, **10**, 42–8.

Royal College of Nursing (RCN) (2003). *Defining Nursing*. London: Royal College of Nursing.

Simon HA (1950). *Administrative Behaviour*. New York: Macmillan.

Further reading

American Nurses Association. Nursing world. www.ana.org.

Hawley G (ed.) (2007). *Ethics in Clinical Practice: An Interprofessional Approach*. Harlow: Pearson Education.
A useful introductory text exploring a wide range of ethical and cultural issues relevant to clinical decision-making.

International Orem Society for Nursing Science and Scholarship. Self-care deficit nursing theory. www.scdnt.com.

Marriner Tomey A and Alligood MR (2006). *Nursing Theorists and Their Work*, 6th edn. St Louis, MO: Mosby.
A valuable resource covering a range of nursing theories and how they relate to nursing practice.

NANDA International. www.nanda.org.

Nursing and Midwifery Council (NMC) (2002). *An NMC Guide for Students of Nursing and Midwifery*. London: Nursing and Midwifery Council.
For readers of this chapter who are also student nurses, this is an essential resource. It clearly explains the responsibilities of student nurses in relation to patient care (Appendix 3).

Roper N, Logan W and Tierney AJ (2000). *The Roper–Logan–Tierney Model of Nursing*. Edinburgh: Churchill Livingstone.
This is the final text from the originators of the most popular nursing model used in the UK. It explains and elaborates on the key features of the model and provides an accessible text from which nurses may continue to understand and apply the useful principles to practice.

Royal College of Nursing. www.rcn.org.uk.

13

Loving nursing: nursing beyond boundaries and the search for well-being

Stephen G Wright

In this life, we cannot do great things. We can only do small things with great love.

Mother Teresa (cited in Kornfield, 1993, p. 14)

Introduction

We teeter always on the existential edge. At any moment our quietly ordered lives can fall into chaos. All the things we have built and created, often in part to protect our lives against disruption, can fall apart. I witnessed this recently after a delayed flight to Australia – suddenly my plans and those of 500 others were thrown into disarray. Connecting flights were missed, important appointments scuppered, long cherished meetings and events would not happen. Passengers responded in varying degrees, from quiet resignation to volcanic fury.

The collapse of order into disorder on that journey was to mirror events in my own life a week later. I was going to begin this chapter with some insights from a study on the nature of nursing I helped to create for *Nursing Standard* a few years ago. The insights then gained from my role as dispassionate observer (Wright, 2004) were brought into sharp focus, and affirmed, as my own predictable existence was plunged into uncertainty when a major health problem arose. Thus by chance, if chance it be, my introductory words shifted from being grounded in theory to the experience of practice as nurses and others did what they had to do to keep me in this world. I was teetering then on the existential edge, watching all my plans disintegrate as a life-threatening heart condition seemed likely to tip my entire being over the edge.

In that emergency department a long way from home, it was the nurses and doctors who were visible in this reality keeping me with them. I bless every one of them, not least for the way they affirmed some core beliefs about nursing that this chapter will seek to explore. In the next few pages we will look at some of the current thinking on the nature of nursing and how we promote well-being. To do this, we will discuss specifically the nature of well-being and the qualities that nurses bring into work and relationships with patients that enhance it. Many words and concepts are used in nursing without us really considering their deeper meanings, and yet they are fundamental to our grasp of nursing work and its impact on well-being. Thus, parts of this chapter will examine what we mean by holism, right relationship, consciousness, spirituality and the sacred, listening and touching skills – these words and the concepts they describe are part of the language of nursing, and yet our understanding of them is sometimes superficial. To begin this chapter, please take a few moments to work though Reflection point 13.1.

Learning objectives

After studying this chapter you should be able to:

- understand the breadth of the concept of well-being;
- grasp what is meant by 'compassion' and see its place within the chaos that can be nursing;
- explore the physical, intellectual, emotional and spiritual components of intelligence;
- define what is meant by 'holism' and understand nurses' and patients' roles within this;

- explore the concepts of right relationships, connection and sacred space;
- see the importance of both touch and listening within your practice.

Reflection point 13.1

We have begun by using the word 'well-being'. What does this mean to you? How is it related to health, healing and wellness, and what, if any, are the differences? Is someone who is dying 'healthy'? Can someone with a chronic debilitating illness experience 'well-being'? Make some notes on your own thoughts about these issues before we proceed.

Now apply these thoughts to yourself, as you are now. Would you say that you are in a state of well-being (as you define it yourself) right now? If not, why not? If you are, then on what basis are you making this judgement? What is it for you that defines your own personal sense of well-being? Think back to the last time you might have considered you were not in a state of well-being – were you sick? Had you had an accident? Were you worried or unhappy about something? What was it like for you?

Humanisers, chaos managers and clear-eyed lovers

Modern psychology sees two particular states of consciousness or ways of being in the world. The first is the everyday conscious realm of our thinking and behaviour that we are aware of. The unconscious realm lies beneath our everyday awareness, and yet it influences the latter in many ways that are unknown to us, until we explore it more deeply. Consciously or unconsciously, we all live with the anxiety of being. Tillich (2000) argues that we fill our lives with all manner of things – possessions, relationships, work, drugs – in order to keep at bay the fear of non-being, of death, of meaninglessness, which bubbles beneath the surface of our psyches, threatening to become exposed and cast us into overwhelming anxiety and despair whenever our ordered existence comes unstuck and is revealed for the fragile thing it is.

This idea of the shadow of death in our unconscious minds means that we create things in order to keep death at bay – not least, our health services. In that sense, says Obholzer (2003), there is no such thing as health or well-being in the unconscious, only the concept of death – and one of the ways we defend against death is to create social institutions such as health services. Indeed, he notes, 'our health service might be more accurately called a "keep death at bay" service'.

Although we don the role of nurses, this does not remove us from our place as human beings like everyone else, subject to the same underlying anxiety of our own existence. At the same time we enter the anxiety of others when health crises threaten well-being. Our desire for well-being, for ourselves and others, is the defence against chaos and disorder that might be precursors to death. Nurses are there in health promotion work in countless ways seeking to stop people falling into the chaos that ensues when even the most minor health problem takes hold. We are there as accompaniers, what Campbell (1984) called 'companions', coming alongside patients when ill health strikes. Like passengers on a journey, nurses and patients come together for a while, and remain together while the journey obtains, and then separate as the need for nursing passes away – perhaps to restoration of health, or the management of disability, or death.

Nurses have very clear rules laid down about how we should behave in this context, and this chapter is written with its roots in the NMC Code (2008) (Appendix 1). That we should 'treat people as individuals and respect their dignity', 'not discriminate' and 'act as advocates' are essential prerequisites to the promotion of well-being. Without these characteristics, nursing is reduced to rote automatism, and people simply do not respond with a sense of well-being when treated in this way. As we shall see in this chapter, the meeting of individual needs lies at the heart of our sense of wellness, and that includes the individual needs of the nurse. All of the assumptions in this chapter are also based on the need to 'use the best available evidence' (NMC Code, 2008). Some of the subjects discussed may seem somewhat difficult at first to underpin with evidence, and yet, as will be indicated in the various sections, evidence there is, especially from emerging research (and not all of it purely nursing) to show that there are firm foundations in practice for the key ethical, practical and moral aspects of modern nursing. There is much in the NMC Code that illuminates the nurse's responsibility to patients and the profession. But it may be curious to note that there is nothing specific in relation to nurses and our own self-care needs. As we shall explore, the right relationship we cultivate with patients, which underpins a sense of well-being, surely sits in parallel with nurses being in the right relationship with themselves. However, the evidence suggests that, in many respects, many nurses are sometimes deficient in promoting their own well-being, let alone that of others (Wright and Sayre-Adams, 2000). Thus, let us look a little more closely at what is meant by 'well-being' and how as nurses we can nurture it in our own lives and the lives of those we serve.

The state of well-being, which dictionaries variously define as being comfortable, contented, healthy and untroubled, is just that – a state, a human condition. Notice it is a 'being' and not a 'doing' word, referring to a condition, a feeling or a perception that explains how we experience ourselves, how we *are* in the world. And, like all such feeling words, it is profoundly subjective – well-being for a dying person might mean they have come to a place of peace and acceptance of their fate, while for another person even the thought of dying might project them into feeling dis-comfited and troubled, knocking them out of their otherwise perceived state of well-being. Well-being is thus not a constant, and because human beings seek well-being (and note also that we call ourselves 'human beings', not 'human doings') and to be in states where harmony prevails, we spend a lot of our lives doing things to promote it – taking in food and drink, exercising, attending to hygiene and so on in order to keep the body healthy, avoiding conflict, seeking lov-ing relationships, finding work that satisfies, spiritually searching, and looking for connection, meaning and purpose in life.

Well-being is related closely to the word 'will' – the capacity to bring control and volition into our lives. Loss of control can mean loss of well-being, whether that loss can be because others are exercising power over us, such as a bullying boss or a kidnapper, or whether some disease takes away our ability to order our own lives. 'Will' and 'well' are also linked linguistically to words such as 'whole', which derives from the Teutonic 'healan' and the Greek 'holos' referring to hale, whole, hearty, healthy, holy. When we are in a state of well-being, we feel whole, at one and at peace with the world and our place in it, and perhaps even to concepts beyond the world – the absolute, the eternal, the divine, how ever and if ever we experience it.

The work of nurses is focused on health and our perceptions of it that contribute significantly to our sense of well-being. For accompanying disease there is invariably dis-ease – the feelings of fear, uncertainty and disharmony that abide with the illness experience. Nursing works as a humanitarian act to protect and maintain well-being specifically in relation to health, and yet health itself is such a broad concept that nurses can be found in countless avenues of life, in car-ing roles that transcend the treatment of disease. The diversity of perceptions and expectations of health is mirrored in the expansion of nursing roles into countless settings where human beings fall into, or risk falling into, suffering. Historically this has led nursing into real difficulties in defining what nursing is. And whole forests have been felled for the paper needed by nursing theorists to do that defining. Yet, a lack of strict definition may paradoxically be of service, for it allows nurses to infiltrate innumerable situations where people suffer and to be of service. These sloppy boundaries can be distressing to nurses and those who sometimes seek to organise us, but they may also set us free to go where the need is. Nurses can be found with the wounded in war zones, feeding refugees, helping the homeless, at the highest levels of politics, taking care of the addicted, giving drugs, policy-making, working in complementary therapies, and so on – what a broad church!

And so to my nurses in that emergency room. What were they doing and being that made their care so effective for me? First of all, in our technologically rich but often spiritually poor health system, they were humanising that system for me. By their humour, their concern, their kindness and their explanations, they made the clinical but soulless setting bearable. In short, they used their expressive, relational qualities to make me feel cared for and cared about, and they made me feel connected, informed and held, especially as my body slipped irrevocably into chaos and my choices of exercising will diminished by the minute until there was no choice but to surrender entirely to the process over which I had no control. Indeed there was a certain relief, a feeling of well-being, that came with having no more choices to make, to putting myself entirely in their and, in my book, God's hands, and trusting the process and that all might be well. It turned out that it was – as my opportunity to write this chapter bears witness.

Second, my nurses were not only holding my hand, making me feel better, accompanying me in my fear. They were also active participants in the chaotic dance that was going on around me and within my body as my heart fell further into dysfunction. This was the 'moderated love', as Campbell (1984) has described it, the agape that transcends love associated with lust or desire for things or people but that is a form of love in which there is sincere loving concern for the well-being of another, indeed for all of humanity. This calls us to move beyond sympathy, where we can understand what another feels and feel it as if it were our own, and beyond empathy, where we can identify with the other person's situation and really feel it as they might feel it themselves. Into compassion, which calls us to combine feeling with action, the heartfelt desire to care, to be of service, to alleviate suffering. Their kindness and attentiveness were not just emotional concern but also practical action. They related but they were also technically skilful. Knowledge and feelings, action and compassion, science and art – all were merging into comprehensive and effective caring. They thus demonstrated the symbiosis of art and science in nursing. A nurse who can relate well to you is pretty pointless if they cannot control the infusion in the emergency room; likewise the nurse who knows the science and has the manual skills but is cold and disconnected inhibits the patient's sense of well-being.

Compassion arises out of the unconditional love that Campbell has described, but goes further for it spurs us to action. But what is compassion? Sogyal Rinpoche says:

> *it is not simply a sense of sympathy or caring for the person suffering, or a sharp clarity of recognition of their needs and pain, it is also a sustained and practical determination to do whatever is possible and necessary to help alleviate their suffering.*

> (Sogyal Rinpoche, 1992, p. 187)

Nursing is about bringing more love and compassion into the world through the relief of suffering and the promotion of well-being. It is compassion without attachment (Ram Dass and Bush, 1992; Longaker, 1998), a way of being in the world that does not exhaust us with the burden of caring for others, but that liberates us to care from a place of resting at home within ourselves.

In the hands of my nurses at this crisis time, I felt this loving concern, backed up with all the actions that they were taking – checking monitors, shaving my chest, administering drugs. It was loving, but it was love in action. And feeling loved is one of the most profound agents of well-being. For nurses to be loving in this way requires numerous elements to be in place, which I discuss later in this chapter.

'Love', however, is not a word that sits easily within much of contemporary nursing dialogue, and many nurses are somewhat diffident about its use in their work (Savage, 1995). But I observed the way my nurses were managing the chaos of my body, and more invisibly the ever present potential chaos of the hospital system and indeed of life all around me. At any moment, the ordered world of the hospital could tip over into chaos – staff sickness, power failures, a mass emergency – all those potential agents of chaos out there, which nurses keep at bay or manage when they arise – with the core intent of keeping the patient safe and well. It crossed my mind as I lay on that trolley that maybe someday there will be an advertisement in the nursing press for 'chaos managers (band 8)'.

Loving compassion, the ability to humanise the system and the ability to manage the forces of chaos were all qualities my nurses were exhibiting that contributed to my safety and comfort and to my sense of well-being. A fourth quality was evident, which I have described in detail elsewhere (Wright, 2005), and you could see it in the eyes. It's that feeling you get in an ordinary conversation when you know the person is either fully attentive to you or is perhaps politely listening while their attention has really drifted off elsewhere. At dinner some years ago, a group of nursing professors, myself among them, were pontificating on the nature of nursing, as professors are inclined to do. The only non-nurse present, the husband of my host, listened with great patience but eventually felt moved to interrupt. 'You've got it all wrong,' he said.' When I was sick in hospital I realised there are only two types of nurses – the glassy-eyed and the clear-eyed.'

My friend went on to describe in layperson's terms what Benner (1984) in her seminal thesis had described as 'presencing'. The glassy-eyed ones came into his room, did all the practical nursing, seemingly as good as any other, 'but you could tell by the glazed look in their eyes, no matter what they were saying to you or you to them, that they weren't really *with* you.' He went on to talk about 'clear-eyed' nurses, who were 'absolutely present' for him. 'You could tell again by the look in their eyes – so clear, so attentive – that nothing else was going on with them. They weren't thinking about the next job or what they did the night before. They were just right there for me, right there.'

The capacity to 'be in the moment' or to 'be here, now' (Ram Dass, 1971) for somebody has a meditative quality to it, an approach to caring where our own agendas and mental 'busyness' are set aside so that we can be fully attentive to the other. The best carers, of whatever sort – doctors, nurses, chaplains, social workers and the rest – are just being present and doing what needs to be done with full attentiveness and awareness. People feel better around such carers and, like my friend, when feeling better they are more likely to get better. He made another interesting observation: that his clear-eyed nurses were just as busy as the others, but it was something about the grace of their presence that made the difference. Thus, a therapeutic relationship may not be dependent on time and the opportunity to get to know someone deeply; it may depend more simply on who we are. Not just doing but also being determines the quality of the therapeutic encounter, however brief. The work of the expert carer is not just built on professional knowledge and skills; it is also dependent on understanding the immense healing power of our uncluttered selves. Modern professional education pays much attention to the former, and arguably the latter is still a barely explored territory.

Reflection point 13.2

Pause in your reading for a moment and think about what it is like for you when you are actually working with patients. Do you find it easy to be fully attentive to them, just dealing with whatever arises at that moment? Do you sometimes find yourself feeling distracted, under pressure to move to the next job, pulled away to another patient who needs you, or worried about something at home? Do you think the patients notice the difference and, if so, how does this affect them? How does this affect you? What do you feel like in those moments when you know you are fully present for the patient before you and their needs, just dealing with what arises. What do you feel like when you are distracted, pulled away, focused on other things?

If we consider the nursing examples cited above, it may be seen that the complexity of nursing being and doing draws on our rich capacity of what it is to be human. In watching one of the nurses caring for me, I counted some 80 different decisions in some 10 minutes, then lost count and was reminded of an earlier opportunity (Wright, 2004) observing the rapid-fire decision-making process of nursing. And all of this was going on in a seamless artful way that belied the underlying intricacy and complexity. The capacity to manipulate equipment in a smooth and efficient manner, talk to the doctor and myself, measure a drug regime, cleanse my skin, watch the monitors, tell a colleague what to do, respond to a request from a nurse beyond the curtain, adjust my clothing – all these are individually simple yet collectively complex decisions, flowing one into the other, a stream of simultaneous decision-making that is quite breathtaking when you really consider it.

The stream was in full flow, yet masked by a matter-of-factness that belies the underpinning synthesis of thought and feeling and action. Such internal processing and external action, being and doing, had come about not by accident but by considered education and training, marrying up many ways of knowing with the inherent personal capacities. In such circumstances, what we see at work here is an integration of knowledge and skill that transforms the work from limited task into complicated craft – yet like all craft, it seems graceful and effortless but leaves you full of wonder about 'where did that all come from?' What is key to nursing work is the *integration* of many levels of knowing, problem-solving and action. Precisely because they are well integrated and appear to flow with ease, then, they often belie to the observer (and those who pay for or appreciate nurses) just how complex the reality of nursing work is. The different domains of intelligence at work are:

- *Physical intelligence*: ways of moving, handling equipment and manipulating things in the environment – such ways of knowing become embodied, there is no conscious effort of 'I must put my hand thus' or 'I turn my head this way'. The information has been learned and internalised and assimilated so that conscious monitoring of every action is unnecessary (without which even the simplest of bodily coordinations would take a long time to complete – thus we always think of the novice nurse as being 'slow' compared with the experienced nurse). Nursing at this level is, literally, like riding a bike – the body and mind have learned what to do in a given set of circumstances so they can just get on with it. At the same time, the inherent physical intelligence of our bodies continues – the autonomic nervous system and other methods of maintaining homeostasis keep our bodies in harmony without having to think about it. Thus we possess a huge range of embodied physical intelligence, some acquired and some inherited, that enable efficient action with harmony beyond conscious control.
- *Intellectual intelligence*: synthesising nursing knowledge of pain control, for example, or how organisations tick, how a patient gets transferred home, what specialist help is available, and

so on, drawing on an infinite well of information, facts and memories to find ways to solve problems, to know what to do and what sort of help is needed. Thus nurses draw on an incredibly deep well of knowledge and experience to make decisions, teach and help. Our capacity to process information at this level is important and the concept of IQ is integral to nursing – for we have various ways of determining whether nurses are of sufficient intellectual intelligence to master the amount of information needed to deliver patient care.

- *Emotional intelligence*: IQ and what might be called PQ (physical intelligence) have traditionally been given much attention in the preparation of nurses. Many early models of nursing education laid great emphasis on physical and intellectual skills. Emotional intelligence (EQ; Goleman, 1995) is the capacity to sympathise and empathise, to 'get inside the patient's skin' and see and feel the world from the patient's point of view, while at the same time having acquired insight and emotional maturity into our own internal emotional processes – to know when a patient is suffering but also to know our own, to experience all the gamut of human emotions because we are aware of them in ourselves too and know how to respond to them in healthy ways; all this is part of emotional intelligence. This is part of the emotional underpinning of caring, an ability to respond at a feeling level to what we and patients experience, and, perhaps more importantly, to be able to do so authentically. There is much debate about whether emotional intelligence can be taught, and it certainly does not respond to a list on a handout about 'how to be kind'. The process of teaching and learning about emotional intelligence is partly the product of our life experiences, but it can also be developed in, for example, group processes or one-to-one work with a therapist, where we can come to know better what makes us and others tick, and how to respond from a place that is sincere. Otherwise, caring becomes a rote, superficial response, where we may appear to be caring, but behind this 'glassy-eyed' actions is the shallowness of the trained customer-relations person who wishes us a 'nice day' or assures us that 'we care about you'. These superficial responses are masks to engage us in some way (usually for profit or cooperation), and yet they rest on the barren landscape of emotional indifference. Caring has to be genuine in nursing, and patients can be quick to spot it when it is not. Emotional intelligence, backed up by a genuine humanity to attend to the well-being of another, kindness, attentiveness, openness, caring – these and other attributes form part of the compassionate caring response, which the best of nursing brings forth but which cannot be manufactured.
- *Spiritual intelligence*: this is, arguably, like EQ, a subject much neglected in the twentieth-century preparation of nurses. Spiritual intelligence (Zohar and Marshall, 2000) is more than the knowledge of when to summon the chaplain or how to get other help for a patient's religious needs. A full exploration of the relationship between spiritual and religious care is beyond the scope of this chapter, but we can see spiritual intelligence as concerning the heartfelt desire to find meaning, purpose and connection in life, even among suffering and dis-ease, and not just joy and happiness. It concerns the capacity to seek beyond ordinary existence for the transcendent, the absolute and (for some) the divine. This is the intelligence of what some cultures call the 'soul' and others the 'true self', and that which binds us and connects us to others and all creation. Historically, nursing has shied away from the exploration of spirituality, other than checking the patient's religion and finding help when needed (Wright, 2005). Yet spiritual care is not something that is the reserve of the religionists. The ability to sit with someone in distress and help them find meaning in it, to listen deeply and to be fully present with another are all the attributes of spirituality.

Scenario 13.1

Mrs Evans is being cared for at home after major surgery. Nurses call in each day to check her dressing and monitor her drug regime. While there, Julia, one of the nurses, realises that Mrs Evans is still feeling very weak and has not been feeding herself well or attending to her personal hygiene. Julia helps Mrs Evans to wash, tidies her hair and later organises a care assistant to call in each day to help with hygiene. When Julia goes back to the GP surgery, she makes some calls to see what help can be organised with meals on wheels and gets in touch with Mrs Evans' family and friends to see what extra help can be given. While changing Mrs Evans' dressing, Julia spends some time telling her how the wound is healing, allaying her fears about infection. Mrs Evans lives alone and loves to have her nurses call in – it's company after all – and Julia senses this. Julia is a busy nurse, like all the rest in her team, but she makes sure that she spends some time with Mrs Evans, making her a cup of tea and so on. They talk about all sorts of things – families, work and reminiscences. Julia knows that sometimes she doesn't need to say very much – Mrs Evans seems content just to chat and be heard. Once Mrs Evans talked about what she wanted to happen if 'things went wrong' – she is often negative about her life. Even though the surgery was routine and the wound infection manageable, Mrs Evans always seems to fear the worst and says things such as 'If it's going to go wrong for anybody, you can be sure it will always be me that gets it.' Julia notices this and sometimes just listens, and sometimes offers facts and advice to counteract Mrs Evans's fears, making a point of holding her hand or giving her a hug. That seems to make Mrs Evans more hopeful and less pessimistic. Sometimes Mrs Evans mentions dying or becoming more disabled. Julia listens. Mrs Evans is probably going to be fine, but there is not much else she can do. Anyway, Julia feels that maybe just being around and listening is enough. Somehow Mrs Evans seems a little lighter after their conversations; in fact she once said that she was glad of her chats with Julia because 'It reminds me that I'm still here and life's not all that bad.' Julia notices that whenever she leaves Mrs Evans, she feels a little lighter and happier in herself too.

Consider this everyday nurse–patient interaction and the four 'intelligences' outlined in the text above. Which of these was Julia using in her work?

The four domains of intelligence flow into, depend upon and affect each other, and their integration is the bedrock of nursing action, the landscape of immense caring opportunity. Such work places great demands upon nurses to make full, caring, compassionate connection to others in the promotion of well-being. Nursing patients towards whole/well-being asks for a parallel whole/wellness of nurses and being in 'right relationship' (Wright and Sayre-Adams, 2000) with those we work with, the organisations we work for, patients and our deepest selves. Nurses who feel more whole in themselves and who work in environments where they feel cared for and about are more likely to be able to put into practice the full gamut of their abilities and to do so more efficiently and effectively at every level (Gooch, 2006). Holistic nursing needs nurses and contexts that nurture a sense of holism, and yet holism has become a profoundly misunderstood word in nursing (Dossey *et al.*, 2000).

Holism

Holism is much more than the limited attempts at description that often appear in health care literature or in common parlance. Holism is sometimes reduced to ideas of giving total care to the patient's biopsychosocial needs. Latterly it has become fashionable to add spiritual needs as well. Holistic care and holism are more than these. Holism encourages us to think of human beings as part of the universe, which is a dynamic web of interconnected and interrelated events, none of which functions in isolation. Healing and holism, as suggested earlier, are closely related words, taking us beyond the absence of disease and beyond the notion of human beings as being no more than products of their biological processes. Modern physicists such as Talbot (1991) and Bohm (1973) have been at the leading edge of our understanding of holism. Bohm, for example, writes:

There has been too little emphasis on what is, in our view, the most fundamentally different new feature of all, i.e. the intimate interconnectedness of different systems that are not in spatial contact . . . the parts are seen to be in immediate connection, in which their dynamical relationships depend, in an irreducible way, on the state of the whole system (and indeed on that broader system in which they are contained, extending ultimately and in principle to the entire universe.) Thus one is led to a new notion of unbroken wholeness which denies the classical idea of analysability of the world into separate and independently existing parts.

(Bohm, 1973, p. 149)

Holism asks us to reach out beyond our limited definitions of what people are, passed down in biological, medical, sociological and psychological models. Everything, absolutely everything, is connected. No system functions in isolation. Martha Rogers (1970) in her nursing theory of 'unitary human beings' was one of the first to bring this new paradigm into a nursing and health care context.

In holistic nursing we are led into the view that nurse and patient can no longer be seen as separate entities when well-being is being sought. We are all caught up in the process, the search for well-being together. Young (quoted in Forder and Forder, 1995) observes this when he says:

There can be a moment in healing when there is perfect balance and all distinction . . . between wounded and healer disappears. It is at this moment that something else can enter and both are transported to a place of mystery. Part of us yearns to return to that place because it is here that we are made whole.

(Young, 1995, p. 138)

Nurses too are healers – drawing wholeness and well-being into the world from countless situations of crisis and chaos associated with the health–illness continuum. This sense of participating together in a process where distinctions merge offers us a perspective on the holistic nature of nursing. It differs markedly from the traditional view that nursing concerns only what one person does to another – injects a drug, applies a treatment, and so on. In the holistic sense, well-being and healing are reached as much with the involvement of the nurse and all that they bring to the caring relationship, as with the patient and the milieu in which the two come together. And the milieu is not just the home or the hospital but the subtle connection and interplay of the whole of creation, of all that is.

Holism challenges the notion embraced by much of Western medico-scientific thinking that we are entirely separate as human beings and who we are can be defined by our biological and psychological limits. An increasing body of research is now lending scientific credence to the holistic paradigm – nurses are part of the healing stream and many recent studies support the holistic notions that we do not end at our skin and that our presence, and more importantly our loving presence, can influence another person even though we are not in physical contact with them. The work of Achterberg and colleagues (2005) and the Institute of HeartMath (2006) have awesome implications for the ways in which nurses work with patients and each other. Achterberg *et al.*, using a magnetic resonance scanner, demonstrated that the healing intention of someone not in physical contact with another (i.e. in a separate room) can be illuminated by changes in the patterns emerging on the scanner – something as yet unexplained but that many in the healing professions have long suggested exists (e.g. Dossey, 1997). Studies on non-local healing – that is, where there is no physical contact with patients, such as prayer and therapeutic touch – have yielded some startling results with profound implications for nursing. It seems that something about our intention and about our presence can directly affect others, even though we are not in direct contact with them. Other work by the HeartMath team indicates that one person's electrocardiogram (ECG) pattern can be mirrored in the electroencephalogram (EEG) pattern of another, again even though they are not touching. We might conjecture: does this give us other clues as to how teams work together when the leader is feeling serene and when they are not? If one person in a team is feeling off centre, are there more ways that they might be influencing patients and colleagues than just the observable behaviour? When we are feeling more 'at one', then, based on these studies, can it be that people are more likely to feel at one around us? I was watching a group of nurses on a dermatology unit recently and the sister in charge, in this extremely busy environment, kept her cool. She was well grounded in herself and radiated a sense of calm and attentiveness that was infectious. People got on with their work in the same way. They responded to her harmony by being the same themselves. I watched how this radiated out to the patients on the unit as well. The workload was high and fast-paced, but you'd barely know it by the quiet presence of the leader and the team members, who just got on with it.

I contrast this with an experience on another unit a few weeks later, which was nowhere near as busy and yet where the staff seemed to be all over the place. The ward leader seemed permanently detached and distracted. The team seemed uncoordinated and disconnected. As a visitor with my sick partner, we both felt the uncertainty, and the nurses seemed to be always somewhere else (glassy-eyed). We did not feel at ease, confident or understood.

If we do not end at our skin, then what is it that might connect us in the holistic web? What is it that we cannot see and yet which seems to allow the well-being of one person to affect another? Is it some form of energy that has yet to be identified? Modern physics recognises only four forms of energy – strong and weak nuclear forces, gravity and electromagnetic. Is that word 'energy', so often bandied around in health and healing work – especially in the new age thinking, real, but as yet unidentified scientifically? Is it something to do, as Dossey (1997) posits, with some unknown ability of consciousness to reach out beyond our own physical nervous system? Is this ineffable consciousness located not only in the functions of the brain but in part of the vast web that connects the universe and connects all things?

Consciousness

Health professionals are trained to use the term 'state of consciousness' to describe a continuum from 'normal' behaviour to pathological or altered states, varying from drug-induced to psychotic states, from metabolic derangement to post-traumatic head injuries. However, much of cutting-edge science in the field of consciousness research is illuminating how very limited this view is. Newman (1986) was one of the first nursing theorists to see health as more than bodily integrity but that true health occurs only as our consciousness expands – the unending learning but understanding of ourselves and our place in the scheme of things, the transformation of the shadows in our unconscious by bringing them into the light of the conscious mind. Furthermore, an increasing body of evidence is pointing to the non-locality of consciousness as suggested above – in other words, consciousness is not just about what we loosely consider taking place in the 'mind' with thought, dreams and ideas. It actually impacts upon our bodies and the wider world in infinitely more complex ways than has hitherto been considered or researched.

The work of Pert in the relatively new field of psychoneuroimmunology shows how our emotions can affect the physical state of the body (e.g. Pert, 1997). To summarise this view: if we take an example of a person given a diagnosis of a serious illness, the anxiety associated with the diagnosis causes the immune system to be depressed just at a time when it is needed to deal with the illness. Thus, nurses working in ways that reassure the patient, and inspire trust, confidence, hope and so on – in other words, that promote a sense of well-being even in the face of adversity – may help the patient to feel more relaxed and able to cope. This relaxation takes the brakes off the immune response produced by fear and allows the patient's own innate capacity to heal and protect against illness to kick in effectively – self-healing emerging from an environment of well-being nourished by nurses. Nightingale (1860) asserted that 'nursing is putting the patient in the best condition for nature to act' – and modern science is now providing evidence in support.

Descartes famously pronounced 'I think therefore I am' (*cogito ergo sum*). Thinking is the realm of the mind, very useful in its own way in acting out our roles and functions in the world. But defining our humanity by our capacity to think can be problematic for nursing – often we are helping people who cannot think or whose capacity to do so is diminished. Are such people less human? Is there a sliding scale based on thinking ability by which we can set points of definition – so this person is human or this person is not? The mental processes that produce thinking may not, as I have suggested, be the sole repository of consciousness. Other systems across the world, such as the chakra approach in India or the chi of China, indicate that there may be other ways of defining consciousness and what makes us human. Or, for that matter, consider the concepts of 'soul' in Western thinking and 'essence' in Middle-Eastern thought, which leads us to the possibility that the soul, while being related to consciousness and our humanity, at the same time transcends it. There is more to us, it seems, than our brainwork, and, if people are also souls or have other levels of consciousness not dependent on the brain, then nursing is not just about patient care – it is also soul care. For some people and in some models of thinking about human beings, our brain chemistry is what we are – there is no 'other', no grander dimension, no consciousness beyond the body – hence, once the brain is dead, humanity ceases. What is left is just a carcass to do with as we will – of no meaning or purpose. Yet nurses work on this existential edge where intuition, subjective feelings, customs, habits and countless other perceptions vie for authority with what science cannot agree is true. Try as we might to be an evidence-based profession, much that is not evidence-based is also the realm of nursing – thus we respect the bodies of the dead, honour rites and customs that do not fit with the evidence of biological function, and respond to people with feelings and the will to act, which go beyond what rational problem-solving about nursing care might dictate. The fact that we do not see the body as all that we are is evidenced, for example, by the way we prepare it for relatives to see after a loved one has died, by the way we talk to a patient diagnosed as brain dead and science would tell us that they cannot possibly hear, or the ethical dilemmas we have over abortion, euthanasia and so on. Often the cruellest acts of nursing, or rather anti-nursing, emerge when, consciously or unconsciously, we see no hope in caring, for the 'thing' we care for has ceased to be human by rational scientific definition. When we lose sight of the humanity of the person, when we make them 'other' instead of seeing them holistically as the same as us, indeed part of us, then we risk imposing all manner of dehumanising acts upon them. The history of nursing is littered with enquiries, disciplinary actions and criminal cases where nurses have abused and neglected patients – and ceasing to see the patient as fully human has invariably been a significant contributor.

Not long ago I attended a conference on brain death during Brain Awareness Week in the UK. It was my lot to follow a well-known scientist who had done much work in the UK and internationally on brain death and coma scales, and his session was deeply appealing to all of the audience. He was so certain. We can feel very assured by certainty in others. The nub of his case was this: the function of the brain can be measured – 'vegetative' (how I loathe that word and all it conjures up about brain-injured people) states can be assessed and given certain criteria, by which we can be assured that the person is really 'dead' and then life support systems can be switched off. I felt disturbed by the seductive simplicity of this argument. Needless to say, my subsequent session where I expressed serious doubts about this approach went down like a lead balloon in some quarters. Any suggestion of uncertainty, of humility in the face of human illness, of reverence for the possibility that we might be more than the sum total of our cerebral atoms and their functions was uncomfortable to many. And it can be seen why; it is, after all, so much easier if you are caught up in the difficult business of caring, and really tough decisions at the end of life, to feel, to need to feel, that our actions are rooted in reason and logic. Introduce the concept of soul, of the possibility of consciousness not being the sole preserve of the brain and its functions, of realms of knowing beyond the body (common to all spiritual traditions, and yet until recently, as in the research cited above, largely ignored or rejected by modern scientific medicine), and then this steady ship of certainty is holed below the waterline.

Reflection point 13.3

I have nursed many patients who have been brain-damaged and who were deeply unconscious, and others who were no longer oriented to ordinary reality, such as people with advanced Alzheimer's disease. At first I found it difficult to connect with people with these problems – the everyday avenues of communication, for example, were shut down. I could not get a full sense of them as people, even when I got to know something of their life histories. However, I often felt a sense that, even though the person had been lost or somehow become invisible, there was always something 'more' there that kept me willingly nursing them – some sense of a 'presence' that did not depend upon my knowing the ordinary personhood that they must have had while fully alert and well. Have you ever experienced this yourself, or does this just seem too odd to you? Does the person cease to exist in your view when the brain no longer functions, in which case are you just nursing the body that is left behind? Or is there something more than this for you, and if so what is it? When does a person cease to be a person to you? What do your beliefs and values tell you about what it is to be human and when, if at all, do we stop being human?

The notion that we may be more than our biology, that we are not so much human beings having a spiritual journey as spiritual beings having a human journey (de Chardin, 1959), runs against the grain of much of modern scientific health care. For example, I have been involved recently in an enquiry where abuse of patients with Alzheimer's disease was a prominent feature. Although the right noises about caring had been made, some terrible things had been done to these patients, and a cardinal feature of the underlying problem was that a significant number of the staff – fairly conventional nurses and doctors – were not facing up to the underlying hopelessness that they felt about their patients. Although much work was going on with 'reality orientation', the only reality accepted was ordinary reality. The patients were seen as ultimately lost causes in their own form of (declining) vegetative state. This shadow in the unconscious was covered up by 'chronic niceness' (Speck, 1994) but ultimately leaked out. Behind the mask of caring lay some deeply uncaring feelings and actions that were not being faced (Obholzer and Roberts, 2003).

Many aspects of modern health care like this suffer because of our limited concepts of what it is to be human – concepts that are now being challenged scientifically, as in the examples I have offered above in the discussions on holism and consciousness. Furthermore, there are signs that calls for change are getting louder, from both patients and professionals, and the change demanded is less about the right roles or systems, and more about the right models on which these are built. The current dominant force that sees 'mind', 'consciousness' and 'personhood' purely as products of the brain is being broken. The reduction of human beings to biological processes, such that who we are is relegated to the outcome of a bunch of neurones and neurochemicals, is being challenged as never before. The idea that, when we break down, we can be rectified if we can be tweaked with the right chemical or psychotherapeutic spanners is increasingly being seen as simplistic. No part of the health care spectrum has escaped the consequences of non-holistic models, and the fulfilment of our part in the promotion of well-being is thereby diminished.

Thus, what Pert's, Achterberg's and other studies cited in the previous section on holism seem to be pointing to is a greater understanding of the nature of consciousness than has generally been considered in orthodox health care, and that has enormous implications for human well-being in the future. It also illuminates the significance of not just what nurses do, but also who we are with patients, our being as well as our doing, and it is through being that we relate to others. The quality of that relating is of profound significance for the sense of well-being of those for whom we care – in relating rightly, we promote well-being.

Right relationships for well-being: feeling better and getting better

I have explored the concept of right relationship in more detail elsewhere (Wright and Sayre-Adams, 2000) and summarised the impacts from the research on staff and patients. As we enter into relationships with others that foster well-being, these are characterised by a

> *harmonious, balanced, attentive, action-orientated way of being in the world. It is built on values of respect and reverence for persons and the whole of creation, seeking to be in relationship with them in patterns which are loving, supportive, available and not hooked on models of power, control, and abuse. It seeks to nourish and aid others to choose and pursue their own life path, to make right choices that are equally loving and nourishing for them, without imposing our will or worldview upon them. Indeed in right relationship, there is no us and them, no separation, but an acknowledgement of the inescapable interconnectedness of all life, all relationships, all creation.*
>
> (Wright and Sayre Adams, 2000, p. 4)

In right relationships we find that the qualities of trust, faith, honesty, authenticity and integrity are embedded in the nursing milieu that nurse and patient enter. Indeed, trust and a belief in the nurse, considering the studies on consciousness and psychoneuroimmunology cited above, appear to be significant factors in triggering the healing response, as is the belief in the patients themselves that they can heal. Well-being is enhanced not just by the 'doing' by nurses – the treatments and practical aspects of our role – but also by the 'being' – the presence and quality of that presence of the nurse with the patient. In feeling better around nurses, all the evidence points to patients getting better too – and, even if dying, they die better.

It can be argued that, if our relationships with our patients, our innermost selves, our colleagues and our employing organisations were harmonious and 'right', then there would be significant increases in patient and staff well-being. The American 'magnet' study (McLure *et al.,* 1983), for example, was one of the early pieces of nursing research correlating staff well-being, patient well-being and organisational effectiveness; it was followed by many others (WHO, 1994; Borrill *et al.*, 1998; Williams *et al.*, 1998; HEA, 1998; CBI, 1999; Hatfield, 1999; Obholzer and Roberts, 2003; RCN, 2005). At every level, the quality of relationships affects well-being of both staff and patients and organisational goals (see the excellent summaries on the websites of the Health and Safety Executive (www.hse.gov.uk) and the RCN (www.rcn.org.uk)).

If the well-being of the patient is at least in part triggered in the relationship with the nurse, interacting in the total environment, and consciously participating in healing, then this begs some questions about the quality of that relationship. What is needed to support right relationships? In the fairy story 'The Snow Queen', Hans is unable to be loving until the splinter of ice is removed from his heart. Icy, heartless nurses are uncommon but not rare. Whether the products of unresolved wounds in our own hearts, or hellish working environments, or cultures that do not value caring (Obholzer and Roberts 2003) – whatever the cause, the heartless unloving nurse's behaviour invariably lies at the root of adverse comments about nurses and nursing.

Many factors in the environment can inhibit feelings of well-being and openheartedness among nurses, from poor staffing levels to poor leadership, from hostile management practices to low pay, as the surveys cited above suggest. It can indeed be difficult to keep our hearts open in hell – staying loving in often hellish contexts of suffering, being compassionate with patients when we can feel unsupported by others, unsure of ourselves and faced with the 'floodgate for a never ending tide of misery' which is before us day and night (Hillesum, 1996). At the same time, many nurses bring unresolved issues into working relationships that distort the possibilities of effective caring (Snow and Willard, 1989; Obholzer and Roberts, 2003). Roberts observes:

> *It is therefore of greatest importance for helping professionals to have some insight into their reasons for choosing a particular kind of work or setting in which they find themselves, and awareness of specific blind spots: their valency for certain kinds of defences, and their vulnerability to certain kinds of projective identification.*

(Roberts, 2003, p. 118)

Reflection point 13.4

So, why did you decide to become a nurse? What is it about the job that brings you greatest satisfaction? What is it about the work that challenges you most? Consider the last time when involved in caring for patients that you felt:

- angry;
- sad;
- hopeful;
- hopeless;
- happy.

Why did you experience these feelings and what was going on in the work, the environment and in yourself that produced them? What do you have in your nursing life that enables you to explore these feelings and actions safely – a mentor, a clinical supervisor, a trusted and wise counsellor?

In other words, part of our process of becoming a nurse involves deepening our insight into our own inner processes, our conscious and unconscious motivations, if we are to become healed and whole within ourselves and fulfil our potential in caring for others without the 'baggage' of our unhealed selves. It is debatable whether nursing as a whole and the organisations we work for pay adequate attention to these issues, not least perhaps because exploration of the inner terrain can be profoundly challenging and the resources and people to support it are not always available.

If we look at the work of the nursing development unit (NDU) movement in the late 1980s and early 1990s, these units were often working harder and doing more, and yet sickness, absenteeism and attrition rates were less, and quality of patient care was higher (Salvage and Wright, 1995). Why? Because the staff in them felt more supportive of each other, had a shared sense of mission and purpose in their work, and had a deeper sense of connection with each other, which made the work culture more soulful, more satisfying. Dis-spirited workforces are a recipe for disaster for the individuals who work in them, for the teams and for those who depend on them for care. Space here does not permit a detailed exploration of the many possibilities that can be drawn upon to promote right relationship among teams and organisations and within ourselves, but the writings cited above offer a vast range of possibilities. Suffice to say at this stage that, in order to enter right relationship with others, it is not possible to bypass the emotional work upon ourselves or the issues in teams and organisations – in an holistic view, each affects the other. Even with recent government policies in the UK encouraging more support to staff in the NHS, it seems that there are still many miles to go. Attrition rates and morale among nurses remain problematic, and application of methods for personal and organisational insight remain patchy.

Well-being, environment and sacred space

Thoreau wrote:

> *It is something to be able to paint a picture, or carve a statue, and so to make a few objects beautiful. But it is far more glorious to carve or paint the atmosphere in which we work, to effect the quality of the day – this is the highest of arts.*
>
> (Thoreau, cited in Donahue, 1985, p. 9)

Although the maturing nurse moves along the trajectory from novice to expert, as Benner (1984) in her classic study illuminated so richly, there may be yet another level beyond excellence. It is the level of art form, when there is a synthesis of knowledge and experience, of inner and outer connection that transcends reduction into rational analysis. A gifted sculptor and good friend was asked once how she drew from blocks of stone her exquisite creations. She replied, 'I don't know, but what I do know is that if I did know I couldn't do it' (Wright, 2006a).

She had a profound love for her work and it was a love that was full of imagination – the capacity to see situations and relationships and not see only what is but what might be. So it is with many nurses. The artist can explain the technicalities but goes a stage further, touching us deeply in ways that defy mere analysis. We can appreciate the skill that goes into the works of Hildegard von Bingen or da Vinci or Eliot, but it is far more difficult, if not impossible, to fully explicate why they move us. Science helps us to understand why things are as they are; art takes us a stage further into feeling what it is like to *experience* them. Nursing is 'the finest of the fine arts' (Nightingale, 1860), but what is the essence, the impetus, that takes it to that level? What is it in the emotional labour of nursing (Smith, 1992), that ability to connect when married to what we do births something unique in each caring encounter? Remember, we are human beings not human doings. When we get it right (and we do not always, as I have suggested earlier), there is a fluid, seemingly effortless flow of heart, mind and body that creates mutual well-being. The emotional labour in the (he)art of nursing is engaged in the creation of right relationship with all that is.

Relationship also takes place in the context of the lived environment. Nursing has a long track record of health promotion, from Florence Nightingale's early efforts to promote better sewage systems in towns to the countless general and specialist roles of nurses associated with diet, smoking, exercise and a wide range of other lifestyle and social issues that affect health. The promotion of well-being is related to but more than the promotion of health. The artistry of nursing is not just concerned with the relationships we have or the actions we take with patients, but also calls upon us to consider the aesthetics of the wider environment. Nightingale (1860) was one of the first to see well-being as related intimately to the design of buildings and the quality of light, air and space – something that much of modern architecture seems to have ignored. Many of our buildings designed for health care are often technically and clinically efficient but aesthetically and spiritually poor. Yet there is abundant evidence to indicate that the built environment has a direct impact upon staff and patient well-being – everything from the decor of rooms in colours that promote healing, to geological energies, access to nature, and views from windows that support recovery from surgery (Andrews, 2003; Galindo and Rodriguez, 2000; Clarke, 2006). Recently more attention has been paid to honouring and developing further that early work of Nightingale (Andrews, 2003; Dossey *et al.*, 2005), showing how nurses have influenced health care settings to bring greater appreciation of aesthetics, the arts, access to fresh air and light and so on to support patient well-being – and further, to show how nurses have reached out to embrace nursing concerns in the well-being of wider communities, of those who are refugees, starving or oppressed, and environmental movements and concerns for the health and well-being of the whole planet. Global nursing – embracing economic, social and environmental concerns – is a natural nursing extension of caring for individuals.

The relationship that we have with the world around us influences our own well-being and that of others. Such a relationship is one of respect, of reverence. The relationship is one that is sacred for, although we are part of it, it is greater than ourselves. In nursing, we bring small sacred acts of love into the world that Mother Theresa spoke of to make even the most hostile of environments and relationships blossom with hope and healing.

There is a Sufi saying that 'You think that by understanding one, you can understand two, for one and one is two. But to understand two, you must first understand "and".' It is in the space between, the sacred space, the place of 'and' where we connect. In connection lies right relationship. In right relationship lies the sacred space of healing. I have explored the concept of sacred space in detail elsewhere (Wright and Sayre-Adams, 2000), but for the purposes of this chapter the subject embraces the whole context in which the search for well-being takes place. The sacred space – of environment and relationships all intermingled in the whole, each influencing the other – is the milieu in which nurses participate in the transmutation of suffering and potential suffering into well-being.

Dependence is also well-being

'Productivity, technology, lucidity, capacity, independence, autonomy, and the supremacy of individual rights and physical perfection measure the spirit of the age' (Hudson, 2003) – Western culture worships youth and independence. Our near obsession with autonomy blinds us to other opportunities that disability, whether by birth, accident, disease or ageing, can bring. So much of nursing is wrapped up in the idea that independence = well-being, but it is worth exploring briefly in this chapter whether this is true. Could dependence be a transforming power, an opportunity for deepening our connection with each other and with our deepest selves? As Ram Dass (2000) points out in his insights into his own ageing and disability, after a lifetime of helping others, he learned that the shadow of his illness was enlightened by the joy of being in relationship with others where they could express their need to help him. Helping is not a linear one-way relationship from A to B; it is a mutual process, with helper and helped gaining. Thus 'autonomy' is something of a limited concept at any age, let alone in old age. A more holistic, well-being approach to dependency from whatever source sees the 'transforming power, or spirit, of *inter*dependence (or heteronomy) over against the prevailing spirit of idealised independence (or autonomy)' (Hudson, 2003).

Negative views of dependency trap carers and cared for in the place of 'being a burden'– which fuels negative perceptions of ageing, the euthanasia debate, and some of the worst aspects of abuse of people who are the most vulnerable (Obholzer and Roberts, 2003; Wright, 2005). The 'being a burden' cry is another assumption that needs to be challenged, for the values around dependency/independency infect our whole culture, as I have suggested above. At almost every level we are given the signal that to be self-caring is good, and to need care is bad. Thus the fear of being a burden is often rooted in internalised feelings of low self-worth, guilt, or the taking on board of cultural norms and views about dependency – feelings and views that nurses who see through the illusions of dependency are ideally placed to challenge. Well-being in dependency can be achieved when patients are helped to make a conscious shift in their perceptions of it, in part through the use of those nursing skills I summarised above that can both change the world and change the way we perceive the world. This is more than adaptation to limitations; it is a deeper shift of consciousness about the whole nature of what it is to be dependent on others and extinguishing its negative influences.

Reflection point 13.5

While visiting a friend in hospital recently, I overheard an elderly woman in a nearby bed talking with her family. She complained endlessly that she wanted to die, wept at the thought that she would need their help at home, and seemed very sad at the thought, as in the above discussion, that she would 'be a burden' on them. Why do you think this woman feels the way she does? If you were nursing her, what sort of things could you say or do to help her see things differently, assuming you think you should? Consider yourself too – at what point do you think, if you were ill or dependent, that you might say that you had 'had enough'? Where is the point for you that you would feel you had become a burden, and what things for you would alleviate this? It's worth considering also, assuming that you are fit and well now, how your views of how you might respond in the event of dependency might change should you actually become dependent.

We are not islands. Independence is an illusion. Our humanity rests upon the connection that we all depend on each other in different ways at different times of our lives. We have need of others when we can't manage alone. But we also have needs to be needed. Our humanity is made real when we connect with each other, when needing help and needing to give help, which all human beings experience, are brought together. Being with others in their suffering can be one of the most demanding of human experiences, but it can also be one of the most rewarding. The tougher path for us is to confront, even in the midst of suffering, the possibility of finding well-being through a shift of consciousness, a shift of values married to practical action that can find well-being out of low expectations or the belief that being dependent is 'bad'.

Touch and well-being

Touch, the means by which we make physical contact with, and sense of, the external world, is but one aspect of a complex way in which human beings connect with ordinary reality. Our skin is the largest sense organ of the body, and touch is the first sense to develop in the human embryo, the one most vital for survival. Much of the infant's first information about the world is gained from the way they are touched during the birthing process, and touch continues to be used to learn about our environment. It is through the skin that knowledge about the external world is communicated to the brain, and in turn people convey to others information about themselves. A piece of skin the size of a British penny contains more than 3 million cells, 4 m of nerves, 100 sweat glands, 50 nerve endings and 1 m of blood vessels. It is estimated that there are about 50 receptors over $100 \, cm^2$, a total of about 900 000 sensory receptors per person (Sayre-Adams and Wright, 2002).

All cultures have developed their own customs and taboos around touching. It has been suggested that Western European culture is one of the most touch-deprived in the world. In one famous study, Jourard (1964) watched pairs of people in coffee shops in Puerto Rico, Paris, Florida and London. He counted the number of times one person touched another during an hour. In Puerto Rico the average was 180 and in Paris 110, but in Florida it was only 2 and in London 0. I grew up in a working-class family in Manchester in the austerity of the post-war period. Being touched and cuddled by my parents and family was a rare phenomenon – so rare that I can remember the occasions when it did happen. Whether Jourard's study would come up with the same findings today is debatable. We live in a culture when touch in all its forms is quite explicit on film and television and invited in popular music, where many programmes encourage physical and emotional expression such as the numerous TV confessionals. However, I am often left wondering whether these apparent attempts at connection are superficial, a kind of faux intimacy where we hear the other's story but maintain a safe distance. Meanwhile New Age touchy-feely approaches are the stuff of the treatment rooms of countless therapists and have exploded into orthodox health care, often to compensate for the sense of disconnection, including the absence of loving physical touch, in an increasingly high-tech scientific medical milieu.

At the same time, our culture seems to be prohibitive about touch in unparalleled ways, where fear of accusations of sexual harassment, molestation or paedophilia feed a caution about the risks of 'inappropriate' touch. Touch is a most profound medium for finding our place in the world, for feeling whole and loved and worthy. Fear of touch drives a wedge through the possibilities and wonder of intimacy, connection and feeling good. Fear of being touched physically often underpins a fear of being touched more intimately at an emotional and spiritual level. At the same time, 'risk management' processes can place carers such as nurses under considerable limitations in order to practice 'safely'. Opportunities for meaningful, helping and healing intimacy and connection are subverted by the superstacking of legislation, professional regulation, risk management and indemnity insurance policies that raise immense barriers to therapeutic human relationships.

Different religious, cultural and social habits and expectations in our society mean that there is huge variation in acceptable forms of touch. What is acceptable for some is unacceptable to others. At the same time, everyone needs touch. Infants cannot survive without it, and studies show that the need for touch does not diminish as people grow older. Indeed, older people may suffer most acutely from lack of touch because of separation from or loss of family and friends. They are also affected by various social stigmas and expectations of how older people should behave, such as assumptions that they should no longer need or desire close physical contact (Marr and

Kershaw, 1998). Yet, touch also functions as an effective communication channel for the older person at a time of life when other forms of communication may be less acute. Touching has always been an integral part of demonstrating that nurses care, intuitively recognising that it promotes well-being long before science demonstrated its significance. But it is the way we touch that determines whether it will be an act of healing or a mechanistic procedural act. Many of us intuitively move forward to hold a hand or to touch an arm as a gesture of reassurance. It is a means of saying, without words, that we care and we understand. Indeed, in situations where words fail, our loving presence indicated by gentle and appropriate touch may be the only 'language' that is left to us or that is necessary. Other, less positive feelings can, however, be indicated. For example, judgemental attitudes are revealed in the way we do or do not touch people. If we seek to use touch in caring ways, we are often called to explore much of our own inner processes, values and motivations if it is to be expressed sincerely and authentically. I know of a hospital chaplain who is deeply homophobic and who, for various reasons, is unable or unwilling to explore that issue beyond stating theological arguments. He believes he can keep it to himself where patients are concerned, and seems oblivious to the subtle, and sometimes not so subtle, ways that he leaks his true feelings. For any kind of touch to be truly effective, it must be given authentically by a warm, genuine, caring individual to one who is willing to receive it. Touch cannot be packaged and dispensed, for insincere or inappropriate touching may be more harmful than none at all.

Evidence of the use of touch as a method of healing can be traced back 15 000 years (Sayre-Adams and Wright, 2002), and the Bible has many references to the 'laying on of hands'. Healing was considered as much part of the early Christian ministry as administering the sacraments. Members of royal families were thought to heal with the 'royal touch'. Currently, many modern 'healers' do so in the name of a spirit guide, a particular guru (dead or alive), or believing they have a special dispensation from God and can transmit, control or channel healing 'energy' through touch. As suggested earlier, modern physics and recent research offer us new dimensions of the significance of touch in the promotion of well-being and the way that touch is not limited to skin-to-skin contact.

A quantum physics perspective, for example, reveals a very different view of the body and the nature of touch and connection; a universe of enormous interchange of energy – the body not so much a solid fixed mass but in constant exchange of energy internally and externally. Part of this 'energy' is consciousness; indeed, some have argued that it *is* the energy. The ancient mystics express their perception that 'all is one' and that consciousness is not only in the body but also in the body in a grander field of consciousness. They share a common ground with modern quantum physicists for whom everything is part of the whole.

Certain approaches to healing touch may work regardless of the techniques, simply because the patient believes in, or has faith in, the therapy and the practitioner, feels good in their presence, and gets a relaxation response (a feature hitherto often dismissed as the placebo response (Pert, 1997)). These alone may be sufficient to switch the patient into healing by boosting the autoimmune response as suggested above. Hippocrates commented that some people recover simply because of their satisfaction with the goodness of the doctor. In the space where we come together – the 'sacred space' (Wright and Sayre-Adams, 2000) – there is an opportunity for it to be filled with the loving consciousness that nourishes well-being. In other words, something about the way we are with people may be as significant as, if not more so than, what we do.

In healing touch, the one therefore does not heal the other, for the process is one of mutuality, of a joint venture into the realms of the unknown.

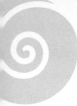
Healing, the emergence of right relationship at, between and among all the levels of human being, is always accomplished by the one healing. No one and no thing can heal another human being (but themselves). All healing is creative emergence, new birth, the manifestation of the powerful inner longing, at every level, to be whole.

(Quinn, 1992, p. 34)

We contribute to this healing environment when we are fully present with the other, indeed let go of notions of 'other'. It is enriched when we are willing to engage fearlessly in the depths of touch, when we are able to transcend notions of humans being only physical entities. Thus those who wish to participate in healing remove barriers to the healing process so that right relationship in the 'sacred space' of healing can be birthed. 'Being with' someone in right relationship may be the switch that triggers the potential of someone to heal themselves, to which Nightingale and Hippocrates, mentioned above, have alluded. Our presence can be the harmonising rhythm that the one in search of healing seeks, for this pulsating field of energy, this underlying reality beneath our solid reality that the mystics and quantum physicists describe, may be one of the sources from which disease arises when we are no longer in harmony with this rhythm. Can it be, therefore, that part of the healing work of nurses arises when we become the strong harmonising rhythm on the sick person who is not in harmony?

Reflection point 13.6

Jocelyn was a middle-aged nurse who came to see me because she was burned out. A lot of problems had occurred at once in her life, and she found herself unable to cope. Indeed, some 'chickens had come home to roost' – some painful things in her childhood had resurfaced at this time that she thought she had long since buried, including sexual abuse by her father and brother. She was married, but her relationship was on the rocks – one reason being that she could not bear for her husband to touch her. Both her children had left home – one was a heroin addict and was very dependent on her for money, and the other was estranged and had left the country and not made contact for several years. She had been accused of bullying and harassment at work and was suspended from her job as a unit manager. She wept copiously and she was in great distress, feeling that she was unloved and indeed never had been loved, and was incapable of loving others. She told me that she never liked to be touched and would avoid close physical contact with people. My heart wanted to reach out to her in her suffering, and I felt a strong desire just to hug and hold her in distress. Would you have done so? What would you see as appropriate touch, if at all? Can you think of some things you might say or do or recommend to help Jocelyn feel connected and loved, to feel whole and a sense of well-being once more? What cautions would you bear in mind when considering the need for and use of touch with Jocelyn?

You may be interested to know that Jocelyn, in her discovery of well-being, began gently to accept touch from myself – first just the holding of her hand after asking her permission, and later a hug on arrival and departure from our meetings. She began to experiment with 'safe' touch – having an aromatherapy massage, for example – and looked at how touch was lacking in her life in so many ways, including contact with her sons. She is now well, has left nursing and is running her own small business. After several years of 'inner work' she has reunited with her husband, her eldest son has been 'clean' for over a year, and she took a break to visit her younger son in Australia; although that meeting was very difficult, he has agreed to return to the UK to celebrate his twenty-first birthday at home.

Some approaches to touch, such as reiki, therapeutic touch, massage and so on, have been grouped loosely in the category of complementary or alternative therapies. Huge numbers of nurses have become involved in this movement, seeking to work independently as therapists or integrating them into their everyday practice (Heelas *et al.*, 2005). There is much controversy over whether these therapies can be shown to 'work' (in terms, for example, of studies using double-blind randomised controlled trials). However, the therapies seem at least to offer degrees of personal attention and comforting that much of the conventional system still lacks – and it is this promotion of well-being that may be of influence in assisting the immune response.

A large body of research has suggested that laying on of hands can increase the rate of wound healing and improve psychological and spiritual well-being (see Sayre-Adams and Wright (2002) for a summary). Touch, physical touch, is part of but not the whole of this process. The contact of skin to skin is but a part of a more complex picture, a catalyst, a medium for a deeper and richer landscape of possibility to be made extant. Touch is, therefore, more than physical contact, although this is an important part of it. It is about deep human connection – right relationship with ourselves and others and perhaps that which lies beyond the self. To be touched deeply demands that we overcome inherent fears of intimacy. Our egos, our personhoods, struggle with intimacy at many levels for, in joining, the independent identity is threatened. Nurses in a state of well-being themselves are an essential key to restoring well-being to others who have lost it.

Deep listening and well-being

We connect by touch at more than physical levels, and when we hear the story of another we are touched in quite different ways. Yet it is so hard to find silence these days. Noise bombards us from every direction and some cannot bear to be without it, preferring the interminable TV or radio backdrop rather than be in silence. Perhaps this is with good reason, for in silence we may hear the loudest and often most unpleasant chatter of all, the incessant sound of our own mind. And it is this sound that often prevents us from really hearing what others have to say, that inhibits our connection with others in ways that feel heartfelt, to engage in 'deep listening' (Wright, 2006b).

In the book of Job (21:1–2) in the Old Testament, Job is assailed by just about every form of suffering imaginable. Friends constantly advise and console him, telling him that it will be all right – 'Job's comforters'. In exasperation he tells them to stop and 'listen to what I am saying, for that is all the comfort I ask of you'. Listening – without leaping in with a desire to fix things or without taking on board the other's anguish in a kind of faux compassion – is an art, and art is part of the he-art of nursing. The distractions of the environment are not the only things that gets in the way of listening deeply; our own inner chorus of mental processes drowns things out too, arising from that fearful place in ourselves that wants to solve and fix and be sure. Nurses can easily get caught up in such fixing roles, and our capacity to really hear what the other is saying to us can thereby be diminished. When we do not hear fully, then we do not connect fully; and when we do not connect fully, we reduce the way of well-being. The connection between people remains forever superficial, artificial, like actors in dialogue – real people are not speaking to each other. When we are really attached to identification with a role ('I am a nurse' versus 'I am a being who happens to work as a nurse'), then the role becomes a trap. Entrapment in this way

alienates us from one another: a social worker and juvenile offender just miss, a nurse and patient seem worlds apart; a priest and parishioner, so distant, so formal. What otherwise would be a profound and intimate relationship becomes ships passing in the night.

(Ram Dass and Gorman, 1990, p. 125)

The potential for healing and compassion, hearing the sound of another's heart as well as the sound of our own, is missed.

Preoccupied with our own stuff, trying to listen while at the same time assessing and framing a reply – these are barriers to deep listening. We cannot do all of these at the same time as well as *really* paying attention to someone in need. Thus, in countless situations, we 'just miss' and an opportunity for human connection is lost. Listening at this deep level does not come easily and is rarely arrived at simply by life experience. It takes courage (coeur-age – to be in the heart) to set aside ourselves and all our 'stuff' and to be fully present for, and attentive to, the other.

Holden (2002) recognises the toughness of this task, for to fully pay attention to another we have to get ourselves out of the way, to get past the masks we offer to the world that hide our fears that we are lacking or flawed in some way. Part of the task is to confront these fears, yet we can be inhibited from doing so because we fear being overwhelmed by them if we do. Holden goes on to point out how we project these feelings on to others, by trying to fix them or control them or receiving communications as if they are an attack upon ourselves – an attack to be defended robustly. Thus we rarely listen deeply because we are already busy with our own interior plans, assessing what to do, how to respond or how to keep control of the situation. It is not possible to listen fully when we are already engaged in preparing a reply. Communications fall into games of mental ping-pong, with the players at a safe distance and never really connecting with each other.

The solution is to encourage the evolving of more aware nurses who can see beyond the masks that we present to each other. This can be done only, in the view of Holden and many other spiritual teachers, by adopting a commitment to spiritual practice and expansion of our consciousness that connects us to the deep peace and safety that lie in our very essence, our hearts and our souls. Without this spiritual maturity we are afraid to operate other than behind our masks and roles, for who on earth would be left if we let them drop even for a little while? We are required, as Pym (1999) suggests, 'to switch off the demanding self' so that we can pay close attention and witness the drama – needing a wholly different way of being for most of us and our workplaces.

When we can confidently set aside our ego agendas, we can get ourselves out of the way. This enables the listener to

> totally switch off his or her own views for the duration of the 'listen'. By doing so he is able to give his total attention to the speaker. In the process he or she will have a brand new experience: by not interrupting or arguing he will hear things that he has never heard before. The speaker too will have a brand new experience. He will be aware that he is being heard by someone who is not going to come back to him with a reply, criticism or opposition. And not only is he heard, he hears himself.

(Pinney, cited in Pym, 1999, pp. 110–11)

Giving space to speak enables the person to feel heard and for the nurse to listen – to hear what is being said but also what is not being said. The use of silence, waiting, getting the self out of the way, and ensuring the space for the other to speak enables a deeper quality of listening to take place that can truly promote understanding, compassion, connection and right action – the essential elements in the promotion of well-being.

Listening deeply is a powerful catalyst for well-being and is a natural part of the repertoire of nursing; it is at the very heart of it. It is a vital means of connection with another, for when our stuff is out of the way, we not only hear the other but hear ourselves as well.

CONCLUSION

The scope for nursing intervention in the promotion of well-being, as it has been explored in this chapter, offers a far grander vista of opportunity than the theme of health promotion, for the latter is but a building brick of the former. Nursing concerns, since the Nightingale era, have reached out into domains of well-being in a vast continuum from the bedside of the patient to the action in planetary well-being. Nurses have a long track record of intervention for well-being for the individual self, communities, environment and now, with the increasing exploration of nursing roles of matters spiritual, the divine or absolute as well (Fisher *et al.*, 2000; Wright, 2005).

Ecologist and philosopher Brian Swimme saw:

> The great mystery is that we are interested in anything whatsoever. Think of your friends, how you met them, how interesting they appear to you. Why should anyone in the whole world interest us at all? Why don't we experience everyone as utter, unendurable bores? Why isn't the cosmos made that way? Why don't we suffer intolerable boredom with every person, forest, symphony, and seashore in existence? The great surprise is the discovery that something or someone is interesting. Love begins there. Love begins when we discover interest. To be interested is to fall in love. To be fascinated is to step into a wild love affair on any level of life.
>
> (Swimme, 1984, p. 84)

The wild love affair that is nursing engages love with action. Sympathy, empathy and loving concern are translated into words and deeds that change the quality of peoples' lives. Tender loving care may have become something of a cliché, yet it is the heart of nursing practice and the core of our work in the birthing of well-being into the world.

References

Achterberg J, Cooke C, Richards T, *et al.* (2005). Evidence for correlations between distant intentionality and brain function in recipients: a functional magnetic resonance imaging analysis. *Journal of Alternative and Complementary Medicine*, **11**, 965–71.

Andrews G (2003). Nightingale's geography. *Nursing Inquiry*, **10**, 270–74.

Benner P (1984). *From Novice to Expert: Excellence and Power in Nursing Practice*. Menlo Park, CA: Addison-Wesley.

Bohm D (1973). Quantum theory as an indication of a new order in physics: implicate and explicate order in physical law. *Foundation of Physics*, **3**, 139–68.

Borrill C, Wall T, West M, *et al.* (1998). *Mental Health of the Workforce in NHS Trusts*. Sheffield: Institute of Work Psychology, University of Sheffield.

Campbell A (1984). *Moderated Love*. Edinburgh: SPCK.

Clarke I (2006). Building with feeling. *Spirituality and Health International*, **7**, 100–105.

Confederation of British Industry (CBI) (1999). *Promoting Mental Health at Work*. London: Confederation of British Industry.

De Chardin PT (1995). *The Phenomenon of Man*. London: Collins.

Donahue M (1985). *Nursing: The Finest Art*. St Louis, MO: Mosby.

Dossey L (1997). The forces of healing: reflections on energy, consciousness and the beef stroganoff principle. *Alternative Therapies in Health and Medicine*, **3**, 8–14.

Dossey B, Keegan L and Guzetta C (2000). *Holistic Nursing: Handbook for Practice*. Aspen, CO: Gaithersburg.

Dossey B, Selanders L, Beck D and Attewell A (2005). *Florence Nightingale Today: Healing, Leadership, Global Action*. Silver Spring, MD: American Nurses Association.

Fisher J, Francis L and Johnson P (2000). Assessing spiritual health via four domains of spiritual well-being. *Pastoral Psychology*, **49**, 133–45.

Forder J and Forder E (eds) (1995). *The Light Within*. Dent: Usha.

Galindo P and Rodriguez J (2000). Environmental aesthetics and psychological well-being: relationships between preference judgements for urban landscapes and other relevant affective responses. *Psychology in Spain*, **4**, 13–27.

Goleman D (1995). *Emotional Intelligence*. New York: Bantam.

Gooch S (2006). Emotionally smart. *Nursing Standard*, **20**, 20–22.

Hatfield D (1999). Gallup organisation: new research links emotional intelligence with profitability. *The Inner Edge*, **1**, 5–9.

Health Education Authority (HEA) (1998). *More than Brown Bread and Aerobics*. London: Health Education Authority.

Heelas P, Woodhead l, Seel B, Szerszynski B and Tusting K (2005). *The Spirituality Revolution: Why Religion Is Giving Way to Spirituality*. Oxford: Blackwell.

Hillesum E (1996). *An Interrupted Life*. New York: Owl.

Holden M (2002). *Boundless Love*. London: Ryder.

Hudson R (2003). The spirit of the age and the spirit of ageing. *Sacred Space*, **4**, 5–11.

Institute of HeartMath (2006). *Science of the Heart: An Overview of Research Conducted by IHM*. Boulder Creek, CA: Institute of HeartMath.

Jourard J (1964). *The Transparent Self: Self Disclosure and Well-Being*. Princetown, NJ: Van Nostrand.

Kornfield J (1993). *A Path with Heart*. New York: Bantam.

Longaker C (1998). *Facing Death and Finding Hope*. London: Arrow.

Marr J and Kershaw B (1998). *Caring for Older People*. London: Arnold.

McLure M, Poulin M, Sovie M and Wandelt M (1983). *Magnet Hospitals: Attraction and Retention of Professional Nurses*. Kansas City, MO: American Academy of Nursing.

Newman M (1986). *Health as Expanding Consciousness*. St Louis, MO: Mosby.

Nightingale F (1860). *Notes on Nursing: What it Is and Is Not*, 1980 edn. Edinburgh: Churchill Livingstone.

Nursing and Midwifery Council (NMC) (2008). *The Code: Standards of Conduct, Performance and Ethics for Nurses and Midwives*. London: Nursing and Midwifery Council.

Obholzer A (2003). Social anxieties in public sector organisations. In Obholzer A and Roberts V (eds). *The Unconscious at Work*. London: Brunner-Routledge.

Obholzer A and Roberts V (eds) (2003). *The Unconscious at Work*. London: Brunner-Routledge.

Pert C (1997). *Molecules of Emotion*. New York: Scribner.

Pym J (1999). *Listening to the Light*. London: Rider.

Quinn J (1992). Holding sacred space: the nurse as healing environment. *Holistic Nursing Practice*, **6**, 26–35.

Ram Dass (1971). *Be Here Now*. New York: Crown.

Ram Dass (2000). *Still Here*. London: Hodder & Stoughton.

Ram Dass and Bush M (1992). *Compassion in Action*. New York: Bell Tower.

Ram Dass and Gorman P (1990). *How Can I Help*? New York: Knopf.

Roberts V (2003). The self-assigned impossible task. In Obholzer A and Roberts V (eds). *The Unconscious at Work*. London: Brunner-Routledge.

Rogers ME (1970). *An Introduction to the Theoretical Basis for Nursing*. Philadelphia, PA: Davies.

Royal College of Nursing (RCN) (2005). *At breaking point? A survey of the Well-Being and Working Lives of Nurses*. London: Royal College of Nursing.

Salvage J and Wright S (1995). *Nursing Development Units: A Force for Change*. London: Scutari.

Savage J (1995). *Nursing Intimacy: An Ethnographic Approach to Nurse–Patient Interaction*. London: Scutari.

Sayre-Adams J and Wright S (2002). *Therapeutic Touch*. Edinburgh: Churchill Livingstone.

Smith P (1992). *The Emotional Labour of Nursing: How Nurses Care*. London: Macmillan.

Snow P and Willard C (1989). *I'm Dying to Take Care of You*. Redmond, WA: PCB.

Sogyal Rinpoche (1992). *The Tibetan Book of Living and Dying*. San Francisco, CA: Harper.

Speck P (1994). Working with dying people. In Obholzer A and Roberts V (eds). *The Unconscious at Work*. London: Brunner-Routledge.

Swimme B (1984). *The Universe Is a Green Dragon*. Santa Fe, NM: Bear.

Talbot M (1991). *The Holographic Universe*. New York: Harpercollins.

Tillich P (2000). *The Courage to Be*. Newhaven, CT: Yale University Press.

Williams S, Mitchie S and Pattani S (1998). *Improving the Health of the NHS Workforce*. London: Nuffield Trust.

World Health Organization (WHO) (1994). *Guidelines for the Primary Prevention of Mental, Neurological and Psychosocial Disorders. 5. Staff Burnout*. Geneva: World Health Organization Division of Mental Health.

Wright S (2004). Deconstructing nursing: from theory to practice – attentive, tuned in, focussed. *Nursing Standard*, **18**, 15–16.

Wright S (2005). *Reflections on Spirituality and Health*. Chichester: John Wiley & Sons.

Wright S (2006a). The heart of nursing. *Nursing Standard*, **20**, 20–23.

Wright S (2006b). The beauty of silence. *Nursing Standard*, **20**, 18–21.

Wright S and Sayre-Adams J (2000). *Sacred Space: Right Relationship and Spirituality in Healthcare*. Edinburgh: Churchill Livingstone.

Zohar D and Marshall I (2000). *Spiritual Intelligence: The Ultimate Intelligence*. London: Bloomsbury.

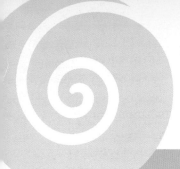

Assessment: the foundation of good practice

Ruth Beretta

14

Introduction

Assessing patients or clients is an essential role of every nurse and may occur on several occasions during the day, whether meeting a patient or client for the first time, reviewing a care plan, or preparing for the patient's transfer or discharge.

Each person is an individual with unique health and social care needs. This means that assessment is a highly skilled activity that requires professional knowledge and a range of well-developed communication and interpersonal skills. With the introduction of single shared assessment between nurses and other professionals involved in the health and social care of patients and clients, such as physiotherapists, occupational therapists and social workers, assessment is now an even more vital activity. The aim of assessment is to ensure that the patient or client receives a seamless episode of care.

Learning objectives

After studying this chapter you should be able to:

- recognise the importance of assessment in establishing a plan of care to meet a person's health care needs;
- establish the importance of multiprofessional working in order to provide shared care by health and social care practitioners;
- identify the skills and knowledge required for accurate assessment;
- explain the importance of using tools for assessment;
- account for the role that nursing models play in guiding and organising care.

What is assessment and why do it?

Assessment begins the nursing process and is about collecting data or information involving the patient or client and their family or carers, in order to identify the patient's or client's needs. However, it must be recognised that the data collected will impact not only on the nursing care plan but also on the care provided by other members of the multiprofessional team, such as physiotherapists, speech and language therapists, occupational therapists and members of the social care team.

The purpose of assessment is therefore to:

- make a judgement about a person's health status: do they need nursing care?
- decide whether there is a need to refer to other members of the care team;
- provide information to plan and deliver individualised care.

The information or data provided by assessment may be objective or subjective. If the information is objective, then it is based on measurement and can be verified by another person, for example temperature or body weight. If the information is subjective, then it is based on the ideas, feelings, values and beliefs of the nurse; for example, the nurse may have identified that the patient talked rapidly and fiddled with their clothes, and then come to the conclusion that the patient is nervous.

The data gathered through assessment identify the strengths and weaknesses of the patient or client and therefore identify their needs. This assists in the formulation of a plan of care; care can then be provided as per plan and evaluated to review its effectiveness. Evaluation of care results in reassessment of the patient's or client's needs (Figure 14.1). Assessment is therefore an ongoing process and is the foundation of good practice.

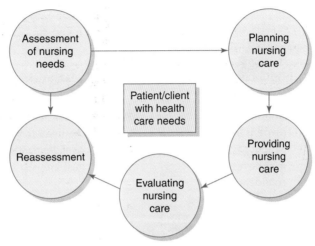

Figure 14.1 Assessment as the first part of the nursing process.

The NMC Standards of Proficiency and assessment

The Nursing and Midwifery Council *Standards of Proficiency* (NMC, 2004) identify the importance of assessment in establishing the foundation of good practice. The specific competencies and their relationship to assessment are identified in Table 14.1.

When should assessment be carried out?

> **Reflection point 14.1**
> Jot down the occasions when you think it is important for the nurse to assess patients or clients.

You may have identified the following occasions:

- An assessment is usually carried out when the nurse first meets a patient or client, which may be on admission to hospital, on a visit to a clinic, or in the patient's or client's own home. As identified earlier, the information obtained helps the nurse to establish a plan of care.
- Assessment may be carried out on a daily basis, to check the relevance of the care plan and to identify whether there is improvement or deterioration in the patient or client. This may mean that the care plan has to be updated in order to accommodate the new information gathered.
- Assessment is usually carried out before a patient or client is discharged home from hospital, in order to identify whether there is a need to continue care when the person is at home. This

may be a joint assessment involving other members of the multiprofessional team, such as the physiotherapist, occupational therapist, social worker and general practitioner (GP).

- Continuous assessment made be required for patients who are critically ill, for instance those requiring intensive care, young children and babies. Clients with mental health problems who are considered to be at risk of suicide also require regular assessment.

In all instances, the important issue is that assessment must take place before planning and delivering care.

Table 14.1 NMC pre-registration standards of proficiency and their relationship to assessment

NMC domain	NMC competency	Relationship to assessment
Professional and ethical practice	Practise in accordance with an ethical and legal framework that ensures the primacy of patient and client interest and well-being and respects confidentiality	In the course of assessment, nurses obtain very personal information; the need to respect patient confidentiality and act in a patient's best interest is paramount
	Practise in a fair and antidiscriminatory way, acknowledging the differences in beliefs and cultural practices of individuals or groups	On assessment, nurses must make sure that they do not allow their personal feelings about a person or their way of life to cloud their judgement about them
Care delivery	Undertake and document a comprehensive, systematic and accurate nursing assessment of physical, psychological, social and spiritual needs of patients, clients and communities	Nurses use their ability to interact with others and a range of assessment tools to identify health and social care needs
	Formulate and document a plan of nursing care, where possible in partnership with patients, clients, their carers, family and friends, within a framework of informed consent	Assessment is the first stage of the nursing process; information collated must reflect the concerns of the patient or client, not just those of the nurse
Care management	Demonstrate knowledge of effective interprofessional working practices that respect and use the contributions of members of the health and social care team	A nursing assessment is unique; however, the information collected completes a package of care with other health care professionals
Personal and professional development	Demonstrate a commitment to the need for continuing personal and professional supervision activities in order to enhance knowledge, skills, values and attitudes needed for safe and effective nursing practice	Assessment should be based on the best available evidence for care

Source: NMC (2004).

Ensuring assessment is effective

As suggested by the NMC Standards of Proficiency (NMC, 2004) and the NMC Code (2008), (Appendix 1) information gained at assessment may need to be shared with other members of the team, providing the patient or client gives consent for this to happen, in order to provide a comprehensive package of care. This may also require referral to a practitioner outside the nursing team whenever it is in the patient's best interests. Across the UK, all health departments are working towards ensuring that older patients and clients are assessed by means of a single assessment process, which was introduced by the Department of Health (DH) in England and the Department of Health, Social Services and Public Safety (DHSSPS) in Northern Ireland in 2002 in response to the *National Service Framework for Older People* (Standard 2 – Person centred care) (DH, 2001). Known in Wales as the Unified Assessment (Welsh Assembly Government, 2006) and in Scotland as the Single Shared Assessment (Scottish Executive 2001), the principle of the single assessment process is that information gained through assessment by any health or social care professional can be used by health and social care organisations so that patients are not asked the same questions more than once and effective use is made of available resources.

Reflection point 14.2
Can you think of examples where it would be helpful to patients or clients if the assessment were shared between other members of the multiprofessional team?

You might have considered some of the following examples:

- An older adult who has had a stroke (cerebrovascular event). As well as needing nursing care, this person may, as a minimum, require:
  - the services of a physiotherapist to help regain mobility;
  - the services of an occupational therapist to assist in supporting independence with daily living activities;
  - the services of a speech and language therapist to provide exercises to regain speech;
  - the assistance of a dietician to provide appropriate diet when unable to swallow properly;
  - the assistance of a social worker when being rehabilitated before discharge home.
- An adult who has depression. This person may:
  - be managed at home with regular visits from the community psychiatric nurse (CPN);
  - have regular visits to the day hospital managed by the community occupational therapist;
  - take prescription antidepressant medication provided by the GP.

Where does the information for assessment come from?

Within the professional and ethical practice domain of the NMC Standards (NMC, 2004), the nurse is advised that patient and client confidentiality is very important and that any information received must be used in the patient's best interest. Nurses must be sure that, if the patient or client is unable to speak for themselves, then there is agreement to having a carer or relative speak on their behalf. Nurses must also be sure that patients and clients are aware that information about them may be shared with other members of the care team and that they give consent for this to take place (NMC Code).

Patient or client
The patient or client is usually a primary source of data. When questioned, most patients are more than happy to provide information to help plan their care.

Questions put to patients and clients can be 'open ' or 'closed '. An open question, such as 'Tell me how your pain has been over the past few days', gives the person an opportunity to give you their side of the story. A closed question elicits a 'yes' or 'no' type of answer, such as 'Are you still in pain?'

However, there may be obstacles to using direct questions.

Reflection point 14.3
What situations might make it difficult to use the patient or client as the primary source of information in assessment?

You may have identified some of the following situations. The person being assessed is:

- in severe pain;
- emotionally upset;
- confused;
- too breathless to speak;
- unable to communicate in your language;
- hard of hearing;
- asleep or unconscious;
- a person with a learning disability who uses sign language to communicate.

This does not mean that the nurse cannot gather information from the patient or client. Methods other than verbal questioning can be used to gain information, such as the following:

- Visually observing the person:
  - How clean and tidy is the person? Have they been caring for themselves?
  - What colour is the person? Do they appear pale, flushed, cyanosed or jaundiced?
  - What does the person's facial expression reveal? Pain? Happiness or anger?
  - Is the person bleeding or losing fluid from anywhere?
  - What does the person's position reveal? Are they holding their stomach because they are in pain?
  - How mobile is the person? Can they walk?
- Using the sense of smell:
  - Does the person have stale breath, suggesting that they have not eaten or taken fluids for some time?
  - Does the person smell of tobacco?
  - Does the person smell of urine?
- Using the sense of touch:
  - How hot or cold is the person?
  - Does the person's skin feel clammy or dry?
- Using the sense of hearing:
  - Does the person have noisy breathing?
  - Does the person have slurred speech?

Carers, family and friends
If the patient or client is unable to give information to nursing staff for assessment, then carers and family members can usually provide useful information relating to the history of the current situation. They will usually also know the person's eating likes and dislikes, hygiene, times of

sleep, and details of the episode that has brought them to seek health care. Older people, people with memory disturbance or dementia, and people with an altered perception of themselves or of reality may need someone to advocate for them and speak on their behalf, but they must remain at the centre of any decision-making about their care (NMC Code).

Patient or client records

The patient or client may have a record of previous hospital admissions or episodes of health care. It can be useful to review this record before meeting the patient or client to see whether the information they give you matches up with what you have read about them.

Patient records are also likely to contain results of investigations such as blood tests and X-rays, a list of current medications that the patient may be taking, and reports from other health care professionals such as physiotherapists and occupational therapists.

How is information for assessment obtained?

Establishing rapport and trust

As considered earlier, the nurse carries out assessments on an almost continuous basis, whether meeting the patient or client for the first time, or reassessing or evaluating a package of care that is ongoing.

Very often, perhaps the patient is admitted to hospital or is being visited by the community nurse at home, the first nurse that the patient sees will be responsible for the patient's assessment and for providing information in order to formulate a plan of care. This means that the relationship between the nurse and the patient must be one where communication can take place easily. Often patients or clients are anxious at the thought of requiring care and may be nervous and unsure of themselves. The nurse needs to come across as professional and assured, easily developing rapport and trust with the patient. This can be difficult to achieve, especially in an emergency situation. Consider Scenario 14.1.

SCENARIO 14.1

José Mendez was very proud of his garden. He spent many hours cultivating his vegetables and regularly won prizes, especially for his garlic and onions. One day, just as he was due to go indoors for tea, he developed severe chest pains. His wife, Maria, frantically rang for the family doctor to visit. However, surgery hours were over and the recorded message advised callers to contact NHS Direct or to dial 999 in an emergency. Uncertain what to do and most concerned at José's continued pain, Maria called for an ambulance.

The ambulance arrived within 10 minutes of the call and the crew told José that he had probably had a 'heart attack', best treated in hospital. Maria immediately started to cry, begging to go in the ambulance with her husband. This was agreed and the ambulance made its way to the local hospital, having radioed ahead.

On arrival at the hospital, José was still in pain. He looked very ill and was becoming breathless. Maria was crying and waving her arms hysterically as she got out of the ambulance. The ambulance crew quickly got José out of the ambulance and into the lift, and they made their way to the coronary care unit (CCU). The nurse in charge, Andy, greeted them.

Andy welcomed José as Mr Mendez and quickly introduced himself. He told the ambulance crew that a bed had been prepared for José just inside the ward and they wheeled him off. In the meantime, he asked Maria to wait in the waiting room with another nurse, Susie, who would bring her a drink. As she drank her tea and calmed down, Susie asked Maria what had happened to José and whether he was taking any medications.

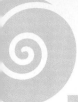
SCENARIO 14.1 (Continued)

On the ward, José had been helped into bed, attached to a cardiac monitor and given medication to relieve his pain. An oxygen mask was also put on to help his breathlessness.

Maria joined José after about 15 minutes, by which time he was feeling much better and the pain was subsiding. Both José and Maria were very impressed and felt confident that all would be well.

Can you identify the ways in which the trust of José and Maria was gained and the assessment process was started?

In Scenario 14.1, you may have identified the following ways in which the trust of José and Maria was gained:

- Andy used good interpersonal skills and greeted José by name. This immediately let José and Maria know that the ward was prepared for him and gave them confidence.
- Although distraught on arrival at hospital, Maria settled down with Susie and was then able to provide information about her husband's condition and his medication, for use in his care plan.
- Andy used his visual observation skills quickly to establish that José was in pain and breathless. This meant that José's treatment started almost as soon as he was made comfortable in bed, and was not delayed by his being asked questions that could have been distressing.

The assessment process was under way even before Andy and the coronary care unit (CCU) nurses had met José and Maria. Andy realised the importance of making a patient feel relaxed and confident, and so he made sure that everything was ready when the ambulance crew radioed him. When he first saw José, he realised from the way he was leaning forward on the trolley that he was breathless and grimacing with pain. Andy knew that Maria would be a useful source of information about her husband but that she was too upset to stay at his bedside. Andy decided that Susie should keep Maria company in the visitors' room. Once José's pain was settled, Andy could gain more information by carrying out his own investigations.

Asking questions

It has already been established that, where possible, the patient or client is the primary source of data for assessment, and that using open or closed questions should provide the necessary information in order for a care plan to be formulated. But would you know what questions to ask?

Reflection point 14.4

Using a friend or a relative, take about 15 minutes to find out as much as possible about their health. Now compare your questions with those that a nursing colleague would have asked.

What questions did you use? Did you find that the questions asked depended on a number of variables, such as the person's age, their experiences of health care, how much they know and understand about health care, and what their expectations are for health?

These variables make asking questions in the process of assessment rather a haphazard affair. However, you may have been guided by the NMC Standard that assessment should be comprehensive, systematic and accurate, taking into account 'physical, psychological, social and spiritual needs of patients, clients and community' (NMC, 2004).

SUMMARY

- Assessment is the first part of the nursing process and assists the nurse in identifying patient or client strengths and weaknesses, and in the formulation of a care plan.
- Information obtained at assessment may be subjective or objective.
- Assessment is carried out when the patient or client first meets the nurse, and is then carried out continuously as care is evaluated.
- Information for assessment may come verbally from the patient or client, or it may come from the use of notes, questioning of family and carers, or using the nurse's senses.
- There are links between the process of assessment, the Standards of Proficiency (NMC, 2004) and the NMC Code, such as the need to respect information gained at assessment as confidential, and the need to ensure that people are informed about how and why information is shared by those who will be providing their care.

Nursing models: a systematic approach to assessment

One way to develop a systematic approach to assessment is through the nursing process, guided by a nursing model. Most models originated in the USA in the 1960s and aimed to describe what nurses do. One description of a nursing model is 'a mental picture of nursing' (Newton, 1991) or a means of guiding, directing and organising care. To describe what nurses do, most nursing models use a framework, or a series of cue questions, to assess and gain information about the patient or client for formulating a plan of care.

Three nursing models with their frameworks for assessment are considered here – those of Roper, Logan and Tierney, of Orem and of Peplau.

Roper, Logan and Tierney's model

This British model, developed in the 1970s, uses as its framework 12 activities of living:

- maintaining a safe environment;
- communicating;
- breathing;
- eating and drinking;
- eliminating;
- personal cleansing and dressing;
- controlling body temperature;
- mobilising;
- working and playing;
- expressing sexuality;
- sleeping;
- dying.

Roper *et al.* (2000) consider that assessing how, why, when and where we carry out the activities of living will produce a comprehensive picture of a person's lifestyle and highlight any 'problems' or 'potential problems' that may require nursing care. This is particularly so if the assessment takes into account how the person carries out the activities of living usually and what they are like now. Alongside this, Roper *et al.* identify that people move along a continuum from conception to death and, depending on the situation, along a further continuum of complete dependence to complete independence, and possibly back again. They also suggest that the activities will be influenced by physical, psychological, sociocultural, environmental and politico-economic factors, so the assessment should be unique to the individual and, therefore, holistic.

A typical assessment sheet for the Roper–Logan–Tierney model is shown in Table 14.2. Note that Roper *et al.* (2000) suggest that it may not be necessary to address every activity of living in every assessment.

Table 14.2 Typical assessment sheet for the Roper, Logan and Tierney (2000) model of nursing

Activity of living	Cue issues	Usual routine	Problems: actual/potential
Maintaining a safe environment	External environment: possible dangers or accidents. Internal environment: homeostasis		
Communication	Speech, hearing, sight, written, intellectual function, language, pain		
Breathing	Ability to breathe, cough, phlegm (sputum)		
Eating and drinking	Likes and dislikes, chewing, swallowing, cooking, resources		
Eliminating	Bowel and bladder habits, continence		
Personal cleansing and dressing	Skin condition, cleanliness, dressing, type of clothing		
Controlling body temperature	Sensitivity to changes in temperature, elderly, very young		
Mobilising	Activity and movement		
Working and playing	Exercise, well-being, how time is spent		
Expressing sexuality	Body image, femininity, masculinity		
Sleeping	Patterns of sleeping and waking		
Dying	Awareness of dying or grieving		

Orem's model

Orem began work on her model in the 1970s, basing it on the concept of 'self-care' (Orem, 2001). 'Self' is seen as physical, psychological, social and spiritual needs and 'care' as the activities that a person carries out in order to maintain life and develop in a way that is normal for that person (Cavanagh, 1991).

In order to assess a person using this model, the eight universal self-care requisites are addressed:

- maintenance of a sufficient intake of air;
- maintenance of a sufficient intake of water;
- maintenance of a sufficient intake of food;
- provision of care associated with elimination processes and excrements;
- maintenance of a balance between activity and rest;
- maintenance of a balance between solitude and social integration;
- prevention of hazards to life, human functioning and human well-being;
- promotion of human functioning and development within social groups in accord with human potential, known human limitations and the human desire to be normal (Orem identifies this as 'normacy').

According to Orem, a person is said to be 'healthy' if they have sufficient self-care abilities to meet universal self-care requisites. However, Orem identifies further self-care requisites, depending on the circumstances that the person is in. These are the *developmental self-care requisites*, which occur at specific periods of human development, such as infancy, adulthood and old age, and the *health-deviation self-care requisites*, which occur when a person becomes ill, is injured or has a disability. It may be that a person is unable to self-care if they have developmental or health deviation self-care requisites to meet. Orem identifies this person as then having a *self-care deficit* and there is a need for nursing care.

The aim of assessment of a person, using Orem's model of nursing, is the determination of the person's abilities to self-care and the identification of self-care limitations or self-care deficit. A typical assessment sheet for the Orem model is shown in Table 14.3.

Peplau's model

Peplau originally published writings on interpersonal skills in the early 1950s, and it is a development of her thinking that is the basis for her model of nursing (Peplau, 1991). She sees the

Table 14.3 Typical assessment sheet for the Orem (2001) model of nursing

Universal self-care requisites	Self-care abilities	Self-care limitations
Maintenance of a sufficient intake of air		
Maintenance of a sufficient intake of water		
Maintenance of a sufficient intake of food		
Provision of care associated with elimination processes and excrement		
Maintenance of a balance between activity and rest		
Maintenance of a balance between solitude and social integration		
Prevention of hazards to life, human functioning and human well-being		
Normacy		

nurse–patient relationship as the most important issue in nursing and believes that, without it, nursing actions would not be effective. Much of the work published identifying the application of Peplau's model to care is related to patients or clients in a mental health setting, although it can be equally suitable for all client groups (Simpson, 1991).

The overwhelming belief within Peplau's model is that the patient or client should be moving towards health, and that the nurse has a number of roles that can educate and empower the person to do this. This will occur within the phases of the nurse–patient relationship (Peplau, 1991).

Phases in the nurse–patient relationship

Peplau sees the nurse and patient or client as passing through four phases of relationship:

1 *Phase of orientation*: this identifies the patient or client entering the unknown, with no knowledge of the new environment, the nursing staff, or the condition that has brought them to seek health care. The nurse can expect the patient or client to be anxious and confused, requiring explanations of procedures and routines. Peplau sees the nurse and patient taking the roles of strangers at this time.

2 *Phase of identification*: this identifies the patient or client finding out more about the reason for health care, the people who can be relied upon for help and advice, and how the patient or client can become more involved in their own care.

3 *Phase of exploitation*: this identifies the patient or client making full use of the resources around them and moving towards healthy behaviour. Peplau sees this as the patient or client moving from dependence towards independence.

4 *Phase of resolution*: the patient or client is preparing to live a healthy lifestyle outside of a health care setting. This is the drawing to a close of the nurse–patient relationship that has been so important in providing support and education to help the patient or client move towards health.

Simpson (1991) considers that each phase can be discrete and observed, or they may overlap, and nurses should be aware of this in order to enable patients and clients to move on.

Roles of nurses

Peplau suggests that, as patients or clients move through these phases, the nurse can adopt a number of roles, dependent on the situation:

- *Stranger*: Peplau sees this as the opportunity to begin the nurse–patient relationship; it should not be based on presumptions about the person being assessed.
- *Resource*: as the person moves through the phases of identification and exploitation, the patient can use the nurse to gain information, skills and resources to help move towards health.
- *Teacher*: the nurse teaches the patient or client how to deal with, for example, a situation, condition or medication.
- *Leader*: this may be a flexible role as the patient or client moves towards health, gradually taking more control.
- *Counsellor*: Peplau suggests that not all nurses can counsel, but sometimes it is helpful to the patient or client for the nurse just to listen and allow the patient to draw their own conclusions on their progress.
- *Surrogate*: this is the nurse acting as a substitute when the person is ill. It is important that, during the phase of resolution, this role is reduced.

Assessment is most likely to occur during the phase of orientation and is about the nurse collecting information. Adopting one or more of the roles may then allow the nurse to make observations of the verbal and non-verbal cues and identify problems for nursing care.

Reflection point 14.5

Using the assessment frameworks of Roper, Logan and Tierney, Orem, and Peplau, carry out an assessment of Manjeet and Samantha in the scenarios identified below.

Manjeet Dhaliwal is admitted to the medical ward with newly diagnosed diabetes. He has recently graduated with a first-class honours degree in fine art and is due to start work as a graphic designer. He has been feeling generally unwell and has lost weight, but he put this down to the stress of his exams.

Samantha Temple is 10 years old and had emergency surgery yesterday for appendicitis. She has twin sisters who are 4 years old, and her father is currently working abroad. Samantha seems to be very quiet today and says she does not want to get up until her mother arrives to look after her.

For Manjeet, you may have identified the issues outlined in Table 14.4 using Roper, Logan and Tierney's model, and for Samantha, those in Table 14.5.

For Manjeet, you may have identified the issues outlined in Table 14.6 using Orem's model, and for Samantha those in Table 14.7.

A possible assessment of Manjeet using Peplau's model is as follows. Phase of orientation – the nurse greeted Manjeet on the ward; he looked very anxious and was leaning forward in his chair as he spoke. The nurse asked whether she could sit with him and ask him some questions. He replied that he wanted to get 'this thing sorted out as quickly as possible' and for him to get on with his life. Manjeet said he was to start his first job next week and could not afford for anything to go wrong. He also told the nurse that he had an uncle who had had diabetes and had died at an early age following a heart attack. The nurse made the following notes:

- Manjeet is very anxious about the diagnosis of diabetes. He is not sure what it is, how to manage it or the impact it will have on his life.
- Manjeet appears to be highly intelligent and is keen to start his first job. He seems to want to be as independent as possible.

Table 14.4 Issues identified in the assessment of Manjeet using Roper, Logan and Tierney's (2000) model

Activity of living	Usual routines	Potential/actual problems
Maintaining a safe environment	Fully independent	Blood sugar is unstable; does not know how to inject insulin
Eating and drinking	Eats 'junk food'; likes to drink socially – about 5 pints of lager a week	Needs to understand a 'healthy diet' in order to maintain diabetic control; fasts each Ramadan
Working and playing	Fully independent; due to start a new job next week; played football in the university league	Very worried that he will not be well enough to start his new job and will not be able to get involved in sport
Expressing sexuality	Independent; has casual girlfriends but 'no one serious'	Worried he will not be able to have a 'normal relationship' with a girl
Dying		Manjeet's uncle died following a major heart attack; he had poorly controlled diabetes

Table 14.5 Issues identified in the assessment of Samantha using Roper, Logan and Tierney's (2000) model

Activity of living	Usual routines	Potential/actual problems
Maintaining a safe environment	Fully independent	Samantha has had an operation and may develop a wound infection; she may haemorrhage
Communicating	Usually independent; likes to read Harry Potter stories	Samantha is quiet and withdrawn; she is shy without her mother present
Eating and drinking	Usually independent; does not like milk unless really cold; prefers to eat white bread	Has an intravenous infusion in place until she starts to drink; has been feeling slightly sick since the operation
Eliminating	Tends to open her bowels three times per week	Bowels not opened since hospital admission
Personal cleansing and dressing	Usually independent; likes to shower	Has refused to wash without her mother
Controlling body temperature	Independent	Had a raised temperature before going to theatre for surgery; still raised
Working and playing	Fully independent; enjoys school	Has been very withdrawn and does not interact with other children

Table 14.6 Issues identified in the assessment of Manjeet using Orem's (1991) model

Universal self-care requisites	Self-care abilities	Self-care limitations
Maintenance of a sufficient intake of air	Usually no difficulties	None
Maintenance of a sufficient intake of water	Usually no difficulties	None
Maintenance of a sufficient intake of food	Eats 'junk food' and drinks 5 pints of lager a week	Fasts each Ramadan; has a knowledge deficit about healthy eating and how to manage during Ramadan
Provision of care associated with elimination processes and excrement	No difficulties	None
Maintenance of a balance between activity and rest	Usually very active; plays football	Has been feeling very tired recently
Maintenance of a balance between solitude and social integration	Usually sociable with active life outside university	Worried about socialising with work colleagues
Prevention of hazards to life, sugar human functioning and human well-being	No difficulties	Does not understand how to inject insulin or check his blood
Normacy	No difficulties	Concerned that he will not be able to have a girlfriend, or that he may suffer an early death like his uncle, who also had diabetes; now worried that his use of alcohol is responsible for his diabetes

Table 14.7 Issues identified in the assessment of Samantha using Orem's (1991) model

Universal self-care requisites	Self-care abilities	Self-care limitations
Maintenance of a sufficient intake of air	No difficulties	None
Maintenance of a sufficient intake of water	No difficulties	Has an intravenous infusion; she is not drinking at present
Maintenance of a sufficient intake of food	No difficulties	Has been feeling sick since her operation
Provision of care associated with elimination processes and excrement	No difficulties; opens bowels three times per week	Bowels not opened since admission
Maintenance of a balance between activity and rest	No difficulties, although prefers to be alone than with her twin sisters	Refuses to get up until her mother arrives
Maintenance of a balance between solitude and social integration	Quite shy; misses her father, who is away on business	Is withdrawn and has not mixed with the other children
Prevention of hazards to life, human functioning and human well-being	No difficulties	Has potential for wound infection, haemorrhage and pain
Normacy	No difficulties	Does not like the company of her twin sisters, because they like playing with dolls; she prefers to be with her father and go fishing

- Manjeet has lost weight; his clothes hang loosely on him.
- Manjeet had an uncle with diabetes, who died of a heart attack. Manjeet is aware of the need to have his diabetes well controlled but has no knowledge of what this will entail.
- Manjeet says he regrets drinking alcohol because, as strict Muslims, his parents would be disappointed in him.

The nurse then went on to write out Manjeet's care plan, identifying how she could take on the roles of teacher, resource person and counsellor as Manjeet moved through the phases of the relationship.

A possible assessment of Samantha using Peplau's model is as follows. Phase of orientation – Samantha was admitted to the children's surgical ward in the evening, complaining of abdominal pain. This was thought to be due to appendicitis. Samantha's mother came to the hospital with her but was unable to stay because her two other daughters were at home, unattended. Samantha's father was working away on business. The staff nurse on the children's ward assessed Samantha and eventually took her to theatre for her operation. He noticed that Samantha was very shy and that her mother answered his questions. The staff nurse was actually quite pleased when Samantha's mother decided to go home, so he could get to know Samantha a little better. He made the following notes about Samantha and her mother:

- Samantha is hot and in abdominal pain. She probably has appendicitis and will require surgery fairly soon.
- Samantha has been vomiting and her mouth is dry.

- Samantha is a bright girl but obviously shy. Her mother is used to speaking for her.
- The family do not seem to be well supported by an extended family or neighbours, as the younger sisters have been left unattended.

Phase of identification – the staff nurse was not on duty the following morning after Samantha's operation, and one of the student nurses tried to strike up a relationship with Samantha. She asked Samantha whether she hurt anywhere and whether she was ready to get up, have a wash and have something to eat and drink. Samantha seemed surprised that she was allowed up, but she refused to move and said she would not have a wash until her mother arrived. The student nurse went to the nurse in charge to report the following:

- Samantha says she is not in pain but she refuses to move, so she probably does have pain.
- Samantha has still had nothing to eat or drink.
- Samantha has not passed urine since her operation.
- Samantha says she will not move or have a wash until her mother arrives, but her mother rang the ward earlier to say she would not be visiting until after lunch.

The nurse in charge used this information to consider the nursing roles that would be needed to move Samantha towards health and through the phases of exploitation and resolution.

Reflection point 14.6
- Which assessment framework did you prefer to use?
- Do you think it is important to have a framework for assessment?
- Which framework makes it easier to be aware of the subjective information available to the nurse at assessment?
- Is there enough specific information identified to be able to formulate a plan of care?

These two scenarios demonstrate some of the issues raised in the NMC Standards (NMC 2004), for example that nurses:

- 'practise in accordance with an ethical and legal framework which ensures the primacy of patient and client interest and well-being'. The nurse will be made aware that Manjeet is a Muslim but that he drinks alcohol when he socialises with his friends from university. His parents would be upset if they were aware of this, so the information is important when educating Manjeet how to manage his diabetes, but it is confidential information;
- 'practise in a fair and anti-discriminatory way, acknowledging the differences in beliefs and cultural practices of individuals or groups'. The nurse may have been shocked and disappointed that Samantha's mother did not stay with her until she went to the operating theatre, or stay overnight with her. The nurse must acknowledge that Samantha's sisters also require attention and must be non-judgemental towards the rest of the family.

However, the scenarios may also serve to highlight a lack of detail in the assessments carried out and that much of the information gathered could not be measured or recorded in any systematic manner.

Reflection point 14.7
Identify the ways in which the assessments of José, Manjeet and Samantha lack in detail and accuracy.

Possible omissions you may have identified are listed in Table 14.8.

It is not possible to provide answers to questions such as those posed in Table 14.8 from the information gleaned using nursing models. Assessment tools, such as recording the temperature, a pain assessment tool, blood sugar testing and a mouth care assessment, may also be required.

Table 14.8 Omissions from the assessments

José	Manjeet	Samantha
How severe was José's chest pain?	How much weight had Manjeet lost?	How hot was Samantha before surgery? Was she the same temperature on return?
How did the nurse in the CCU know it was resolving?	How different from the 'normal' was Manjeet's blood sugar level to cause him to be diabetic?	How much pain was she in, and is that the reason for her not wanting to move?
How breathless was José?	How will he know how much insulin he requires?	How dry was her mouth?
Did the oxygen make his breathing better or worse?		How much did she vomit?
How did the nurse know which medication to give?		How much fluid had she received by the infusion?

SUMMARY

- Nursing models assist in providing a framework to enable a comprehensive assessment of physical, psychological, spiritual and social needs of patients and clients.
- Nursing models may enable you to learn what is the usual behaviour of the patient or client, how this differs from their behaviour when they are ill, or whether they can be taught to manage their own health condition.
- It is not sufficient to gather information with nursing models alone; assessment tools are also required to allow the gathering of objective information.

Tools for assessment

Tools for assessment should be able to provide a valid and reliable measure of the patient's or client's problem or potential problem. Many of the tools used form part of a strategy to minimise the risk that a patient or client faces during their period of hospitalisation or when in receipt of health care.

An example of one of the tools used in many acute ward areas to support the early recognition of patients at risk of critical illness is an early warning system (EWS). The EWS illustrated in Table 14.9 was devised as a result of a study conducted by Hogan (2006), who found that patients on many wards have respirations counted as a routine part of clinical observations as

Table 14.9 Example of an early warning system

Score	3	2	1	0	1	2	3
Temperature (°)		<35.0	35.1–35.9	36–37.5	37.6–38.9	>39	
Blood pressure (mmHg)	<70	71–80	81–100	101–199		>200	
Heart rate (/min)	<40		40–50	51–100	101–110	111–129	>130
Respiratory rate (/min)		<8		9–14	15–20	21–29	>30
Central nervous system			New agitation, confusion	Alert	No response to voice	No response to pain	Unconscious

Source: Hogan (2006).

little as 50 per cent of the time, which means that vital signs of a patient's potential deterioration are missed.

In the example shown in Table 14.9, the scores are added; the higher the score, the greater the risk to the patient. If the score triggers a warning, then the appropriate support is provided for the patient or the alarm is raised for medical help.

Scenarios 14.2 and 14.3 are used to give examples of how other tools can be used.

SCENARIO 14.2 Alexander Ziolkowski

Alexander Ziolkowski arrived in Britain from Poland during the Second World War. He settled in the Midlands, where he met and married his wife, Nora. They raised four children, with Alexander working in the coal mining industry for many years. Nora and Alexander's children have now all married and moved away.

Alexander retired at the age of 63 years, already suffering with chronic lung disease, probably related to his years in the mines. He has bought his house from the colliery, but he is now looking for a bungalow, as climbing stairs makes him breathless. On his last hospital admission, he refused to allow the occupational therapist to accompany him home to assess his living circumstances, but now he is wishing he had.

Alexander is admitted to the medical ward with an acute exacerbation of his chronic obstructive pulmonary disease (COPD). He is too breathless to talk on admission, and he appears cyanosed and sweaty. He is wearing an oxygen mask attached to a small cylinder. He refuses to get into the prepared bed, preferring to sit upright in a high-backed chair.

Nora accompanies her husband and tells the nurses on the ward that Alexander has not been downstairs for a week because of his breathlessness. He has been using his oxygen a lot and sometimes gets confused. She says he has not eaten or drunk for several days, and she thinks he is losing weight. Nora also says that her husband is a practising Roman Catholic and would like to have last rites performed by Father Joseph if he is going to die.

The nurse allocated to care for Alexander is Mary, who knows him from previous admissions to the ward. She winks at Alexander when he arrives and gives his arm a friendly squeeze, telling him she has a student nurse working with her today and that they will soon 'sort him out'. Mary tells the student they will be using the Roper–Logan–Tierney model of nursing to plan care.

SCENARIO 14.3 Simon Cooper

Simon is a 22-year-old man who lives at home with his mother. He works as a casual labourer at the garden centre. He loves the plants and the aquatic section of the garden centre. As part of his work, he often helps customers carry compost and gravel to their cars. Simon has Down's syndrome.

Simon was admitted to the surgical ward and underwent surgical repair of a right inguinal hernia earlier today. He returns to the ward drowsy but rousable and has received pain relief in theatre.

After completing a full set of postoperative observations on Simon, including pulse, blood pressure, respirations, and checking his dressing for leakage, your main concern is to keep him comfortable and free from pain.

Prioritising the assessment

You will recall that assessment is not a one-off process, but one occurring continuously. However, with patients as ill as Alexander in Scenario 14.2, it is vital to gain key pieces of information to start the care package, and then to make a more detailed assessment later.

Reflection point 14.8

Imagine you are the nurse admitting and assessing Alexander. What information do you need to have straight away in order to provide care?

You may have considered using the 'ABC' approach – that is, A for airway, B for breathing and C for circulation. This is a useful strategy in emergency situations and prompts you to make sure that the patient or client is able to survive until a more detailed assessment can be undertaken.

Mary has already noted that Alexander opted to stay in the chair and that he is using oxygen, so she knows his condition is serious. However, she can also see that his breathlessness has not exhausted him completely and that she will have some preliminary information to offer medical staff when they arrive to prescribe medications. The key activity of living for priority assessment is breathing (Prigmore, 2005). Mary asks the following questions:

- Can Alexander breathe?
- Is his airway clear? Is he producing sputum (phlegm) and can he cough it up (expectorate)?
- Is his breathing deep or shallow? Is it noisy?
- How rapid is his breathing? Does he have tachypnoea or bradypnoea?
- Is he becoming confused because of a lack of oxygen to the brain (hypoxia)?
- Is he in a comfortable position to maintain his breathing, or does he need support with more pillows? Does he have dyspnoea or orthopnoea?
- Does he have an acute exacerbation of his condition because of a chest infection?
- Does he have a raised temperature because of infection?
- Does he have a raised pulse because of infection and the extra effort required in breathing? Does he have tachycardia or bradycardia?
- Is he having the right amount of oxygen?

To answer these questions, Mary may already have started to use some tools to produce measurements and an accurate assessment:

Assessment of sputum

Mary is aware that patients with COPD regularly produce sputum, especially first thing in the morning. She is particularly interested in the colour and consistency of any sputum produced, as a change in colour to yellow or green, and becoming more sticky and viscid, could indicate infection.

Assessment of breathing rate and depth

The normal adult respiratory rate (rate of breathing) is 10–15 breaths per minute (Simpson, 2006). Mary is aware of this when recording the number of breaths per minute taken by Alexander, and that rapid breathing (in excess of 24 breaths per minute) is tachypnoea and bradypnoea is a slow rate (less than 10 breaths per minute) (Simpson, 2006). The respiratory rate should always be counted for at least half a minute by observing the rise and fall of the chest. The patient should be unaware that the respirations are being counted, as there is an involuntary tendency to change the breathing pattern. In any patient, an increase in the resting respiratory rate of five breaths per minute can be a serious indicator of respiratory distress, which requires attention (Hogan, 2006). The depth of respiration relates to the volume of air moving in and out of the lungs and the position adopted by the patient for breathing. Mary notes that Alexander is having difficulty in breathing (dyspnoea) but also that he is able to breathe only while sitting upright, supported by pillows (orthopnoea).

Assessment of level of oxygen that the patient is receiving

Mary checks the oxygen mask that Alexander is wearing and notes that 24 per cent oxygen is being delivered to him. However, he still appears to be cyanosed and confused at times, which could be due to hypoxia. Mary decides to carry out pulse oximetry, which checks the oxygen saturation level of arterial blood (SpO_2) (Higgins, 2005). Pulse oximetry is carried out by attaching a probe to the body (usually the fingertip or earlobe is used) and a light detector in the probe detects the amount of oxygen absorbed by the haemoglobin, which is usually 95–100 per cent. An SpO_2 of less than 90 per cent may demonstrate a serious respiratory problem. It is possible to keep a pulse oximetry probe in place for several hours and therefore to monitor the oxygen saturation levels continuously. This is useful for patients such as Alexander.

Assessment of body temperature

In order to assess whether Alexander is breathless due to infection or whether the increased activity of breathing rapidly is causing an increase in metabolic rate and raised body temperature, his temperature is recorded. Mary is aware that the usual body temperature is within a range of 36–37.6 °C (Docherty, 2006) and that raised temperature is known as 'pyrexia' and lowered body temperature as 'hypothermia'. Body temperature may be recorded at a number of sites, most commonly the mouth, axilla (armpit) and tympanic membrane (eardrum). In Alexander's case, the tympanic route is preferable as he does not need to be disturbed and a reading can be obtained within approximately 10 seconds.

Assessment of heart rate (pulse)

The pulse rate is the number of heart beats in a 60-second period. The normal heart rate for an adult is 60–100 beats per minute (Docherty, 2006). A pulse below 60 beats per minute is identified as 'bradycardia' and above 110 beats per minute as 'tachycardia'. Mary expects Alexander's pulse rate to be higher than usual because of his infection, which causes metabolic rate to rise, and because of the extra effort required to breathe.

Already Mary has a significant amount of information, gained from carrying out vital signs and visually observing Alexander, from talking to Nora and from reading the GP's letter that accompanied him (Table 14.10).

Alexander's immediate assessment identifies a number of issues related to his ability to breathe, which have to be addressed immediately. However, further issues in relation to other activities of living can be assessed as his condition stabilises; these are identified under the activities of eating and drinking, personal cleansing and dressing, and mobilising. The condition of

Table 14.10 Assessment of Alexander using the Roper, Logan and Tierney (2000) model

Activity of living	Usual routines	Potential/actual problems
Maintaining a safe environment	Has difficulty in negotiating stairs; he has been confused over the past week and unable to manage hot drinks safely; has home oxygen and uses it regularly	Confused at times and needs to be observed regularly
Communicating	Usually independent; wears glasses for reading	Too breathless to speak at present; he can use a picture board easily
Breathing	Gets out of breath on exertion; does not smoke; uses oxygen at home for at least 6 hours/day	Respiratory rate 24 beats/minute; SpO_2 93 per cent; receiving oxygen at 24 per cent; producing green sputum (sample collected)
Eating and drinking	Usually independent but not much of an appetite; has full set of dentures	Mouth is dry – to be assessed later; nutritional assessment later
Eliminating	Has used a bedside commode for past week; usually constipated	Bowels not opened since hospital admission – for further assessment
Personal cleansing and dressing	Daily assisted wash with help of Nora; weekly shower with aid of community helper; cannot put on socks – too breathless	Appears very sweaty on admission; pressure areas not yet assessed
Controlling body temperature	Usually independent	Temperature 37.8 °C on admission, pulse 98 beats/minute; fan in situ
Mobilising	Has not been out of the house for a month or downstairs for a week; usually manages stairs	Appears immobile; pressure area risk is high – for assessment later
Working and playing	Retired miner; enjoys watching snooker and football on TV; has no exercise	
Expressing sexuality	Has four children all living away; uses electric shaver; does not use deodorant spray – makes him cough	Unable to wash and dress with privacy at home
Sleeping	Sleeps with four pillows; has slept in a chair for the past two nights	Rests in a chair; appears drowsy
Dying	Practising Roman Catholic; aware that he is seriously ill	Has asked Father Joseph to be called for last rites if necessary

Alexander's dry mouth, his state of nutrition and his pressure areas, with associated risk of developing pressure sores, can be assessed with specific tools:

Oral assessment

Alexander's mouth was said to be dry when he was admitted to the ward. Nora told Mary that her husband had not eaten or drunk for several days. He is receiving oxygen via a facemask, which also has the effect of drying his mouth and putting him at risk of developing an oral infection (NT Skills Update, 2003), further deterring him from eating and drinking. Therefore, assessing

Alexander's oral status is important, preferably with an assessment tool that will objectively measure how dry or dirty his mouth is.

Reflection point 14.9

Consider the way you start your day: how soon after you get up do you clean your teeth or take a drink to freshen your mouth?

Most of us take a clean, moist and healthy mouth for granted. When assessing patients or clients, nurses should be observing for:

- a pink moist tongue, oral mucosa and gums;
- teeth/dentures clean and free from debris;
- well-fitting dentures;
- adequate salivation;
- smooth and moist lips;
- no difficulties in eating or swallowing.

If some of these features are absent, and there are added complications of treatment such as medications, and other diseases such as diabetes or anaemia, the person may be at risk of oral problems. An oral risk assessment tool is identified, where the higher the score of the person assessed, the greater the risk of oral problems and the need for mouth care to be included in the care plan (Table 14.11).

Table 14.11 Oral risk indicator tool

Mental status		Food/fluid intake		Teeth/dentures/jaw	
Alert	0	Good	0	Clean and free from debris	0
Apathetic	1	Inadequate diet	1	Debris present	1
Sedated	2	Fluids only	2	Denture present top/bottom (delete)	2
Uncooperative	3	No intake	3	Limited jaw mobility	3
Lips		Tongue		Saliva	
Smooth and moist	0	Pink and moist	0	Present and watery	0
Dry and cracked	1	Coated	1	Thick	1
Bleeding	2	Shiny/red	2	Insufficient/excess	2
Ulcerated	3	Blister/cracked	3	Absent	3
Mucous membranes		Patient's age (years)		Airway	
Pink and moist	0	16–29	1	Normal	0
Red and coated	1	30–49	2	Humidified oxygen	1
White areas	2	50–69	3	Nebulised therapy	2
Ulcerated	3	70+	4	Open-mouth breathing or non-humidified oxygen	3
				Endotracheal/oral intubation	4
Additional scores		Risk indicator			
High-dose antibiotics	4	Score 30+	High		
Steroids	4	Score 24–29	Medium		
Radiotherapy	4	Score below 23	Low		
Diabetes	4				
Anaemia	4				
Cytotoxic drugs	4				
Immunocompromised	4				

Source: University Hospitals of Leicester (2000).

Nutritional assessment

Alexander has not eaten or drunk for several days, due to his breathlessness. Patients who are breathless, and particularly those with chronic lung disease, are known to be at risk of malnutrition (Shuttleworth, 2005). When he is well enough, it would be appropriate to weigh Alexander and compare this weight with what is known to be his usual weight. However, completing a nutritional assessment can be useful, especially if Alexander is to be referred for specialist dietetic support, such as high-protein or high-calorie drinks because of his difficulty in managing solid food. Leicestershire Nutrition and Dietetic Services (1998) developed the nutritional screening tool shown in Table 14.12. The risk of poor nutrition is calculated and a care plan devised accordingly.

Table 14.12 Nutritional screening tool

Body weight for height		Ability to eat	
Acceptable (BMI 19–25)	0	Able to eat independently	0
Overweight (BMI >25)	2	Ill-fitting dentures/chewing problems	3
Recent significant weight loss	3	Swallowing problems	3
Underweight (BMI <19)	4	Needs to be fed	4
		Complete dysphagia	5
Skin type		*Symptoms*	
Healthy	0	Nausea	2
Dry and flaky	2	Vomiting	2
Oedematous	3	Constipation	2
Poor wound healing	4	Diarrhoea	2
Pressure sore/leg ulcer (all grades)	5		
Appetite and dietary intake		*Psychological state*	
Normal appetite/intake	0	Fully oriented	0
On special diet, e.g. supplements	2	Confused	2
Reduced appetite/intake	3	Depressed/anxious/apathetic	4
Appetite and dietary intake		*Psychological state*	
No appetite/very poor intake/nil by mouth/clear fluids for 7 days or more	5		
Age		*Total*	
Over 65 years	2		

Patients or clients scoring 10 or above are recommended to be referred for detailed nutritional assessment.
BMI, body mass index.

Source: Leicestershire Nutrition and Dietetic Service (1998).

Pressure risk assessment

In reviewing the initial assessment of Alexander using the Roper–Logan–Tierney framework (see Table 14.10), you will note that, under the activities of living of 'personal cleansing and dressing' and 'mobility', pressure areas are mentioned. Pressure damage can occur when skin and other tissues are compressed between bone and another surface for a period of time (Pellatt, 2001). This causes the blood supply to the tissues to be reduced or cut off, resulting in damage to the skin. The usual result is skin breakdown and the development of a pressure ulcer (bedsore). Alexander has found difficulty in mobilising because of his breathlessness, and so could be at risk. He has also been sleeping in a chair, putting extra pressure on his sacral area and this again could put him at risk of a pressure ulcer.

Apart from direct pressure, pressure ulcers (sores) can occur by the forces of shearing and friction (Gould, 2001). Shearing occurs when tissues are wrenched in opposite directions, e.g. when a patient 'slides down the bed' or the chair. Friction occurs when the skin surface rubs against another surface. Alexander's elbows may be particularly at risk from friction as he uses his elbows to push himself up in the bed or chair to assist his breathing. The sacrum, heels, elbows, hips, knees and ankles pose the greatest risk (Pellatt, 2001), but any area under pressure can be damaged. Previous assessments of Alexander's physical condition and his nutritional state also place him at great risk of pressure damage, according to some authors (Waterlow, 1998). Several pressure risk assessment tools have been devised, one of the earliest being the Norton scale (Norton *et al.*, 1962), originally for use with older adults (Table 14.13).

Table 14.13 The Norton scale

Physical condition		Mental state		Activity		Mobility		Incontinence	
Good	4	Alert	4	Ambulant	4	Full	4	Not	4
Fair	3	Apathetic	3	Walks with help	3	Slightly limited	3	Occasionally	3
Poor	2	Confused	2	Chair-bound	2	Very limited	2	Usually urine	2
Very bad	1	Stuporous	1	Bedfast	1	Immobile	1	Double	1

Assessment of risk: less than 14 = at risk.

Source: Norton *et al.* (1962).

Reflection point 14.10
It has been suggested that the Norton scale is actually subjective and difficult to score. Can you identify any problems with this scale?

You may have identified the lack of specifics within the scale; for example, what is the difference between a 'fair' and a 'poor' physical condition? How 'occasional' does incontinence need to be before it is used as part of the score? If the patient is catheterised for incontinence of urine, does this give them 'full' continence?

The Waterlow risk assessment (Waterlow, 1998) was originally devised in 1985 and aims to provide much more specific detail about the risk of developing a pressure ulcer (Table 14.14). It gives much more detail and includes factors that the Norton scale does not, for example the patient's gender, risk of alterations to the circulation that could be affected by smoking or the effect of anaemia on the skin, and body mass. You will note also that, according to Norton, the patient is at greater risk of pressure damage in bed than when sitting in a chair, while the Waterlow scale considers the chair-bound person to be at greater risk and hence has a greater score.

Reflection point 14.11
Using the Norton and Waterlow scales, what scores would you allocate to Alexander? Is he at risk of pressure damage? Do both scales place him at equal risk? Which scale is easier to use?

Table 14.14 Waterlow risk assessment

Build/weight for height		Skin type/visual risk areas		Sex/age (years)		Special risks		
Average	0	Healthy	0	Male	1	Tissue		
Above average	1	Tissue paper	1	Female	2	Malnutrition		
Obese	2	Dry	1	14–49	1	Cachexia	8	
Below average	3	Oedematous	1	50–64	2	Cardiac failure	5	
		Clammy (temperature)	1	65–74	3	PVD	5	
		Discoloured	2	75–80	4	Anaemia	2	
		Broken/spot	3	≥ 81	5	Smoking	1	
Continence		*Mobility*		*Appetite*		*Neurological deficit*		
Complete/catheterised	0	Full	0	Average	0	Diabetes, MS	4	
Occasional incontinence	1	Restless/fidgety	1	Poor	1	CVA	–	
Incontinent of faeces	2	Apathetic	2	NG tube/fluids	2	Paraplegia	6	
Double incontinence	3	Restricted	3	only		Major surgery/trauma	5	
		Inert/traction Chair-bound	4	Nil by Mouth/	3	Medication	4	
			5	anorexic				

Score: 10, at risk; 15, high risk; 20, very high risk.

CVA, cerebrovascular accident; MS, multiple sclerosis; NG, nasogastric; PVD, peripheral vascular disease.

Source: Waterlow (1998).

Identifying a score for the risk of pressure damage is the first part of the assessment process. Appropriate pressure-relieving devices should be used, depending on the score obtained. For example, Waterlow (1998) advocates the use of a foam mattress for a score of 10 and an alternating-pressure mattress for a score of 20. Pressure-relieving equipment should also be used in the patient's chair or wheelchair, bearing in mind the increased risk when sitting.

Pressure risk assessments should be evaluated regularly and documented in the patient's plan of care.

Assessing patients for pain

Can you describe what 'pain' is? We all find it difficult, yet most of us have experienced pain at some time of our lives. The International Association for the Study of Pain (IASP, 1992) suggests that pain is 'an unpleasant sensory and emotional experience associated with actual or potential tissue damage or described in terms of such damage'.

Experiencing pain is a subjective phenomenon and many factors influence the way it is experienced, including the following:

- Lack of information about what pain is, how it is caused, and how it will be relieved, and lack of control over pain, all tend to increase pain.
- Families and society often socialise people into ways of behaving when in pain, e.g. the British 'stiff upper lip' contrasts with the Mediterranean wailing.

- The context in which pain is experienced may influence the pain. For example, many women expect to have pain in childbirth, whereas patients recovering from a hip replacement following arthritis of the hip frequently experience no pain because the surgical pain is less than the previous arthritic pain.

Many patients are now taught to manage their own pain after a surgical operation, using patient-controlled analgesia (PCA), whereby they deliver a dose of a drug to themselves in response to pain or before carrying out movement.

Reflection point 14.12
Make a note of the ways you would assess and identify whether Simon is suffering pain.

You may have identified some of the following:

- lack of movement;
- groaning;
- facial grimaces;
- lack of sleep;
- rapid pulse.

Simon may exhibit some of these typical pain responses. However, it may be more appropriate to identify pain in a more systematic and objective manner, using a pain assessment scale, such as the verbal rating scale (Table 14.15) or visual analogue scale (in which patients are asked to place a mark on a line drawn between the numbers 0 and 10, which represents the intensity of pain – the higher the score, the greater the pain).

Table 14.15 Verbal rating scale

Rating of pain	Score
None	0
Mild	1
Moderate	2
Severe	3

Reflection point 14.13
- From the patient's or client's point of view, what might be the advantages of using a pain assessment tool?
- From the nurse's point of view, what might be the advantages of using such a tool?
- Are there any patients or clients who would have difficulty in using such a scale?

You may have identified the following:

- From the patient's viewpoint, using a rating scale means that every nurse on duty will interpret the pain in the same way rather than subjectively. It also means that if the pain relief does not take effect within half an hour and the patient is still in pain, then there may be the opportunity to review the treatment and find an alternative that will work (evaluation of pain relief).

- From the nurse's viewpoint, this is a means of obtaining an accurate record of what causes pain, how severe the pain is, and what helps to relieve the pain. The score that the patient reports may have an impact on the way in which other activities of living are carried out.
- Patients such as Simon, who has a learning disability, may have difficulty in using a rating tool such as those discussed. Elderly people, very young people, and people who are confused or partially sighted may also have a problem using such scales.

SUMMARY

- Assessment tools are useful because they allow specific measurements to be made and provide accurate and objective data for assessment.
- Assessment tools can be quite simple, e.g. temperature recording, or sophisticated, e.g. pressure sore risk, nutrition assessment, pain scales and the amount of oxygen carried by the blood.
- Using such tools to measure, assess and evaluate the needs of a patient or client enables the use of best evidence or research to inform the nursing care that the patient or client receives.

CONCLUSION

Assessing patients and clients is a fundamental nursing skill and vital to meeting the needs of patients and clients. Assessment is the first stage of the nursing process and provides the opportunity to reflect the patient's or client's views and concerns about their need for nursing care, not just those of the nurse. This is particularly important, as the information gained through assessment may help to formulate a plan of care used not only by nurses but also by other members of the multiprofessional health and social care teams.

Assessment may be the first time that the nurse and patient or client meet, and so it is clearly important to develop a trusting and good working relationship from the outset (do not forget: the patient or client will also be assessing you!). This means that the nurse needs to have excellent interpersonal and communication skills. Asking the right questions is clearly important, but so is the ability to listen to what is being said and how it is said, particularly when the client may have a communication difficulty. Subjective or objective data may be revealed by assessment. To assist in data-gathering, a nursing model with a framework for assessment may be used. This may be used in conjunction with assessment tools, enabling accurate measurement. Using evidence-based tools for assessment means that the same information is available to all members of the multiprofessional team and can ensure that the care provided is based on the most up-to-date and research-based care.

Following the principles for assessment identifies that it really is the foundation of good practice.

References

Cavanagh SJ (1991). *Orem's Model in Action*. Basingstoke: Macmillan.

Department of Health (DH) (2001). *National Service Framework for Older People*. London: Department of Health.

Docherty B (2006). Homeostasis. Part 3: temperature regulation. *Nursing Times*, **102**, 20.

Gould D (2001). Pressure ulcer risk assessment. *Nursing Standard,* **11**, 43–9.

Higgins D (2005). Pulse oximetry. *Nursing Standard,* **101**, 34.

Hogan J (2006). Why don't nurses monitor the respiratory rates of patients? *British Journal of Nursing,* **15**, 9, 489–92.

International Association for the Study of Pain (IASP) (1992). *Management of Acute Pain: A Practical Guide.* Seattle, WA: International Association for the Study of Pain.

Leicestershire Nutrition and Dietetic Services (1998). *Nutritional Screening Tool.* Leicester: Leicester Royal Infirmary.

Newton C (1991). *The Roper–Logan–Tierney Model in Action.* Basingstoke: Macmillan.

Norton D, McLaren R and Exton-Smith AN (1962). *An Investigation of Geriatric Nursing Problems in Hospital,* 1975 edn. Edinburgh: Churchill Livingstone.

Nursing and Midwifery Council (NMC) (2004). *Standards of Proficiency.* London: Nursing and Midwifery Council.

Nursing and Midwifery Council (NMC) (2008). *The Code: Standards of Conduct, Performance and Ethics for Nurses and Midwives.* London: Nursing and Midwifery Council.

NT Skills Update (2003). NT skills update: oral hygiene. *Nursing Times,* **99**, 29.

Orem DE (2001). *Nursing: Concepts of Practice.* St Louis, MO: Mosby.

Pellatt G (2001). Caring for the person with impaired mobility. In Baillie L (ed.). *Developing Practical Nursing Skills.* London: Arnold.

Peplau HE (1991). *Interpersonal Relations in Nursing: A Conceptual Framework of Reference for Psychodynamic Nursing.* New York: Springer.

Prigmore S (2005). Assessment and nursing care of the patient with dyspnoea. *Nursing Times,* **101**, 50.

Roper N, Logan W and Tierney AJ (2000). *The Roper–Logan–Tierney Model of Nursing: Based on Activities of Living.* Edinburgh: Churchill Livingstone.

Scottish Executive (2001). Guidance on the Single Shared Assessment of Community Care Needs. Circular no. CCD 8/2001. Edinburgh: Scottish Executive.

Shuttleworth A (2005). Palliative care for people with end stage non-malignant lung disease. *Nursing Times,* **101**, 48.

Simpson H (1991). *Peplau's Model in Action.* Basingstoke: Macmillan.

Simpson H (2006). Respiratory assessment. *British Journal of Nursing,* **15**, 484–8.

University Hospitals of Leicester (2000). *Oral Risk Indicator Tool.* Leicester: Leicester Royal Infirmary.

Waterlow J (1998). Wound care: the history and use of the Waterlow card. *Nursing Times,* **94**, 63–7.

Welsh Assembly Government (2006). *National Service Framework for Older People in Wales.* Cardiff: Welsh Assembly Government.

Further reading

Aggleton P and Chalmers H (2000). *Nursing Models and Nursing Practice,* 2nd edn. Basingstoke: Palgrave.
This book identifies the value of using a framework such as a model for nursing following patient assessment.

Baillie L (2005). *Developing Practical Nursing Skills,* 2nd edn. London: Arnold.
The focus of this book is to develop skills for practice. It uses a problem-based approach with scenarios for each branch of nursing. Many of the tools for assessment are used in the case studies, and the book is well referenced and illustrated.

Watson D (2006). The impact of accurate patient assessment on the quality of care. *Nursing Times,* **102**, 34.
This article explains clearly the importance of nursing assessment in formulating a plan of care to be used by all member of the care team.

Catherine Lawrence

Introduction

This chapter is aimed at familiarising students with the notion of competencies in children's nursing. Competency-based practice has become a fundamental aspect of care delivery in child health settings for both student and registered nurses. In terms of nursing education, a competency-based framework was developed by the United Kingdom Central Council for Nursing, Midwifery and Health Visiting (UKCC, 1999a), now adopted by the Nursing and Midwifery Council (NMC), and was implemented at national level. This NMC competency framework has been used to structure this chapter, as it reflects the changes that have taken place in nursing education. The first part of the chapter briefly addresses the following three key questions:

- What is competency-based practice?
- How were the competencies developed for children's nursing?
- Is children's nursing different?

The remainder of the chapter uses explicit examples from children's nursing practice to illustrate how competency-based practice can be achieved within the child health context. We challenge you to reflect upon your experiences when caring for children and families in a variety of settings and relate those experiences to the achievement of the competencies in children's nursing.

Competency-based practice is a relatively new concept within pre-registration nursing courses and, although the term 'competence' has been used widely within nursing for a long time, the notion of competence is now central to the pre-registration programmes as set out in the document *Fitness for Practice* (UKCC, 1999b). Understandably, the general public expects that a qualified professional, from whatever area of work, will be competent in carrying out normal professional tasks and duties (Eraut, 1994). The NMC Code (2008) (Appendix 1) makes explicit the need for individual practitioners to maintain and improve professional knowledge and competence. Additionally, there is a requirement for nurses to acknowledge any limitations in knowledge and competence and to decline to perform duties unless they are able to perform them in a safe and skilled manner. Therefore, the aim of competency-based practice in pre-registration nursing is the achievement, by the student on qualification, of the 'skills and ability to practice safely and effectively without the need for direct supervision' (UKCC, 1999a, p. 35).

The current 3-year pre-registration programme consists of a 1-year foundation programme and a 2-year branch programme, both of which are assessed using generic NMC competencies. In the initial development phase of this programme, it was recognised early on that the generic NMC competencies (now 'standards of proficiency') required adaptation in order to reflect a child and family focus. Children are different from adults physiologically, emotionally and cognitively, and within our society children have different rights and legal status compared with adults (Doyle and Maslin-Prothero, 1999). It can be argued, therefore, that children's needs are different and, if these needs are to be met, then the education of children's nurses must focus specifically upon them achieving the core skills and competencies (NBS, 2000) that will meet the needs of the child and family. Therefore, a project was established in anticipation of this programme to develop clinical competencies for the child branch. Using nominal group techniques and expert panels that involved practitioners in children's nursing, the NMC competencies were made relevant to this specific branch. This has resulted in clinically relevant outcomes in the four domains of practice, as well as the inclusion of a fifth domain, considered by participants in the project to be essential to capture the essence of children's nursing.

The specialised training for nurses caring for children has been recognised since 1888 (Bradley, 1999) and the attributes required by nursing students in 1888, such as having acute observational skills and being able to communicate and play with children, are comparable with the standards of proficiency required by the NMC today. The continued existence of the child branch is currently testimony to the fact that nurses caring for children require a different educational preparation. The routes leading to a different registration would imply that the competencies required to be entered on to the Register should be different for a children's nurse when compared with other nurses: if the sphere of practice (caring for children) and the educational preparation (child branch) are different, then the result must be different in terms of outcomes and competencies. In reality, this has not been the case until now. Linked to this, there is an assumption that there are specific qualities, knowledge, skills and attitudes in nurses who care for children. The development of clinical competencies in the pre-registration programme has provided an opportunity to celebrate what is different in children's nursing. Rather than simply adding client group to every generic competency in order to make them specific to the care of children, the identification of specific child health-focused outcomes has helped to produce a clinical assessment document that is relevant and appropriate to assess the real world of children's nursing practice.

Learning objectives

After studying this chapter you should be able to:
- appreciate proficiency-based practice in children's nursing;
- understand how the generic NMC standards of proficiency can be achieved in children's nursing practice through using vignettes taken from practice;
- reflect on your own personal practice and consider how your experiences have helped to develop your competencies.

How to use this chapter

This chapter explores all five domains in children's nursing, providing an explanation of the importance of the identified competency in children's nursing and the outcomes to be achieved.

The aim is for students to familiarise themselves with the standards of proficiency. By reading the examples of evidence, which are snapshots from children's nursing practice, you are encouraged to make the link between the reality of practice and the proficiency statement and outcomes. It is important to note that pseudonyms are used throughout in order to protect the children's confidentiality.

Suggested pre-reading has been given to help you complete the reflection questions in an informed way. The questions are designed to challenge you to utilise your experiences of caring for children and families and to identify how you have achieved or can achieve the proficiencies within your own practice.

Domain 1: ethical practice

Proficiency statement A

'Manage self, one's practice and that of others, in accordance with the NMC Code, recognising own abilities and limitations.' The responsibility and accountability of the nurse is central to their professional practice. In terms of children's nursing, the NMC Code has to be applied to the context of caring for the child and the family. Safety is a key concept that underpins the practice of children's nurses. Respecting the confidentiality of the child and family is crucial to the professional relationship that is built up between a children's nurse and the family.

Outcome criteria

- Practise in accordance with the NMC Code.
- Practise safely, adhering to professional standards of practice, e.g. in administration of medication.
- Identify when nursing care requires expertise beyond own current scope of competence and consult with registered nurse.
- Consult with other health care professionals when the needs of the child and family fall outside the scope of nursing practice.

Example of evidence

I arrived on duty one morning and found that there were two staff nurses off sick and I was the most senior member of staff on duty. However, even as a third-year student nurse I felt that it would be unsafe to take charge of the ward, and the agency night nurse who had been in charge of the night shift was unwilling to stay. By applying my knowledge of accountability I contacted the senior nurse immediately and a staff nurse from another ward was sent to take charge. However, she did not know any of the children and families and I acted in a responsible manner by assisting her throughout the day as I was familiar with the care of each child and family. I also supervised a first-year student nurse so as to ensure a safe standard of practice was maintained. The staff nurse and I discussed the ward staffing problems with the doctors and they agreed to cancel admissions to the ward that day, thus demonstrating that a safe collaborative approach had been taken by all the health professionals involved.

Reading

Bristol Royal Infirmary Inquiry (2001). *The Report of the Public Inquiry into Children's Heart Surgery at the Bristol Royal Infirmary 1984–1995: Learning from Bristol – the Recommendations*. London: The Stationery Office.

Nursing and Midwifery Council (NMC) (2002). *An NMC Guide for Students of Nursing and Midwifery*. London: Nursing and Midwifery Council.

Nursing and Midwifery Council (NMC) (2007). *Standards of Proficiency for Entry to the Register*. London: Nursing and Midwifery Council.

Reflection point 15.1

Reflect on your practice and consider whether you feel you have ever been asked to perform a task that was beyond your capability. This may have been a 'simple' task such as measuring a patient's blood pressure or recording fluids on a chart.

- Did you feel unsafe?
- Were you able to voice your concerns to the supervising nurse?

Can you relate your experiences to the NMC Code? For example, do you feel that you have always respected your patients as individuals, always obtained consent before giving care and always maintained confidentiality?

Proficiency statement B

'Practise in accordance with an ethical and legal framework that ensures the primacy of patient/client interest and well-being and respects confidentiality.' Ethical and legal principles are the foundations on which children's nursing practice is based. Children's nurses are legally accountable since the implementation of the Children Act (DH, 2004) and, therefore, all children's nurses need to be familiar with this Act and how it applies to the practice area. Furthermore, children are considered to be a vulnerable group and thus open to exploitation and abuse. Ethical principles require the children's nurse to uphold the rights of the child and to act as the child's advocate when necessary. Children's nurses also apply ethical principles when supporting parents.

Outcome criteria

- Demonstrate knowledge of legislation relevant to nursing practice.
- Ensure confidentiality and security of information acquired in a professional capacity.
- Demonstrate knowledge of the complexities that arise out of ethical issues and legal dilemmas experienced in practice, e.g. informed consent, resuscitation issues, children's rights.
- Uphold and promote the interests and well-being of children and families at all times.

Example of evidence

I was allocated to care for a baby whose mother was suspected of causing a physical non-accidental injury. I was aware of my professional role in terms of child protection by always ensuring that I stayed in the room with the mother when she visited her child, and I accurately documented her activities during those visits. I read the hospital trust's policy on child protection and contacted the nurse specialist for child protection, who was able to give me support and advice. I tried to maintain a professional and non-judgemental relationship with the mother, but I found this difficult at times, due to the realisation that the trust between a nurse and parent is undermined by a child protection issue. I liaised with the social worker and organised a time when she could come and see the mother.

Reading

Alderson P (2000). *Young Children's Rights: Exploring Beliefs, Principles and Practice*. London: Jessica Kingsley Publishers; pp. 22–48.

Charles-Edwards I (2001). Children's nursing and advocacy: are we in a muddle? *Paediatric Nursing*, **13**, 12–16.

Dimond B (2002). *The Legal Aspects of Nursing*, 3rd edn. London: Pearson Longman; Chapter 13.

Department of Health (DH) (2004). *The Children Act*. London: Department of Health.

Reflection point 15.2

Reflecting on your experience, can you identify an incident from practice when you used your ethical knowledge? This may have involved you in upholding the rights of a parent who felt ill informed regarding a medical or nursing decision or being involved in the care of a child who was 'not for resuscitation'.

Consider how 'routine' procedures, such as taking a blood sample from a child, relate to the issue of informed consent. Are you aware of when a parent must give consent and/or at what age a child may consent to their own care?

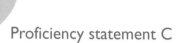

Proficiency statement C

'Practise in a fair and antidiscriminatory way, acknowledging the difference in beliefs and cultural practices of individuals or groups.' The UK is a multi-cultural society where children's nurses care for children and families from a variety of ethnic and cultural groups. Children's nurses therefore need to be familiar with the cultural practices and religious beliefs of the community in which they practise. The children's nurse needs to use a non-judgemental approach to care and make efforts to understand cultures that are different from their own. When working with children and families, decision-making should be seen to reflect fairness and should not discriminate against vulnerable or minority individuals or groups.

Outcome criteria

- Maintain, promote and represent the rights of children and families in the health care setting.
- Respect the values, customs and beliefs of children and families.
- Provide care that demonstrates sensitivity to the child's and family's diversity.

Example of evidence

While I was on my community practice placement with a community children's nurse (CCN), we visited a 7-year-old boy called Billy who had asthma. He was from a travelling family and lived in a council flat with basic sanitary conditions. The flat was very dirty and smelt strongly of urine and body odour, and throughout our visit the extended family was present. The CCN wanted to do some health promotion with Billy's main carers (mother and grandmother), so she asked me to try and develop a relationship with Billy.

I was rather anxious as to how I was going to proceed and decided to play with Billy and, by talking to him, to try and understand how he lived. He told me that he did not go to school on a regular basis and felt that it was not important to be able to read or write. He told me about his family and friends and how much he liked living with all his relatives. He explained that in the summer the family 'went on the road' and gradually some of the extended family members joined in the conversation. I began to understand the importance of the extended family to Billy and how suspicious they were of authority figures such as us. I felt that, by the end of the visit, I had gained the family's trust and had begun to understand the caring beliefs of travelling families.

Reading

Dimond B (2002). *The Legal Aspects of Nursing*, 3rd edn. London: Pearson Longman; Chapter 13.

Richardson J (2006). Cultural aspects of children's nursing. In Glasper A and Richardson J (eds). *A Textbook of Children's and Young People's Nursing*. Edinburgh: Churchill Livingstone.

Spires A (2002). Managing cultural diversity in care. In N Kenworthy, Snowley G and Gilling CM (eds). *Common Foundation Studies in Nursing*, 3rd edn. Edinburgh: Churchill Livingstone.

Valentine F and Smith F (2000). Clinical governance in acute children's services. *Paediatric Nursing*, **12**, 6–8.

Reflection point 15.3

Can you identify a family that you have cared for that had a different cultural or religious background from your own?

- How did you feel when you were asked to care for this family?
- How did you develop non-discriminatory attitudes towards the family?

Consider the questions above and reflect upon how you would meet the needs of a Muslim child, a Sikh child, a Jewish child and a Christian child in relation to religion, diet and dress.

SUMMARY

- Children's nurses must always practice in accordance with the NMC Code and provide a safe and secure environment for the children and families.
- Every nurse should be aware of their own knowledge and abilities and should not practise beyond their current scope of competence.
- Children's nursing practice must be underpinned by legal and ethical principles that uphold and promote children's rights in partnership with the family.
- The same care should be delivered to all children and families, regardless of their ethnic origin, and differing beliefs in relation to health, illness, diet and religion must be respected.

Domain 2: care delivery

Proficiency statement D

'Engage in, develop and disengage from therapeutic relationships through the use of appropriate communication and interpersonal skills.' The importance of effective therapeutic communication with children and families cannot be underestimated within the process of quality nursing, and the achievement of the above competency is at the centre of every relationship that the children's nurse will engage in. To communicate effectively within a relationship with children and families requires the nurse to use conversations as a goal-directed tool related to the health and well-being of the child. The children's nurse must use age-directed, culturally specific language that matches the language of the child and family.

Creating a therapeutic relationship with children and their families is not always easy and requires you to develop effective verbal and non-verbal communication skills and techniques, as well as a range of interpersonal skills. With children, it is important to give them time; to speak to them clearly and honestly using simple language and a quiet, unhurried and confident voice; and to use transitional objects when, and if, appropriate in order to convey the message effectively. When communicating with families, it is important to encourage them to talk, to listen to them actively, to be empathetic, and to convey acceptance of the uniqueness of each family unit.

Outcome criteria

- Make effective use of a range of interpersonal and communication techniques.
- Ensure that verbal and non-verbal communication is compatible and appropriate, taking account of age, gender, language, values, culture and sensory differences.
- Maintain professional caring relationships that focus on meeting the child's and family's needs.
- Understand the boundaries of the professional caring relationship and how relationships are formed, maintained and completed.

Example of evidence

On a previous shift I admitted a 4-year-old Asian girl, called Saira, with her mother, who was being admitted for minor surgery. Saira's mother said that her English was not very good but that she did

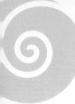

not need an interpreter. As I talked to Saira's mother I used open-ended questions and lay vocabulary, which she seemed to understand. I actively listened to her and showed interest through trying to maintain eye contact. However, Saira's mother rarely looked at me when talking, which I respected as being culturally specific behaviour. From her facial expressions I could see that she was anxious and sometimes found it difficult to express herself, but I tried to use silence positively to give her time.

Throughout the shift I continued to build upon my relationship with Saira and her mother. Because she was only 4 years old, Saira was initially very wary of me while she evaluated me as a stranger, but I gave her time and waited till she trusted me and then, using play with her favourite doll, I helped to prepare her for surgery. I felt it was important that they had time together as a family, especially when her father visited.

Reading

Betts A (2002). The nurse as communicator. In N Kenworthy, Snowley G and Gilling CM (eds). *Common Foundation Studies in Nursing*, 3rd edn. Edinburgh: Churchill Livingstone.

Matthews J (2006). Communicating with children and their families. In Glasper A and Richardson J (eds). *A Textbook of Children and Young People's Nursing*. Edinburgh: Churchill Livingstone.

Wong D and Hockenberry M (2003). *Nursing Care of Infants and Children*, 7th edn. St Louis, MO: Mosby; Chapter 6.

> **Reflection point 15.4**
> From your experiences, identify your learning related to:
>
> - greeting the child and family on admission, e.g. it is essential to state your name and who you are;
> - communicating with a frightened child, e.g. being gentle, taking your time and gaining the child's trust;
> - dealing with an aggressive or rude parent, e.g. maintaining a calm and professional approach;
> - avoiding blocks to communication, e.g. identifying the cause and solving the problem such as by using an interpreter or using play to communicate.
>
> Consider how differently you use your communication and interpersonal skills with people from different age groups, e.g. an infant, a toddler, a school-aged child and an adolescent. Which interpersonal skill do you use predominantly with each group?
>
> Consider the non-verbal channels of communication, such as touch, proxemics, posture, kinesics, facial expression and gaze, and think of examples from your practice where the culture of the child and family has positively or negatively affected your ability to communicate using these channels.

Proficiency statement E

'Create and utilise opportunities to promote the health and well-being of patients/clients and groups.' A healthy child is not simply a child who does not have an injury or a disease, but a child who is enabled to develop optimally and to achieve a state of physical, mental and social well-being. As a dependant, a child is reliant on their parents or carers to provide a safe environment in which the child can flourish, which includes accessing the available health services and utilising welfare and economic information appropriately. Until children become self-caring and independent, adults mediate for the child between the child and the child's environment.

As a teacher, supporter and referrer, the children's nurse can promote the health of the child by focusing on health and well-being alongside clinical care. The nurse is in an ideal situation to use health education, in partnership with the child and family, as a tool to achieve health or illness-related learning. This may be to produce changes in knowledge and understanding, such as why the child's compliance with a specific diet is essential, or it may be to facilitate the acquisition of an essential skill, such as suctioning a tracheostomy tube or nasogastric tube feeding.

Outcome criteria

- Consult with the child, family and relevant groups in order to identify the whole range of needs for the child's health and well-being.
- Provide relevant and current health, welfare and economic information to individual children and families in a way that increases their knowledge.
- Provide support and education to children and families in order to develop and maintain their life and independent living skills.
- Demonstrate an understanding of the principles of education, empowerment and social inclusion.

Example of evidence

During my community experience I was allocated to a day nursery that admitted children from 6 months to 5 years of age. While I was there I involved myself with learning how the health and well-being of this age group was promoted by the staff. With the parents of the infants and toddlers, the immunisation programme was addressed and a record of each of the child's immunisations was recorded; if the child had not been immunised, the dangers of this were discussed with the family, and appropriate resources and leaflets were provided.

The children were taught to wash their hands as soon as they were physically able to do so. They were taught that dirty hands had germs on them and that when they had been playing outside, before and after they had their meals, and after going to the toilet they had to wash their hands. They were supervised doing this so that they were protected from the hot water. In the oldest group the children used play to learn about healthy eating, and they had cooking and baking sessions to prepare some of the food. This enabled them to learn which foods were 'healthy' and they could eat a lot of, and others that they could eat only some of.

Reading

Department of Health (DH) (2001). *Reference Guide to Consent for Examination and Treatment.* London: Department of Health, pp. 16–19.

Hall D and Elliman D (2003). *Health for All Children*, 4th edn. Oxford: Oxford University Press.

Moules T and Ramsay J (1998). *The Textbook of Children's Nursing.* Cheltenham: Stanley Thornes; Part 1, Module 3, nos. 5 and 6.

Naidoo J and Wills J (2002). *Health Promotion: Foundations for Practice*, 2nd edn. London: Baillière Tindall; Section 3 (13).

Reflection point 15.5
Reflect upon your experiences at school and make a list of the topics of health education that you were taught, for example healthy diet, sexual health practice and dental care.

Consider this list and think about how you have, or could have, promoted the health of the children and families you have cared for recently in relation to those topics.

How would you increase a child's or young person's ability to make choices about the things that affect their health? This could be by providing resources such as informative literature and videos or DVDs.

A young mother cannot decide whether to breast-feed or bottle-feed her first-born preterm infant. What advice would you give? For example, it would be important to highlight the benefits and disadvantages of each method.

Proficiency statement F

'Undertake and document a comprehensive, systematic and accurate nursing assessment of the physical, psychological, social and spiritual needs of patients, clients and communities.' The assessment of a child is an ongoing process that commences when the child and family first require nursing care and support and subsequently continues throughout the whole time that the child is receiving care, whether in hospital or in the community, until the child is discharged. The data to be collected are directed by an assessment tool that is underpinned by the overarching concepts of the model, framework or pathway that is used in that particular setting (e.g. Casey, 1995; Smith *et al.*, 2002). Whichever assessment tool is used, the collection of information is all directed towards identifying the health and well-being of the child through identifying their needs and problems.

Essentially, the assessment stage is fundamental to the planning of holistic, good-quality care; in order to assess a child effectively, the children's nurse requires many skills. To collect information, the nurse requires a sound knowledge base, effective interpersonal and interviewing skills, and skills of observation and measurement, together with the ability to interpret the results accurately in order to plan the care.

Outcome criteria

- Select valid and reliable assessment tools for the required purpose.
- Use interviews, interactions, observations and measurements systematically to collect data regarding the health and functional status of the child and family.
- Analyse, interpret, record and communicate data accurately to inform nursing care and to take appropriate action.

Example of evidence

During a shift I admitted an 8-year-old boy called James who had suspected appendicitis. He was accompanied by his mother and father. Using the ward assessment tool, which was formulated and underpinned by the Partnership Model (Casey, 1995), I assessed James's physical, psychological, social and spiritual needs. The verbal information I collected was mainly from his anxious parents because James was very upset and in a lot of pain. I observed James's behaviour and non-verbal communication and measured his vital signs and urinalysis. I assessed his pain as being quite severe, because he looked pale and shocked, he was guarding his abdomen and, using a self-report pain assessment tool, he assessed his rating to be 8 on the Wong/Baker Faces Scale (Wong and Hockenberry, 2003). He was being extremely brave but was very anxious and needed and received comfort from his parents.

When I felt I had collected all the essential information, I documented it on the appropriate forms and charts and discussed his plan with my supervisor. As the shift progressed I continued to observe and monitor James closely as I delivered his preoperative care.

Reading

Casey A (2006). Assessing and planning in partnership. In Glasper A and Richardson J (eds). *A Textbook of Children and Young People's Nursing*. Edinburgh: Churchill Livingstone; Chapter 7.

Downer P (2002). Nursing theory and nursing care. In N Kenworthy, Snowley G and Gilling CM (eds). *Common Foundation Studies in Nursing*, 3rd edn. Edinburgh: Churchill Livingstone; pp 365–90.

Smith L, Coleman V and Bradshaw M (eds) (2002). *Family-Centred Care*. Basingstoke: Palgrave.

Wong D and Hockenberry M (2003). *Nursing Care of Infants and Children*, 7th edn. St Louis, MO: Mosby; Chapter 26.

Reflection point 15.6

Explore the different models, frameworks and pathways that you have used in practice and compare the assessment tool in each case. For example, compare the Roper–Logan–Tierney assessment tool (Roper *et al.*, 2000) with that of Orem (2001).

From your experiences to date, consider how you welcome and greet the child and family when you meet as strangers at the admission assessment, in order to provide a reassuring and secure environment, for example the tone of your voice and your facial expression.

List the other assessment tools (e.g. pain assessment tools) that you have used for observation and measurement during the assessment of the child. Do you feel this improved the quality of your assessment data?

Proficiency statement G

'Formulate and document a plan of nursing care, where possible in partnership with patients, clients, carers and significant others within a framework of informed consent.' Although different approaches may be taken to planning care for children, owing to the wide variety of settings in which they are cared for, care should be planned in partnership with the child (dependent on age) and the family. Whether care plans are computerised, preprinted or handwritten, the nurse, child and family should plan individual, achievable, realistic short- or long-term goals collaboratively in order to enable the child to restore and maintain his or her optimal level of health and well-being.

The nurse is required to plan a variety of evidence-based actions in order to help and support the child to achieve his or her goals. Identifying appropriate actions should be undertaken in discussion with the child and family, in order to negotiate and consent to their involvement and participation in the provision of self-care/care and to promote and ensure the maintenance of the family unit. Planning appropriate, evidenced-based care can be a complex process, requiring a sound knowledge base, and you should undertake this in discussion with your supervisor.

Outcome criteria

- Together with the multiprofessional team, establish priorities in collaboration with the child and family, based on the assessment of their needs and the resources available.
- Formulate and document plans of care collaboratively with the child, family and other professionals.
- Demonstrate an awareness of the principles of informed consent when planning care with the child and family.
- Identify expected outcomes, including a timeframe for achievement and/or review.

Example of evidence

During three concurrent 12-hour shifts, I admitted and cared for a 2-year-old child with bronchiolitis and his resident mother. Following his admission assessment and identification of his needs and problems, David's mother and I planned and discussed his care together. The short-term goals of David – restoring his usual breathing rate and oxygen requirements (Huband and Trigg, 2006), as well as maintaining his optimal fluid requirements – were seen as a priority. His mother wanted to be involved as much as possible in providing care for David and agreed that initially she would continue to undertake all of his usual care, for example washing, toileting and comforting, as well as some basic nursing care, such as maintaining his position for optimal air entry. I kept her informed of the results of my observations and measurements and ensured that the doctors and physiotherapist informed her of David's progress. As she became more confident and less anxious, through teaching and support from me, she willingly undertook more of David's nursing care. Throughout the time I cared for them I continued to record and document David's progress accurately towards his identified goals and update the care plans as required.

Reading

Dimond B (2002). *The Legal Aspects of Nursing*, 3rd edn. London: Pearson Longman; Chapter 13.

Department of Health (DH) (2001). *Reference Guide to Consent for Examination and Treatment*. London: Department of Health; Chapter 3, pp. 16–19.

Glasper A and Richardson J (2006). *A Textbook of Children and Young People's Nursing*. Edinburgh Churchill Livingstone.

Huband S and Trigg E (2006). *Practices in Children's Nursing*, 2nd edn. Edinburgh: Churchill Livingstone.

Reflection point 15.7

Take a blank sheet of paper and formulate a hypothetical care plan, including problem statements, goal statements and list of actions, for one of the following children and the compare your plan with those formulated by Wong and Hockenberry (2003):

- a 9-month-old infant admitted with acute diarrhoea (p. 1215);
- a 10-year-old boy admitted with an asthmatic attack (p. 1402);
- a 15-year-old girl admitted with an inflamed appendix (p. 1436).

List the difficulties and problems that you have with care-planning, e.g. the difference between a problem and a goal statement and how to make it patient-centred, and seek advice from your mentor, supervisor, link tutor or personal tutor.

Proficiency statement H

'Based on best available evidence, apply knowledge and an appropriate repertoire of skills indicative of safe nursing practice.' The primary goal of planning and delivering care for children and their families is to provide care that is underpinned by the best available evidence in the pursuit of safety and quality. Safe, high-quality care is dependent on best evidence, and the introduction of the concept of clinical governance within the NHS (Valentine and Smith 2000) is a mandate for children's nurses to access, understand, appreciate and use the best evidence in their practice.

To understand what is best evidence requires the ability to review evidence critically in all forms, such as primary research and clinical guidelines, appreciating the core value that best evidence is fundamental to the best interests of the child and family. Using the evidence appropriately requires a wide range and variety of skills, which, once learnt, will enable the children's nurse not only to evaluate confidently and justify their own practice but also to challenge the practice of others.

Outcome criteria

- Identify and evaluate current interventions viewed as best practice and apply these safely in a range of settings.
- Identify recent developments in research and ensure that this knowledge is reflected in your own practice and shared with colleagues.
- Discuss different forms of knowledge and methodologies applied to research.

Example of evidence

Through teaching by qualified staff and reading journal articles and ward protocols, I have learnt about evidence-based nursing care for children with diabetes while on this placement. I have cared for several adolescents with diabetes and feel that I have been able to plan and deliver safe, quality care, based on the best available evidence. Under supervision I have been able to provide for their physical needs in relation to monitoring their blood sugar levels and the administration of insulin, meet their psychological needs in relation to information and compliance with treatment, and help them, through discussion, to cope with living with a chronic illness and their adolescent lifestyle. Using the available evidence I have been able to provide a sound rationale for the care I have given and been able to share this with colleagues.

Reading

Callery P, Neill S and Feasey S (2006). The evidence base for children's nursing practice. In Glasper A and Richardson J (eds). *A Textbook of Children and Young People's Nursing*. Edinburgh: Churchill Livingstone.

Craig J and Smyth R (eds) (2002). *The Evidence-Based Manual for Nurses*. Edinburgh: Churchill Livingstone.

Hamer S and Collinson G (2005). *Achieving Evidence-Based Practice: A Handbook for Practitioners*, 2nd edn. Edinburgh: Ballière Tindall.

Ireland L and Glasper EA (eds) (2000). *Evidence-Based Child Health Care: Challenges for Practice*. Basingstoke: Macmillan; Chapters 5 and 15.

Reflection point 15.8
Choose one aspect of care that you undertake on most shifts, such as tube-feeding or giving parents and children information, and analyse and identify the evidence that supports your practice. For example, what evidence is available to support the placement testing of a nasogastric tube?

From your current placement, choose one child and family and undertake a literature search on one new aspect of care that you have been involved with in delivering to them, such as handwashing, pin site care, kangaroo care or mouth care. Share your results with your colleagues.

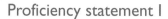

Proficiency statement I

'Provide a rationale for the nursing care delivered that takes account of the social, cultural, spiritual, legal, political and economic influences.' The provision of nursing care for children and families is a complex process and the decisions made must take a variety of influencing factors into account. Social, spiritual and cultural issues can create challenges in everyday practice, as can wider legal, political and economic forces. When prescribing nursing care to meet the desired outcomes for the child and family, a sound justification must be sought. Considering the scarcity and rationing of resources in the NHS today, a knowledgeable and thoughtful team approach should be taken in order to provide equity and fairness in the pursuit of successful outcomes of care.

Outcome criteria

- Identify, collect and evaluate information to justify the effective use of resources in order to achieve planned outcomes of nursing care.

Example of evidence

Over the past few weeks on this placement I have been caring for an 18-month-old child who required tube-feeding because he was unable to maintain an adequate oral intake. The mother was desperate to take the child home because she was a single mother and had another school-aged child. Apart from being tube-fed, there was no reason for the child to be hospitalised at this moment. Therefore, over the past week, with the help of the dietician, I have been able to teach Gavin's mother to pass a tube and to tube-feed him, for which she has shown her competence, and he is ready to go home. I contacted the community paediatric nurse, who visited her in hospital, will order and provide the necessary resources for her at home, and has arranged to visit her until she feels she can cope adequately. I have also contacted the general practitioner (GP).

Reading

Department of Health (DH) (1996). *The Children's Charter*. London: Department of Health.

Kenworthy N, Snowley G and Gilling C (eds) (2002). *Common Foundation Studies in Nursing*, 3rd edn. Edinburgh: Churchill Livingstone; Chapter 5.

Terry L and Campbell A (2006). Legal aspects of child health care. In Glasper A and Richardson J (eds). *A Textbook of Children and Young People's Nursing*. Edinburgh: Churchill Livingstone.

Trigg E and Mohammed T (eds) (2006). *Practices in Children's Nursing: Guidelines for Hospital and Community*, 2nd edn. London: Churchill Livingstone.

> **Reflection point 15.9**
> Can you identify a situation in your community or hospital practice where decisions have been influenced by legal, political or economic forces? For example, do you know who has parental responsibility for a child?
>
> On your current allocation, ask your ward manager how the ward resources are managed in relation to staff, finances and equipment in order to enable the planned outcomes of care to be achieved. Review the current off-duty on your placement and discuss the principles of how this is formulated with the manager.
>
> Identify experiences from your practice where the provision of social, cultural or spiritual care for children and families has created a challenge for practitioners, for example prayer times, special diets and playrooms.

Proficiency statement J

'Evaluate and document the outcomes of nursing and other interventions.' As the last phase of the nursing process, the aim of evaluation is to determine the effectiveness of care and to decide whether the goals of nursing care have been achieved. Evaluating care is as essential as all the other phases of the nursing process and should be straightforward if all the other steps have been undertaken to the highest quality. Evaluation will enable the children's nurse either to determine the child's achievement of the goals of care or to provide the child with the information required for reassessing needs and revising the care plan. Through the continuous evaluation of the care delivered, nurses will increase their knowledge to be able to predict that certain actions are more likely to be effective, based on experience and choice. A clearly written, accurate and unambiguous statement of the outcome of care must be documented appropriately.

Outcome criteria

- Review and evaluate the child's and family's progress towards planned outcomes of care.
- Document changes in nursing outcomes and nursing interventions.

Example of evidence

Whilst on this placement I cared for a 1-year-old boy called Ahmed who was admitted with a 2-day history of diarrhoea and vomiting. He was severely dehydrated, had a very sore bottom and was extremely miserable. The priority goals of care were to restore his hydration, retrieve the integrity of his anal skin and recover his normal, happy disposition. I delivered the prescribed actions listed in the care plan to meet the stated goals of care and, through observations, measurements and discussion with his mother, I evaluated the effectiveness of the care I had delivered and revised the care plans where appropriate, in discussion with my supervisor. I recorded my judgements of the value of the care delivered to Ahmed in relation to his predicted goals, informing the relevant team members of his progress.

Reading

Downer P (2002). Nursing theory and nursing care. In N Kenworthy, Snowley G and Gilling CM (eds). *Common Foundation Studies in Nursing*, 3rd edn. Edinburgh: Churchill Livingstone; Chapter 13.

Nursing and Midwifery Council (NMC) (2005). *Guidelines for Records and Record Keeping*. London: Nursing and Midwifery Council.

Wong D and Hockenberry M (2003). *Nursing Care of Infants and Children*, 7th edn. St Louis, MO: Mosby; Chapter 1.

Reflection point 15.10

Make a list of the sources of data that inform your evaluation of care, e.g. observation chart records, child and family feedback or child behaviour.

From your experiences in caring for children, identify one aspect of care where you have learnt that there is more than one solution to a problem, e.g. pin site care or behavioural programmes.

When evaluating care for children who have undergone day-care surgery, what would you say are the main criteria for discharge? Consider tolerance to oral fluids, passing urine and realistic pain levels.

Proficiency statement K

'Demonstrate sound clinical judgement across a range of differing professional and care delivery contexts.' Achieving the above competency is about demonstrating the ability to undertake a variety of roles while being able to rationalise and justify safe, sound decisions. Caring for children and their families requires a wide knowledge base, ranging from physiology, child development and social care provision to the professional, ethical and legal issues that provide the basis on which decisions are made. Flexibility and adaptability are required in order to provide family-centred care that upholds the best interests of the child and family and values the diversity of their beliefs and the contexts and circumstances where care is provided.

Outcome criteria

- Use evidence-based knowledge from nursing and related disciplines when choosing and individualising nursing actions.
- Demonstrate the ability to transfer skills and knowledge to a variety of circumstances.
- Recognise the need to adapt your nursing practice to varying circumstances and respond safely to meet your duty of care.

Example of evidence

During this current placement I cared for a 12-year-old girl called Lisa who was undergoing treatment for leukaemia. She had been prescribed oral medication but hated it intensely, and when I attempted to administer the drug on this occasion she refused to take it. She said she had had enough but on discussion she agreed she would take it if it could be given by another route. I was aware that she was old enough and mature enough to understand the implications of her treatment and also that it was in her best interests to have this medication. So I contacted the SHO, who came to the ward and agreed to change the prescription. I feel that I fulfilled my duty of care while acting in Lisa's best interest.

Reading

Brykczynska G (2000). Not quite the judgement of Solomon. *Paediatric Nursing*, **12**, 6–8.

Caulfield H (2002). Legal issues. In N Kenworthy, Snowley G and Gilling CM (eds). *Common Foundation Studies in Nursing*, 3rd edn. Edinburgh: Churchill Livingstone; pp. 123–4.

Dimond B (2002). *The Legal Aspects of Nursing*, 3rd edn. London: Pearson Longman; Chapter 13.

Glasper A and Richardson J (2006). Ethics in children's nursing. In Glasper A and Richardson J (eds). *A Textbook of Children and Young People's Nursing*. Edinburgh: Chuchill Livingstone.

Reflection point 15.11
Make a list of the forms of consent you usually obtain from:

- a 3-year-old child;
- a 10-year-old child;
- a 15-year-old child;
- the child's parents.

There are three forms of consent: oral, implied and that given in writing.

Domain 3: care management

All children and young people who are patients in hospital or in the community are owed a duty of care. What does this mean? A duty of care is owed once the nurse or other professional undertakes to perform certain tasks for the child.

Can you think of any circumstances where you may feel that to promote family-centred care may not be in the child's best interests, for example in certain cases of physical or sexual abuse.

SUMMARY

- Effective interpersonal and communication skills are essential in order to initiate and maintain a professional caring relationship.
- Children's nurses have a key role in promoting health and must be proactive in empowering children and families through information, support and education.
- The skills to undertake and document an accurate, reliable and holistic assessment are essential in order to identify the needs and problems of the child and family.
- The formulation of individual care plans/critical pathways should reflect collaboration and partnership with the child, parents and multiprofessional team, as should the evaluation of the care delivered.
- Research and evidence-based practice must be used to guide the delivery of up-to-date, adaptable and safe care for the children and families.
- Justifying the utilisation of scarce resources in the delivery of optimal care for children and families should be a priority.

Domain 3: care management

Proficiency statement L

'Contribute to public protection by creating and maintaining a safe environment of care through the use of quality assurance (QA) and risk management strategies.' Quality assurance is now an essential aspect of nursing practice, and for children's nurses QA related to safety has a particular relevance. Children are potentially exposed to more hazards within the hospital environment and community setting than adults, due to their limited awareness of hazards and inability to protect themselves from harm. Policies and procedures are therefore written to protect the child and to guide safe nursing practice. Some knowledge of clinical governance is highly relevant to senior student nurses, as an understanding of how practice is managed safely within the community or hospital trust is crucial on registration.

Outcome criteria

- Understand and apply the principles of QA to ensure the maintenance of a safe environment.
- Identify, eliminate and prevent environmental hazards where possible.
- Use risk management strategies that best meet the needs of the child, family and public.

Example of evidence

During the course of the shift I assisted the staff nurse in the administration of an intramuscular (IM) injection to a child. I was aware of the hospital policy related to the role of students regarding the administration of drugs and the guidelines provided by the NMC (2004). We followed the

333

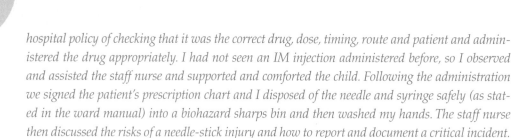

hospital policy of checking that it was the correct drug, dose, timing, route and patient and admin-
istered the drug appropriately. I had not seen an IM injection administered before, so I observed
and assisted the staff nurse and supported and comforted the child. Following the administration
we signed the patient's prescription chart and I disposed of the needle and syringe safely (as stat-
ed in the ward manual) into a biohazard sharps bin and then washed my hands. The staff nurse
then discussed the risks of a needle-stick injury and how to report and document a critical incident.

Reading

NHS Modernisation Agency (2003). *Essence of Care*. London: NHS Modernisation Agency.

Nursing and Midwifery Council (NMC) (2004). *Guidelines for the Administration of Medicines*. London: Nursing and Midwifery Council.

Valentine F and Smith F (2000). Clinical governance in acute children's services. *Paediatric Nursing*, **12**, 6–8.

Watson J (2006). Ensuring quality and the role of clinical audit. In Glasper A and Richardson J (eds). *A Textbook of Children and Young People's Nursing*. Edinburgh: Churchill Livingstone.

Reflection point 15.12

Reflect on your own practice experience and identify a protocol or policy that has enabled you to practice safely, e.g. passing a nasogastric tube or drug administration.

Can you recall an incident during a clinical placement when you felt that 'unsafe' practice had taken place? Try to explore why you felt it was unsafe and how risk management strate-gies may have improved quality assurance. For example, a poor patient–staff ratio may require agency staff cover.

Proficiency statement M

'Demonstrate knowledge of effective interprofessional working practices that respect and utilise the contributions of members of the health and social care team.' Interprofessional care is a rap-idly developing theme within the arena of childcare services and being able to work collabora-tively is an essential skill for all children's nurses. Demonstrating an awareness of the various roles of the members of the health and social care teams, and valuing and respecting the knowl-edge and contribution of other professionals, are central to good nursing practice. Liaison skills are a prerequisite for all children's nurses on qualification.

Outcome criteria

- Establish and maintain collaborative working relationships with colleagues.
- Work with colleagues in the decision-making process concerning the child and family.

Example of evidence

A 6-month-old infant called Jamie arrived on the ward from the accident and emergency depart-
ment with a suspected non-accidental injury. I admitted Jamie and gathered information from
Jamie's mother about her health visitor and GP. The staff nurse in charge then suggested that I
should contact the staff liaison health visitor, who liaises with the local community care teams, and
the duty social worker, who arranged to visit Jamie and his mother. On arrival the social worker
asked the staff nurse and myself to accompany her while she interviewed Jamie's mother. During the
discussion the mother stated that she had been under stress and had unintentionally harmed Jamie.

The social worker then explained to Jamie's mother what would happen and that the nurses would supervise her care of Jamie. The liaison health visitor contacted the family's local health visitor and GP, and they both confirmed that Jamie's mother had recently sought professional help for stress. A case conference was organised for the following day and the hospital and community-based health professionals met to discuss Jamie's future. Jamie was eventually allowed home, but he was placed on the at-risk register and support was given to Jamie's mother from the community care team.

Reading

Burr S (2001). Learning from Bristol: acting to improve a Cinderella service. *Paediatric Nursing,* **13**, 19–22.

Munro R (1999). Together we can do it. *Nursing Times,* **9**, 27.

Schobar M and McKay N (2000). *Collaborative Practice in the 21st Century.* Geneva: International Council of Nurses.

Soothill K, Mackay L and Webb L (eds) (1999). *Interprofessional Relations in Health Care.* London: Arnold.

Reflection point 15.13

During the course of a day spent on a clinical placement, note how many health care professionals, such as nurses, doctors, a physiotherapist or a radiologist, are involved in the care of one child and family.

Consider the information passing between the children's nurse and other members of the multiprofessional team. What role does the nurse have? The nurse's availability at the bedside means that the nurse is the coordinator of care and needs to liaise with the multiprofessional team.

Proficiency statement N

'Delegate duties to others, as appropriate, ensuring that they are supervised and monitored.' The ability to delegate is a complex skill and is developed over time. The ability to assess the competence of other staff demands insight and reasoning, and being able to take responsibility for your decisions and actions requires knowledge and confidence. Accountability is central to this dimension of professional practice, and children's nurses are accountable, on registration, not only to the profession but also to the child and family.

Outcome criteria

- Demonstrate the ability to coordinate care, taking into account the role and competence level of the staff involved in the delivery of care.
- Recognise and understand the scope of your own accountability and responsibility when delegating aspects of care to others.

Example of evidence

During my final ward, as a third-year student nurse, I was encouraged by the ward sister to take charge of the ward for an 8-hour shift under the supervision of a staff nurse. I took the handover report from the night staff and then allocated the nurses to the children, ensuring that all of the student nurses were being supervised by a trained member of staff. I assessed the capabilities of each nurse and confirmed that each student felt able to cope with the workload. I instructed the staff to feed back details of the care they were giving and any changes that were occurring in the condition of their patients. As the day progressed, I felt able to make decisions such as contacting the doctors when a child's condition deteriorated, and I liaised with members of the multiprofessional team, such as the physiotherapist and dietician.

Three hours into the shift I had to re-evaluate the workload of one student when a sick child's condition deteriorated. Following a discussion, I felt she was competent to 'special' the child and delegated her other patients to the supervising staff nurse.

I organised the lunchtime breaks without compromising the safety of the children's care and continually encouraged the junior nurses, giving positive feedback when appropriate. By the end of the shift I felt that I had coped with running a busy ward and felt in control of the care delivered to each child.

Reading

Marquis B and Huston C (2006). *Leadership Roles and Management Functions: Theory and Application*, 5th edn. Philadelphia, PA: Lippincott, Williams & Wilkins.

Murphy W (2001). Leadership and community children's nurses. *Paediatric Nursing*, **13**, 36–40.

Tomey A (2004). *Guide to Nursing Management and Leadership*, 7th edn. St Louis, MO: Mosby.

> **Reflection point 15.14**
>
> Reflect on your clinical experiences and consider how the care of children is organised. Then, although you may not have had the opportunity to manage a ward yet, reflect on how you have managed care for a group of patients.
>
> Can you identify the criteria used to delegate a certain group of patients to your care? Think of your stage of training, competence and confidence.
>
> - Had you cared for some of the patients previously? Familiarity with the care usually breeds confidence.
> - How sick were the children, and how challenging was their care? Were you assessed by your supervisor as being able to provide the required care?
> - Was the presence of a parent a factor in how patients were allocated? Did the parent provide the majority of the care?
> - Was skill mix a factor? How were junior nurses supported? Were the ill children cared for by the most experienced staff?

Proficiency statement O

'Demonstrate key skills.' Key skills underpin the practice of all nurses. For children's nurses, competence in literacy, numeracy and problem-solving are essential for safe practice. Without the skills of literacy, the children's nurse would be unable to document accurately the care given to the child and family and to articulate this clearly and concisely. Numeracy and the ability to calculate medicines and fluids accurately are essential, while problem-solving enables the children's nurse to make clinical decisions on behalf of the child when necessary.

Outcome criteria

- *Literacy*: interpret and present information that can be clearly understood by others and that adheres to the principles of record-keeping.
- *Numeracy*: use numeracy skills to calculate and interpret data and to understand the significance for care delivery, e.g. administration of medication and fluid balance.
- Demonstrate the application of information technology within the delivery of care and adhere to the Data Protection Act.

- Demonstrate problem-solving skills as part of making clinical decisions within the delivery of care.

Example of evidence

When caring for a patient one day, I demonstrated each of the key skills. Zoe was admitted to the ward as a booked admission for routine day-case surgery. I read the doctor's notes and passed on the relevant information to the nurse in charge, which included the child's diagnosis and previous admissions to hospital. I also accessed the clinical computer system to obtain Zoe's blood, urine and electrolyte results for the doctor to review on clerking. I devised a care plan, ensuring that I signed it and had it countersigned by a registered nurse, and throughout the day I made sure that the care I gave to Zoe was accurate and legibly documented. Following surgery Zoe was in pain and required the administration of analgesia. I was able to calculate the dose accurately and I administered the drug following the hospital drug policy. At the end of the day I evaluated Zoe's care and completed her discharge planning record.

Reading

Baillie L (ed.) (2001). *Developing Practical Nursing Skills*. London: Arnold.

Gatford JD and Anderson RE (2006). *Nursing Calculations*, 7th edn. London: Churchill Livingstone.

Nursing and Midwifery Council (NMC) (2004). *Guidelines for the Administration of Medicines*. London: Nursing and Midwifery Council.

Nursing and Midwifery Council (NMC) (2005). *Guidelines for Records and Record Keeping*. London: Nursing and Midwifery Council.

Reflection point 15.15

Think about how you record the care given to the children that you care for, and consider whether the language you use is appropriate. Are there any vague statements recorded that give little information about the care given, and is any information missing?

Consider how numeracy is used in areas of practice other than drug administration, for example fluid calculations and height and weight measurements.

Explore a clinical dilemma where decisions need to be made, such as when to discharge a child and family home or whether to carry out a clinical procedure. Try to identify the various decisions that could be made and how the final decision is reached. For example, has the child met the criteria for discharge or what are the options that could be taken for a 2-month-old baby who is not sucking his feed?

SUMMARY

- Quality assurance and risk management strategies should be used to guide the delivery of care and the maintenance of a safe environment.
- Effective communication between children's nurses and the multiprofessional team should create the probability that optimal, seamless care is delivered to the child and family.
- The delegation of duties must take the roles and competence levels of staff into account because nursing activities require specific knowledge, skills and attitudes.
- Literacy, numeracy, information technology and problem-solving are the key skills that underpin the practice of nursing and the achievement of the competencies.

Domain 4: personal and professional development

Proficiency statement P

'Demonstrate a commitment to the need for continuing professional development and personal supervision activities in order to enhance knowledge, skills, values and attitudes needed for safe and effective nursing practice.' The professional practice of children's nursing takes place in a context of continuous change. Children's nurses cannot expect to practise safely and effectively unless they engage in continuing professional development activities to maintain and update the knowledge base that underpins their practice. They must also facilitate the regular and ongoing monitoring and evaluation of their own practice with supervision, reflecting in and on practice, with the maintenance of a professional portfolio playing a significant part. The achievement of this competency is at the centre of lifelong learning and career development.

Outcome criteria

- Use reflection in and on practice in order to identify your personal professional development needs.
- Discuss with colleagues the additional knowledge and skills required to manage professionally challenging situations.

Example of evidence

On a previous shift I was caring for an 11-year-old boy, James, who had been admitted that day in a sickle cell crisis: his mother was present with him, and his father was at work. I was working with a senior staff nurse, who was also my supervisor for that shift.

I had never looked after a patient with sickle cell disease before and I was grateful for the comprehensive handover from a staff nurse. Following handover, the senior staff nurse and staff nurse agreed to check and administer intravenous (IV) drugs to James while I spent some time familiarising myself with his care plan and medical notes. I popped my head in to speak to James and his mum. As I talked with James and his mum I realised that they were very knowledgeable about the treatment he was being given.

I took the opportunity early on in my shift to identify a haematology textbook in the ward library and read up what I could on sickle cell disease. On reflection, when reading about the therapeutic management during a crisis, I realised that in fact I understood quite a bit already, as I had previously cared for children receiving blood transfusions, intravenous therapy and antibiotics, oxygen therapy and IV morphine. Throughout my shift I was able to observe interactions between the senior staff nurse and James's mum. On one occasion she was explaining about a new antibiotic and how this differed from other antibiotics James had received. This highlighted to me how practice is constantly changing and how important it is to keep one's knowledge up to date. This was also an example where a nurse and parent were sharing their knowledge and experience, an outcome that would benefit James and his mum, as they would have the knowledge to manage this change in his pattern of care.

Reading

Hinchliff S (1998). Lifelong learning in context. In Quinn F (ed.). *Continuing Professional Development in Nursing: A Guide for Practitioners and Educators*. Cheltenham: Stanley Thornes; pp. 34–58.

Johns C (2004). *Becoming a Reflective Practitioner*, 2nd edn. Oxford: Blackwell Science.

Rolfe G, Freshwater D and Jasper M (2001). *Critical Reflection for Nursing and the Helping Professions: A Users Guide – Models of Critical Reflection*. Basingstoke: Palgrave.

Reflection point 15.16

Can you think about other situations and the approaches that you took to ensure that you had sufficient knowledge to deliver safe and effective care, such as caring for a child with an unfamiliar clinical condition or receiving treatments that are new to you.

Think about situations where parents or carers are very knowledgeable about their child's care and how you, as a student, can make the most of their knowledge while remaining confident in your caring role.

Think about how you use reflection on action to assess your own performance. Take some time to write about the steps you are taking to manage your own professional development.

Proficiency statement Q

'Enhance the professional development and safe practice of others through peer support, leadership, supervision and teaching.' Children's nurses do not work in isolation. They are part of a team and, as such, much can be gained through the giving and receiving of peer support. This is just one aspect of creating and maintaining an environment that is conducive to learning. Role modelling, teaching, preserving a questioning approach to all aspects of clinical care, and seizing learning opportunities as they arise are other facets of personal and professional development that must be kept alive throughout the career of a children's nurse. The achievement of this competency is central to children's nurses accepting responsibility for the role they play in the maintenance of safe and effective nursing practice.

Outcome criteria

- Contribute to creating a climate conducive to learning.
- Act as a positive role model to others by demonstrating safe practice.
- Demonstrate effective teaching skills.
- Demonstrate effective leadership through the delivery of safe nursing practice.

Example of evidence

I have been working on the haematology and oncology unit for 6 weeks. In that time I have been caring consistently for children receiving chemotherapy and have, as a result, observed registered nurses and parents undertaking mouth care.

On a previous shift I admitted an 8-year-old boy called Tom. Tom was diagnosed as having acute myeloid leukaemia, for which he was prescribed chemotherapy. Three days following his admission I was caring for Tom and assessed that he was now well enough to undertake his own mouth care. I discussed the mouth care Tom would require with one of the staff nurses and described the approach I would take to teaching Tom and his dad about his new mouth-care regimen. My plan for teaching was to be practice-based with some supporting literature. The staff nurse was able to supervise my teaching and asked if I would mentor a new student joining us: Tom and his dad were happy for there to be a small group of us participating in the process.

I taught Tom and his dad about the importance of mouth care and stressed the need to clean his teeth twice a day. I talked them through the tool we use on the ward to assess Tom's mouth on a daily basis and used the tool to highlight the problems that Tom might experience, such as mouth ulcers, dry lips and bleeding gums. Through questioning, it was clear that Tom's dad had a good grasp of the problems that may be encountered. I stressed the need to look in Tom's mouth every day and why it was important to respond to any complaints of oral problems. I observed Tom cleaning his own teeth and taking the antifungal agent, reinforcing how good his technique was. Together we looked through the mouth-care information booklet and talked about care at home and the importance of dental check-ups. I took the opportunity to talk about general oral health for the whole family and the need to use sugar-free drinks and medicines where possible. Tom's dad asked me a number of questions, all of which I was able to answer. I documented Tom's mouth-care regimen in his parent-held record and care plan, noting that Tom and his dad had been taught mouth care.

Following the teaching session we took the opportunity to talk about different children on the unit and the reasons why their mouth-care regimen might be different. The staff nurse shared her knowledge and a group discussion ensued, which I was able to contribute to. The staff nurse taught myself and the student about the various treatments for oral problems and we discussed different approaches to teaching, for example with a younger child, where mouth care was not already part of daily care and where there was some resistance to undertaking the role. Our responsibility to role-model safe practice and teach from an informed background was explored. I then had the opportunity to supervise the new student undertaking mouth care on another child.

Reading

Antrobus S and Kitson A (1999). Nursing leadership: influencing and shaping health policy and nursing practice. *Journal of Advanced Nursing*, **29**, 746–53.

Hinchliff S (ed.) (2008). *The Practitioner as Teacher*, 4th edn. London: Ballière Tindall.

Johns C and Freshwater D (eds) (2005). *Transforming Nursing through Reflective Practice*, 2nd edn. Oxford: Blackwell Publishing.

Marquis B and Huston C (2006). *Leadership Roles and Management Functions: Theory and Application*, 5th edn. Philadelphia, PA: Lippincott, Williams & Wilkins.

Reflection point 15.17

From your experience, think about situations that have challenged your abilities to teach a new skill, such as a frightened child, a parent who was anxious, or a family whose first language was not English.

Take a few minutes to think about what supervision means to you and then outline the key skills of supervision.

How do you support the colleagues you work with? Detail the approach you take in sharing knowledge.

Think about health care professionals that you have worked with and write down the leadership skills that they have used to promote effective and efficient child health care.

SUMMARY

- Each individual nurse must accept the responsibility for their continued professional development and personal supervision activities in order to develop their competency within the sphere of children's nursing practice.
- Each nurse should contribute proactively to the development and progression of all team members through peer support, leadership, supervision and teaching.

Domain 5: children's nursing and child health

Proficiency statement R

'Have knowledge of cognitive, social and emotional development and impact of health, illness and environment.' Growth and development are complex processes: many changes occur during a lifetime and are influenced by numerous factors. The achievement of the above competency is central to children's nurses understanding the physical changes that take place during development and the special needs generated by these changes. Ill health can have a dramatic effect on development, as can social and emotional factors. Promotion of normal development and enabling the child to realise their full potential rests on the children's nurse being fully conversant with all the stages of growth and development. Recognising alterations from the child's norm and working with the child and family to establish realistic future goals is an important role for the children's nurse in the many areas in which health care is delivered.

Outcome criteria

- Identify normal and abnormal development in a range of settings.
- Understand normal physical, psychological and social development and use this knowledge to inform their practice.
- Create an environment that promotes development.
- Understand the impact of illness on the developing child.

Example of evidence

On a previous shift I was caring for Claire. Claire is 8 years old and has learning difficulties. She had been admitted for a tonsillectomy and adenoidectomy. Claire's mum and dad were with her and they were both anxious about the forthcoming surgery. They had attended a pre-admission clinic, where, through the use of therapeutic play, Claire had started to be prepared for the surgery. A play specialist had spent time with Claire showing her the mask and playing with syringes. Both parents were concerned about how far that preparation had helped Claire, as her learning difficulties prevented her from being able to express her understanding of what had taken place. My assessment of Claire, using observation and toys, revealed that Claire had retained some of the information from the clinic meeting. This was confirmed when Claire recognised the play specialist who had been working with her at the clinic.

Claire herself did not appear to be anxious, as long as both parents were present with her. I realised very quickly that I would need to spend a lot of time with Claire and her family to be able to support Claire through the procedure, allowing enough time for explanation, to use toys and pictures to encourage understanding. Through the relationship that Claire had with her parents, they were able to facilitate this communication process, so it was a team approach. I was able to use the knowledge of both parents to help me to prepare Claire. We used favourite toys to help in the process and relied very much on visual descriptions. Claire had been previously admitted to hospital with a broken leg, and so with the help of her parents we were able to use that experience of how she coped to help in our preparations. I felt it was important to engage with Claire, to use myself in the process of communication, and with the help of Claire's parents and the play specialist draw on all my creative skills as a children's nurse to ensure that Claire was prepared for surgery within the context of her developmental and needs.

Reading

Berk L (2006). *Child Development*, 7th edn. Boston, MA: Pearson.

Glasper A and Richardson J (2006). *A Textbook of Children and Young People's Nursing*. Edinburgh Churchill Livingstone.

Trigg E and Mohammed T (eds) (2006). *Practices in Children's Nursing: Guidelines for Hospital and Community*, 2nd edn. London: Churchill Livingstone.

> **Reflection point 15.18**
> Think about a nurse that you consider to be an expert children's nurse. What makes them an expert in your eyes? Try to share this with your other colleagues so that you start to develop a picture of what it is to be a children's nurse.
>
> Think of examples from your practice where a child's development has been affected by their health, social, emotional or environmental factors, and then consider the ways in which you and the rest of the health care team worked with the child and family to maximise the child's potential to progress in their development.
>
> Spend some time focusing on a chronic illness and the effect that may have on a child's developmental progress. Consider how the illness may have an effect on the child's family, school, interactions with peers and future employment.

Proficiency statement S

'Demonstrate knowledge and awareness of the child in the context of the family and society (the wider context).' Developing a collaborative approach to working with families is necessary to facilitate them in the role of carer and to promote the health and well-being of the whole family. The achievement of this competency is central to the children's nurse delivering truly family-centred care. To involve families in their child's care requires the nurse to have an understanding of the child and family, to support the individuality of each, and to be comfortable and familiar with maintaining professional boundaries.

Outcome criteria

- Show an awareness of the changing nature of the family in society and how it contributes to maintaining the integrity of the family unit.
- Recognise and respond to the effect that an ill child has on the family unit.
- Practise the principles of partnership, negotiation and sharing the care with the child and family.

Example of evidence

On a previous shift I was caring for Ali, a 2-year-old Bangladeshi boy who had been readmitted with diarrhoea following a bone marrow transplant for an immunological condition (severe combined immunodeficiency). Ali's mother was resident with him and undertook the role of main carer. Ali's paternal grandmother visited daily. Although Ali's mother spoke English, his grandmother spoke very little English but appeared to understand a little more. On this particular day Ali was receiving all his care from his grandmother.

Throughout the shift I worked with Ali's grandmother to deliver care to Ali. At first I thought it would have been quicker to do the care myself, as I was not sure how much his grandmother understood what I was saying. I was busy with two other patients and did not know how I was going to remember to check on Ali and his grandmother. Ali needed frequent nappy changes, his nappies needed to be weighed and output recorded; a skin care regimen was to be followed. Ali's mother was confident and competent in doing all these aspects of care. I was not sure about the grandmother's role and how far she wanted to be involved in assisting in the nursing care. Yet Ali responded to his grandmother's involvement in a positive way. When she changed his nappy he was less distressed and much more cooperative. Grandmother was clearly an important person in Ali's life and her involvement in his care was natural.

We very quickly set up a way of working, with his grandmother changing his nappy. On the first occasion I showed her what we were cleaning his bottom with and applied the cream. I showed her where to store the nappies for me to weigh; his grandmother was to ring the call bell and let me know when there was a nappy there to be weighed and recorded. I observed his grandmother doing his care and was confident in her competence. I felt it was important to maintain the family structure and involve his grandmother where I could. Although negotiating roles was made complex because of the language barrier, we quickly developed a relationship using simple language and hand signs, resulting in us being able to share in caring for Ali.

Reading

Ball J and Bindler R (2006). *Child Health Nursing: Partnering with Children and Families*. Upper Saddle River, NJ: Pearson.

Brace O'Neill J (1998). Professional boundaries in pediatric nursing practice. *Journal of Pediatric Health Care*, **12**, 225–7.

Casey A (1995). Partnership nursing: influences on involvement of informal carers. *Journal of Advanced Nursing*, **22**, 1058–62.

Darbyshire P (2003). Mothers' experiences of their child's recovery in hospital and at home: a qualitative investigation. *Journal of Child Health Care*, **7**, 291–312.

Soanes L (1997). Effect of conflict on the successful formation of nurse–parent relationships. *Journal of Cancer Nursing*, **1**, 191–6.

Reflection point 15.19
Think about society today and the variety of family structures that a children's nurse works within. Reflect on your own beliefs and values and consider the different approaches you use to ensure that families are involved in care through a successful process of negotiation.

Consider some of the relationships that you have witnessed in practice. Can you identify both positive and negative relationships and explore the reasons for these outcomes in relation to family structures, beliefs held by nurses and other health care professionals, and approaches to family-centred care?

Textbooks refer to 'professional boundaries'. Can you describe what this means to you in relation to how you care for families?

SUMMARY

- In order to enable every child to realise their full potential, every children's nurse must have knowledge of the cognitive, social and emotional development of children and the impact that health, illness and the environment may have on this.
- Understanding the child in the context of the family, and with a clear focus on children's services, is fundamental to the achievement of true family-centred care.

CONCLUSION

The aim of this chapter has been to facilitate learning and understanding about competency-based practice in children's nursing. Following a brief explanatory background of what competency-based practice is and how the generic NMC competencies were developed to capture the essence of children's nursing, the reality of children's nursing practice has been captured through using vignettes that provide examples of how the competencies can be achieved.

It is hoped that the reader has been stimulated to reflect on their own practice and consider how experiences have led to competency development.

Acknowledgement

We would specifically like to acknowledge the hard work undertaken by our colleagues in the Department of Children's Nursing, London South Bank University, in developing the competencies for the child branch programme. Permission has been granted by the university to publish the competencies in this chapter.

References

Bradley S (1999). Catherine Wood: children's nursing pioneer. *Paediatric Nursing*, **11**, 15–18.

Casey A (1995). Partnership nursing: influences on involvement of informal carers. *Journal of Advanced Nursing*, **22**, 1058–62.

Department of Health (DH) (2004). *The Children Act*. London: Department of Health.

Doyle KA and Maslin-Prothero S (1999). Promoting children's rights: the role of the children's nurse. *Paediatric Nursing*, **11**, 23–5.

Eraut M (1994). *Developing Professional Knowledge and Competence*. London: Falmer Press.

Huband S and Trigg E (2006). *Practices in Children's Nursing*, 2nd edn. Edinburgh: Churchill Livingstone.

National Board for Nursing, Midwifery, and Health Visiting for Scotland (NBS) (2000). *Children's Nursing: Core Skills and Competencies*. London: National Board for Nursing, Midwifery, and Health Visiting for Scotland.

Nursing and Midwifery Council (NMC) (2004). *Guidelines for the Administration of Medicines*. London: Nursing and Midwifery Council.

Nursing and Midwifery Council (NMC) (2008). *The Code: Standards of Conduct, Performance and Ethics for Nurses and Midwives*. London: Nursing and Midwifery Council.

Orem D (2001). *Nursing: Concepts of Practice*. St Louis, MO: Mosby.

Roper N, Logan WW and Tierney A (2000). *The Roper–Logan–Tierney Model of Nursing Based on Activities of Living*. Edinburgh: Churchill Livingstone.

Smith L, Coleman V and Bradshaw M (eds) (2002). *Family-Centred Care*. Basingstoke: Palgrave.

United Kingdom Central Council for Nursing, Midwifery and Health Visiting (UKCC) (1999a). *Nursing Competencies Second Stage*. Annexe 1 to JEC/00/01. London: United Kingdom Central Council for Nursing, Midwifery and Health Visiting.

United Kingdom Central Council for Nursing, Midwifery and Health Visiting (UKCC) (1999b). *Fitness for Practice*. London: United Kingdom Central Council for Nursing, Midwifery and Health Visiting.

Valentine F and Smith F (2000). Clinical governance in acute children's services. *Paediatric Nursing,* **12**, 6–8.

Wong D and Hockenberry M (2003). *Nursing Care of Infants and Children,* 7th edn. St Louis, MO: Mosby.

Further reading

Action for Sick Children. www.actionforsickchildren.org/index2.html.

Alderson P (2000). *Young Children's Rights: Exploring Beliefs, Principles and Practice.* London: Jessica Kingsley Publisher.
A useful and concise text that gives the reader an excellent grasp of the rights of children of all ages. An invaluable resource for practitioners, as it refers to issues of involving children in decisions and explores levels of involvement and the skills required to achieve that. The notion of acting in a child's best interest can be realised only when practitioners have a clear understanding of what that means and how important it is to respect children's rights; this book is well able to guide practitioners in this area.

Bristol Royal Infirmary Inquiry (2001). The Inquiry into the Management of Care of Children Receiving Complex Heart Surgery at the Bristol Royal Infirmary. www.bristol-inquiry.org.uk.

Bristol Royal Infirmary Inquiry (2001). *The Report of the Public Inquiry into Children's Heart Surgery at the Bristol Royal Infirmary 1984–1995: Learning from Bristol – the Recommendations.* London: The Stationery Office.
This is a large document – the report runs to over 500 pages and has 198 recommendations – but is essential reading for all health care professionals. The recommendations aim to produce an NHS in which patients' needs are at the centre and in which systems are in place to ensure safe care and to maintain and improve the quality of care. This is compelling reading and reveals how organisations can fail families. Readers are forced to consider their own practice and to reflect on their organisation. Recommendations reinforce best practice and therefore practitioners need to be conversant with the report and its findings if they are to play any part in ensuring that quality of care continues.

Department of Health. www.dh.gov.uk.

Darbyshire P (1994). *Living With a Sick Child in Hospital: The Experiences of Parents and Nurses.* London: Chapman & Hall; pp. 120–64.
A seminal text that is a must for all children's nurses. This text explores the complex pressures of a child's hospitalisation and the relationship between the parents and nurses. This is gripping and revealing reading, allowing the reader to reflect on their own practice, and the practice of others, when creating partnerships in care.

Dimond B (1996). *The Legal Aspects of Child Health Care.* London: Mosby.
The Children Act 1989 led to an increased recognition of the legal rights of the child. An understanding of these rights is crucial in relation to practice, research and teaching. This book explains the law and legal issues that help practitioners to work within the law and facilitate decision-making in situations where ethical issues are not clear-cut.

Huband S and Trigg E (eds) (2000). *Practices in Children's Nursing.* Edinburgh: Churchill Livingstone.
This book is a useful reference for those working with children, both in hospital and in the community. It discusses a wide variety of child-focused clinical nursing practices, identifying the special needs and problems of infants and children within the context of family-centred care.

Ireland L and Glasper EA (eds) (2000). *Evidence-Based Child Health Care: Challenges for Practice.* Basingstoke: Macmillan.
The contributors in this edited text provide a wide range of topics, including clinical practice, management, research and education in the child health arena, and in so doing share a variety of experiences of the everyday challenges of child health care.

Kenworthy N, Snowley G and Gilling C (eds) (2002). *Common Foundation Studies in Nursing*, 3rd edn. Edinburgh: Churchill Livingstone.
Although this text was produced for the common foundation year of all 3-year pre-registration courses, it contains a holistic overview of the theory and principles of practice that can provide a valuable resource for children's nurses well into the branch programme.

Le May A (1999). *Evidence-Based Practice.* London: NT Books/EMAP.
This is an authoritative and concise publication that will be an invaluable resource to nurses in practice. It provides an overview and guides the reader to other useful reading. Includes some useful tables that summarise the key issues.

Moules T and Ramsay J (1998). *The Textbook of Children's Nursing.* Cheltenham: Stanley Thornes.
This book is valuable to children's nurses in that it explores many different aspects of children's nursing and increases the learning potential by involving and encouraging the reader to participate in the learning process by undertaking various activities. It clearly highlights the essential roles of the nurse.

Naidoo J and Wills J (2000). *Health Promotion: Foundations for Practice.* London: Baillière Tindall.
This book provides nurses, as health promoters, with a theoretical framework to enable them to be clear about the intentions and outcomes of interventions designed to promote the health of their patients and clients. Although not child-focused, it provides a wide range of principles and practices that can be readily applied to the care of children and their carers.

National Board for Nursing, Midwifery, and Health Visiting for Scotland (NBS) (2000). *Children's Nursing: Core Skills and Competencies.* London: National Board for Nursing, Midwifery, and Health Visiting for Scotland.
An excellent, easy-to-ready document that summarises core skills of children's nurses. A useful tool when considering individual roles and the skills required being competent. Also useful for students when thinking about generalist and specialist practice, and the context of skills within holistic care.

Nursing and Midwifery Council. www.nmc-uk.org.

Rolfe G, Freshwater D and Jasper M (2001). *Critical Reflection for Nursing and the Helping Professions: A Users Guide – Models of Critical Reflection.* Basingstoke: Palgrave.
This text offers a guide to all aspects of reflective practice. It offers structured approaches that will guide students through the realities of 'actually doing it'. Supervision, reflective writing and reflective research are also addressed with interactive writing exercises, and points for discussion make this a very useful text for group and individual learning.

Royal College of Nursing. www.rcn.org.uk.

Victoria Climbié Inquiry. The Victoria Climbié Inquiry: Report of an inquiry by Lord Laming. www.victoria-climbie-inquiry.org.uk/finreport/finreport.htm.

Wong D, Hockenberry-Eaton M, Winklestein M, Wilson D and Ahmann (1999). *Nursing Care of Infants and Children*, 6th edn. St Louis, MO: Mosby.
This weighty tome has always been viewed as an excellent teaching text for children's nurses because of the enormous range of information that it provides about the health and illness of infants, children and young people. Each new edition offers extensive revision and up-to-date evidence-based practice.

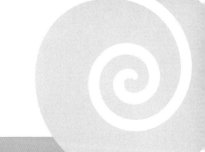

16 The needs of young people

Marcelle de Sousa

Introduction

This chapter aims to explore and extend your knowledge about the young people who need your care. It examines the developmental period of adolescence and the impact that illness has on this time of transition, and it highlights the lack of health care provision that currently exists for this group of young people who have specific needs. It also discusses the role that health care professionals can play to help young people deal with the issues that arise from the conflict of being an adolescent and coping with illness. The chapter also discusses the current shortfall in education for nurses who care for this client group and provides some recommendations.

Health promotion is essential for young people, who need help to maintain a healthy lifestyle; however, discussion of this, apart from a brief look at how nurses, and particularly school nurses, can influence well-being in this population (Bekeart, 2002), is beyond the scope of this chapter.

The terms 'adolescent', 'young person' and 'teenager' are used interchangeably to describe this specific group.

Learning objectives

After studying this chapter you should be able to:

- understand that adolescence is a period of intense and rapid development;
- appreciate the specific health care needs of adolescents;
- understand the relationship between development and risk-taking behaviours;
- recognise the impact of chronic disease on adolescent development.

Background

What is adolescence?

The World Health Organization (WHO, 1989) defined adolescence as the period between 10 and 19 years of age, but changes in the socioeconomic climate may have extended this period beyond age 19 years. Poor health, unemployment and a lack of financial security may all contribute to this.

Adolescence is a transition from childhood to adulthood. There is change, both mental and physical, adaptation to new concepts and thinking, and great learning and preparation for a new role as an adult. Whether or not you agree that, at the end of this period, a mature adult emerges is a topic of endless debate.

Adolescence was not a well recognised or much used term before the nineteenth century (Conger and Galambos, 1997). Interestingly, however, Aristotle spoke of the young being 'passionate, irascible and apt to be carried away by their impulses' (Conger and Galambos, 1997). Many would agree that this holds true today. Many theories have been put forward about this intense period of transition and development (Box 16.1). Some authors thought that the search for identity – that of formation versus confusion – was what the period of adolescence was all about (Erikson, 1968). Elkind (1968) called the egocentric behaviour that presents in adolescence as the 'imaginary audience and personal fable'. Freud (cited in Conger and Galambos, 1997) spoke about the dominance of hormonal changes and developing sexuality. A useful guide to adolescent development is given in the *ABC of Adolescence* (Viner, 2005).

BOX 16.1 Theories of adolescence

- *Hall*: storm and stress/feelings and emotions.
- *Erikson*: search for identity formation/confusion.
- *Elkind*: search for self-imaginary audience/egocentric.
- *Schave and Schave*: younger versus older adolescent thinking.
- *Freud*: sexual/hormonal dominance.
- *Piaget*: concrete/formal cognition.

Schave and Schave (1989) postulated that adolescence could be separated into two distinct phases. Early adolescence, between the ages of 11 and 14 years, was different from late adolescence because of specific changes, including the pubertal, hormonal, social and physical changes that cause the young adolescent to 'become vulnerable to shifting and volatile states of mind' and so act differently. Young adolescents were seen as unable to accept responsibilities for their actions. The late stage of adolescence, from 15 to 18 years, was when 'due to a consolidation of changes in cognitive thinking, an integration of self occurs'.

Piaget's theory centred on stages of development; the two that are relevant to the period of adolescence are the stage of 'concrete operations' (age 7–11 years) and 'formal operations' (age 12 years onwards). Some have argued that Piaget's work does not truly represent adolescent development (Coleman and Hendry, 1999), but the majority still find it useful in assessing how adolescents might use knowledge to make decisions.

Hall, a psychologist, was the first in the Western world to theorise about a time of 'stress and storm' (Conger and Galambos, 1997). He postulated that adolescents continually fluctuate between extremes of feelings and emotions. This was a view acknowledged by many theorists, psychologists and the public, but it has been seriously challenged by the contrary view that the majority of young people do not have a stormy time but adjust very well (Conger and Galambos, 1997; Coleman and Hendry, 1999).

This phase of growing encompasses great physical and psychosocial change for the young person. Puberty, with its huge rise in hormonal levels, growth spurts, spots and relationships, has a profound effect on the developing adolescent. Acne, for instance, if not treated properly, can have a profound effect on the young person (Greener, 2002).

Adolescence is often a period when young people are perceived as 'difficult'. Unfortunately, this is often the view of adults who appear to have forgotten their own adolescence. The media further compounds this negative image of young people. However, the majority of young people go through this period of development without any problems and in good health. Adolescents need information and advice given in a non-judgemental manner and that respects them as individuals with a right to confidentiality and an ability to make decisions about their lives.

Adolescence can, however, be a very distressful time for some, which may account for the high rates of depression, suicide and anxiety-related illness (Coleman and Hendry, 1999). Suicide is rare in teenagers under the age of 15 years, but 7 per cent of 11- to 15-year-olds will self-harm at some point (Hawton and James, 2005) The rates of attempted suicide, although high, are reported to be falling, particularly among young males (Coleman and Schofield, 2007). However, there has been an increase in the numbers of adolescents who present with anxiety-induced illnesses, and there is very little understanding of, or resources to deal with, this issue (Mallinson *et al.*, 2001). A detailed look at the reasons why adolescents harm, hurt or kill themselves is available in the report published by the Office of National Statistics (2001).

Health care provision

The number of adolescents in the UK is growing and is projected to reach 6.5 million in 2012 (Macfarlane, 1996). The area of health care services specific to adolescents has, however, largely been neglected by the UK government and health care providers until now (Ministry of Health, 1959; DH, 1976).

Despite the UK signing up in 1993 to the United Nations Convention on the Rights of the Child (UN, 1989), there has been little focus on the rights of children and young people as individuals or on the care that they receive. Kurtz and Hopkins (1996) eloquently confirm this by commenting that

> *children and young people have always been targeted by health care programmes, more in the spirit of charity or in the interest of adult society than of entitlement by rights.*

A focus on the health care needs of young people and their general well-being is long overdue (NHS Executive, 1996). Government programmes such as those that have focused on teenage pregnancy, for which the UK has the highest rate in Western Europe (Coleman and Hendry, 1999), have been welcomed, but more is needed for this group with distinct needs. Tackling the rising levels of underage drinking (90 per cent of 15-year-olds have tried alcohol, and a third drink alcohol more than once a week; DH, 2007) and obesity (18 per cent of boys and 17 per cent of girls aged 11–15 years are classified as obese; Craig and Mindell, 2008) in this age group are the new targets of the Department of Health's agenda (DH/DfES, 2007b). It is good news that adolescent health is finally on the national agenda. Standard 4 of the Children's National Service Framework (NSF) has focused on the needs of adolescents. England has finally got its own commissioner for children's services. Children and young people now have a champion at government level.

User views are an essential component of the clinical governance agenda in the modern NHS, and it is particularly welcome that children and young people are beginning to be consulted about the service that they receive. (See the work of the Social Policy Unit, University of York, and the National Children's Bureau (NCB).) The Hospital Standard Document (DH, 2003), which is the first module of the NSF, recognises the unique need of adolescents in hospital. Perhaps adolescents, who previously have been at a distinct disadvantage, will finally have their voices heard and receive health care by suitably qualified professionals in dedicated clinical settings.

McKinney and colleagues (1977) list developmental tasks that adolescents have to achieve in order to reach maturity. This can be used as a framework to try to understand the specific health care needs of adolescents:

- achieving independence from parents;
- acquiring the social skills required of an adult;
- achieving a sense of oneself as a worthwhile person;
- developing the necessary academic and vocational skills;
- adjusting to a rapidly changing physique and sexual development;
- achieving an internalised set of guiding norms and values.

Relevant competencies

The relevance of the following competencies from the NMC Code (2008) (Appendix 1) to the care of young people will be looked at in the discussion below:

- Make the care of people your first concern, treating them as individuals and respecting their dignity.
- Work with others to protect and promote the health and well-being of those in your care, their families and carers, and the wider community.

SUMMARY

You should now:
- be able to define the period of adolescence;
- be familiar with some of the issues that adolescents face today;
- have some knowledge about the history of poor provision of services for adolescents;
- understand the issues that adolescents face today.

Considerations in caring for adolescents

Risk-taking behaviour

Young people experiment and indulge in risk-taking and antisocial behaviour. Offending behaviours peak at the age of 17 years in boys and 15 years in girls (Coleman and Schofield, 2007). However, in the period 1995–2005, there was a marked decrease in the number of offences committed by young people (Coleman and Schofield, 2007). This may be due to recent youth justice reforms.

In 1992, injuries were the most common cause of death in 15- to 18-year-olds (Macfarlane, 1996). Adolescents are also vulnerable and often quite frightened people. Acts of bravado may often be attempts to cover their insecurity. Some adolescents consume alcohol with little regard to the side effects or long-term effects, and public health messages such as 'smoking causes cancer' have very little effect on young people as they know that their friends who smoke do not have cancer.

Risk-taking is often seen in young people who do not comply with medical regimes (Kyngas, 2000a,b,c), such as taking medication or physiotherapy. Graft rejection with graft loss in young people who have had a renal transplant and who do not comply with their immunosuppressive therapy is well documented and continues to be an immense problem (Watson, 2002). Nurses who work in accident and emergency (A&E) departments are all too familiar with the diabetic teenager who presents with diabetic ketoacidosis, often in a coma as a consequence of not adhering to a medical regime that is seen as restrictive. Attitudes such as 'It won't happen to me' and 'I haven't taken my medicines, but I feel fine' pose a challenge to health care professionals working with such adolescents (Watson, 2002). Consider Scenario 16.1.

SCENARIO 16.1

Tracy is a 16-year-old girl who has been admitted to the paediatric ward from the A&E department with a fracture. She has also consumed alcohol. She needs to wait until it is safe for her to go to theatre for an operation on her fractured dislocated elbow, which she sustained when she fell over in the street. You have to connect and care for her intravenous infusion, which she needs to rehydrate her. She wants you to take away the infusion. She is angry and abusive and refuses to stop swearing. Some of the parents of the other children on the ward are beginning to complain about her language. She tells you that she has just left her foster home and was out celebrating, but now she is worried about her future.

Reflection point 16.1

Take a moment to reflect on Scenario 16.1 and think of how you might apply the following aspect of the NMC Code: 'Make the care of people your first concern, treating them as individuals and respecting their dignity.'

You need to make sure that Tracy is safe and that the infusion is connected and patent. You might want to move her into a side room, if one is available, away from the young children and where you can talk to her quietly or simply stay with her until she calms down. By removing her from the main ward, you can change the atmosphere that has arisen. If no cubicles are free, then you can draw the curtains around her and sit with her until she has calmed down or fallen asleep. When Tracy is sober you might consider giving her advice on the dangers of binge drinking. There is a need to involve social services and the expertise of the multiprofessional team if you work with one.

Involving parents

Parents must be involved and informed of all aspects of care. They must also be educated, supported and encouraged to help their child towards achieving independence, taking ownership of their disease and becoming autonomous in decision-making.

Consent and decision-making

The issue of consent continues to be an item of great debate. The Family Law Reform Act (1969), Section 8 allows a young person who is aged 16 years or older to consent to treatment. This consent applies only to treatment and does not include consenting to blood or organ donation (Dimond, 1996); however, adolescents under the age of 16 years may consent to treatment if they are deemed to be Gillick competent – that is, have sufficient maturity and understanding. Young people cannot refuse treatment, as this can be overruled by their parents or the courts. Practitioners need to be aware of the differences in age of consent across the UK: 16 years in England and Wales, 12 years in Scotland and 17 years in Northern Ireland. The DH has produced an excellent document regarding good practice in consent (DH, 2001).

> **Reflection point 16.2**
> Thinking back to Scenario 16.1, can you think of anything else you might do for Tracy in accordance with the NMC Code? Would you obtain her consent for the infusion? Do you need to? Do you think you will see her on the ward again?

The subject of how children learn, think and make decisions can be traced back to Ancient Greece (Wood, 1998). As health professionals, we often seem unable to respect the decisions that young patients make about their treatment or their life. Young children are deemed incompetent, and even those over the age of consent may have their decision overruled by the courts. However, Article 16 of the UN (1989) convention states that 'young people have a right to information'. Nurses can play an important part in decision-making by acting as advocates for the young person. Nurses are in the unique position of ensuring that the young person receives the correct information and has the time to reflect on that information before making a decision.

Piagetian theory (Lefrancois, 1992) suggests that children are unable to make logical decisions until they are adolescents (formal operational). However, several studies suggest that even infants can display sophisticated powers of reasoning and understanding of human relationships (Alderson, 1996). By the age of 5 years, children are developing a sense of identification with their parents and a sense of responsibility for their own actions (Erikson, 1987).

The Children Act (1989) states that 'children and young people must be consulted and kept informed about actions taken and participate in decisions about them'. Children who have been seriously ill for a long period of time have been shown to have a 'profound and mature understanding and can cope with and discuss complex and painful knowledge' (Alderson, 1996). The author has personal experience of this. A teenager who had been ill for a long period of time decided quite calmly and clearly that she did not wish to continue with treatment. She was 18 years old. The only people who initially had difficulty accepting her decision were the members of the medical and nursing team.

Children in Western society are usually seen as being dependent on their parents, probably until they leave home or go to university. However, this view is changing – for example, the current climate has seen a change in the grant status for students and so dependence continues. How difficult must it be to try and make truly independent choices while you are still financially dependent on your parents for your education, even though you may be living away from home?

Reflection point 16.3
How do young people who are dependent on their families for care achieve independence? Think about further education, relationships and careers.

An example of young people who have the burden of responsibility are young carers who care for a parent who is chronically ill or disabled at home. They have to assume great responsibility for caring, but they are not asked whether this is what they want to do and often they have no voice in the decision-making processes, whether about themselves, their quality of life or their sick parent (Dearden and Becker, 1998). Many of these young people find it difficult to visualise an independent care-free future.

Alderson (1996) cites cases of children becoming more responsible for their actions if they are called as witnesses in criminal cases or they are on trial for the crime. Remember the case of the murder of the toddler Jamie Bulger? The two people found guilty of his murder were children.

If we are to believe what the theorists say about the cognitive abilities that are beginning to blossom in a child from the age of 7 years, then adults should listen closer to what they say. Do parents of well children do this? At best a child's view is listened to, but in the end the adult makes the final decision in 'the best interest of the child'. Adults assume that it is their right to make the decision because they 'know best'.

'The need for adults to feel in control can also serve as a barrier to listening to children' (Alderson, 1996). Alderson believes that adults fear that listening seriously to children will commit them to supporting unwise choices that the child might make or, worse, let children 'run rings round them' or 'stop respecting them'. Alderson sees setting limits as a licence for adult power. This is a powerful statement and is one that the majority of adolescents would agree with but one that a large number of adults would find offensive. This is summed up well by the following quote: 'What is best for the child is often only best understood 20 years after childhood' (Lansdowne, 1998).

Reflection point 16.4
Think about adolescents who have survived because their parents made treatment decisions when they were children. There is no right or wrong, but there is a debate about decision-making.

Erikson (1987) reminds us that development takes place because of the experiences a child gains through a series of conflicts. Piaget alludes to the infant's world here and now – that is, whoever feeds and keeps the infant warm will be the most significant. This of course develops into the next phase, when a baby is able to identify their mother. So, when do children begin to decide? The familiar scenario of a toddler having temper tantrums because they cannot get their own way may not be acceptable to many adults as it is an indication that the toddler is making up their own mind. However, it must represent the start of the decision-making process, which will become more finely tuned with the acquisition of knowledge. Erikson (1987) puts forward the theory that, from the age of 18 months, children learn that they can be autonomous and that their intentions can be realised. This stage progresses until about the age of 3 years, and then the child begins to develop a sense of self and a responsibility for their own actions. Does this imply that children who fall ill at this age worry that they may be responsible for their illness?

Nurses can also become emotive when difficult decisions have to be made for their patients, and they need to be familiar with the law governing this area. It is not easy to find the answers to some questions that arise when caring for young people in a clinical setting. How do you measure competency? Who is available to do so? Why can you consent but not refuse?

Consider the case of Re W (1992) (see Dimond, 1996), which concerned a young girl who had a long history of being in care and who had developed anorexia. She was being tube-fed. The local authority decided that she needed specialist treatment and that she should be moved to a specialist unit. At the age of 16 years, she consulted her solicitor and decided that she should not be moved to a specialist unit for treatment without her consent. The court overruled her, stating that she was not able to make a competent decision as she had anorexia, which would impair her mental capacity, and that unless she had the specialist treatment at the new unit her condition would deteriorate.

Now consider the case of Mrs Gillick who challenged the health authority about her daughter getting contraceptives without her mother's permission. The law lords upheld for the health authority and gave us 'Gillick competent', whereby a young person under the legal age of consent can consent on their own if they are competent and mature enough to be able to understand. This represented a milestone for all health care professionals who care for young people; but remember that a young person under the age of 16 years can consent to treatment but they cannot refuse treatment as they can be overruled by their parents or the courts. This is always done in the best interest of the child or young person. Consider Scenario 16.2.

SCENARIO 16.2

Neil is 17 years old and has just been diagnosed with non-Hodgkin's lymphoma. He needs to start chemotherapy. The doctor has given Neil and his parents information about the drugs, their side effects and why Neil must commence treatment soon. He has been told that he has a good chance of making a complete recovery if he has treatment. Neil, after some deliberation, decides that he will not consent to the treatment. His parents, although very upset, are determined that Neil must consent for treatment to commence.

Reflection point 16.5
In Scenario 16.2, do you think Neil has made the right decision? What has influenced or guided your answer? Why do you think his parents are not making the decision to treat? After all, he is still a minor. Do you think that Neil is competent to make the decision? What can you do to help Neil and his parents?

Neil has an illness that has a good prognosis if treated. He is worried about the side effects of the treatments. He is still in shock after hearing the diagnosis. He has cancer. He needs time and someone to talk to both him and his parents. His parents need support to help Neil make the right decision. Giving them all time and more information informs their decision. Young people also have a right to advocacy services and to have legal representation in matters relating to decisions that they have made. Where a patient has refused a particular intervention, you should ensure that the patient realises that they are free to change their mind and accept treatment later. Where delay may affect their treatment choices, they should be advised accordingly (DH, 2001).

Attitude to death and dying

Young people often have a curious attitude to dying and death. This might relate to themselves dying or anyone close to them dying. A belief in the personal fable can be damaging, as adolescents may be reluctant or refuse to accept that they may have a potentially life-threatening disease (Eiser, 1993). Adolescents often avoid learning, or are reluctant to know, about long-term effects of disease.

The author has worked in the late effects service for survivors of childhood cancers. These teenagers were treated with chemotherapy and radiotherapy for oncological problems when they were children. They have survived and now have issues that are important to them. Some mention that they were never really involved in the decision to have treatment. They talk of 'not owning their cancer'. Most are glad to be alive and extremely grateful that their parents made all the decisions, but some say that the treatment was so painful and unpleasant that, had they known beforehand, they 'would not have agreed to it'. This is said even with the knowledge that, without the treatment, they would have died. Many of these teenagers are sterile, impotent and short in stature and have the added onus that they may develop a secondary malignancy (Wheeler *et al.*, 1998). Many of these side effects were not made clear when treatment options were offered. This action is defended by the argument that there is a limit to what you take in when you are in shock. However, practice is changing to accommodate the questions that young people have. Today, young people do not have to rely on adults 'telling them things'. Information can be accessed via the Internet and television programmes and magazines that cater to the teenage market.

Developing a relationship and trust

A predominant preoccupation with self often irritates all who come into contact with adolescents, and this can make it difficult to form relationships with them. Unfortunately, this also applies in the health care setting, making it problematic for young people to access health care.

Adolescents take time to form relationships with health care providers. A common complaint from parents and other adults is the adolescent who 'grunts' or is 'monosyllabic'. Teamworking to deliver a comprehensive package of care is often difficult when caring for young people who may appear not to want help.

Adolescents who are asked questions about themselves rarely answer truthfully. Trust has to be established before real information is divulged. So, for example, if a young person is asked whether they smoke, they will often answer untruthfully. This has potential risks if the adolescent is being admitted for surgery. It is vital that the nurse gets the right information, and achieving this is a skill that comes with practice. Treating the adolescent with respect and dignity enables the nurse to gain the adolescent's confidence. Consider Scenario 16.3.

SCENARIO 16.3

You have been asked by the nurse in charge to admit and carry out an assessment for care-planning on a 15-year-old girl, Kirsty. She is being admitted for investigations. Her mother has had to return home but will be in later to answer any questions. Kirsty tells you that she smokes 'only a few' when she is with friends. Her mother does not know and 'will kill her if she finds out'.

Reflection point 16.6
How will you carry out your task? Do you think you will receive the information you need? What will you do about the information that Kirsty gave you that is sensitive and that she does not want her mother to know? What advice will you give Kirsty?

In the one dedicated adolescent medicine service in the UK, information obtained during the admission process by nurses is shared with the multiprofessional team at the weekly meeting. The issue of a young person smoking is taken on board not only by their nurse but also the school teacher, youth worker, doctor and play specialist; each has a different approach and advice. The team does not always divulge information to parents unless it is in the best interests of the young person. This is where the crucial difference between paediatric and adolescent care lies. As a nurse you have a duty to discourage any behaviours that may harm health. You must be able to give adolescents information that will help them stop these behaviours.

Reflection point 16.7

Is there a difference between caring for a child and an adolescent? Why is there a difference? When do you break a confidence? What role do parents play when you are caring for their teenager?

Concern with image

It is interesting to note that adolescents are less concerned with issues around smoking, drugs and alcohol intake (Coleman and Hendry, 1999) than they are about their image – weight, acne, and how they interact with peers and form relationships. Adolescents who have had renal and endocrine disease may be very concerned by their short stature; teenagers who have diabetes find the high-calorie diets difficult to adhere to because of the associated weight gain. Nurses who care for young people have a professional duty to offer health advice and information that deals with all these issues.

Reflection point 16.8

Think about an adolescent who is physically disabled. What do you think are the issues for them? Is it easy for them to form relationships with able-bodied peers? Do they challenge boundaries?

SUMMARY

You should now understand:
- the differences between caring for adolescents and caring for children;
- issues of consent in young people;
- issues of confidentiality;
- the role that the nurse can play in delivering public health messages to young people.

Addressing the health care needs of adolescents

As discussed above, adolescents have been ignored as a client group with specific care needs. This applies not only in clinical settings but also in the community. Young people often receive postcode care in the community. This is dependent to some extent on current resources but more on who should deliver care to whom and up to what age care is received. Health visitors usually provide a service to children up to the age of 12 years. District nurses usually care for adults and rarely have the time for adolescents who are at home. In some areas where there are paediatric community nurses, they provide the care needed by young people at home. School nurses have always been the providers of care and health advice to adolescents and are probably the most important group of providers, as they have contact with large numbers of teenagers. Practice nurses are an underused resource for meeting the health care needs of young people; this deserves investment.

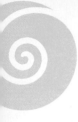

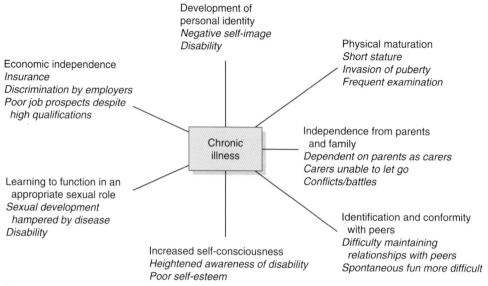

Development of
personal identity
Negative self-image
Disability

Physical maturation
Short stature
Invasion of puberty
Frequent examination

Economic independence
Insurance
Discrimination by employers
Poor job prospects despite
  high qualifications

Chronic
illness

Independence from parents
  and family
Dependent on parents as carers
Carers unable to let go
Conflicts/battles

Learning to function in an
  appropriate sexual role
Sexual development
  hampered by disease
Disability

Identification and conformity
  with peers
Difficulty maintaining
  relationships with peers
Spontaneous fun more difficult

Increased self-consciousness
Heightened awareness of disability
Poor self-esteem

Figure 16.1 Impact of disease on development.

The impact of disease on normal development is illustrated by Figure 16.1. Young people find medical regimes to be restrictive and to interfere with daily living. Frequent hospital admissions, clinic visits, therapy and blood tests that are essential to maintaining health may hamper socialisation with peers and school life (Eiser, 1993). Clinics that are held after school, less frequent hospital visits, more shared care with local clinicians, and a negotiation with young people about therapy can have two positive outcomes – less emphasis on the sick adolescent and more emphasis on being normal, and perhaps a better adherence with medication and therapy. Adolescents have been shown to favour drop-in clinics where the visit to the GP remains confidential.

Adolescents like being seen by the nurse they know (Norwich Union, 2002). Nurse-led clinics and nurse specialists or practitioners can develop good relationships with young people and help them to prepare for transition and transfer to adult services (see below).

Much work is needed to change current methods of treatment, which are often paternalistic. Involving the young person in negotiating treatments, giving them ownership and encouraging decision-making is a way forward.

Dedicated clinical areas

Teenagers continue to be cared for in inappropriate clinical settings, such as adult or paediatric wards, despite their views on how and where they should be cared for (Norwich Union, 2002). When health authorities were surveyed about current and future provision for adolescents, the majority had no plans for separate provision for adolescents (Viner and Keane, 1998).

Henderson *et al.* (1993) analysed admission rates in the Oxford region of adolescents between the ages of 10 and 19 years. Most admissions were for surgical rather than medical reasons. The single most common reason for male adolescents to be admitted was head injury and for female adolescents to give birth or to have a termination of pregnancy. These admissions were significant in that, with increasing age, the adolescent was likely to be admitted to adult specialty areas such as obstetrics. This confirmed the view held by the National Association for the Welfare of Children in Hospital (NAWCH, 1990) (now known as Action for Sick Children) that it may be difficult to place these patients according to age in a suitable ward. A dedicated clinical area is the answer.

The argument that there are insufficient numbers of adolescents in any hospital to warrant separate facilities is one that is convenient but not true (Audit Commission, 1993; Viner and Keane, 1998). One survey has demonstrated that nurses find it difficult to care for young people and to respect their individual needs when they are surrounded by either young children or old people (Norwich Union, 2002).

Clinical settings dedicated to adolescents would be able to address the most important areas of care, such as the following:

- privacy;
- confidentiality;
- promoting autonomy;
- dignity and respect;
- holistic approach to care;
- education;
- leisure;
- information and advice.

It could be argued that all patients deserve this. The only dedicated adolescent medicine service unit in London that has addressed these needs for young people, despite the obstacles, deserves praise. If a unit is to cater to the needs of young people, then it must incorporate the views of young people (de Sousa, 1999). Adolescent units must have a charter, so that young people know what to expect from the team that cares for them, and house rules, so that they know what is expected of them as inpatients (Baker, 1996).

The multiprofessional team

Teamwork is essential for an holistic approach to health care. The ideal multiprofessional team for adolescent care consists of:

- a doctor dedicated to adolescent medicine;
- nurses (trained in both child and adult nursing, and in mental health as a bonus);
- psychologists, psychiatrists and psychotherapists;
- teachers;
- youth worker;
- activity coordinators;
- dedicated physiotherapists and occupational therapists.

All members of the multiprofessional team should be able to contribute to the care of the adolescent.

When working as a member of a team, you remain accountable for your professional conduct, any care you provide and any omission on your part.

Disclosure of information

The NMC Code instructs us that the health care record must be used as a tool of communication within the team and that it should be written with the involvement of the patient whenever this is practical. At the specialist unit in London mentioned above, nurses have devised a questionnaire and assessment tool that is completed by the adolescent and then checked by the nurse. This has been found to be extremely useful in getting difficult information from young people. The adolescent then signs a contract of care that has been jointly planned by the team and the young person.

Where there is an issue of child protection, you must act at all times in accordance with national and local policies. Unfortunately, there will always be occasions when an adolescent discloses information that must be shared with people outside the immediate team. This may happen in the acute situation in an A&E department or on the ward. There is a direct association between self-harm and abuse, including sexual abuse (Coleman and Hendry, 1999). Therefore, any adolescent who presents to an A&E department with self-harm needs to have counselling and psychiatric help in order to find out whether there is any history of abuse. Abuse, whether it is sexual or physical, must be investigated further. There is mandatory training for all members of staff who care for young people so that they can recognise the signs, help the young person and know when to refer on. Also, as young people are vulnerable, police checks on all staff members who care for them are mandatory.

This is where interagency working comes into its own. A hospital-based nurse will never have the information that is held in the community. Sharing of essential information, while not breaking the rules of confidentiality, is now mandatory (Lord Laming, 2003).

The sexual act is illegal in Britain under the age of 16 years, and when a young person discloses that they are sexually active the nurse must seek advice to help clarify the situation, so that the young person may be protected. All NHS trusts, both hospital- and community-based, must have a designated safeguarding nurse and doctor.

Reflection point 16.9
Are you aware of local and national policies about safeguarding? Why do you think it is important for all nurses to be aware of policy regarding safeguarding?

Transition from paediatric to adult services

The American Society of Adolescent Medicine defines transition as 'the purposeful, planned movement of adolescents and young adults with chronic and medical conditions from child centred services to adult oriented health care systems' (Blum *et al.*, 1993).

Adolescents who live with chronic illness, such as renal disease or cystic fibrosis, face a further hurdle: making the transition to adult services (Viner, 1999). Greater numbers of children now survive such illnesses, often with a disability or signs of long-term effects of medication. Transferring these young people to large adult services, which often have scant resources and, in some areas, a lack of expertise in paediatric disease processes (de Sousa, 1998; Viner and Keane, 1998; Esmond, 2000), is sometimes a daunting task.

All of these young people will have been cared for by expert paediatric teams, with few financial constraints. Patient numbers are small in paediatric practice compared with adult practice. Paediatric teams focus on growth and education, and adopt an holistic approach to care, but, as Viner (1999) points out, they neglect the development of autonomy and increasing adult behaviour. In contrast, adult services focus on reproduction and autonomy but not on growth and family concerns.

Transition is now an issue, and various programmes for preparation for transition have been developed. Greater resources and training of all health care professionals are needed to ensure that transition is a smooth, successful process for young people and their families. The issue of transition needs to be part of nursing, medical and allied profession education so that helping and supporting children, adolescents and young adults to make the transfer becomes part of care.

The government is now supporting transition programmes and has identified transition champions to help in this project (DH/DfES, 2007a).

Adult doctors are perceived to be reluctant to accept adolescents with chronic disease into their services, and paediatricians may be reluctant to let them go (Schidlow and Fiel, 1990; White, 1997; Viner, 1999). There may be several reasons for this: many adult doctors may be unfamiliar with the pathology of congenital diseases, and there may be a reluctance to accept patients who have expensive treatment regimes and medication, such as frequent physiotherapy or growth hormone replacement therapy injections. Adult nurses may feel uncomfortable in the presence of questioning parents who have a greater understanding and knowledge about the disease process and treatments than they do.

Walford (1996) accused paediatricians of, in the process of making life easier for their patients and families, putting their patients at risk of potential problems and failing to adapt to the long-term effects of their illness. Adult physicians have the resources and ability to discuss fertility and genetic issues, which paediatricians do not offer to the adolescent. Post-transition groups who were interviewed indicated that they found it easier to talk to adult doctors about contraception, children and marriage (Pownceby, 1996).

Influence of school

Adolescents with a chronic disease may spend long periods in hospital, and this can interfere with normal development. The adolescents are isolated from their 'well' peers at school and home, and missing school can impede the development of independence and autonomy. McGinty and Fish (1996) point out that, of the many transitions that an individual makes in a lifetime, the one from school through adolescence is the most important.

Adolescents who are moved to adult care while still in full-time further education may not be able to access teachers and tutorials, as the staff who provide education are not part of adult health care systems. Primary school teachers may often extend their role to covering secondary education when a teenager is a patient on a paediatric ward. This is despite the recommendations from the Department of Education and the National Health Executive (1994), which 'stressed the need for continuity in education for the sick or injured child'. Parents may also have negative views about education in the light of chronic life-threatening illness; in a study of chronically ill children, parents expressed serious concerns about their children's prospects for successful adult roles following interrupted periods of schooling (Luft and Koch, 1998). However, the 'importance of school for children with chronic disease cannot be underestimated, it is often the yardstick by which the impact of the disease is assessed' (Eiser, 1993, p. 46).

Fiorentino *et al.* (1998) reviewed the importance of schooling for disabled teenagers. Many viewed their school as their main source for socialisation. This study commented on the abrupt end of this important part of their lives when they reached school-leaving age. Unlike their non-disabled peers, teenagers with special needs continue to have these needs in adulthood. Stevenson *et al.* (1997) reported on the lack of continuation of this service. Very often there is no provision for normal adolescent activity for teenagers with a disability and, as a result, many of this group are often not only less mature but also less confident and not equipped to deal with adult-oriented dilemmas (Eiser, 1993). In addition, teenagers with a disability or chronic disease often miss out on work experience, as treatment regimes and lack of mobility may prevent them from taking part in this (White, 1997).

Health promotion

You must promote the interests of patients and clients. This includes helping individuals and groups gain access to health and social care information and support, relevant to their needs.

(NMC Code, 2008)

Smoking, drinking alcohol and teenage pregnancy continue to be issues among young people (Coleman and Schofield, 2007). The government has promised to provide more education and advice in order to reduce and prevent adolescents from indulging in behaviours that pose a risk to their health. Nurses have a crucial role to play in helping adolescents to maintain a healthy life style. Nurses who work in the community, particularly school nurses and nurses in general practice, are best placed to address the health needs and risk behaviours of young people. Good practice such as drop-in clinic services for schools (Stansfield, 2001) must be supported and replicated. As mentioned earlier, the health of young people is now a major item on the UK government's agenda: to help young people to lose weight, to stop substance misuse and to continue to lower the high rate of teenage pregnancy.

The Adolescent Health Forum of the Royal College of Nursing (RCN) calls for nurses in the primary sector to:

- recognise the unique difficulties young people have in accessing services and seek creative alternatives for its provision, ensuring youth-friendly environments;
- ensure public health and health promotion activities are inclusive of diversity, for example gender, ethnicity, disability, sexuality, refugee status and socioeconomic status;
- support multi-agency partnerships;
- receive training that explores attitudes, develops skills and increases knowledge of this age group relevant to the school, home or practice setting;
- support the development of health and social care research that identifies gaps in service provision and 'best practice' (RCN, 2002).

Nurse education in adolescent care

Current nursing curricula do not address adolescence. In the author's own practice, only nurses who have undergone the mental health (RMN) programme are well equipped to care for adolescents. The author constantly meets nursing students and newly registered nurses who do not understand the issues that arise when caring for adolescents. In a survey carried out by the Adolescent Health Forum (RCN, 2008a), a big gap in knowledge was identified by nurses who care for young people. In response to the findings of the survery the Adolescent Health Forum (RCN 2008b) has published a guide for nurses caring for young people. The DH has decided to try to address this gap for all health care professionals and will launch an e-learning programme in 2008 (DH and RCPCH, 2008). Perhaps the time is right for institutes of learning to look at this omission and address it. Nurses who have trained on the adult branch often care for adolescents in the A&E department, but they do not receive any formal education or training that focuses on adolescence. There is also an opinion that all health care professionals may need specific training so that they can care for this distinct group (de Sousa and Needham 2002).

Many universities have developed modules that do address this gap in nurse education. This is not the answer, however, as these modules are costly and difficult for nurses to access, particularly if the trust they work for does not view such training as a priority. Adolescent development, and its related issues, must be included in the curriculum for both child and adult branch education. A pathway to the first adolescent health degree in the UK has been launched. This is good news for nurses who wish to focus on the care of young people.

CONCLUSION

This chapter has tried to engage the reader in the interesting world of adolescents. It is hoped that, after reading this, young people will not be dismissed as non-adherent or difficult. They have distinct health care needs, which have largely been ignored. Adolescents should not be cared for inappropriately on paediatric or adult wards; they deserve dedicated clinical settings. They deserve nurses who have had specific training to recognise their needs and development. To understand their concept of health, this intense challenging period of development must be taken into consideration. Young people need to be respected, and given more information and time, so that they can become autonomous and make sensible decisions about their health and lives. Nurses need to recognise the legal aspects of caring for young people. This area of caring is dependent on a multiprofessional team approach, and services must be seen to be accessible, friendly, non-judgemental and confidential.

References

Alderson P (1996). Sociological aspects of adolescent health and illness. In Macfarlane A (ed.). *Adolescent Medicine*. London: Royal College Of Physicians.

Audit Commission (1993). *Children First: A Study of Hospital Services*. London: HSMO.

Baker C (1996). Young people's unit. In Macfarlane A (ed.). *Adolescent Medicine*. London: Royal College of Physicians.

Bekeart S (2002). Sexual health workshop. *Paediatric Nursing*, **14**, 22–6.

Blum RWM, Garrell D, Hodgman CH, *et al.* (1993). Transition from child-centered to adult health-care systems for adolescents with chronic conditions: A position paper of the Society for Adolescent Medicine. *Journal Of Adolescent Health*, **14**, 570–76.

Coleman J and Hendry LB (1999). *The Nature of Adolescence*. London: Routeledge.

Coleman J and Schofield J (2007). *Key Data on Adolescence*. Brighton: Trust for the Study of Adolescence.

Conger JJ and Galambos NL (1997). *Adolescence and Youth: Psychological Development in a Changing World*. New York: Longman.

Craig R and Mindell J (eds) (2008). *Health Survey for England 2006*. Vol. 2: Obesity and other risk factors in children. Leeds: The Information Centre.

Dearden C and Becker S (1998). *Young Carers in the UK*. London: Carers National Association.

Department of Education and the National Health Executive (1994). *The Education of Sick Children*. Circular no. 12/94. London: The Stationery Office.

Department of Health (DH) (1976). *Fit for the Future*. London: HSMO.

Department of Health (DH) (2001). *Good Practice in Consent: Implementation Guide – Consent to Examination and Treatment*. London: HMSO.

Department of Health (DH) (2003). *Getting the Right Start: National Service Framework for Children*. London: Department of Health.

Department of Health (DH) (2007). *Long-Term Ambition on Obesity*. London: Department of Health.

Department of Health (DH) and Department for Education and Skills (DfES) (2007a). *Transition: Getting It Right for Young People*. London: The Stationery Office.

Department of Health (DH) and Department for Education and Skills (DfES) (2007b). *Choosing Health for Children and Young People*. London: The Stationery Office.

Department of Health (DH) and Royal College of Paediatrics and Child Health (RCPCH) (2008). *E Learning in Adolescent Health*. London: Royal College of Paediatrics and Child Health.

Department of Health (DH), Home Office, Department for Education and Skills (DfES) and Department for Culture, Media and Sport (2007). *Safe Sensible Social: The Next Steps in the National Alcohol Strategy*. London: The Stationery Office.

De Sousa M (1998). Making the transition from paediatric to adult care. *Cascade*, **26**, 4–5.

De Sousa M (1999). *Setting Up an Adolescent Unit: An Emergent Strategy – the Nurse as a Strategist*. London: RCN Institute.

De Sousa M and Needham J (2002). Generation gap. *Nursing Standard*, **16**, 96.

Dimond BD (1996). *The Legal Aspects of Child Health Care*. London: Mosby.

Eiser C (1993). *Growing Up with a Chronic Disease: The Impact on Children and their Families*, 2nd edn. London: Jessica Kingsley Publishers.

Elkind D (1968). Egocentrism in adolescence. *Child Development*, **38**, 1025–34.

Erikson E (1968). *Youth and Crisis*. London: Faber & Faber.

Erikson E (1987). The human life cycle. In Schlein S and Erikson EH (eds). *A Way of Looking at Things: Selected Papers from 1930 to 1980*. New York: Norton.

Esmond G (2000). Cystic fibrosis: adolescent care. *Nursing Standard*, **13**, 47–52.

Fiorentino L, Phillips D, Walker D and Hall D (1998). Leaving paediatrics: the experience of service transition for young disabled people and their family carers. *Health and Social Care in the Community*, **6**, 260–70.

Greener M (2002). Hit the spot. *Nursing Standard*, **16**, 18.

Hawton K and James A (2005). Suicide and deliberate self harm. In Viner R (ed.). *ABC of Adolescence*. London: BMJ Books.

Henderson J, Goldacre M and Yeates D (1993). Use of hospital in patient care in adolescence. *Archives of Disease in Childhood*, **69**, 559–63.

Kurtz Z and Hopkins A (eds) (1996). *Services for Young People with Chronic Disorders in their Transition from Childhood to Adult Life*. London: Royal College of Physicians.

Kyngas H (2000a). Compliance of adolescents with chronic disease. *Journal of Clinical Nursing*, **9**, 549–56.

Kyngas H (2000b). Compliance of adolescents with diabetes. *Journal of Pediatric Nursing*, **15**, 260–67.

Kyngas H (2000c). Compliance of adolescents with rheumatoid arthritis. *International Journal of Nursing Practice*, **6**, 261–7.

Lansdowne R (1998). Listening to children: have we gone too far (or not enough)? *Journal of the Royal Society of Medicine*, **91**, 457–61.

Lefrancois G (1992). *Of Children: An Introduction to Child Development*. Belmont, CA: Wadsworth.

Lord Laming (2003). *Report into the Death of Victoria Climbié*. London: Department of Health.

Luft P and Koch LC (1998). Transition of adolescents with chronic illness: overlooked needs and rehabilitation considerations. *Journal of Vocational Rehabilitation*, **10**, 205–17.

Macfarlane A (ed.) (1996). *Adolescent Medicine*. London: Royal College of Physicians.

Mallinson P, Connell H, Bennett MS and Eccleston C (2001). Chronic musculoskeletal and other idiopathic pain syndromes. *Archives of Disease in Childhood*, **84**, 189–92.

McGinty J and Fish J (1996). Educational aspects of transition. In Kurtz Z and Hopkins A (eds). *Services for Young People with Chronic Disorders*. London: Royal College of Physicians.

McKinney JP, Fitzgerald HE and Stommen EA (1977). *Developmental Psychology: The Adolescent and Young Adult*. Homewood IL: Dorsey Press.

Ministry of Health (1959). *Welfare of Children in Hospital*. London: HSMO.

National Association for the Welfare of Children in Hospital (NAWCH) (1990). *Setting Standards for Adolescents in Hospital*. London: Action for Sick Children.

NHS Executive (1996). *Hospital Services for Children and Young People*, 5th report. London: House of Commons, Health Committee, Minutes of Evidence.

Norwich Union (2002). *The Views of Adolescents and Nurses on the Provision of Healthcare in Hospitals*. Eastleigh: Norwich Union Healthcare.

Nursing and Midwifery Council (NMC) (2008). *The Code: Standards of Conduct, Performance and Ethics for Nurses and Midwives*. London: Nursing and Midwifery Council.

Office of National Statistics (2001). *Children and Adolescents Who Try to Harm, Hurt or Kill Themselves*. London: HMSO.

Pownceby J (1996). *The Coming of Age Project*. Bromley: Cystic Fibrosis Trust.

Royal College of Nursing (RCN) (2002). *Caring for Young People*. London: Royal College of Nursing.

Royal College of Nursing (RCN) (2008a). *The Report of an RCN Survey into how Nurses Support Young People in Health Care Settings to Inform the Development of a Guide*. London: Royal College of Nursing.

Royal College of Nursing (RCN) (2008b). Adolescence Boundaries and Connections. London: Royal College of Nursing.

Schave D and Schave B (1989). *Early Adolescence and the Search for Self: A Developmental Perspective*. New York: Praeger.

Schidlow DV and Fiel SB (1990). Life beyond pediatrics: transition of chronically ill adolescents from pediatrics to adult health care systems. *Medical Clinics of North America*, **74**, 13–20.

Stevenson CJ, Pharoah POD and Stevenson R (1997). Cerebral palsy: the transition from youth to adulthood. *Developmental Medicine and Child Neurology*, **39**, 336–42.

Stansfield G (2001). Drop in services for schools: health promotion. *Journal of Community Nursing*, **15**, 13.

United Nations (UN) (1989). *Convention on the Rights of the Child*. Geneva: United Nations.

Viner R (1999). Transition from paediatric to adult care: bridging the gap or passing the buck? *Archives of Disease in Childhood*, **81**, 271–5.

Viner R (ed.) (2005). *ABC of Adolescence*. London: BMJ Books.

Viner R and Keane M (1998). *Youth Matters*. London: Action for Sick Children.

Walford S (1996). The approach of consultant physician. In Kurtz Z and Hopkins A (eds). *Services for Young People with Chronic Disorders*. London: Royal College of Physicians.

Watson AR (2002). Rejection, recurrence, or non-adherence. *Lancet*, **359**, 1997.

Wheeler K, Leiper A, Jannoun L and Chessells J (1998). Medical cost of curing childhood acute lymphoblastic leukaemia. *British Medical Journal*, **296**, 162–6.

White PH (1997). Success in the road to adulthood: issues and hurdles for adolescents with disabilities. *Pediatric Rheumatology*, **223**, 697–707.

Wood D (1998). *How Children Think and Learn*. Oxford: Blackwell.

World Health Organization (WHO) (1989). *The Health of Youth*. Geneva: World Health Organization.

Further reading

Allmark P (2002). Pregnant minors: confidentiality issues and nurses' duties. *British Journal of Nursing*, **11**, 257–60.
Pregnancy in minors is a complex issue. This useful guide helps nurses in a challenging situation.

Department of Health (DH). www.dh.gov.uk.
All policies regarding adolescent health can be downloaded from this site.

European Training in Effective Adolescent Care and Health (EuTEACH). www.euteach.com.
This is an excellent site. All teaching materials from the summer school can be downloaded.

Royal College of Paediatrics and Child Health (RCPCH) (2003). *Bridging the Gaps: Health Care for Adolescents*. London: Royal College of Paediatrics and Child Health.
This is a comprehensive look at how services should be provided for this age group.

Shelley M (1993). Adolescent needs in hospital. *Paediatric Nursing*, **5**, 16–18.

Steven D (1992). Lump it or like it. *Nursing Times*, **88**, 30.
Real-life story of what it is like to be a teenager on a children's ward.

Teenage Health Freak. www.teenagehealthfreak.com.
This site discusses what is important and what worries young people.

Viner R (ed.) (2005). *ABC of Adolescence*. London: BMJ Books.
A succinct and easy-to-read guide to adolescence.

17 The needs of the acutely ill adult

Jacqueline Elton and Hayley Reading

Introduction

This chapter aims to explore some of the fundamental issues that influence the care delivered to acutely ill adults. Through the examination of three scenarios, the reader can examine the care provided to patients in clinical practice.

Pre-registration nurses are required to care for people of all ages and nationalities, who experience a wide range of health and illness. Following registration, nurses may decide to specialise in one particular field of nursing, often determined by either medical pathology or age. This chapter focuses on the care provided to acutely ill adults of any age. The issues and conditions examined within the chapter are likely to be encountered at any point in the nurse's training in almost any specialty. The chapter also demonstrates how the guiding principles and competencies of the Nursing and Midwifery Council (NMC, 2004) requirements for pre-registration nursing programmes have direct application in clinical practice.

Learning objectives

After studying this chapter you should be able to understand:
- changing patterns of health care;
- care of a patient with myocardial infarction;
- care of a patient with chronic obstructive pulmonary disease;
- care of a patient following an overdose;
- communication as it applies to both patients and colleagues;
- the importance of confidentiality and appropriate consent;
- the meaning of illness;
- care of patients from diverse ethnic backgrounds;
- health education applied to the patients discussed in this chapter.

The student will be able to relate these issues to the competencies for entry to the register (NMC, 2004; see Appendix 2).

The acutely ill adult

This chapter concerns the care of the acutely ill adult. Individuals, regardless of age, are unique, having different life experiences, different care requirements, and different expectations of their care when they come into contact with the health and social care services.

We will, briefly, examine the demographic and governmental factors influencing nursing care and the way in which it is delivered. Three typical but diverse patient scenarios are used in this chapter to consider not only physical care but also the psychosocial and cultural factors that impact on care.

Many nurses care for patients who may be the age of their parents, friends or even themselves. In the past, the need for professional detachment was much discussed. We now talk in terms of holistic care and of becoming more involved in patients' experiences. However, the need for a degree of detachment is still relevant: if we overidentify with patients, it may not be possible to give the best advice or treatment, as we become too close to the problem. Professional distance is not to say that nurses do not care; it is about being able to engage in, and then disengage from, an appropriate therapeutic relationship that will benefit both the patient and the nurse. This is clearly identified in the NMC Code (2008) (Appendix 1) under the subheading 'Maintain clear professional boundaries'.

Changing patterns of health care

Ideally, the provision of treatment within the National Health Service (NHS) is both equitable and equal. In other words, all people, irrespective of who they are and where they live, will have the same level of, and access to, high-quality services. Unfortunately, this is not always the case. The inverse care law (Tudor Hart, 1971) postulated that the greater the need for care within a given population, the poorer the provision of and access to care.

A new classification of social class was introduced in 2001. The National Statistics socioeconomic classification (www.statistics.gov.uk) replaces the Registrar General's classification shown in Table 17.1. However, the findings of the following study were based on the earlier classification.

Table 17.1 Registrar General's classification of social class

Class	Example
I Professional	Doctor
II Managerial	Senior manager
III Skilled manual/non-manual	Secretary
IV Semiskilled	Assembly-line worker
V Unskilled	Labourer

Source: OPCS (1980).

The Independent Inquiry into Inequalities in Health (Acheson, 1998) noted that death rates fell among men and women over the past 20 years across all social groups. However, the difference between class 1 and class 5 (see Table 17.1) has widened, with shorter life expectancy for both men and women in social class 5 compared with social class 1. It also noted that premature mortality (before age 65 years) is higher among individuals from lower social classes. The report identified that people from many ethnic minority groups have higher than average mortality rates; for example, mortality rates are twice as high in infants of mothers born in Pakistan and the Caribbean compared with the UK national average. The Acheson Inquiry is now 10 years old but is still central to government health policy (Flint, 2005), where its key findings are still seen as having relevance. The National Service Frameworks (NSFs) for both coronary heart disease (DH, 2000a) and diabetes (DH, 2001d) also clearly indicate inequalities in both mortality and morbidity.

In addition to these inequalities, the demographic shift must inevitably affect the service. Put simply, the UK population is ageing: the overall population grew by 8 per cent over the past 30 years, from 55.9 million in 1971 to 60.6 million in mid-2006. Importantly, however, this growth is not spread evenly across all age ranges: the number of people aged over 65 years grew by 31 per cent over this same period. The number of people aged 85 years and over grew by 69 000 in the year to 2006 to reach a record 1.2 million. Over the past 30 years, the median age of the UK population rose from 34.1 years in 1971 to 38.8 years in mid-2005 (see www.statistics.gov.uk). This ageing population, with more people living to a greater age outside the extended family, will increase demands on health and social care services. At the same time, the percentage of the working population who are paying taxes towards health and social care services becomes proportionately smaller. By 2021, 20 per cent of the population will be over the age of 65 years.

Health care is also becoming more technological, with interventions that would have been impossible 20 years ago now being seen as commonplace; for example, surgery can now be undertaken to correct cardiac abnormalities in utero. Such advances are costly and are an additional pressure for health care providers.

Government initiatives

The NHS Plan (DH, 2000b) has been the most recent major plan for investment in, and reform of, the NHS. It outlined a long-term vision for health care provision in England and Wales in the twenty-first century. The comparable plan for Scotland was set out in the document *Our National Health* (Scottish Executive, 2001).

The NHS Plan highlighted a number of key initiatives that impact on the care that nurses and medical staff are expected to deliver. Some of the key areas are now well developed and include the following:

- *New hospital-building programme*: with the private finance initiative, a number of major rebuilds have been completed. Under such an initiative, private money is used to support the financing of new hospitals.
- *Introduction of the modern matron*: a visible assertive figure who supports ward sisters in delivering services and to whom the public can turn for help and support.
- *Better hospital food*: this is in response to the public request for better hospital food, coupled with research indicating that malnutrition can occur when patients are in hospital (Wise, 1997; Age Concern, 2006).
- *More nurse training and medical school places*: this is to meet the current shortfall in trained nurses and doctors. However, although there has been an increase in the number of training places, financial constraints have limited the amount of recruitment that has been possible in some areas, with nurses seeking employment outside the NHS (Rose, 2007).
- *Modern information technology (IT) systems*: the NHS currently runs a wide variety of information technology systems. New schemes from NHS Connecting for Health (www.connecting-forhealth.nhs.uk) support the NHS to deliver better, safer care to patients, linking general practices and community services to hospitals. It is envisaged that patients will be able to choose and book their appointments online, and information systems will be able to provide details of patients' community care when they are admitted to hospital.
- *New skills and roles for nurses*: this includes the new nurse consultant role, the introduction of the modern matron (see above) and the Chief Nursing Officer's ten key roles.
- *Initiatives to standardise and raise services to a minimum acceptable level*: an example of an initiative to raise standards is the National Service Frameworks. At the time of writing, these include the *NSF for Coronary Heart Disease* (DH, 2000a), the *NHS Cancer Plan* (DH, 2000c), the *NSF for Paediatric Intensive Care* (DH, 1998), the *NSF for Mental Health* (DH, 1999), the *NSF for Older People* (DH, 2001b), with the second phase *A New Ambition for Old Age* launched in 2006 (DH, 2006), the *NSF for Diabetes* (DH, 2001d), the *NSF for Long-Term Conditions* (DH, 2005), the *NSF for Renal Services* (DH, 2004) and the *NSF for Chronic Obstructive Pulmonary Disease* (DH, 2008). Comparable initiatives in Scotland include the *Scottish Diabetes Framework* (Scottish Executive, 2002a) and the *Coronary Heart Disease and Stroke Strategy* (Scottish Executive, 2002b).

- *Greater public and patient involvement in health care*: this has led to the establishment of patient advocacy and liaison services (PALS) in all trusts. These have undergone a number of changes since their establishment, but they still act to advise patients if they are having difficulty using health care services.

Within the NHS Plan, the National Institute for Health and Clinical Excellence (NICE) has the remit to examine the evidence for the efficacy and efficiency of NHS treatments and to recommend their use, or otherwise, within the NHS. This should address the inconsistencies within, for example, prescribing patterns. One of the inconsistencies within prescribing is the so-called 'postcode lottery', which means that a person who lives in one area of the country can get certain forms of treatment, while a person who lives in a different, but nearby, area may not access the same treatment.

This apparent inconsistency is more noticeable if one travels around the country. The introduction of devolution means that the various countries of the UK now determine health policy in response to the needs identified within that country. For example, personal care is provided free in Scotland but is means tested in England.

Reflection point 17.1

How would you address the issue of a patient, or a patient's family, wanting to know why the patient cannot receive a treatment that medical staff have indicated would be beneficial but are unable to prescribe within your geographical location?

Remember that you are not in a position to prescribe. If the health authority has taken this decision about treatment, then there is nothing you can do to alter the intervention. Instead, concentrate on advising the patient about their rights and the avenues of influence that may be open to them, such as pressure groups. Also consider who would be most appropriate to speak with the patient.

The NHS Plan for England (DH, 2000b) includes the Chief Nursing Officer's ten key roles, which relate to expanding the role of the nurse to better meet the needs of patients. These ten key roles are:

- to order diagnostic investigations such as X-rays and pathology tests;
- to make and receive direct referrals to, for example, a therapist or a pain consultant;
- to admit and discharge patients within agreed protocols;
- to manage certain patient caseloads;
- to run certain clinics;
- to prescribe medicines and treatments;
- to carry out a wide range of resuscitation procedures;
- to perform minor surgery and outpatient procedures;
- to triage patients, using the latest IT, to the most appropriate health professional;
- to take a lead in the way local health services are organised and run.

As a nurse, it is important for you to consider the possible implications of these changes for the patterns of health and illness. However, in the majority of cases, patients are unlikely to consider these aspects of society, health and illness. Most patients will be more concerned with the more immediate effects of their condition. Patients wish to have access to services when they become ill, and to be treated in comfortable, clean surroundings by staff members who have time for them and their problems or anxieties. Patients want to be cared for by nursing and medical staff who have good technical knowledge and good interpersonal skills, who can engage with them, and who are competent to 'do a good job'.

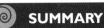

SUMMARY

Nursing is delivered within an ever-changing environment. Key changes within society are:
- the demographic shift;
- changing public expectations.
  The key government documents that currently guide service change are:
- the NHS Plan (DH, 2000b);
- Our National Health (Scottish Executive, 2001);
- National Service Framework for Mental Health (DH, 1999);
- National Service Framework for Coronary Heart Disease (DH, 2000a);
- National Service Framework for Older Persons (DH, 2001b);
- National Service Framework for Diabetes (DH, 2001d);
- Scottish Diabetes Framework (Scottish Executive, 2002a);
- Coronary Heart Disease and Stroke Strategy (Scottish Executive, 2002b);
- National Service framework for Long term conditions (DH, 2005).

There follow three scenarios. Each considers, in broad outline, the physical care requirements and then, in more detail, the core elements that determine the patient's experience. These cases have been selected to represent a range of typical and yet diverse patients and their families. By considering the individual, both in hospital and in the primary care setting, a wide range of issues can be examined. However, it should be noted that most of the issues examined will have a degree of application in all of the scenarios outlined.

Scenario 17.1: Mrs Patel

What is a myocardial infarction?

A myocardial infarction (MI) is one type of coronary heart disease and is commonly referred to as a 'heart attack'. Although the heart may stop beating during a heart attack (cardiac arrest), this is often not the case, although some patients believe that a heart attack and a cardiac arrest are the same thing.

Coronary heart disease kills more than 110 000 people a year in England; of these, 41 000 are under the age of 75 years. Around 300 000 people have an MI each year (DH, 2000a). Death from coronary heart disease is three times more likely in unskilled working men than in men in professional or managerial occupations. As such, coronary heart disease can be seen to reflect the inequalities in health outlined earlier in this chapter. There is also ethnic variation in the incidence of heart disease: people from the Indian subcontinent have a disproportionately higher

SCENARIO 17.1

Mrs Patel is a 56-year-old Asian woman who has lived in the UK for the past 5 years in a traditional household, where she has very little contact outside the family and local Asian community. She speaks no English, but she is fluent in three Asian languages. She is married and lives within an extended family consisting of her husband, grandparents and three children.

She has been admitted to the coronary care unit (CCU) and diagnosed as having had an anterior myocardial infarction. She has no previous cardiac history. Her recovery is uneventful. She is transferred to a general medical ward after 48 hours and discharged home at 7 days, with follow-up by a cardiac rehabilitation nurse.

mortality, with the death rate being 38 per cent higher for men and 43 per cent higher for women than for the UK as a whole.

An MI causes tissue within the heart to be damaged due to an interruption of the blood supply to that area. This results in the heart beating less effectively while recovery takes place. If the damage is extensive, scar tissue forms in the muscle of the heart so that it may not regain its former efficiency.

Predisposing factors for myocardial infarction

The predisposing factors are believed to include the increasingly processed high-sugar, high-fat diets and increasingly sedentary lifestyle many individuals lead in the UK, which can lead to obesity. Smoking is also a major contributory factor in heart disease. The Coronary Heart Disease National Service Framework (DH, 2000a) sets out clear targets to help individuals who wish to give up smoking.

Symptoms of myocardial infarction

The symptoms at onset are typically pain in the central chest and radiating down the left arm; the patient may describe the pain as 'crushing'. Signs of shock, with rapid irregular pulse, falling blood pressure and shortness of breath, may accompany the pain. For a diagnosis of MI to be made, there will also be changes in the patient's electrocardiogram (ECG) and raised cardiac enzymes. At least two of these three symptoms need to be present for the diagnosis to be confirmed; importantly, some people have an MI without complaining of any central chest pain. Some patients report feeling as though they have indigestion.

Physical care

The key points for the immediate physical care of an individual admitted with an MI are for analgesia, stabilisation of the condition, possible thrombolysis, and rest to relieve the work of the damaged myocardium. Thrombolysis involves the administration of 'clot-busting' drugs to treat a thrombus that has caused the MI. The diagnostic tests include:

- ECG (Box 17.1);
- cardiac enzymes;
- urea and electrolytes (U&Es) (Table 17.2);
- full blood count (FBC).

The ECG indicates where the cardiac damage has occurred and gives an indication of the degree of damage. It is not 100 per cent diagnostic, however, and changes may not occur until some time after the event.

Cardiac enzymes are enzymes released when cells are damaged. There is a marked increase in cardiac enzymes when an MI has occurred. It is noteworthy that some cardiac enzymes are less specific and are elevated in the event of other trauma, including bruising and physical trauma. Cardiac enzymes are typically assessed on admission, at 6 hours and at 24 hours. The troponin I test is more cardiospecific and shows an increase only in the event of the myocardium being affected; a level of less than 0.06 ng/mL indicates that it is unlikely that there has been a cardiac event, while a level above 0.06 ng/mL indicates an intermediate risk of the person having had an MI.

U&Es and FBC are standard blood tests that measure the levels of the various components within the blood. Variation in these test results may give information about the cause of a cardiac or other irregularity. As a nurse, it is important that you have knowledge of the typical values of

BOX 17.1 The electrocardiogram

The 12-lead electrocardiogram (ECG) is carried out on the ward or on the coronary care unit (CCU) in the event of suspected myocardial infarction (MI) or a patient developing chest pain.

An ECG is a graph of the electrical activity within the heart. As the muscles of the heart contract, a small electrical current is detectable; this is what is recorded by the ECG. In order to perform an ECG, the leads are attached to the limbs and chest, as shown in Figure 17.1. It is important to ensure good adhesion of the electrodes, otherwise a poor-quality trace will result. For the same reason, it is important that the patient remains still and is as relaxed as possible, as muscle activity from anywhere in the body will be detected by the ECG.

The leads give a trace that is a two-dimensional representation of the three-dimensional heart. This requires skill to interpret. The trace illustrated in Figure 17.2 is a normal heart rhythm. The key feature that the non-specialist looks for is regularity – that is, does the trace look the same all the way through?

Each part of the trace indicates electrical activity within the heart. This electrical activity results in muscle activity, so for depolarisation read 'contraction':

- *P wave*: depolarisation of the atria.
- *QRS wave*: depolarisation of the ventricles.
- *R wave*: repolarisation of the ventricles (getting ready to contact again) The repolarisation of the atria is masked by the *QRS complex*.

Lead positions

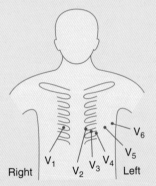

V_1 – 4th intercostal rib space (right)
V_2 – 4th intercostal rib space (left)
V_3 – over 5th rib (left)
V_4 – 5th intercostal rib space (left)
V_5 – 5th intercostal rib space axilla line (left)
V_6 – 5th intercostal rib space mid axilla line (left)

The limb leads are attached to each leg and arm as indicated on the leads

Figure 17.1 Lead positions in the electrocardiogram.

A normal sinus rhythm

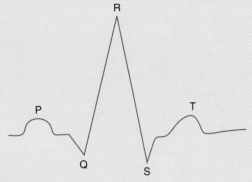

Figure 17.2 Normal sinus rhythm.

Table 17.2 Normal ranges for full blood count (FBC) and urea and electrolytes (U&Es)

FBC	U&Es
Hb: 11.5–18 g/dL	Sodium (Na): 133–142 mmol/L
White cells: 4–11 × 10^9/L	Potassium (K): 3.3–5.3 mmol/L
Platelets: 150–400 × 10^9/L	Urea: 2.5–6.5 mmol/L
Neutrophils: 40–75%	Creatinine: 60–120 μmol/L
	Glucose: 3.5–5.5 mmol/L

Hb, haemoglobin.

the commonly used blood tests in a given clinical area. The nurse usually spends more time than the medical staff with the patient, and thus the nurse is in a better position to observe changes in the patient's physical condition, which can then be related to the investigations. It could be argued that such knowledge is part of the doctor's remit rather than that of nursing, since it typically requires a medical intervention to initiate treatment. However, such knowledge is an illustration of NMC competency 2h, noting the need to be able to use and recognise knowledge from other disciplines for the benefit of patient care.

In the immediate period after admission, a number of interventions are likely:

- rest;
- constant monitoring of heart rate and rhythm;
- analgesia;
- oxygen.

Analgesia is important and is likely to include an opiate, such as diamorphine, in the first instance, in order to give rapid pain relief. Since nausea is a common side effect of opiates, an antiemetic is often also administered. Glyceryl trinitrate (GTN) may be given to reduce cardiac workload, thus reducing pain. If the patient is not already receiving aspirin, they may be given aspirin on arrival in the accident and emergency (A&E) department or CCU, not as an analgesic but for its antiplatelet activity. Typically, the dose of aspirin is 300 mg on admission, and thereafter 150 mg daily, reducing to 75 mg daily on an ongoing basis.

Psychological care

It can be argued that to consider physical and psychological care separately is unreasonable, given that nurses strive to achieve a holistic approach to care. In this chapter, they are developed separately to allow development of themes and ideas, but nevertheless they are inextricably linked. It is worth noting that psychological adjustment to a diagnosis of coronary heart disease is often problematic. Lewin (1997) reports literature establishing that 15–25 per cent of people with MI remain depressed for long periods after their MI. Lewin *et al.* (1998) note that relationship and sexual problems are reported in 20–58 per cent of patients studied.

When Mrs Patel arrives in the hospital, she is likely to be in pain. She has never been in hospital before. Her pain, the new environment and being unable to speak English will increase her level of anxiety and possibly that of her family.

In order to care adequately for Mrs Patel, it is vital for the nurses to be able to communicate effectively. Without communication, how do we obtain her consent for procedures? How do we provide access to rehabilitation? At the very basic level, how does Mrs Patel make her needs known and how do we determine whether or not she is in pain?

Reflection point 17.2

How would you facilitate communication with Mrs Patel? How would you obtain her consent for a procedure such as insertion of a peripheral cannula?

Communication

The need to communicate is central to effective delivery of health care and is implicit within all the competencies for entry to the register (NMC, 2004; see Appendix 2). Without communication, many aspects of assessment, planning and evaluation of care are impaired. For example, how is it possible to know whether the nurse is respecting the patient's cultural and spiritual needs? Communication can be both verbal and non-verbal. Verbal communication is the spoken word, but even this is not straightforward. It is important to take note of the patient's background when considering the language that is used. For example, consider the contrast between professional language and everyday language: the author has previously asked patients whether they have 'passed stool', but patients may not recognise this term – less technical language is needed to elicit whether the patient has opened their bowels.

It is important to identify the patient's first language. Even if the patient appears to understand some English, it would be inappropriate to assume full and clear understanding.

Non-verbal communication should also be considered, as this component often has more meaning and significance than the spoken word. An example is asking the patient whether they are feeling well or whether they have any problems. The patient may say, 'Yes, I feel fine, Nurse – no problems', but if they are sitting with their arms and legs tightly crossed, avoiding eye contact with the nurse and growling the response, then there is a clear difference between their verbal and non-verbal cues. Generally non-verbal cues are taken to be the accurate indicator of what the person means.

Reflection point 17.3

With a partner, face each other and have a short conversation. The subject matter is irrelevant – it can be your next holiday if you wish. Ask a third person to watch the conversation and keep notes of the body language displayed by both participants. At the end of the conversation, feed this back. Repeat the exercise, switching roles.

Next, repeat the exercise using inappropriate body language, for example avoiding eye contact and shuffling. Afterwards, discuss how the different body language made you respond to one another.

Another good exercise is to observe someone you regard as a good communicator to see how they use body language to put someone at ease – for example, making eye contact, placing themselves on the same level as the patient, and reflecting back the patient's statements. It is also interesting to watch a poor communicator and see what it is that makes their communication skills ineffective.

To communicate with Mrs Patel, it is necessary to gain access to an interpreter. This service may not be readily available in the language required; and even if it is accessible, it is unlikely to be available 24 hours a day and at short notice. If Mrs Patel wants a cup of tea or to go to the toilet, there is a temptation to use her family or other hospital staff as interpreters. However, this may create difficulties by causing embarrassment for all parties and raising issues of confidentiality and consent.

As nurses, we have a duty to respect the confidentiality of patient information gained. The section 'Respect people's confidentiality' in the NMC Code sets out the nurse's duty of confidentiality, and there have been a number of cases of nurses losing their registration for divulging patient information inappropriately.

Reflection point 17.4

Which, if any, of the following three circumstances would represent a breach of confidentiality by the nurse?

- Mrs Patel's son asks you to explain his mother's condition and prognosis.
- You discuss Mrs Patel's case with a friend who is also a nurse.
- In an unrelated case, a former patient of yours is arrested and charged with an offence, which the police believe he may have discussed with you. The police request information from you that you gained in the course of looking after the patient.

It could be argued that a breach of confidentiality has occurred in all three cases. Mrs Patel's son has no right to access information about his mother's condition, unless she gives her consent. In the event that Mrs Patel has given consent for her son to receive information, then how has that consent been obtained? If the nurse has asked Mrs Patel, via her son, whether she minds the information being given out, what certainty is there that the translation and its feedback have been relayed accurately by her son? At ward level, practicality often means that family members are used to interpret, but this must always be approached with a degree of caution.

If the nurse in the second situation is working in the same area and you are discussing professional management issues, then it may be argued that it is a continuation of care for Mrs Patel. However, any discussion of a patient with an individual not related to their care is a breach.

In the third instance, the issue is less clear-cut. Referring back to the NMC Code, you must disclose information if you believe someone may be at risk of harm, in line with the law of the country in which you are practising. As a practising nurse, the safest course of action may well be to refer the issue to your senior manager or the trust's legal department.

Informed consent

Consent can be verbal, non-verbal or written. Implied consent may be assumed if, for example, the patient holds out their arm for a blood sample to be taken. Even in such circumstances, however, care needs to be taken – for example, had the patient been expecting to have their blood pressure checked rather than a blood sample taken?

Guidance from the Department of Health identifies the following factors as being required for a patient's consent to be valid. The patient must:

- be competent to take that decision;
- have sufficient information to take that decision;
- not be acting under any duress (DH, 2001c).

An important point to emphasise is that a signature on a consent form is *evidence* that the patient has given consent, but it is not *proof* of valid consent.

In obtaining consent from Mrs Patel for any intervention, in the absence of a professional interpreter, family members or other members of hospital staff are commonly used. The guidance from the Department of Health states that it is inappropriate for children to act as interpreters

(DH, 2001c). In addition, the use of a family member could violate the duty of confidentiality, although if Mrs Patel assents to the use of the family member, then it could be argued that she has given implied consent to the practice. When using a family member, there is no form of quality control, and, as such, we are unable to establish whether translation is accurate.

When considering consent, it is important always to remember that *any competent adult has the right to refuse treatment* and that if the nurse is to advocate effectively for the patient, the nurse may need to support the patient in this refusal, sometimes in the face of criticism from other health professionals.

The meaning of illness

As Mrs Patel recovers from her MI, she may benefit from access to a cardiac rehabilitation programme. These programmes vary widely around the country (British Heart Foundation, 2007), but generally such a programme will include information on regaining former activity levels, preventing a further MI, and general health education relating to diet and exercise. The World Health Organization (WHO, 1993) recommends that cardiac rehabilitation programmes should include exercise training, relaxation and secondary prevention and pay attention to the patient's psychosocial adjustment. The WHO also recommends that the patient's partner and other family members be included. It should, however, be noted that West (2004), in a multicentre randomised controlled trial, found little evidence of the effectiveness of cardiac rehabilitation as currently practised in the UK.

There is evidence that individuals from ethnic minorities are less likely to access cardiac rehabilitation programmes (Thompson *et al.*, 1997) and that lack of interpreter services, among other factors, means that the needs of patients from some ethnic minorities are not met fully (Tod *et al.*, 2001). To be most effective, such interventions need to be tailored to the needs of the individual patient and to the patient's understanding of illness. For some people, illness is seen as fate; it may be viewed as a punishment from a higher power, or it may be seen to be the result of a poor lifestyle. Unless the nurse becomes familiar with the implications of transcultural nursing and understands the meaning of illness for that patient, it will not be possible to provide optimal care.

SUMMARY

- Communication is central to care. Where communication is impaired by, for example, a language barrier, the patient may be disadvantaged.
- Consent is a complex issue, and the nurse must always be aware that *any competent adult* has the right to refuse any intervention.
- Illness can mean different things to different people, this being determined by experience, culture and background.

Scenario 17.2: Mrs Smith

What is airways disease?

Asthma is a chronic condition in which narrowing of the airways occurs in response to, for example, infection, allergy, exercise or an unknown stimulus. Although asthma is chronic, acute exacerbations are common. In this scenario, we consider an acute-on-chronic condition. When the airways narrow, breathing becomes increasingly laboured, with expiration being particularly difficult, giving a typical

SCENARIO 17.2

Mrs Smith is a 42-year-old woman with long-standing asthma who works in a textile factory. She smokes five to ten cigarettes per day and has done so since the age of 15 years. Over the past 5 years, her asthma has worsened and chronic bronchitis has been diagnosed. She is currently taking inhaled steroids in addition to regular bronchodilators. She is a single parent with a 12-year-old son.

She has not previously required hospitalisation, but she has been admitted to a general medical ward, via the medical admissions unit, with an exacerbation of her chronic obstructive pulmonary disease due to a chest infection.

On arrival from the admissions ward, she is receiving 40% oxygen with humidification, has regular nebulisers prescribed, is expectorating thick yellow-green sputum and is receiving intravenous antibiotics.

wheezing sound on expiration. In the early stages, this narrowing is reversible using bronchodilators, such as salbutamol. A bronchodilator is a medication that works by dilating the smooth muscle in the airways, thus making breathing easier. However, if the condition progresses, the airways become permanently thickened and narrowed, reducing the effectiveness of bronchodilators. The next line of treatment is the addition of an inhaled steroid (e.g. beclometasone), which reduces inflammation and makes the airways less sensitive to the stimulus, thus reducing the likelihood of an asthma attack. Typically both a bronchodilator and an inhaled steroid are prescribed.

As the condition progresses, the degree of reversibility decreases and the loss of function becomes permanent. This is chronic obstructive pulmonary disease (COPD), also known as chronic obstructive airways disease (COAD).

There are a number of recognised risk factors for COPD. Occupational risk factors include working in mines and furnaces and working with grain. Additional risk factors include:

- smoking;
- childhood respiratory tract infections;
- low birth weight;
- low socioeconomic status;
- airway hyper-reactivity;
- passive smoking (GOLD, 2001).

Of these risk factors, smoking is the most important. In England and Wales in 2004, there were a total of 500 755 deaths of adults aged 35 years and over; of these, an estimated 88 800 were caused by smoking (Information Centre, 2006). Smoking is identified as the main cause of COPD. The disease is rare in non-smokers, and approximately 80 per cent of deaths from COPD can be attributed to cigarette smoking (Health Education Authority, 1998). The prevalence of COPD in men in the UK appears to have peaked, but the incidence in women continues to increase, possibly linked to the continued increase in smoking in women. It has also been noted that children of smoking patients have more respiratory diseases than children of non-smokers (Cook and Strachen, 1997).

The NHS Plan included a major expansion of smoking-cessation services, with the aim of making help to give up smoking more widely available. This includes increasing the availability of nicotine replacement therapy and requesting NICE guidance on the most appropriate and cost-effective prescribing regimes for smoking cessation. The target is that, by 2010, at least 1.5 million people in Britain will have given up smoking. There is strong and ongoing evidence that active interventions from health care professionals can increase smoking-cessation rates (Lancaster *et al.*, 2000; Information Centre, 2006).

Physical care

Mrs Smith will require humidified oxygen until her condition improves. High-percentage oxygen is given, as both the COPD and the superimposed infection compromise oxygen exchange. It is possible for her to become hypoxic – that is, a low oxygen level in the tissues. Hypoxia may potentially impair mental functioning and cause further tissue damage. Oxygen needs to be prescribed, since it is not without potential hazards, especially in individuals with COPD. Humidification of oxygen keeps secretions loose to aid their expectoration. If high-percentage oxygen is not humidified, then drying of the upper airways can result, leading to mucous plugs, leading to poorer gas exchange and impaired respiration.

When assessing Mrs Smith's breathing, there are a number of observations that can be undertaken:

- *Respiratory rate*: a healthy individual generally has a respiratory rate of 12–14 breaths per minute; if the respiratory rate is much higher (a rate above 20 breaths/min is not uncommon), this can be an indication of serious respiratory distress. The rate needs to be checked regularly, possibly every 4 hours to begin with, as an increase in rate could indicate that the patient's condition is deteriorating.
- *Saturation*: this is measured using a pulse oximeter and indicates the level of oxygen in the blood by means of an external probe. A healthy non-smoker generally has a saturation of 96 per cent or higher; if the saturation is below this, then monitoring is required. Some individuals with COPD have saturations in the mid- to high-eighties but are quite well, as their physiology has adapted to them being chronically hypoxic.
- *Accessory muscles*: are the accessory muscles being used to support respiration? If the patient is finding it particularly difficult to breathe, then they may adopt the orthopnoeic position – sitting forward, with their arms resting on their knees or the bed table. The accessory muscles are not normally used in breathing but come into play when breathing is difficult. The orthopnoeic position increases the available respiratory volume.

As part of the assessment of Mrs Smith's physical needs, it is important to establish how she sleeps, both in hospital and at home. Many patients with chronic respiratory difficulties sleep with three or more pillows in an upright position. While Mrs Smith is acutely short of breath, she will certainly benefit from being nursed sitting upright.

Reflection point 17.5

Using a basic anatomy text, identify the locations and insertion points of the accessory muscles. This will enable you to recognise whether the accessory muscles are being used, which will form part of your assessment in any patient with respiratory difficulties.

A central part of the assessment process is to determine what degree of help Mrs Smith needs with her activities of daily living. She is likely to require assistance with hygiene and elimination in the short term, as any exertion may exacerbate her breathlessness. It is important to remember that, for an individual with a respiratory problem, a large part of their energy is spent on the physical act of breathing, and they will not be able to function as they did before the acute episode of the illness.

Since Mrs Smith has a chest infection, she is receiving antibiotics, which are medications effective against bacterial infection. She may be pyrexial, in which case paracetamol will help to lower her temperature and keep her more comfortable. There are also various non-pharmaceutical methods for lowering temperature, including reducing the amount of clothing that the patient is wearing, ensuring good ventilation (not always easy in a ward bay, where other patients may be feeling cold) and providing a fan. Tepid sponging may be used if her pyrexia becomes more pronounced. It is worth noting that patients with an increasing temperature often report feeling cold or have rigors. This is because the part of the hypothalamus (the body's 'thermostat') that regulates body temperature has been temporarily 'reset' to a higher than normal temperature, which means the body activates mechanisms such as muscle tremors to reach the temperature dictated by the brain. The patient will report feeling hot only when the hypothalamus is set back to normal temperature and the body recognises that the core temperature is too high. At this point, the patient will state they feel hot, sweat and look flushed.

It is important to be aware that Mrs Smith is likely to have a very dry mouth, both from the oxygen and because she is likely to be mouth-breathing. She may be eating very little as she is feeling unwell and it is difficult to chew and swallow when needing to breath with the mouth open.

The nurse needs to offer frequent drinks and easily swallowed food, such as ice-cream. Cold drinks are likely to be very welcome.

Monitoring Mrs Smith's temperature will indicate whether the infection is beginning to settle. Regular monitoring of the respiratory rate gives an early indication of any change. Observation of the sputum is also important, as changes in its appearance or volume may indicate a change in the patient's condition. In cases of severe chest infection, there may be blood in the sputum. Infected sputum may be viscous and yellow-green in colour. Care should always be taken when handling any body fluid, due to the potential risk of infection. If the patient is using a sputum pot, it should always have a lid, which should be removed only briefly to observe the contents of the pot. The sputum pot should be changed at least daily and the used pot disposed of according to the hospital's clinical waste policy, for example by incineration. It is probable that sputum will be requested for culture and sensitivity (C&S). This laboratory test indicates which antibiotics the infective organism is sensitive to, thus ensuring that the patient is prescribed the correct antibiotics. Other conditions that may be indicated by observation of the sputum are heart failure (in which case, the sputum may be frothy and white), severe chest infection and neoplasm (which may be indicated by bloodstaining).

Monitoring peak flow readings or spirometry may give an indication of the degree of airway reversibility and the overall function. A peak flow recording gives a measure of the lung elasticity; the individual is required to exhale as rapidly as possible, giving a reading of litres/minute exhaled.

As the infection resolves, Mrs Smith will discontinue oxygen and revert to her normal medication with a view to returning home as soon as she is well enough. During this recovery phase, it is important not to push Mrs Smith to do more than she is physically capable of doing. She is likely to be keen to go home as soon as possible, as she has a child and her job to return to. In many cases, patients simply want to go home because hospitals are usually noisier than their own home, the food is not what they are used to, and there is little to occupy them.

Psychological care

As with Mrs Patel, the factors discussed here are linked inextricably to the physical care outlined previously.

Dignity and privacy

This is one of the benchmarks covered in the *Essence of Care* documents (DH, 2001a, 2007b). These documents aim to promote the improvement of practice in delivery of the fundamentals of care. In the case of Mrs Smith, she is a normally independent lady who, for at least a few days, will need help washing, dressing and going to the toilet and who is also producing large amounts of sputum.

There is a tendency to regard the privacy curtains around hospital beds as being soundproof, but they are not. Not only will Mrs Smith's neighbours hear what you say to her (see the previous discussion on confidentiality) but they will also hear when she uses the commode. In some individuals this leads, unsurprisingly, to constipation as they will not be able to open their bowels when they know others can hear them. If Mrs Smith's breathlessness permits, it is far preferable that she is wheeled to the toilet. In either case, it is important to give her the opportunity to wash her hands afterwards. Even if she does not normally take laxatives, it may be necessary to prescribe them now – constipation needs to be prevented, as straining to open her bowels could increase her breathlessness.

Health education

In the case of a patient with a chronic chest condition, there are a number of areas of health education that can be considered, some of which are more practical than others.

In common with other public buildings in the UK, British hospitals are non-smoking areas, with no or very limited (and possibly inaccessible for unwell patients) areas available for smokers to use. The target set for trusts was for all NHS hospitals to be non-smoking by the end of 2006 (Health Development Agency, 2005), however the *Chief Executive Bulletin* (DH, 2007a) records that many areas have made excellent progress; implicit in this is that the target has not yet been met.

As Mrs Smith smokes, we can recommend strongly that she stops, but we cannot force her to. However, in line with the smoke-free hospital policy, she can be offered support with smoking cessation while she is an inpatient, such as providing nicotine replacement patches or gum to reduce the stress of withdrawal, and offering support from the smoking cessation advisers based in hospitals and health centres (NICE, 2006). It can be argued that the stress of being hospitalised makes it a particularly difficult time for a person to give up smoking; however, if no facilities for patient smoking are available, then it needs to be explained firmly that smoking on the ward is forbidden. Some patients may still attempt to smoke covertly in the hospital. There is a clear risk management issue if a patient smokes around oxygen, since although oxygen itself is not flammable, it encourages other flammable substances to burn more easily.

The involvement of the multiprofessional team is vital for Mrs Smith, as she may benefit from pulmonary rehabilitation, which is run in some centres. In the same way that a cardiac rehabilitation programme includes a number of factors, a pulmonary rehabilitation programme enables the individual to move towards the best possible health condition to maximise their potential. Gibson and colleagues (1998) note that self-management education for individuals with asthma improves their health outcome.

Lifestyle changes

It is important not to judge patients' lifestyles and not to expect that you can make them change their way of living. Nurses can advise on areas that may be deleterious to health and encourage change, but that is all. There are a number of aspects of Mrs Smith's lifestyle where health education may improve her health.

Mrs Smith works in a textile factory. This is likely to be a high-dust environment, which is not helpful for an individual with COPD. It may be worth discussing with Mrs Smith the possibility of her changing her job, as leaving the textile factory may improve her health. However, Mrs Smith is a lone parent, and therefore it is probable that she needs to work to support both herself and her son. She may be unqualified for a job elsewhere. If she has worked in the same area for some years, it is probable that the majority of her friends and social acquaintances also work in the textile factory. By recommending that she changes her job, we could be asking her to lose her social support network. Leidy and Haase (1999) describe the difficulty some patients with COPD have when facing the challenges of maintaining their personal integrity and making changes in lifestyle and health that the disease forces on them.

Moving to a warm, dry climate helps many people with chronic chest conditions. We can certainly suggest this idea to Mrs Smith and her son, but the previous concerns about losing her social network would still apply. The expense of moving house and emigrating with a young child who is in school may not be feasible. Such cases can be difficult for the health care professionals involved, as the best advice for health may be unachievable, even if the patient would like to follow the advice.

The NMC (2004) competencies clearly identify the need to utilise appropriate opportunities to promote the health and well-being of patients and clients. The dilemmas presented by Mrs Smith's case are very real. Health education and suggestions for lifestyle changes can be seen clearly as being in the patient's best interest, but such changes are not always practicable. Nurses need to be aware of these potential limitations and conflicts.

Changes in self-image

In addition to her lifestyle, Mrs Smith will have certain perceptions about her self-image, all of which will have been affected by her acute-on-chronic condition. She has seen her own condition deteriorate over the past 5 years to the point where it is not curable and she has had to learn to live with it.

Having experienced this deterioration, Mrs Smith may be asking herself 'What next?' and wondering whether she will get worse. Such questions are not easy to answer. The NMC Code and the registered nurse competencies discuss recognising one's own abilities and limitations. The nurse needs to be able to offer something constructive but, importantly, if the nurse is asked such a question and is unsure of the answer, they must refer it to a more senior professional. Far more damage is done by giving an inaccurate or badly handled answer than by saying 'I don't know, but I will get someone else to come and talk to you'.

It is possible that Mrs Smith may undergo a form of bereavement reaction. Consider the four stages of grieving (Parkes, 1986):

- shock and alarm;
- searching;
- anger and guilt;
- gaining a new identity.

These stages identify a possible model to understand the phases that an individual goes through when they, or a loved one, are dying. This can be applied to chronic illness where the loss of function and abilities are beyond the control of the individual or their family.

Again, the answer may lie in accessing another member of the multiprofessional team, for example a psychologist or a counsellor, who can help Mrs Smith to accept changes in her body image and lifestyle.

Effects on children

Mrs Smith's son will perceive that his mother is different from other children's mothers if she becomes breathless when they play or she is unable to run with him. As Mrs Smith is a lone parent, her son will have to be cared for by someone else while she is in hospital. This may be a friend, a member of her family, or foster care arranged through social services. For any child, this leads to a degree of uncertainty. Mrs Smith's son may ask 'Will this happen again?' and 'Is my mum going to be all right?' Zahlis (2001) examined the effects of parental ill health on children in relation to breast cancer and found that the child tries to understand the situation and wonders what may happen in the future to them and the rest of the family. Brandt and Weiner (1998) studied families in which one parent had multiple sclerosis; they found that children in households with less adequate finances and more discord were at greater risk of mental ill health than children in families with better finances and better relationships.

The nurse needs to facilitate the child visiting if his mother is unable to arrange this. From a risk management point of view, it is not appropriate for ward staff to fetch the child. It would, however, be entirely appropriate for nursing staff to liaise with friends, relatives or the voluntary sector to facilitate visiting.

Possible community concerns

Within NMC competency 1 (professional and ethical practice – see Appendix 2), the need to recognise one's own abilities and limitations is noted. NMC competency 3 (care management) notes the need to utilise contributions of the health and social care team. Both of these competencies clearly apply in relation to Mrs Smith's future planning, in that it may be advisable to ask her whether she wishes to access a social worker. If her condition causes her to change her employment or affects how she is able to care for her child, then the social worker can advise Mrs Smith on the benefits and services available.

Although it may not be required yet, there is the possibility that Mrs Smith may require oxygen at home at some point in the future. This is usually ordered via the general practitioner (GP) and can take the form of either cylinders (if oxygen is for fairly short periods each day) or an oxygen concentrator (if it is required for longer periods). If Mrs Smith does require oxygen at home, then work needs to be carried out with her to explain the dangers of smoking and oxygen. Support is also required, as patients on home oxygen therapy can experience physiological and psychological difficulties (Ring and Davidson, 1997).

It is important to remember that a patient has a life both before and after they leave nursing care. Sometimes the choices that the patient makes do not concur with the recommendations of the nurse. However, this is the right of the patient, providing that they have been given all relevant information and accompanying explanations so that they can make an informed choice as to whether or not to take the advice. If the nurse has provided the information in a form that the patient is comfortable with and can understand, then, whatever the patient's decision, it can be argued that the nurse has discharged their responsibilities appropriately.

SUMMARY

- In both acute and chronic illness, the effects on the individual extend beyond a single episode of care.
- Illness can change how both the individual and others regard themselves.
- Health education should always be made available with access to accompanying explanation and clarifications, but it may be refused or ignored.
- The effects of parental ill health on children should always be considered.

Scenario 17.3: Mr Jones

SCENARION 17.3

Mr Jones is a 20-year-old student in the second year of a sociology degree at university. He has been admitted following an overdose. According to the history he gave to the admitting nurse, he took most of a bottle of 50 paracetamol tablets 8 hours before arriving at the hospital. He was accompanied to the hospital by his flatmate, who returned home to find Mr Jones semi-conscious, with a bottle of pills and an empty vodka bottle at the side of the bed. His flatmate called the ambulance.

By the time Mr Jones arrives on your ward, he has gone through the emergency department and is receiving intravenous acetylcysteine. Acetylcysteine is a drug that augments glutathione reserves (depleted by toxic paracetamol metabolites) in the body and, together with glutathione, binds directly to toxic metabolites. These actions serve to protect the cells in the liver (hepatocytes) from toxicity due to paracetamol overdose.

Mr Jones insists that what has happened was an accident, that he is going to leave the ward shortly, and that he does not want to talk to anyone. He also insists that he does not want his parents (his legal next of kin) to be informed of his admission.

What is an overdose?

A drug overdose is the accidental or intentional use of a drug or medicine in an amount that is higher than is normally used or prescribed. All drugs have the potential to be misused, whether they are prescribed by a doctor, purchased over the counter from a pharmacist, or bought illegally on the street.

Paracetamol is the most common drug taken in overdose in the UK, accounting for 48 per cent of all poisoning admissions to hospital and an estimated 100–200 deaths per year (Wallace *et al.*, 2002).

It is possible to take an overdose of paracetamol by mistake as many over-the-counter cold and flu remedies contain this drug. If the person does not read or follow the instructions on the packet carefully, they may take the recommended dose of paracetamol (1 g up to four times daily) and then additionally take a cold remedy containing paracetamol. Some common analgesic preparations also contain paracetamol, such as co-codamol (codeine and paracetamol).

An intentional overdose may be taken as a deliberate attempt to commit suicide or as a 'cry for help', where there is no real intention to cause long-term self-harm. Paracetamol can be particularly hazardous in this respect. Nearly all paracetamol overdoses are taken knowingly, although in some cases the expectation is not to die but to become unconscious and then recover (Hawton and Fagg, 1992).

Patients who have taken an intentional overdose highlight an aspect of nursing care that brings nurses face to face with moral questions of life and death. It is perhaps unsurprising that nurses may react with anger and frustration and with tactics of avoidance towards such patients

Reflection point 17.6
Assessment using activities of daily living (Roper *et al.*, 2000) is discussed in Chapter 14. Using Roper and colleagues' activities of daily living, assess this patient. What are the key problem areas that you identify?

(McLaughlin, 1994). Meeting the patient's physical needs is only one part of the nursing care required in cases of intentional overdose, as such patients are psychologically vulnerable.

Mr Jones is a 20-year-old student, and many of the nurses caring for him, particularly the student nurses, are of a similar age and going through similar experiences at university. It is possible that student nurses involved in Mr Jones's care may overidentify with him, seeing some aspect of themselves in another student. It is important that the nurses remember that, although there are clearly points of common reference, they do not know what else is happening to Mr Jones that has led to his admission.

Patients' lack of communication with health care professionals can prove very challenging. It is imperative, however, that the nursing response is to interact with the patient in a kind, caring and respectful manner (Wiklander *et al.*, 2003). It is important not to become anxious about knowing the solution to the patient's problems. The nurse should not moralise but should encourage the patient to talk about their difficulties and explore possible coping strategies.

Why do people take overdoses?

An intentional overdose is usually an attempt to stop suffering. Any person has the potential to consider overdose if they perceive their suffering to be intolerable, interminable and inescapable (Chiles and Strosahl, 1995). The presence of a psychiatric disorder does not itself predict suicidal behaviour, and the vast majority of psychiatric patients never attempt suicide (Mann, 2002). In fact, half of patients who overdose intentionally have no specific psychiatric disorder (Chiles and Strosahl, 1995).

Most patients explain their overdose as a reaction to being in a 'terrible state of mind', dealing with an 'unbearable situation', feeling a loss of control, wanting to die, or wanting to 'escape' (Schnyder *et al.*, 1999). Most deny that the overdose was intended and state that it was designed to manipulate others, to make people understand how desperate they were feeling, to seek help from someone or to make things easier for others (Schnyder *et al.*, 1999).

Treatment for paracetamol overdose

Although paracetamol can be bought without prescription, the drug can be extremely hazardous if taken in higher than the recommended dosage. As little as 10 g of paracetamol can produce fatal hepatotoxicity. The maximum recommended dose of paracetamol is 8 g in 24 hours.

It is often assumed, even by many health care professionals, that drinking alcohol with paracetamol increases the effect of the overdose and contributes to death. Although this is the case with many medicines used in overdose, alcohol does not increase the effect of overdose of paracetamol. In a normal healthy adult, alcohol taken with paracetamol does not increase the injury to the liver; in fact, as alcohol and paracetamol compete for the same metabolic pathways, there may even be a protective effect from the alcohol.

Following an overdose of paracetamol, there are four recognisable stages:

- *First 24 hours*: the patient experiences anorexia, nausea, vomiting and sweating. Results of biochemical tests are often normal.
- *24–72 hours*: the patient may become asymptomatic or may experience upper right quadrant pain.
- *72–96 hours*: there is clinical deterioration, with gastrointestinal bleeding, coagulopathy (deranged blood clotting), hypoglycaemia, renal failure and electrolyte imbalance. This is due to liver failure, and is the stage when death can occur.
- *After 96 hours*: recovery.

Mr Jones will be given an antidote to paracetamol. Antidotes include methionine and the more commonly used acetylcysteine (Parvolex®). Acetylcysteine protects against liver damage if it is given within 8 hours; it reacts with the toxic breakdown products of paracetamol, thus preventing them from damaging the liver. There have been no deaths among patients given acetylcysteine within 16 hours of paracetamol ingestion (Hersh *et al.*, 2000). Acetylcysteine can also be administered beyond 24 hours, although the effect then may not be as beneficial (Hamm, 2000).

According to the history taken in the emergency department, Mr Jones took the paracetamol 8 hours before admission. If he has taken all 50 tablets from the bottle, then he has ingested a total of 25 g of paracetamol (over three times the maximum daily dosage). On arrival he would have blood taken for paracetamol levels and international normalised ratio (INR), among other tests; he would also be commenced on acetylcysteine in advance of the test results (University Hospitals of Leicester, 2005).

The INR is a measure of blood clotting time. It is the ratio of the patient's clotting time against a control clotting time – if the control sample clots in 10 seconds and the patient's sample clots in 20 seconds, then the INR is 2.0. The factors within the blood that control clotting times are manufactured within the liver, and therefore an extended clotting time (shown by a raised INR) is an early indication of liver damage. Mr Jones will then need blood tests at least daily while he is an inpatient to determine whether liver damage has occurred.

Potential long-term consequences of paracetamol overdose

Paracetamol in the recommended dosage is a safe and effective analgesic. However, an overdose can have serious long-term consequences, as the function of the liver can be affected to the point where hepatic failure requiring liver transplant is required.

Mr Jones insists that his overdose was accidental. Nurses have to use interpersonal skills and clinical judgement to determine the veracity of this claim. On balance, it may be difficult to argue that 50 tablets and a bottle of spirits are taken by accident. It is, however, possible that Mr Jones may not be aware of the possible consequences of what he has taken.

Cries for help versus attempted suicide

Regardless of whether it is determined that the overdose was a genuine attempt of Mr Jones to kill himself, it is important that the nurse's personal values are not allowed to affect how care is delivered. Many religions identify suicide as a sin. If the nurse believes that Mr Jones has committed a mortal sin by attempting to kill himself, then it would be inappropriate to make this apparent to the patient. It is the duty of the nurse to be non-judgemental, and actions and behaviours that are guided by personal beliefs, including religious tenets, should not be made overt to the patient. For many nurses, the reality of this is asking a patient whether they wish to see a religious advisor.

In most cases where an attempt has been made at self-harm, the patient is referred to the deliberate self-harm team or a psychiatrist if there is not a specific team. Patients who have taken a decision to harm themselves by taking an overdose are referred for advice and counselling, which may be from specialist nurses trained in deliberate self-harm counselling.

Control and restraint

Mr Jones had made clear from the outset his intention to leave the ward. Such situations can be difficult for the nurse. Most general nurses have neither the training nor the experience to restrain a patient safely and legally. In the event that a patient physically assaults another patient, a visitor or a member of staff, it is acceptable for physical force to be used to restrain the individual. However, it is less clear-cut whether a patient who is threatening to leave an area against medical advice can be restrained. There are guidelines within hospitals that must be adhered to, but the general principle is that, in law, nurses have no right physically to prevent a patient from leaving a ward. Reasoning and discussion are to be encouraged, however. A highly relevant piece of legislation is the Mental Capacity Act (2005), which gives clear guidance as to when an individual does and does not have the capacity to make their own decisions.

Confidentiality

Mr Jones has stated clearly that he does not want his next of kin to be informed of his admission. As he is over the age of 18 years, and therefore an adult, nurses are professionally bound to comply with his request.

Reflection point 17.7

You are caring for a patient, and both you and the patient are aware that he is terminally ill. The patient asks you to promise not to tell anyone and then informs you of his intention to commit suicide upon discharge from hospital. He intends to do this because he wishes to die with dignity at a time of his choosing rather than risk pain and loss of dignity. How would you respond?

Under the NMC Code, you have an obligation to respect the patient's confidentiality. However, it is illegal to assist in a suicide, and potentially you could be implicated in his death if he commits suicide after informing you of his intention. The advice of a senior member of staff should always be sought in such situations, and you should avoid promising the patient confidentiality under such circumstances.

SUMMARY

- To provide effective care, the multiprofessional team needs to work across health and social care boundaries.
- When caring for a patient with a terminal (or any other) prognosis, the nurse must remember their own needs for support.
- Ethically, it is not always possible to meet the requests that patients may make.

CONCLUSION

As can be seen from these scenarios, caring for patients creates many challenges – not only those presented by the physical condition of the patient, but also those presented by the psychosocial condition of the patient and the demands of differing cultural expectations.

It is important to note that although each of the patients in the scenarios above required very different care, some general principles apply to every patient that the nurse has cared for and will care for:

- the need for comprehensive and ongoing assessment;
- the need for evidence-based care, i.e. why are we doing this?
- the effective working of the multiprofessional team;
- planning for the patient's discharge from the point of admission.

This chapter has examined how the nurse meets the needs of the patients in the scenarios and related this to the competencies required for entry to the nursing register. Each of the competencies

CONCLUSION (continued)

applies in each of the scenarios, either implicitly or explicitly. The competencies act as a framework within which practice develops.

Applicability of the NMC competencies to practice

Each of the competencies can be applied to each of the patients, and the following makes the relationship between practice and the competencies explicit.

NMC competency 1 requires that a nurse act in accordance with the NMC Code – that the nurse recognises her own limitations. The scenarios show clearly that there is a need to hand elements of the patient's care over to other professionals when the knowledge required is not that of nurses. Also apparent in the scenarios is the necessity of acknowledging limitations within nursing practice or knowledge. There is no harm in saying 'I don't know, but I'll find out', whereas mishandling a communication or a procedure can do irreparable harm. The need to maintain confidentiality and act in the patient's interest appears clear-cut when written down, but, as demonstrated by Mrs Patel's scenario, the situation can be less clear when applied to a person in real life. The need to practise in fair and antidiscriminatory ways, and to acknowledge differences in belief and culture, can also be more difficult in reality. The majority of trained nurses within the NHS are white, but in some areas of the UK the patient caseload can be very different; for example, in the city of Leicester 25.7 per cent of the population is of Indian origin (OPCS, 2001). To this end, it is important that nurses take the opportunity to study the culture of the communities for which they care.

NMC competency 2 concerns care delivery, with each of the eight categories being interdependent. The need to develop a therapeutic relationship is central to all the scenarios in this chapter. In some cases, the nurse may find that an effective therapeutic relationship eludes them. It would be wrong for the nurse automatically to assume that they are a poor nurse; rather, they should consider whether they could have tried a different approach and review whether other patient interactions are more effective. (If none of the nurse's interactions leads to an effective therapeutic relationship, then possibly the problem lies with the nurse and urgent clinical supervision or guidance needs to be sought.)

The need to promote well-being and health is central to Mrs Smith's care in Scenario 17.2. The information can be provided and advice given, but the nurse can only advise, not compel. By providing a supportive, non-threatening environment when caring for the patient, by building up the therapeutic relationship and by providing practical help (e.g. advice on how to obtain nicotine replacement patches), advice for health promotion is more likely to be received positively by the patient.

The need for accurate assessment, care-planning and documentation is central to effective care delivery for all patients (see also Chapter 14). Accurate documentation not only facilitates the effective delivery of care by the members of the multiprofessional team but also permits retrospective assessment of care provision. Such retrospective examination of documentation may be for audit or research purposes or to facilitate investigation of a complaint.

The use of evidence-based nursing practice and sound clinical judgement are key elements of patient care in all three scenarios in this chapter, since, without the evidence base and the clinical judgement, how is it possible for the assessment and care-planning process to take place?

NMC competency 3 concerns care management. The four elements within this category are interdependent. The provision of accurate documentation, across interprofessional boundaries, is also an example of risk management.

Demonstration of the key skills of literacy and numeracy is central to effective communication. The best care plan in the world is of no use if the nurse taking over care provision cannot read it.

NMC competency 4 concerns personal and professional development. These areas are not explicit in the scenarios in this chapter, however; for a professional nurse, such ongoing development should be implicit in all interactions in the workplace. Nursing is about caring for and working with people; each person is unique, which makes each interaction slightly different. Because of this uniqueness, there is an opportunity to learn and reflect – perhaps by asking whether a situation

CONCLUSION (continued)

have been handled any differently. Much of this reflection is informal but nonetheless is an opportunity to develop.

The utilisation of a clinical supervisor is to be recommended, as this provides the option of more formalised reflection while maintaining the confidentiality of the patient–nurse interaction.

Leadership is not the domain of the ward sister or the matron. Leadership is a characteristic that every registered nurse can display. The nurse provides leadership and learning opportunities to the patient, if that is what the relationship requires. Also, the nurse provides leadership and guidance to health care assistants and students in a team and helps to create an environment that is conducive to learning and caring.

Although the competencies inform and underpin the practice of every registered nurse, it is the unique personal and professional characteristics of that nurse, their interpersonal skills, their enthusiasm and their ability to care about the work that they do that patients will respond to. In short, it is about wanting to do a good job and enjoying the work.

References

Acheson D (1998). *Independent Inquiry into Inequalities in Health*. London: HMSO.

Age Concern (2006). *Hungry to be Heard*. London: Age Concern.

Brandt P and Weiner C (1998). Children's mental health in families experiencing multiple sclerosis. *Journal of Family Nursing*, **4**, 41–64.

British Heart Foundation (2007). *Cardiac Rehabilitation . . . Recovery or By-Pass: The Evidence*. London: British Heart Foundation.

Chiles JA and Strosahl KD (1995). *The Suicidal Patient: Principles of Assessment, Treatment, and Case Management*. Washington, DC: American Psychiatric press.

Cook DG and Strachen DP (1997). Review: parental tobacco smoke increases the risk of asthma and respiratory symptoms in school age children. *Evidence-Based Nursing*, **3**, 86.

Department of Health (DH) (1998). *Paediatric Intensive Care: A Framework for the Future*. London: HMSO.

Department of Health (DH) (1999). *National Service Framework for Mental Health*. London: HMSO.

Department of Health (DH) (2000a). *National Service Framework for Coronary Heart Disease*. London: HMSO.

Department of Health (DH) (2001a). *The Essence of Care: Patient-Focused Benchmarking for Health Care Practitioners*. London: HMSO.

Department of Health (DH) (2000b). *The NHS Plan*. London: HMSO.

Department of Health (DH) (2000c). *NHS Cancer Plan*. London: HMSO.

Department of Health (DH) (2001b). *National Service Framework for Older People*. London: HMSO.

Department of Health (DH) (2001c). *Good Practice in Consent Implementation Guide: Consent to Examination or Treatment*. London: HMSO.

Department of Health (DH) (2001d). *National Service Framework for Diabetes*. London: HMSO.

Department of Health (DH) (2004). *National Service Framework for Renal Services*. London: HMSO.

Department of Health (DH) (2005). *National Service Framework for Long-Term Conditions*. London: HMSO.

Department of Health (DH) (2006). *A New Ambition for Old Age: Next Steps in Implementing the National Service Framework for Older People*. London: HMSO.

Department of Health (DH) (2007a). *Chief Executive Bulletin, 8 February*. London: Department of Health.

Department of Health (DH) (2007b). *Essence of Care: Benchmarks for the Care Environment*. London: HMSO.

Department of Health (DH) (2008). *National Service Framework for Chronic Obstructive Pulmonary Disease*. London: HMSO.

Flint C (2005). Speech by Caroline Flint MP, Parliamentary Under Secretary of State for Public Health: UK EU Presidency Summit: Tackling Health Inequalities – Governing for Health 18 October 2005. www.dh.gov.uk/en/News/Speeches/Speecheslist/DH_4124219.

Gibson PG, Coughlan J, Wilson AJ, *et al*. (1998). Review: self management education for adults with asthma improves health outcomes. *Evidence-Based Nursing*, **1**, 117.

Global Initiative for Obstructive Lung Disease (GOLD) (2001). The Phase III Gold Initiative. www.goldcopd.com.

Hamm J (2000). Acute acetaminophen overdose in adolescents and adults. *Critical Care Nurse*, **20**, 69–74.

Hawton K and Fagg J (1992). Deliberate self poisoning and self-injury in adolescents. *British Journal of Psychiatry*, **161**, 816–23.

Health Development Agency (2005). Guidance for Smokefree Hospital Trusts. www.nice.org.uk/aboutnice/whoweare/aboutthehda/hdapublications/guidance_for_smokefree_hospital_trusts.jsp.

Health Education Authority (1998). *The UK Smoking Epidemic: Deaths in 1995*. London: Health Education Authority.

Hersh EV, Moore PA and Ros GL (2000). Over-the-counter analgesics and antipyretics: a critical assessment. *Clinical Therapeutics*, **22**, 500–48.

Information Centre (2006). Latest NHS Stop Smoking Figures. www.ic.nhs.uk.

Lancaster T, Stead L, Silagy C and Sowden A (2000). Review: advice from doctors, counselling by nurses, behavioural interventions, nicotine replacement therapy and several pharmacological treatments increase smoking cessation rates. *Evidence-Based Nursing*, **4**, 13.

Leidy NK and Haase JE (1999). Patients with chronic obstructive pulmonary disease experienced ongoing challenges of preserving their personal integrity. *Evidence-Based Nursing*, **2**, 135.

Lewin R (1997). Psychological guidelines for cardiac rehabilitation. In Thompson DR, De Bono D and Hopkins A (eds) (1997). *Guidelines for Cardiac Rehabilitation*. London: National Institute of Nursing and the Royal College of Physicians of London.

Lewin R, Ingelton I, Newens AJ and Thompson DR (1998). Adherence to cardiac rehabilitation guidelines: a survey of rehabilitation programmes in the United Kingdom. *British Medical Journal*, **316**, 1354–5.

Mann JJ (2002). A current perspective of suicide and attempted suicide. *Annals of Internal Medicine*, **136**, 302–11.

McLaughlin C (1994). Casualty nurses' attitudes to attempted suicide. *Journal of Advanced Nursing,* **20**, 1111–18.

National Institute for Health and Clinical Excellence (NICE) (2006). *Brief Interventions and Referral for Smoking Cessation in Primary Care and Other Settings.* London: National Institute for Health and Clinical Excellence.

Nursing and Midwifery Council (NMC) (2004). *Requirements for Pre-Registration Nursing Programmes.* London: Nursing and Midwifery Council.

Nursing and Midwifery Council (NMC) (2008). *The Code: Standards of Conduct, Performance and Ethics for Nurses and Midwives.* London: Nursing and Midwifery Council.

Office of Population Censuses and Surveys (OPCS) (1980). *Classification of Occupations 1980.* London: HMSO.

Office of Population Censuses and Surveys (OPCS) (2001). *General Household Survey England and Wales.* London: Office of Population Censuses and Surveys.

Parkes CM (1986). *Bereavement.* London: Penguin.

Ring L and Davidson E (1997). Patients' experiences of longterm home oxygen therapy. *Journal of Advanced Nursing,* **26**, 337–44.

Roper N, Logan W and Tierney AJ (2000). *The Roper Logan–Tierney Model of Nursing: Based on Activities of Living.* Edinburgh: Churchill Livingstone.

Rose D (2007). Nurses leave for Australia in thousands as NHS halts recruitment. *The Times,* 17 February 2007.

Schnyder U, Valach L, Bichel K and Michel K (1999). Attempted suicide: do we understand the patients' reasons? *General Hospital Psychiatry,* **21**, 62–9.

Scottish Executive (2001). *Our National Health: A Plan for Action, a Plan for Change.* Edinburgh: Scottish Executive.

Scottish Executive (2002a). *Scottish Diabetes Framework.* Edinburgh: Scottish Executive.

Scottish Executive (2002b). *Coronary Heart Disease and Stroke Strategy.* Edinburgh: Scottish Executive.

Thompson DR, Bowman GS, Kitson AL, de Bono DP and Hopkins A (1997). Cardiac rehabilitation services in England and Wales: a national survey. *International Journal of Cardiology,* **59**, 299–304.

Tod AM, Wadsworth E, Asif S and Gerrish K (2001). Cardiac rehabilitation: the needs of south Asian cardiac patients. *British Journal of Nursing,* **10**, 1028–33.

Tudor Hart HJ (1971). The inverse care law. *Lancet,* **1**, 405–12.

University Hospitals of Leicester NHS Trust (2005). *Clinical Guidelines.* Leicester: Medical Directorate, University Hospitals of Leicester NHS Trust.

Wallace C, Dargan P and Jones A (2002). Paracetamol overdose: an evidence based flowchart to guide management. *Emergency Medicine Journal,* **19**, 202–5.

West R (2004). *Rehabilitation after Myocardial Infarction: Multicentre Randomised Controlled Trial.* London: Department of Health.

Wiklander M, Samuelsson M and Asberg M (2003). Shame reactions after suicide attempt. *Scandinavian Journal of Caring Sciences,* **17**, 293–300.

World Health Organization (WHO) (1993). Cardiac rehabilitation and secondary prevention: long term care for patients with ischaemic heart disease. Briefing letter, regional office for Europe, Copenhagen, Denmark.

Wise J (1997). Patients go hungry in British hospitals. *British Medical Journal*, **314**, 399.

Zahlis EH (2001). The child's worries about the mother's breast cancer: sources of distress in school-age children. *Oncology Nursing Forum*, **28**, 1019–25.

Further reading

Dimond B (1999). Patient confidentiality. *British Journal of Nursing*, **8**, 9–18.
A series of articles that address many of the issues raised by patient confidentiality. The author is a barrister and makes a complex area intelligible.

Dougherty L and Lister S (2004). *The Royal Marsden Hospital Manual of Clinical Nursing Procedures*, 6th edn. London: Blackwell Science.
This manual gives the latest evidence-based procedures for high-quality patient-focused care. A valuable resource for both the student and the experienced nurse.

Hampton JR (2003). *The ECG Made Easy*, 6th edn. Edinburgh: Churchill Livingstone.
A slim but useful volume, which really does make the ECG easy.

Tortora GJ and Derrickson B (2006). *Principles of Anatomy and Physiology*, 11th edn. Hoboken, NJ: John Wiley & Sons.
A thorough grounding in aspects of both anatomy and physiology applied to clinical practice.

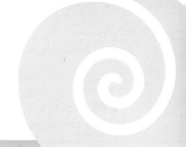

Long-term health needs and rehabilitation

18

Jacqueline Elton and Judith Evans

Introduction

This chapter considers long-term health and rehabilitation needs by comparing and contrasting the needs of a younger and an older individual following a stroke. The two scenarios follow the care of an older couple and a younger family. Through these two families, the chapter examines how government policy affects the service that these individuals receive and explores the physical and psychological care that they require.

It is important to be aware that, although chronic disability affects predominately elderly people, younger individuals may also have chronic disability. Stroke can affect individuals of any age, including fetuses.

The care needs of the two families will be linked to the competencies required of the registered nurse (NMC, 2004) (Appendix 2).

Learning objectives

After studying this chapter you should be able to:
- identify the number of people with long-term needs and the numerous health, social and financial problems that they and their families face;
- understand the importance of being able to communicate effectively;
- understand the importance of interdisciplinary teamworking in relation to care management;
- gain an insight into how a balance between risk and safety impacts on rehabilitation potential;
- understand the importance of carer support;
- identify the difference between rehabilitation and intermediate care;
- understand the impact of government policy and legislation on patient care and the difficulties faced by the agencies involved in commissioning care;
- explain how and why readmission to hospital can and should be avoided.

Government policy and long-term conditions

When considering any aspect of long-term care and rehabilitation, it is important to place it in the context of our ageing population. In 2007 there were more people over the age of 65 years than under the age of 18 years, and people aged over 85 years form the fastest-growing segment of the population, set to double by 2020 (DH, 2006a). Older people also make up the largest single group of people using the national health service (NHS). People aged over 65 years account for two-thirds of hospital patients and 40 per cent of all admissions (DH, 2000).

It is against these pressures and those identified in Chapter 17 that the NHS Plan (DH, 2000, 2002) and the National Service Framework (NSF) for Older People (DH, 2001b) have been produced to improve and raise standards of care and service for older people. The document *A New Ambition for Old Age* (DH, 2006a) has been produced to continue the changes identified within the original NSF for Older People.

In addition to this, in 2005 the Department of Health (DH) launched the *National Service Framework for Long-Term Conditions* (DH, 2005). This NSF aims primarily to address the long-term needs of patients with neurological conditions. However, the NSF makes explicit that stroke for people of all ages is covered by the NSF for Older People and, although the NSF for Long-Term Conditions focuses on people with neurological conditions, much of the guidance contained within it can be applied to anyone with a long-term condition. A list of other publications related to care for people with long-term conditions can be found on the DH website (www.dh.gov.uk).

The NHS Plan (DH, 2000) notes the need to ensure dignity, security and independence in old age and intends to do this by the following means:

- *Assuring standards of care*: the National Care Standards Commission (NCSC) targets standards of care within domiciliary and residential care, while the NSF for Older People sets out standards for services including stroke, falls and mental health problems (all of which could be relevant to any person with a long-term condition). The NSF for Older People is intended to be a 10-year programme to address the needs of older people.
- *Extending access to services*: this includes individuals being able to access extended health screening in order to identify potential problems. It also includes the introduction of the single assessment process; this process consists of producing one joint assessment for each individual with complex needs, to include both health and social care requirements, and which, in theory, will streamline and speed up the process whereby each person's needs are addressed. Currently the introduction of the single assessment process is not universal. There will also be greater involvement of carers in the care-planning process. The personal care plan will be held by the patient or client, or their carer, and will hold details of both the health and social care aspects of the package.
- *Promoting independence*: the plan identifies the need for people to be able to maintain independence with good-quality ongoing support at home rather than moving into institutional care. The plan also identifies both the finance and the need to extend intermediate care and rehabilitation services. Intermediate care is non-acute care, where the patient has no acute illness requiring medical intervention but needs intensive nursing or therapy interventions over a short period to enable them to regain an improved level of functioning. It is typically nursing- or therapy-led. Such interventions can reduce so-called 'bed-blocking' – when a person with no acute medical or nursing requirements occupies an acute bed because, for example, they are waiting for equipment to be fitted at home or to be offered a place in a residential home or community hospital.
- *Ensuring fairness in funding*: if an individual needs to go into a residential or nursing home, the situation regarding funding (i.e. who pays) has long been confusing and complicated. For example, a person receiving nursing care in an NHS hospital does not pay for that care, but they would have to pay for the same care in a residential or nursing home. The plan will make the system fairer by ensuring that all nursing care is funded – although individuals may still have to fund personal elements of care, unless they qualify for social services funding. To assist social services in establishing and commissioning the amount and type of care needed, an assessment known as a 'registered nurse care contribution' (RNCC) is undertaken. Completion of the RNCC assessment establishes whether full nursing care may be required, either at home or in a nursing home. This triggers a second assessment known as a 'continuing health care' (CHC) assessment, which identifies whether the person is entitled to have this care funded by the NHS.

The *NSF for Older People* is a key document that enables elements of the national plan to become a reality. It specifically addresses those conditions that are significant to older people and that have not been addressed by other NSFs. The *NSF for Older People* has eight standards:

- *Standard 1 – rooting out age discrimination*: NHS services will be provided, regardless of age, on the basis of clinical need alone. Social care services will not use age in their eligibility criteria or policies to restrict access to services. The DH (2007) notes that hospitals and social services have reviewed policies and procedures to ensure that they are non-discriminatory but that changing implicit rather than explicit discrimination is a longer-term issue.
- *Standard 2 – person-centred care*: NHS and social care services treat older people as individuals and enable them to make choices about their own care. This is achieved through the single assessment process, integrated commissioning arrangements and integrated provision of services, including community equipment and continence services. At this point, progress against the standard is variable (DH, 2007).
- *Standard 3 – intermediate care*: older people will have access to a range of new intermediate care services at home or in designated care settings in order to promote their independence by providing enhanced services from the NHS and councils to prevent unnecessary hospital admission and providing effective rehabilitation services to enable early discharge from hospital and thus prevent premature or unnecessary admission to long-term residential care. The DH (2007) notes that there has been an increase in the provision of intermediate care facilities.
- *Standard 4 – general hospital care*: older people's care in hospital is delivered through appropriate specialist care and by hospital staff who have the right sets of skills to meet their needs. Almost three-quarters of hospitals have specialist multiprofessional teams for the elderly (DH, 2007).
- *Standard 5 – stroke*: the NHS will take action to prevent strokes, working in partnership with other agencies where appropriate. People who are thought to have had a stroke have access to diagnostic services, are treated appropriately by a specialist stroke service, and subsequently, with their carers, participate in a multiprofessional programme of secondary prevention and rehabilitation. This standard shows progress in a number of areas, with a decreased average length of stay. There has also been an overall increase in the number of specialist stroke units, although only 36 per cent of patients who have had a stroke spend time on such a unit (DH 2007).
- *Standard 6 – falls*: this states that the NHS will work in partnership with councils in order to take action to prevent falls and reduce resultant fractures or other injuries in their populations of older people. Older people who have fallen will receive effective treatment and, with their carers, receive advice on prevention through a specialist falls service. There is some progress against this standard, but, again, it is identified as being patchy (DH, 2007).
- *Standard 7 – mental health in older people*: older people who have mental health problems have access to integrated mental health services, provided by the NHS and councils, to ensure effective diagnosis, treatment, and support for them and their carers. The DH (2007) identifies patchy progress against this standard, noting a serious lack of suitable care homes.
- *Standard 8 – promotion of health and active life in older age*: the health and well-being of older people are promoted through a coordinated programme of action led by the NHS, with support from councils.

For the purpose of this chapter, standard 5 relating to stroke care is most directly applicable.

Case studies of two families

Scenarios 18.1 and 18.2 are an amalgam of many individuals whom the authors have nursed rather than specific individuals. The progress of the families over the period covered within this chapter will enable the reader to appreciate the complexities that can ensue as illness becomes chronic and the ability of the family unit to function is impaired or ceases. As nurses, we typically see a person in one setting (e.g. hospital) for a fixed period of time, at which point either the patient or the nurse moves on. It is important to realise that patients whom the nurse meets for a single episode of care have a life both before the nurse meets them and (we hope) after leaving the nurse's care.

SCENARIO 18.1

Mr and Mrs White have been married for 60 years, Mr White is a retired bus driver and is 79 years old. Mrs White is 78 years old; she used to work as a secretary in the 1950s but has not had regular paid work outside the family home since then. Mrs White has always performed all of the housework, cooking and cleaning; Mr White believes that such tasks are the woman's and declares that he is unable even to boil an egg. They own their own two-bedroom semi-detached house that has the bathroom and toilet upstairs, adjacent to the master bedroom.

They have two children. Their son, Tony White (aged 53 years), lives 40 miles away, is married with a 10-year-old daughter and works in sales. Their daughter, Grace Smith (aged 55 years), is married with three young children and lives locally (a 20-minute drive away).

SCENARIO 18.2

Mr and Mrs Black have been married for 16 years. Mr Black is 41 years old and works as a travelling salesman. Mrs Black is 38 years old and works part time as a teacher. They have two children, a daughter, Sadie, aged 13 years, and a son, James, aged 9 years. Mr and Mrs Black share the domestic and childcare duties. Mr Black often takes James to the local football ground, where they are both supporters and where James plays for the local junior team.

They have a large mortgage on a four-bedroom house, with a toilet and shower room downstairs and a bathroom and en suite shower upstairs.

Mrs Black's elderly parents live 8 miles away, and the Blacks visit them regularly. Mr Black's parents both died from coronary heart disease when he was a child.

Month 1: Mrs White

Mrs White collapses one evening while doing the washing up. Several hours before collapsing, she complained to her husband that she was feeling dizzy and had a headache, but she put the symptoms down to getting a cold.

Mr White called an ambulance. Mrs White was admitted to the stroke unit at their local hospital following assessment in the accident and emergency (A&E) department, where a left cerebrovascular accident (CVA) resulting in a right-sided hemiplegia was diagnosed.

Mrs White's speech and swallowing were unaffected, but on arrival at the stroke unit she was incontinent of urine, had no movement in her right arm and had only a small amount of movement in her right leg.

Month 1: Mr Black

Mr Black had recently been suffering intermittent bouts of chest pain, which he put down to indigestion due to stress, erratic eating patterns and poor diet.

One evening, while Mrs Black was marking papers in the study, she heard a noise. On investigation, she found Mr Black collapsed on the floor in the lounge.

Mrs Black called an ambulance. She arranged for her neighbour to come in to sit with the children while she accompanied Mr Black to the hospital. He was also diagnosed with a left CVA resulting in a right-sided hemiplegia. Mr Black's speech and swallowing were unaffected and he had a small amount of movement in his right leg.

What is a stroke?

A CVA, or stroke, occurs when the blood supply to part of the brain is interrupted, causing damage and death to an area of the brain. There are two major types of stroke – ischaemic and haemorrhagic.

In an *ischaemic stroke* the blood supply to part of the brain becomes occluded or blocked. The ischaemia or blockage may be due to either thrombosis or embolism. In a *thrombotic ischaemic stroke*, the blood vessel within the brain becomes blocked, often due to atherosclerosis. In an *embolic stroke*, the blood clot travels from elsewhere in the body and blocks the vessel in the brain; for example, the patient may have a pulmonary embolus (blood clot in the lung), part of which breaks away from the main clot and travels to the brain, causing the stroke.

Haemorrhagic stroke occurs when a vessel within the brain ruptures, causing leakage of blood into the brain (intracerebral haemorrhage) or into the membranes surrounding the brain (subarachnoid haemorrhage).

Stroke is the biggest single cause of severe disability and the third most common cause of death in the UK (DH, 2001b). Each year in England and Wales, 130 000 people have a stroke; there are 87 700 first strokes and 53 700 recurrent strokes – the equivalent of someone having a stoke every 5 minutes (Office of National Statistics, 2001). Although CVA affects predominately older people, it also affects a significant number of younger people: every year, 10 000 people under the age of 55 years and 1000 people under the age of 30 years have a CVA (DH, 2001b).

The degree of damage and eventual disability caused by the CVA depends on the area of the brain that is affected. It is important to remember that the right side of the brain controls the left side of the body, and vice versa (Tortora and Derrickson, 2006). Stroke arguably has a greater disability impact than any other chronic disease (Adamson *et al.*, 2004).

Risk factors

A large number of risk factors increase the risk of having a stroke, including:

- atherosclerosis;
- hypertension;
- transient ischaemic attack;
- atrial fibrillation;
- diabetes;
- previous stroke;
- increasing age;

- positive family history;
- smoking;
- obesity (Hickey, 1992).

Note that this list is not exhaustive.

Diagnosis

The diagnosis of stroke is made by medical staff. When Mrs White and Mr Black arrive in A&E, they will have baseline observations (blood pressure, temperature, respiratory rate, pulse) taken, and routine blood tests such as urea and electrolytes (U&E) and full blood count (FBC) (see Chapter 17). A complete physical examination will be undertaken by the doctor to reveal the extent of the neurological deficit and to give the initial diagnosis of stroke.

The National Clinical Guidelines for Stroke (RCP, 2004) recommend that brain imaging (computed tomography (CT) scanning) should be undertaken as soon as possible after the onset of symptoms in all patients, and within 24 hours at most, unless there are good clinical reasons for not doing so. This is in order to confirm the diagnosis and to determine both the location and the extent of the damage. On some occasions, CT scanning will not detect the stroke, in which case a magnetic resonance imaging (MRI) scan may be undertaken.

Assessment and care

The only medication that is prescribed routinely in stroke is aspirin 300 mg, provided that the medical staff decide that the stroke is unlikely to be haemorrhagic in origin. In the early stages of the admission, much of the assessment and care are aimed at both stabilising the patient's condition and establishing the degree of resulting disability. The nurse will need to fully assess the patient's needs using a recognised assessment tool or set of criteria.

The nurse on the stroke unit assesses Mr Black's and Mrs White's condition using the Roper–Logan–Tierney Activities of Daily Living (ADL) model (Table 18.1, p. 398–9) (Roper, 2000; Roper *et al.*, 1996). Following this assessment, the nurse will need to ensure that both nutritional status and risk factors for pressure area breakdown are assessed formally.

Continence care

Neither patient had continence problems before their stroke. It is important that a full assessment is carried out in order to identify the type and, if possible, cause of any incontinence in order that it can be treated appropriately. *The National Clinical Guidelines for Stroke* (RCP, 2004) state that management of both bowel and bladder problems should be seen as an essential part of the patient's rehabilitation and recommend that all qualified nurses should be able to assess incontinent patients and know who to contact for advice and support. It is important that this problem is addressed promptly as there is considerable evidence that incontinence has a negative effect on a person's social and emotional well-being (Norton, 1986; Grimby, 1993; Harris, 1999; Lee, 2004).

When a patient is admitted to hospital, it is usual to test their urine, because many potential or actual problems can be detected. When the nurse obtains the sample, it should be checked visually. Is it clear or cloudy, pale or dark? Cloudy urine may indicate infection, while very dark urine may indicate highly concentrated urine, which may be due to dehydration or poor renal function. Does the urine smell? A fishy odour is a good indication of infected urine. The urine is usually tested with a urine dipstick that changes colour in the presence of, among others, glucose (indicating possible diabetes), ketones (indicating possible diabetes or prolonged fasting), nitrates and leucocytes (indicating possible infection) and blood (indicating possible infection – for females, it is important to ask whether they are menstruating before assuming infection). If a potential infection is indicated, a sample (midstream sample of urine; MSU) is sent for culture and sensitivity – the microbiology department attempts to grow bacteria from the sample and, if they do grow, to identify the bacteria and determine which antibiotics they are sensitive to in order to facilitate effective treatment.

Mrs White's urine sample did not indicate any infection, and she did not report any discomfort on passing water (another potential indicator of infection). She knows when she needs to go to the toilet, and thus it is probable that her loss of mobility is preventing her from getting to the toilet and causing her incontinence. This type of difficulty is referred to as 'functional incontinence', because the problem is in the physical act of getting to the appropriate place and removing clothing in order to urinate appropriately rather than with the urinary tract itself.

As with any other form of incontinence, a complete assessment to establish the cause of the functional incontinence is required (Vickerman, 2002). Once it has been established clearly that the difficulty is due to the loss of mobility, then steps need to be taken to manage the problem in a way that is acceptable to both Mrs White and her family. There are a number of ways to manage urinary incontinence, including:

- catheterisation;
- relevant aids, e.g. pads, convenes or special underwear;
- bladder retraining.

Arguably it is likely to be easier to manage any functional incontinence for Mr Black than for Mrs White because he can use a urinal. Female urinals are available, but they are more difficult to use successfully.

Catheterisation involves passing a thin tube, or catheter, into the bladder (usually via the urethra). Such a device can be temporary and removed as soon as the bladder has been emptied, or it can be longer term, being held in place by a small balloon at the tip of the catheter, which is inflated to prevent it from falling out. Catheterisation is still a relatively common practice in hospitals, but it should be avoided wherever possible because of the associated risks of infection. Urinary tract infections (UTIs) represent 19.7 per cent of all health-care-associated infections, and some 60 per cent of these are related to catheter insertion (Smyth, 2006). Even more alarmingly, 1–4 per cent of catheterised patients with UTI develop bacteraemia, of whom 13–30 per cent die (Ward *et al.*, 1997).

Relevant aids include the following:

- *Absorbent pads*: these can be worn inside adapted underwear to hold both urinary and faecal soiling. Many pads have a gel core that draws the fluid away from the skin, thereby reducing the risk of skin breakdown and containing both odour and fluid. They come in a wide variety of sizes and absorbencies; the smaller sizes are relatively unobtrusive.
- *Convenes*: these devices may be used by male patients. A convene is a sheath that is placed over the penis and attached to a urine bag by a tube.
- *Underwear with built-in continence pads*: these items can be washed in a washing machine. They are easier for the patient to manipulate, but they may not be as effective as disposable pads.

Bladder retraining can be used if the problem is one of habit or muscle weakness. In Mrs White's case, the cause is due to her lack of mobility; it would not be appropriate to pass a

Table 18.1 Nursing assessments for Mrs White and Mr Black

Activity of living	Mrs White		Mr Black	
	Usual routine	Actual/potential problems	Usual routine	Actual/potential problems
Communication	Says she usually wears glasses and that her hearing is excellent	Mrs White is alert, oriented and responding to questions appropriately; speech does not seem slurred	Says he wears glasses only for reading and driving and has no problems with hearing	Mr Black is alert, orientated and responding to questions appropriately; speech does not seem slurred
Breathing	Says she sometimes has a touch of bronchitis in the winter; she is a non-smoker	Respiratory rate 12/min; no coughing; does not appear distressed	Says he does not have a history of respiratory problems but smokes 40 cigarettes/day	Respiratory rate 16/min; has cough on waking; may need assistance to give up smoking
Eating and drinking	Says she has a good appetite: cereal for breakfast, sandwich at dinner and cooks hot meal for her and her husband in the evening; no alcohol; she is overweight	Speech and swallowing are unaffected, as this was formally assessed in the A&E department	Says he does not eat breakfast, has lunch in transport cafes and has cooked meal with his family in the evening; has a glass of wine with his evening meal and another 6 units of alcohol with friends on weekend; he is obese	Speech and swallowing are unaffected, as this was formally assessed in the A&E department; may benefit from dietary advice
Eliminating	Usually fully continent; has to get up to use the toilet to pass water twice a night; bowels open three to four times a week	She is incontinent of urine, although she says she is aware of needing to go to the toilet; routine ward urine test is negative for signs of infection	Usually fully continent; no prostate problems; does not get up to pass urine at night; bowels open every morning	He is incontinent of urine, although he says he is aware of needing to go to the toilet; routine ward urine test is negative for signs of infection
Personal cleansing and dressing	Has a shower every morning at home	The condition of her skin is good, with the skin over all pressure areas intact	Has a shower every morning at home	The condition of his skin is good, with the skin over all pressure areas intact; has ruddy complexion
Body temperature	Reports her hands get very cold in the winter; otherwise no difficulties	On arrival on the ward, her temperature was 36.8°C	Does not experience any problems with body temperature	On arrival on the ward, his temperature was 36.5°C

Activity				
Mobilising	Usually walks independently around the house and upstairs; uses no walking aids and walks to the local shops twice a week (about half a mile each way)	She has no movement in her right arm and only minimal movement in her right leg: she can flex her hip and knee slightly but has no movement in her ankle and toes; she cannot lift her leg from the bed; her sitting balance is poor: she is flopping to the right	Walks independently; takes very little exercise; gets out of breath easily on exertion	Mr Black has no movement in his right arm and only minimal movement in his right leg: he can flex his hip and knee slightly and has slight movement in his ankle and toes; he cannot lift the leg from the bed; his sitting balance is variable
Working and playing	Usually plays bingo once a week when she goes to the local shops; enjoys pottering around the garden	Worried that she will not be able to help her husband with the garden	Works full time as a travelling salesman; earns basic wage plus commission; worried his employer may not keep his job open; worried about extra stress on wife; usually takes son to football on Wednesday evenings and matches on weekends; goes out for meal and drink with wife and friends on Saturday evenings	Does not appear to have considered the possibility of being unable to return to work yet; financial implications; worried he will not be able to take son to football and that this may affect their relationship; worried about how friends will view him
Expressing sexuality	Married for 60 years	Mr White is with his wife and she is expressing concerns about how he will cope at home – he is 'useless in the kitchen' and they have not spent a night apart since 1982	Mr Black is concerned to know whether the illness will affect his abilities to have sex with his wife	Mr Black is still a young man with an active sex life; once his abilities in this area are known, he may require advice and education on changes that he and his wife will need to consider in order to maintain intimate relations
Sleeping	Usually has a broken night as gets up to pass water a couple of times each night; does not take any night sedation; usually goes to bed at 10 p.m. and gets up at about 6 a.m.	Worried that her husband will not get to sleep with her away from home; concerned that the hospital will be too noisy for her to sleep	Sleeps soundly; has got used to sleeping away from home because of his job; goes to bed at 11.30 p.m. and gets up at 5 a.m.	Jokes that he could do with a rest
Dying	Says her friend, Mrs Mullins, had a stroke and died a few months later			Says that if he doesn't recover enough to go back to work, then he will be no use to his wife and family and would be better off dead, as he is well insured and at least they would have the insurance money

catheter, since if her medical condition is stable she can be assisted out of bed on to a commode or toilet, using a hoist until her mobility improves. Likewise, Mr Black can be given or assisted to use a urinal. These are examples of least intervention being the best.

Reflection point 18.1

You are a student on a general medical ward. The staff nurse you are working with tells you that she is going to catheterise a patient who is incontinent because it is going to be easier than taking her to the toilet.

How might you respond? What evidence could you use to try to persuade the staff nurse that there is another option?

Mobility

In both cases, a full manual handling assessment would be carried out by the ward nursing staff to address issues of safety for Mrs White and Mr Black and for the nursing staff. If the patient is not moved appropriately, then it is possible to cause further injury to the affected limbs, for example dislocation. Inappropriate manual handling can also cause injury to the nursing staff, with back injury being particularly prevalent.

A physiotherapist and occupational therapist will be involved as part of the multiprofessional team from the start of Mrs White's admission. The physiotherapist works on mobility issues, such as sitting balance, standing, transferring and walking. The occupational therapist works with Mrs White and her family to help her relearn the everyday tasks of self-care, teaching her how to get washed and dressed and how to prepare meals.

In addition to assessing and treating patients in hospital, physiotherapists and occupational therapists assess patients and then recommend and order equipment and adaptations that the patients need to ensure their safety and independence after discharge. Some of these aids are readily available; for example, most hospital physiotherapy departments can supply walking sticks to take home. Other equipment, such as hospital beds and raised toilet seats, have to be ordered, while home adaptations, such as an access ramp or a stair lift, require specific details and the involvement of the family or social services, thus making the process much more time-consuming (DH, 2006b).

The role of the nurse looking after Mrs White and Mr Black will be to continue to assist the patients as required and to monitor their medical conditions and ongoing abilities. This includes recording their vital signs, helping them to eat and drink, accurately recording their food and fluid intake, observing and recording their swallowing abilities, mood and eyesight, and assisting with and recording their abilities to carry out the therapeutic regimes that the physiotherapist and occupational therapist have initiated. For example, the occupational therapist assessed Mrs White for washing and dressing and found that she can wash her front with her left hand, but requires help to wash her back and legs.

If the nurse has a considerable workload in the morning, it can be tempting to wash Mrs White rather than help her to do so herself, as it is quicker. This is wholly inappropriate since, both the nursing competencies and the NMC Code (2008) (Appendix 1) are explicit that the nurse needs to work as part of a team and to act in the patient's best interest. If the nurse takes away the independence that the patient is attempting to regain, this is a clear breach of the spirit and the word of both documents. It is of paramount importance to ensure that clear communication occurs between staff, patients and families; phrases such as 'minimal assistance' do not help anyone to understand a patient's abilities.

Psychological care

Mrs White and Mr Black and their families require a great deal of support. As can be seen from their assessment, Mrs White's previous experience of stroke is limited to a friend who died, and Mr Black is concerned about being a burden rather than a provider for his family. Mrs White is concerned about spending time apart from her husband and is worried about his ability to cope in her absence. Mr Black is concerned about caring for his family financially. The NMC Code states that, as a registered nurse or midwife, you must 'work with others to protect and promote the health and wellbeing of those in your care, their families, and the wider community'. It could be argued that this means that the nurse also has a duty to ensure that Mr White's and Mrs Black's needs are met. The nurse will need to liaise with both families to see what help is available within the family and what assistance is required. In some cases, the nurse needs to ensure that a social worker becomes involved to arrange emergency care or financial advice for individuals when the main carer is taken ill.

Mr and Mrs White's daughter Grace is happy to visit her father each day and check he has food in the house that he can prepare. It is important for Mrs White's psychological well-being that she is confident that her husband can manage without her at home.

Mrs Black is able to arrange childcare and process the necessary claims to ensure their financial commitments are met. This will prevent Mr Black from worrying about losing his home.

Although Mrs White has not asked directly whether she will die, she will require reassurance that everything that can be done is being done. Likewise, Mr Black will need reassurance that he can still be a useful member of his family. This need for information extends to the rest of her family, but the nurse must remember that their duty of confidentiality lies with the patient. As such, it is appropriate to gain permission from Mrs White and Mr Black before speaking in depth to their relatives. The need to ensure that patients and relatives receive accurate information in a form that they can understand is explicit in the competencies.

Mr Black has a great need for psychological support, but its nature is likely to be different to that required by Mrs White and her family. The Black family have a large mortgage, which may or may not be covered while Mr Black is not working, depending on whether they have insurance. If the family have appropriate critical illness cover, then their mortgage may be paid off; if they do not have such cover, then there they may be anxious about continuing to pay for the house. Mr Black is likely to have only limited access to sick pay and therefore the household income will be drastically reduced.

Mr Black may be worried that he will lose his job if he is unable to return to work. He may need vocational rehabilitation advice (DH, 2005). Mrs Black will be trying to support her husband while he is in hospital and still maintain a normal routine for their children. In addition, she may be concerned that she is unable to visit and support her parents. The impact of parental ill health on the children must be considered; in this case, it is important to note that the illness is a sudden change and not something that the children have grown up with.

For both patients, communication is not a major issue as their speech has not been affected by the stroke. For many individuals who have had a stroke, however, particularly if the injury is to the left side of the brain, the ability to communicate is seriously impaired, further increasing the patient's isolation. It is important that the nurse does not assume that a patient who cannot speak also cannot hear or cannot understand. Each patient needs careful assessment, as patients who have had a stroke can develop expressive or receptive dysphasia. A patient with receptive dysphasia cannot understand what is being said to them, but they know what they want. A patient with expressive dysphasia knows what they want to say and understands what is being said to them but cannot find the words to respond appropriately. Mitchell (2002) describes graphically the experience of being aware but being unable to make herself understood.

It is important to realise that the psychological issues discussed above do not apply only to patients with stroke – they could equally apply to any person with a chronic condition.

What is the multiprofessional team?

Following admission, the multiprofessional team working with Mr Black and Mrs White and their families will assess their physical and psychological needs. The standard within the NSF identifies the need for care to be provided within a specialist stroke unit by appropriately trained individuals. *The National Clinical Guidelines for Stroke* (RCP, 2004) identify the need for a coordinated multiprofessional team and for staff with a specialist expertise in stroke and rehabilitation.

These guidelines are based on evidence of the effectiveness of specialist care within stroke units (Stroke Unit Trialists' Collaboration, 2004). The multiprofessional team within such a setting would typically consist of a stroke physician, nurses, physiotherapists, occupational therapists, a speech and language therapist, a dietician, a social worker and possibly a clinical psychologist.

The nurse plays a central role within the team by having the greatest degree of contact with the patient, but all members of the team are equally important. A small-scale study by Pound and Ebrahim (2001) noted that patients with stroke who were treated in a stroke unit had a better outcome than those treated in a general ward area but that the patients on a stroke unit received less personal care than those on an elderly care unit. A possible explanation for this is that the members of the multiprofessional team on the stroke unit did not see themselves as equals, thus creating tension. The care management competencies for the register note the need for effective interprofessional working practices and risk management strategies, both of which can be seen in the care that Mrs White and Mr Black and their families receive.

What is rehabilitation?

Rehabilitation is defined in the NSF for Long-Term Conditions as a 'multidisciplinary process which supports the individual to achieve their maximum potential to function physically, socially and psychologically through support and intervention' (DH, 2005). Many people are confused by the differences between rehabilitation and intermediate care. The main differences are shown in Table 18.2.

Table 18.2 Differences between rehabilitation and intermediate care

Rehabilitation	Intermediate care
Usually occurs in hospital	Occurs in hospital, patient's own home or other residential setting
Discharge destination is not known until near discharge date	Discharge destination is known at outset
Length of time not known	Time limited to 6 weeks or less
Does not include admission-avoidance schemes	Normally includes admission-avoidance schemes
Care identified and commissioned before discharge	Bridges the gap between hospital and home, so care may need to be stopped or arranged on completion

Source: DH (2001a,b).

Rehabilitation and intermediate care (also known as 're-enablement') help people to adapt to changes in their life circumstances, with the ultimate goal being to maximise the social well-being of the individual. This concept can be applied to an individual of any age and concerns enabling the person to regain their maximum quality of life. According to the Royal College of Nursing (RCN, 1997), rehabilitation needs to involve all of an individual's daily activities and has three main focal points:

- enhancing and maintaining quality of life;
- restoring physical, psychological and social functioning by recognising the health potential of each individual;
- preventing disease and illness.

In addition, the RCN (1997) identifies five role functions that the nurse engages in while working with older people in a re-enabling setting:

- *Supportive functions*: providing psychosocial support and emotional support.
- *Restorative functions*: aimed at maximising independence.
- *Educative functions*: teaching self-care.
- *Life-enhancing functions*: relieving pain and ensuring adequate nutrition.
- *Team functions*: the range of administrative and supervisory functions of the nurse.

In order for rehabilitation to be effective, the various members of the multiprofessional team must work with the patient to determine realistic and shared goals for the rehabilitation process. If shared and realistic goals are not agreed, then disappointment for the patient is the likely outcome. For example, the multiprofessional team may believe that to transfer independently from bed to chair is the greatest level of mobility that the patient will achieve, but the patient may expect to walk into their local village unaided. The nurse is typically the member of the multiprofessional team with the greatest contact with the patient; as such, the nurse is in a unique position to facilitate understanding and agreement with the patient on what they hope to realistically achieve.

Mrs White and Mr Black were fully independent before their stroke. The intention of the patients and their families is for them to return home with suitable support. Mr Black's intention is also to return to work. *The National Clinical Guidelines for Stroke* (RCP, 2004) advise that early discharge from the stroke unit back into the community should be considered only if there is a specialist community stroke rehabilitation team and if the patient is able to transfer safely from bed to chair. The Guidelines also state that:

i. *Carers should have received all necessary equipment and training in manual handling so they can safely transfer the patient at home*

ii *Patients and families are prepared and fully involved in the discharge*

iii *GPs, the primary healthcare team and community social services are fully aware*

iv *All necessary equipment and support is in place*

v *Any continuing community based treatment continues without a break after discharge*

vi *The patient and family have information about appropriate statutory and voluntary agencies.*

(RCP, 2004)

In a Canadian study, Mayo *et al.* (2000) found that patients with stroke who had early discharge with appropriate home-based rehabilitation had better physical health and reintegration into the community at 3 months than did patients who continued with hospital-based rehabilitation. Interestingly, however, Anderson *et al.* (2000) found that the early discharge with home-based rehabilitation did not improve (or worsen) health or quality of life for patients with stroke in a study in Australia. Griffiths (2000) argues that both of these studies required participants to be relatively independent and therefore the results can not be generalised, noting also that both studies were relatively small scale. Further work needs to be undertaken to examine both the effects on caregivers of early discharge and how best to deliver the coordinated multiprofessional rehabilitation that clearly improves the outcome for patients with stroke.

Month 2

Mrs White is discharged home following an 8-week stay on the stroke unit. Her family have arranged for private home care to visit twice daily, once to help Mrs White get up in the morning and again to put her to bed in the evening. Mrs White still has a fairly dense right hemiplegia affecting her arm more severely than her leg. She has no useful function in the arm, she is able to stand with the aid of her stick, and she can walk around the ground floor of her house and in the garden. She has a hospital bed downstairs in the front room and a commode. Her husband helps her by adjusting her clothing when she needs to use the toilet.

She is happy to be home and says she will teach her husband to cook.

Mr Black is discharged home after an 8-week stay on the stroke unit. He still has a dense hemiplegia affecting his arm, but he has full function back in his affected leg. He is mobile around the house. He is able to get up and down the stairs and he uses the shower. Mrs Black then helps him to dry and dress himself.

He is worried that his sick pay will run out in another couple of months and that he will not be able to return to his job as he is not able to drive. He did not want to be discharged as he was expecting to be 'fully functional' before discharge.

It could be argued that this phase of care for the White family has been successful. Mrs White is back home, she has identified a goal for herself that will help with her self-esteem, and adequate support appears to be in place. Such careful planning for discharge is an important part of attempting to limit readmission to hospital. Munshi *et al.* (2002) studied readmission of older people to acute medical units and noted that about 40 per cent of readmissions were avoidable and that unsorted medical and social problems accounted for 62 per cent of all readmissions. The same paper identified that intermediate care provision may play a crucial role in preventing readmission to acute medical services.

Although Mrs White and Mr Black have gone through very similar experiences, the meaning and the effects of these experiences are different for each of them both. Mrs White seems to consider that things have gone fairly well and that she is home. In part, this may be because her peer group is likely to be experiencing increasing ill health and disability; therefore, her expectations are possibly more realistic.

Mr Black does not consider the fact that he is home and mobile a success. It is probable that he will not have people within his peer group who have any similar experiences. In addition, referring back to his initial assessment, we can see that he had multiple concerns about relationships both within and without the family. He works as a travelling salesman but clearly he cannot drive again yet. The Driver and Vehicle Licensing Authority (DVLA) will need to be notified regarding his stroke, since he still has loss of function 1 month after the event (DVLA, 2005). He may be able to drive again following assessment, possibly with adaptation to the vehicle, but he cannot drive at this time. If he were to drive without declaring the stroke, he would be breaking the law and therefore his insurance would be invalid. Based on his assessment, it appears that his social life centres around going out with work colleagues and taking his son to football. As both of these activities are likely to require him getting to a destination, his ability to drive a car is likely to be important to him.

Mr Black had concerns about how colleagues would view him, but in addition there is the issue of how he views himself. Before the stroke he was the main earner for his family, he is a member of a group of work friends, he is a father who takes his son to football, he enjoys a few pints with friends, and he is the husband and lover of his wife (remember that sexual functioning can be affected by stroke).

Month 11

The Whites' daughter Grace visits two or three times a week. She checks that the freezer is well stocked with meals that Mr White can prepare with minimum effort, as Mrs White has been only partially successful in teaching Mr White to cook.

One day, as she hurries to get out of bed, Mrs White overbalances and falls to the floor. She complains of severe pain in her left shoulder. Mr White calls an ambulance and Mrs White is taken to A&E. She is admitted to hospital with a suspected fractured humerus; however, the confirmed diagnosis is severe bruising but no fracture. She is unable to use her left arm due to the bruising and pain, and her right arm has been affected by the stroke.

Mrs White is admitted to a residential intermediate care facility, where her pain is addressed, the reasons for her fall are explored, and education is given to prevent a reoccurrence.

Mr Black still has a degree of weakness in his affected arm. He is able to wash and dress independently, although still with some difficulty. He is well enough to work now, but he has not been able to get his driving licence back; therefore, he is unable to return to work as a travelling salesman.

Mrs Black is working part time, but she is concerned that her husband has cut himself off from his contacts outside the family. She is also concerned that her children have stopped bringing their friends home with them.

She confides to her friends that she feels she is looking after an old man and that her life has stopped.

The Disability Discrimination Act

Although Mr Black has had to surrender his driving licence, this should not mean that he automatically loses his job. Under the Disability Discrimination Act (2005), Mr Black's employer should make reasonable efforts to adapt the environment and allow him to continue to work. If a person has become disabled (classified disabled), then the company has a legal obligation to make all reasonable adjustments to allow that person to continue in gainful employment. However, where adjustment cannot be made, and redeployment is offered but refused (for example, a disabled manual worker such as a carpenter is offered redeployment into a desk job), then the company may be able to dismiss on grounds of incapability.

The falls National Service Framework

Standard 6 of the NSF aims to prevent falls and to treat them effectively when they do occur. Falls are a major problem in the UK; they are a major cause of disability and death in people over the age of 75 years. Up to 14 000 people a year die in the UK as a result of osteoporotic hip fracture. This is the equivalent of 35 fully laden jumbo jets crashing and killing all on board every year – if this were to happen, then there would likely be a public outcry, with questions being asked in Parliament and the press.

Care

Mrs White does not have a fracture, but she has fallen and is unable to use her 'good arm'. Intermediate care is covered by standard 3 of the NSF (DH, 2001b) and would be ideal for Mrs White under these circumstances – she is not medically unwell, but she requires further rehabilitation following her fall. Equally as important, she is likely to have lost confidence as a result of her fall, which may prevent her from regaining her former level of mobility. Within the intermediate care setting, Mrs White will receive intensive nursing and therapy input to facilitate her return home as soon as possible.

There are a variety of programmes and aids to prevent falls and injury. Robertson *et al.* (2001) identified that a home-based, nurse-delivered exercise programme concentrating on muscle strengthening and balance retraining was effective in reducing falls and serious injury in people over the age of 80 years. In the evaluation of a nurse-led falls-prevention programme, Lightbody *et al.* (2002) found that patients receiving nurse-led interventions had fewer falls, had fewer hospital attendances and spent less time in hospital; the patients were also more functionally independent 6 months after the original fall.

The use of hip protectors to reduce the risk of injury has also been examined. Parker *et al.* (2001) identified that the use of hip protectors reduces the level of hip fractures in elderly people living in institutional or supported home care environments. These findings are supported by Campbell (2001).

The rehabilitation dilemma

Mrs White requires further rehabilitation in order for her to regain her maximum level of functioning and return home. This can, however, present the health care team with a dilemma: rehabilitation has a certain level of risk – Mrs White has fallen once, and if the multiprofessional team, physiotherapists, nurses and medical staff encourage and enable her to walk, there is a danger that she may fall again and sustain further injury. If the health care team were to prevent Mrs White from undertaking or attempting activities independently, then her risk of falling may be reduced – but at what cost? Mrs White would be hindered in her recovery and thus may not regain her maximum possible level of independence.

Reflection point 18.2

You are approached by the relatives of an elderly woman who was admitted from rehabilitation and fell and fractured her hip while walking accompanied to the toilet. The woman is usually fully mobile using only her walking stick. When admitted to the ward, she was unable to transfer from her bed to a chair without the help of two nurses; she is now able to independently walk the length of the ward using a walking frame and is fiercely determined to fully regain her independence. Her family members are very angry that she was allowed to walk around the ward without a nurse, and they are demanding that the nurses on duty are disciplined for negligence.

How might you respond in such a situation?

Carers

The strain on carers is often not fully recognised. If the family is being nursed holistically, then the needs of the whole family should be taken into account. Although all of the practical aspects of providing for Mrs White have been addressed, it could be argued that the less tangible need for support for the family unit has not been taken into account. Both the NSF (DH, 2001b) and the stroke clinical guidelines (RCP, 2004) note the need for contact with local voluntary and statutory agencies. This does not seem to have happened in Mrs White's case. If Mr White were invited to the local carers support group, he could meet with others in a similar position to him and gain support. If Mrs White were to attend a day centre, that would give Mr White one day to himself each week. The following information might be useful for the family:

- local service directories;
- information about local day centres;
- leaflets from the Stroke Association;
- leaflets about social security benefits;
- information on local carers groups (Exall and Johnston, 1999).

Hall (2002) notes that carer support groups provide a focus for health education and should be an integrated part of service delivery, while acknowledging that such groups do have limitations.

Informal carers provide an estimated 80 per cent of community-based long-term care. There are around 6.8 million carers in the UK (OPCS, 1990); about 13 per cent of carers are over the age of 65 years. For carers there are implications for lifestyle change – not only the act of providing the care, but also potentially the financial implications of such caring.

The Whites' son Tony is driving 80 miles a week to visit his parents; this is potentially expensive and time-consuming. As the Whites' daughter Grace is visiting them twice a day, the possibility of her taking paid employment is greatly reduced; there are also potential implications in terms of the care she can provide to her own children. The Whites' house may eventually be sold to pay for long-term nursing or residential care, and thus any expected financial windfall from the parents' will is lost.

Month 12

Mr Black's employer has offered him a job in the office coordinating the salespeople's visits and processing their orders. A colleague who lives nearby has offered Mr Black a lift to and from work in exchange for sharing the travelling costs.

This has improved Mr Black's self-esteem. Since returning to work, he has agreed to visit some close friends. He ordered a taxi to enable them to fully enjoy the evening.

Mrs Black is looking forward to her evening out and is optimistic that her husband is now slowly reforming his contacts outside of the family.

Month 13

Tony and Grace are concerned that their father Mr White is becoming increasingly forgetful. They have come to visit and found the front door unlocked. Mrs White tells them that her husband has been putting the kettle on and forgetting it, so it boils dry. Following a number of similar occurrances, Tony and Grace ask the GP to visit.

Tests show that Mr White has dementia, with resultant risks to himself and his wife.

Lifestyle changes

The social functioning of Mr and Mrs White has undergone great change over their lifetime. They have moved from being workers to retired people, from being parents to care recipients, from being active members of the local community to being outside the community due to physical and mental disability. In the same way, the roles of Grace and Tony have reversed: they have moved from being care recipients as children to being care providers for their dependent parents. There is also the possibility that Grace, as the local carer, may find the social stigma of mental illness affects how others act towards her.

If Mr and Mrs White decide that they will go into care together, it needs to be remembered that it is not always possible for a couple to be placed together, especially if only one partner may needs care. For couples who have been together for many years, separation is difficult. In a small study, Sandberg *et al.* (2001) identified four stages in the process of separation:

1 *Pretending*: the carers tell themselves that this is a trial separation and not permanent.
2 *Dawning*: a growing awareness that the placement is permanent.
3 *Putting on a brave face*: showing the world that everything is all right.
4 *Seeking solace*: attempting to discuss feelings with friends or relatives.

In Sandberg and colleagues' study, a theme that ran through all the stages of separation was that of trying to keep the relationship with the spouse.

It is important that the nurse does not underestimate the effect of the separation for a couple who may have been together for 60 years. The nurse should also be aware that it can be difficult for people to get residential care that is funded by social services if they have not previously had a package of care at home.

Mr and Mrs Black have undergone many similar lifestyle changes. Mr Black has made an effective recovery and is now back at work. The family is readjusting to the new situation. If Mr Black had needed placement in a residential or nursing home, he may have experienced the financial difficulties and separation issues described above; he may also have had difficulty finding a suitable home caring for people of his age group, resulting in him being placed in a care home with people many years older. In this sense, although the NSF for Older People, which covers stroke, makes explicit that it is not acceptable to practise in a manner that is discriminatory, in the case of people such as Mr Black, they are being discriminated against on the grounds of age.

CONCLUSION

It is important for the nurse to realise that anyone, of any age, may move from being a fit and well individual to being a person requiring long-term care or rehabilitation. The nurse must always be aware that such a change in lifestyle and health status affects not only the individual but also their family, and the nurse must respond to this appropriately. Throughout the course of an individual's admission to the health services, it is likely that nursing staff will have the greatest level of input and thus have the greatest opportunity to make a real difference to the individual.

References

Adamson J, Beswick A and Ebrahim S (2004). Stroke and disability. *Journal of Stroke and Cerebrovascular Diseases*, **13**, 171–7.

Anderson C, Rubenach S and Mhurchu C (2000). Early discharge plus home based rehabilitation reduced length of initial hospital stay but did not improve health related quality of life in patients with acute stroke. *Evidence-Based Nursing*, **3**, 127.

Campbell AJ (2001). Purity, pragmatism and hip protector pads. *Age and Ageing*, **30**, 431–2.

Department of Health (DH) (2000). *The NHS Plan: A Plan for Investment, A Plan for Reform*. London: Department of Health.

Department of Health (DH) (2001a). *Intermediate Care*. London: Department of Health.

Department of Health (DH) (2001b). *The National Service Framework for Older People*. London: The Stationery Office.

Department of Health (DH) (2002). *Delivering the NHS Plan: Next Steps on Investment, Next Steps on Reform*. London: Department of Health.

Department of Health (DH) (2005). *National Service Framework for Long-Term Conditions*. London: Department of Health.

Department of Health (DH) (2006a). *A New Ambition for Old Age: Next Steps in Implementing the National Service Framework for Older People*. London: Department of Health.

Department of Health (DH) (2006b). *Supporting People with Long-Term Conditions to Self Care: A Guide to Developing Local Strategies and Good Practice*. London: Department of Health.

Department of Health (DH) (2007). *National Service Framework for Older People and System Reform*. London: Department of Health.

Driver and Vehicle Licensing Authority (DVLA) (2005). *A Guide to Driving Ordinary Vehicles (Group 1) Following a Stroke, TIA, Ministroke, Cerebral Thrombosis or Amaurosis Fugax*. Swansea: Driver and Vehicle Licensing Authority.

Exall K and Johnston H (1999). Caring for carers coping with stroke. *Nursing Times*, **95**, 50–51.

Griffiths P (2000). Commentary. *Evidence-Based Nursing*, **3**, 126–7.

Grimby A (1993). The influence of urinary incontinence on the quality of life of elderly women. *Age and Ageing*, **22**, 82–9.

Hall J (2002). Assessing the health promotion needs of informal carers. *Nursing Older People*, **14**, 14–18.

Harris A (1999). Impact of urinary incontinence on the quality of life of women. *British Journal of Nursing*, **8**, 375–80.

Hickey JV (1992). *The Clinical Practice of Neurosurgical Nursing*, 3rd edn. Philadelphia, PA: Lippincott.

Lee JJ (2004). The relationship between gender and the psychological impact of urinary incontinence on older people in Hong Kong: an exploratory analysis *Ageing and Society*, **24**, 553–66.

Lightbody E, Watkins C, Leathley M, Sharma A and Lye M (2002). Evaluation of a nurse led falls prevention programme versus usual care: a randomised controlled trial. *Age and Ageing*, **31**, 203–10.

Mayo NE, Wood-Dauphinee S and Cote R (2000). Prompt hospital discharge with home care improved physical health and community reintegration and reduced initial length of hospital stay after acute stroke. *Evidence-Based Nursing*, **3**, 126.

Mitchell J (2002). The slow road back. *Health Service Journal*, **112**, 25.

Munshi SK, Lakhani D, Ageed A, *et al.* (2002). Readmissions of older people to acute medical units. *Nursing Older People*, **14**, 14–16.

Norton C (1986). *Nursing for Continence*. Beaconsfield: Beaconsfield Publishers.

Nursing and Midwifery Council (NMC) (2004). *Requirements for Pre-Registration Midwifery Programmes.* London: Nursing and Midwifery Council.

Nursing and Midwifery Council (NMC) (2008). *The Code: Standards of Conduct, Performance and Ethics for Nurses and Midwives.* London: Nursing and Midwifery Council.

Office of National Statistics (2001). Stroke incidence and risk factors in a population based cohort study. *Health Statistics Quarterly,* **12**, 18–26.

Office of Population Censuses and Surveys (OPCS) (1990). *General Household Survey.* London: HMSO.

Parker MJ, Gillespie LD and Gillespie WJ (2001). Hip protectors for preventing hip fractures in the elderly. *Cochrane Database of Systematic Reviews,* (2), CD001255.

Pound P and Ebrahim S (2001). Patients in stroke units have better outcomes, but receive less personal nursing care. *Evidence-Based Nursing,* **4**, 128.

Robertson MC, Devlin N and Gardner MM (2001). A home based, nurse delivered exercise programme reduced falls and serious injuries in people 80 years of age. *Evidence-Based Nursing,* **5**, 22.

Roper N (2000). *Models for Nursing: Based on Activities for Living.* Edinburgh: Churchill Livingstone.

Roper N, Logan W and Tierney A (1996). *The Elements of Nursing: Based on a Model of Living,* 4th edn. Edinburgh: Churchill Livingstone.

Royal College of Nursing (RCN) (1997). *What a Difference a Nurse Makes: An RCN Report on the Benefits of Expert Nursing to Clinical Outcomes in the Continuing Care of Older People.* London: Royal College of Nursing.

Royal College of Physicians (RCP) (2004). *The National Clinical Guidelines for Stroke,* 2nd edn. London: Royal College of Physicians.

Sandberg J, Lundh U and Nolan MR (2001). Spouses who placed partners in care homes experienced emotional reactions to separation and made efforts to maintain their relationship. *Evidence-Based Nursing,* **5**, 32.

Smyth ETM (2006). Healthcare acquired infection prevalence survey 2006. Presented at the 6th International Conference of the Hospital Infection Society, Amsterdam, 2006. (Preliminary data available in Hospital infection Society: The Third Prevalence Survey of Healthcare Associated Infections in Acute Hospitals 2006, www.his.org.uk.)

Stroke Unit Trialists' Collaboration (2004). Organised inpatient (stroke unit) care for stroke (Cochrane Review). In *The Cochrane Library,* issue 1, 2004. Chichester: John Wiley & Sons.

Tortora GJ and Derrickson B (2006). *Principles of Anatomy and Physiology,* 11th edn. Hoboken, NJ: John Wiley & Sons.

Vickerman J (2002). Thorough assessment of functional incontinence. *Nursing Times,* **98**, 58–9.

Ward V, Wilson J, Taylor L, Cookson B and Glynn A (1997). *Preventing Hospital Acquired Infection: Clinical Guidelines (Public Health Laboratory Service).* London: HMSO.

Further reading

Burnard P (2005). *Counselling Skills for Health Professionals*, 4th edn. Cheltenham: Stanley Thornes.

This book deals with the theory and practice of counselling within the context of health care environments. The book gives useful guidance on the elements necessary in order to have an effective therapeutic relationship, even if not in a formal counselling relationship.

Dougherty L and Lister S (eds) (2004). *The Royal Marsden Hospital Manual of Clinical Nursing Procedures*, 6th edn. Oxford: Blackwell.

This book gives a comprehensive and evidence-based approach to, among others, the procedures mentioned in this chapter.

Fawcus R (ed.) (2000). *Stroke Rehabilitation: A Collaborative Approach*. Oxford: Blackwell Science.

This book has contributions from doctors, nurses, speech and language therapists, physiotherapist and others. It gives a thorough grounding in the important contributions that all the disciplines can make to a patient recovering from a stroke.

Mohr JP, Choi DW, Grotta JC, Weir B and Woolf PA (2004). *Stroke: Pathophysiology, Diagnosis and Management*, 4th edn. New York: Churchill Livingstone.

A massive and detailed book that provides in-depth information on most aspects of stroke.

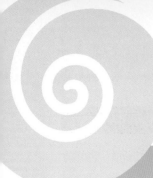

The needs of older people

19

Sue Davies and Mike Nolan

Introduction

Within this chapter we aim to explore experiences of ageing and consider how nurses can work most effectively with older people and their families to maintain their health and well-being. This requires a discussion of the structures and values that determine the life experiences of older people in the UK and their access to health and social care at times of need. We consider the wider environment and society in which older people live and receive care from health and social care practitioners, including the cultural, political and social values that influence the status of older people and their participation in society. Recurrent concerns about the quality of care received by older people will be highlighted, together with new approaches that have been developed to help nurses create effective partnerships with older people and their families. We also highlight the importance of supporting staff and providing them with a stimulating and challenging work environment. In writing this chapter, we have drawn heavily on recent research and other sources of evidence, believing, as does the NMC Code (2008) (Appendix 1), that nurses 'must deliver care based on the best available evidence'.

Learning objectives

After studying this chapter you should:

- be aware of the range of factors influencing experiences of ageing;
- understand the nature of transition in later life and the main transitions that bring older people into contact with nurses and other health and social care practitioners;
- recognise historical concerns about the quality of care received by older people and the role of new frameworks for practice in achieving change.

What is ageing?

The subject of human ageing is complex, and there is no single model that explains how, why and at what rate ageing takes place. Instead, there are many theories embracing the different disciplines that study human life and social interaction. An explanation of these theories is beyond the scope of this chapter, but, if you are interested in these ideas, we have listed some useful further reading at the end of the chapter. In simple terms, the process of ageing involves time-dependent changes in living organisms. These changes affect every aspect of a person's life: physical, psychosocial and emotional. It is important, however, to recognise that chronological age is not a precise marker for the changes that accompany ageing. Indeed, there are dramatic variations in health status, participation and levels of independence among people of the same age (WHO, 2002).

What is important to note is that, the longer a person lives, the more unique they become, as each individual is a product of their biology and life experiences. This means that experiences of later life are hugely diverse, and it is this diversity that makes working with older people and their families so stimulating and challenging.

Some commentators suggest that old age is a social construct; in other words, it is determined by a generally accepted view of what it means rather than an absolute definition. Victor (2006), for example, suggests that the number of years used to define old age is rarely biologically or physiologically based but is rooted in the cultural values and norms of each society. Given the diversity of the population, it is important to recognise that what is considered 'older' will also vary between ethnic groups. Indeed, recognising and responding to such diversity is a key element of the NMC Code.

Reflection point 19.1
Can you think of ways in which chronological age is used in order to determine access to services and opportunities for older people? What are the implications of this?

Points you might have considered include the difficulty for older people of securing travel insurance above a certain age (80 years is the usual cut-off point for many companies) and the need for older drivers in the UK to renew their licence annually. Chronological age is often used to determine access to screening services, and we will revisit this point later in the chapter. The impact of such rigid distinctions is that older people may be excluded from activities that would enhance their well-being and quality of life.

Demographic changes and challenges

Consistent with countries across Europe, the average age of the population of the UK has been increasing steadily. The long-term trends of lower birth rates, improvements in health status and rising longevity have combined to produce a constant growth in the proportion of the population who are aged 60 years and over (Kalache *et al.*, 2006). Similarly, life expectancy at all ages has shown a steady increase, although healthy life expectancy demonstrates a levelling off, suggesting that people are living longer with chronic illness and disability (Figure 19.1). The most rapid changes in life expectancy are apparent among those aged 80 years and over. It is this latter group who generally have far higher levels of disability secondary to multiple chronic diseases, and who

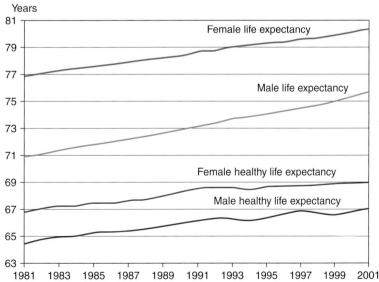

Figure 19.1 Life expectancy and healthy life expectancy at birth by sex, Great Britain 1981–2001 (Office for National Statistics, 2004).

are most in need of care and support, which presents potential challenges to health and social care systems.

Despite this, it is important to recognise that even very frail older people are able to continue to live in the community, often with family support. In 2006, for example, the chance of living in a long-stay hospital or care home was 0.85 per cent for people aged 65–74 years, rising to 17.1 per cent for those aged 85 years and over (Laing and Buisson, 2006). Furthermore, the development of new technologies is increasingly allowing older people to remain in their own homes for longer (Fisk, 1999; Cheek *et al.*, 2005). Nonetheless, an ageing population does present a series of challenges for health and social care practitioners, partly because of the association between disability (including dementia) and advanced old age, and partly because of changes in the household situation of older people.

The way in which people live together has a fundamental implication for patterns of giving and receiving care. The growth in solitary living, the decline in co-residence between generations, and the increase in women's employment outside the home are all impacting on families' ability to provide informal networks of support for older people who need help to remain in the community (Lowenstein, 2006). Most importantly, the trend towards smaller family size has resulted in a reduced number of potential caregivers compared with those needing care. Changes in family structure, resulting from increased geographical mobility and the impact of divorce, are also influencing the availability of family support (Lowenstein, 2006; Victor, 2006). Consequently, families are facing the prospect of caring for older relatives for longer, with fewer potential family members to help. Without adequate support, these caring relationships are likely to break down, resulting in increased demand for formal care services. Developing more effective ways of working in partnership with older people and with family carers is therefore crucial, and this is an area in which nurses can make a significant difference. The NMC Code acknowledges that nurses need to 'work with others to protect and provide the health and well-being of those in your care, their families and carers and the wider community'. However, in order to create such partnerships, it is essential to understand and appreciate what it is like to age.

SUMMARY

- Definitions of ageing are usually based on chronological age, and this may exclude older people from certain activities and services.
- Most nurses will come into regular contact with older people in their day-to-day practice, and it is important to appreciate an individual's experience of ageing.
- Demographic changes and challenges mean that new models of care must be continually developed and evaluated.
- Practitioners need explicit frameworks to help them to develop partnerships with older people and their families.

Experiences of ageing and nursing responses

It is important to keep in mind that everyone's experience of growing older is different. Although there may be common themes, an older person's experience of ageing will be unique to that person. Learning techniques that allow you to appreciate the full range of experiences is an important part of developing the skills to help each older person in their unique situation. It is also important to be aware of each older person's values, which are determined by historical and social influences within the context of their lifespan. This is essential in order to 'treat people as individuals and respect their dignity' (NMC Code). In some situations, it may be appropriate to use a biographical or life-story approach as a way of finding out about the older person's needs as they perceive them. For example, Amanda Clarke and colleagues used a life story method to plan appropriate care for older people within an intermediate care ward (Clarke *et al.*, 2003).

Some experiences of ageing are shown Box 19.1.

BOX 19.1 How older people feel about being old

I am a bit of a fatalist. I say what is to be, will be . . . Mind you, you have to move yourself haven't you? You have got to try – well do the best you can with things, you know, if something does happen. Like – I think the worst thing with getting old – I should imagine everybody will tell you the same – is your health . . . But you try and keep your mind active, as I said before, reading the paper, doing crosswords, you don't want to start sitting in the corner. But you could easily do it you know.

(Fay, aged 80 years)[*][†]

I do my exercises . . . It is probably a vanity thing. I think it is vanity, yes I do . . . I don't like the weight.

(Sophie, aged 78 years)[*][†]

Oh, either you feel that your brain is going you know. I just can't remember things. How you look. How your skin is aging. How you get lines like those which you would love to get rid of. And you sort of think to yourself I don't like old age you know. You can't rush anywhere, you can't do the things you used to do that you used to take for granted. When you are young you take them for granted. Apart from that, once you have got over that problem, once you have thought to yourself, well everyone gets old, so we are all going to be in the same boat one day, you just get on with it and make the best of it.

(Gill, aged 70 years)[†]

That is when you start thinking, God, I must be getting old. I looked in the mirror when I was out with Sam getting the suit, and I thought who is that old guy behind Sam, and of course it was me. But inside you don't feel the age you are. I still think like a 20- or 30-year old. Well I think I do. But it is not until I look at things like that – the skin and everything else . . .

(John, aged 66 years)[†]

[*]*Source: Martin (2006).*

Source: [†]Martin W (2007). *Embodying 'Active' Ageing: Bodies, Emotions and Risk in Later Life.* Unpublished thesis. University of Warwick. Reused with permission.

These views reflect those of the majority of people who are in the later years of their lives – that it is not how old you are in chronological terms that matters, but your capacity to do things. Research projects using interview methods to explore experiences of ageing, such as the one from which these quotes are taken, are a useful source of information. Fictional and autobiographical accounts of the experience of ageing can also contribute a great deal to your understanding of ageing and older people's lives; some examples are given in Box 19.2. It is important to recognise, however, that these represent personal and individual accounts and may not reflect the experiences of all older people.

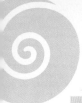
BOX 19.2 Accounts of ageing in literature, drama and films

Memoirs and reflections
- *Precious Lives* by Margaret Forster
- *Lark Rise to Candleford* by Flora Thompson
- *Force of Circumstance* by Simone de Beauvoir
- *The View in Winter* by Ronald Blythe
- *Writing Home* by Alan Bennett (includes the long essay 'The lady in the van')

Poems
- 'Do not go gentle into that good night' by Dylan Thomas
- 'Growing old' by Mathew Arnold
- 'Warning' by Jenny Joseph
- *While We've Still Got Feet* (a book of poetry) by David Budbill
- *I'm Too Young to Be Seventy and Other Delusions* (a book of poetry) by Judith Viorst

Biography and autobiography
- *White Cargo* by Felicity Kendal
- *My Name Escapes Me: The Diary of a Retiring Actor* by Alec Guinness
- *Daddy, We Hardly Knew You* by Germaine Greer

Novels
- *Travels with My Aunt* by Graham Greene
- *The Prince of West End Avenue* by Alan Isler
- *Have the Men Had Enough?* by Margaret Forster

Plays
- *Death of a Salesman* by Arthur Miller
- *Krapp's Last Tape* by Samuel Beckett
- 'Talking Heads' by Alan Bennett (in particular, *The Telegram*)

Films
- *On Golden Pond*
- *Driving Miss Daisy*
- *Ladies in Lavender*
- *The Notebook*
- *Iris*
- *About Schmidt*

Source: Davies (2007, pp. 33–34).

Accounts and representations of ageing reveal the diversity in ageing experiences. Old age can be a time of adventure and new discoveries, for consolidating experiences, focusing on relationships and gaining new wisdom. It can also be a time of adjustment and loss, requiring resilience and coping skills if a good quality of life is to be achieved. A particular challenge for many older people is the number of changes or transitions that take place in later life, and it is to these that we now turn.

Transitions in later life

Older people experience many transitions in life. Most of these are inherently linked to the older person's health and well-being, and it is often a transition that brings an older person into contact with professional nursing. Helping individuals to manage life transitions has been identified as a key function of nursing (Schumacher and Meleis, 1994; Meleis *et al.*, 2000), with transition defined as 'The passage or movement from one state, condition or place to another' (Chick and Meleis, 1986, p. 237).

It is essential that nurses who work with older people appreciate the nature of transitions in later life and the ways in which nurses can support older people to make adjustments and regain stability in order to promote their health and well-being. We now briefly consider three types of transition that affect most older people at some stage and can impact on their health and well-being: retirement, bereavement and moving home. We pay particular attention to the experience of moving to a care home, as this is an area where research has provided a number of pointers for nursing practice.

Retirement

Research exploring the impact of retirement has generally been guided by two perspectives. One perspective views retirement as a stressful and traumatic event, with the potential to generate distress and emotional and physical illness, whereas the other perspective suggests that retirement is an opportunity for growth and development, in which individuals attain a new freedom of choice and the opportunity to create a better quality of life for themselves (Nuttman Schwartz, 2004). Most individuals report high levels of life satisfaction in the period immediately following retirement (Kim and Moen, 2002), although this reduces with advancing age (Pinquart, 2001).

The degree of control over retirement seems to be important to health outcomes. A longitudinal study by Gallo *et al.* (2000) found significant negative effects on mental and physical health after being involuntarily retired. In contrast, older workers who were made redundant and then found new employment demonstrated improvements in their mental and physical health, independently of how long they had been out of work (Stuart-Hamilton, 2006).

Findings of numerous studies support the view of retirement as an important life transition (Nuttman Schwartz, 2004; Kunemund and Kolland, 2007), characterised by anxiety at the beginning and followed by its gradual alleviation. Retirement is also likely to impact upon significant relationships within an older person's life. However, as with many transitions, anticipation of and preparation for the event can help to smooth the passage and limit any negative health effects.

Reflection point 19.2
In whatever context you work with older people, you are likely to come into contact with adults who are approaching retirement or who are recently retired. Think about your role in helping older people to prepare for retirement. Search the Internet or your local library for resources that will enable you to support people experiencing this life transition. These may be general resources, such as self-help guides, or more locally based information, for example about a retirement preparation programme. Make a resource folder that you will have available when the opportunity arises to support someone at this stage in their life.

Bereavement and loss

For many people, old age becomes a time of accumulated loss. These losses can include:

- death of a loved one;
- divorce or separation;
- loss of health or physical abilities (and therefore possibly loss of independence);
- loss of role (e.g. at work or within the family as a spouse, parent or grandparent);
- loss of a pet;
- loss of home.

Grieving can take place after any sort of loss but is usually most powerful after the death of a loved one, as this is one of the most distressing and shocking events that most of us have to deal with. In particular, the loss of a spouse is generally regarded as one of the most stressful of life events. Bereavement is an important and well-established risk factor for depression, with at least 10–20 per cent of widows and widowers developing clinically significant depression during the first year of bereavement. Neimeyer and Werth (2006) highlight the accumulating evidence that the stress of bereavement is associated with a 40–70 per cent increase in mortality among surviving spouses in the first 6 months following the loss. Consequently, nurses and other health care professionals have important roles in caring for older people who have been bereaved. Carroll and Dill Linton (2007) suggest that appropriate support might include the following:

- providing information and education, with sensitivity to what significant others want to know;
- offering emotional support;
- clinical recognition of dysfunctional grieving;
- management and appropriate referral to mental health resources;
- legitimisation of the occurrence of death, so that the bereaved person is assured that all appropriate measures were attempted.

In addition to identifying older people at risk, health and social care professionals can assist bereaved older people to cope with both the short-term and long-term challenges of loss. In the short term, the bereaved person may benefit from coaching in symptom managements skills such as relaxation skills and thought-stopping to interrupt distressing imagery (Neimeyer and Werth, 2006). In the longer term, providing opportunities for self-expression and a deeper processing of the significance of the loss for their ongoing lives may be helpful.

Support groups are one way in which nurses caring for older people can enable older people to make the transition through bereavement. Based on his work with bereavement groups involving older people, Cohen (2000) identified the following benefits of participation: hope, acceptance, less social isolation, new identity and meaning in life, support, catharsis, amelioration of fears, education, help in dealing with painful or intense feelings, and an opportunity to help others. Many older people make the decision to move to new accommodation following bereavement, which is another form of transition.

Moving to new accommodation

According to Oswald and Rowles (2006), there are two broad groups of people who move in older age. Some people move soon after retirement because of social networks and environmental preferences; for example, one-third of such moves are to be nearer children. However, relocation within familiar community boundaries remains the most popular move in old age (Krout *et al.*, 2002). The second group of people move as a result of a deterioration in health or a sudden health crisis (Oswald and Rowles, 2006). After an extended period of frailty, many older people, often reluctantly, make the decision to move into sheltered accommodation or a long-term care facility. In both sets of circumstances, it is important to regard relocation from a life-course perspective and to place emphasis on understanding the processes involved in successfully re-establishing a sense of place attachment following relocation.

Some of the most common reasons that older people start to consider moving home are:

- health decline;
- access or mobility problems;
- home maintenance worries;

- financial concerns;
- feeling lonely, isolated or unsafe;
- living in a home too large for their needs;
- bereavement (HOPDEV, 2006).

There are an increasing number of strategies and assistive technologies that can help older people to 'stay put' if this is what they want. In a large survey (Heywood *et al.*, 2005), older people identified aids and adaptations such as stair-lifts and wheelchair ramps as the most effective means to enable them to remain in their own homes. A further significant change towards securing independence for older people in their homes is the ongoing development of new technology. A common use of technology designed to be supportive to older people is the community alarm system. Nurses are often involved in helping older people to access the resources that will enable them to retain their independence. However, it is essential that older people maintain control over decisions about the use of such technology and are provided with all the relevant information to enable them to make the right choice.

Reflection point 19.3
If you were asked, would you be able to advise an older person about how they could obtain technology to enable them to continue living safely in their own home?

The community alarm scheme is one example of such technology. Most local authorities have information about the community alarm scheme on their websites. The organisation Carers UK is another useful source of information (www.carersuk.org). Home improvement agencies (HIAs) help vulnerable people to maintain their independence, mainly through the repair or adaptation of the person's home. Help is available to homeowners and social housing tenants. Further information can be found at www.foundations.uk.com.

When an older person does decide to move, the nurse can play an important role in helping them to adjust and make a smooth transition. An important aspect of this is being aware of the impact of relocation for the individual. A number of tools are available to assist older people and their carers to determine whether a move would be beneficial for their health and well-being. For example, the charity Elderly Accommodation Counsel (EAC) has developed a brief questionnaire entitled Housing Options for Older People (HOOP). This questionnaire covers nine broad domains:

- size and space;
- independence;
- cost;
- condition;
- comfort and design;
- security and safety;
- location;
- managing;
- quality of life.

You can access the HOOP assessment tool at www.hoop.eac.org.uk/hoop/start.aspx.

The move to a care home

I'd known for years that I would need to go into a care home but held on until I was unable to manage. I don't think it's good to go on expecting family and friends and neighbours to do things for you forever. They're going to get tired of doing it and have other pressures in their lives.

(Alex Thompson, care home resident, quoted in Owen and NCHRDF, 2006, p. 25)

There is no doubt that the move from one's own home to a care home remains a major, and often final, life transition (O'May, 2006). As with many major life decisions, however, with appropriate planning and support the transition can be managed in a way that improves the person's quality of life.

Care homes for older people are now categorised by the type of care they provide – nursing or personal. Care homes (personal) provide board and personal care only, whereas care homes (nursing) are intended for people who need regular or constant nursing care (Froggatt, 2004; O'May, 2006). Choosing the most appropriate type of home can be a bewildering experience for older people and their families. Davies and Nolan (2003) identified three ways in which older people and their relatives reach a decision about care home entry:

- *Making the decision*: there is a relatively proactive and planned approach to deciding that placement is needed.
- *Reaching the decision*: the decision is not made on a planned and rational basis, but rather is reached following a period of indecision.
- *Realising the inevitable*: the decisions is precipitated by a crisis and the decision to admit is neither made nor reached, but rather is accepted.

In interviews with relatives, the first pattern of gradual decision-making was associated with the most positive experiences of the move, but this was described by only a small number of participants in the study. Even when entry to a nursing home was part of a long-term strategy planned by the older person and their family, the actual admission usually took place within the context of a crisis, often following hospitalisation.

The move to a care home can be particularly difficult for spouse caregivers; approximately 7–10 per cent of residents in care homes have a partner living in the community (O'May, 2007). A proactive approach, involving frequent and sensitive exploration of the views of all parties, is likely to ease the transition, and this is a key advocacy role for nurses working with older people, who can encourage, foster and facilitate open communication between older people and their carers.

There is some disturbing evidence to suggest that the older person is not always involved in the decision about the move to a care home, particularly when they are perceived to be cognitively frail (Davies and Nolan, 2003). In some cases, the older person may be transferred to a care home without even having had the opportunity to visit the home beforehand. In a large survey, it was found that only 57 per cent of older people who moved into a care home believed that they had any choice about moving there, and only half had seen the home before moving in (HOPDEV, 2006).

Based on the findings of a number of research studies, Nolan *et al.* (1996) developed a typology describing the admission process to a care home:

- *The positive choice*: the move is viewed by the older person as desirable and they are a partner in the decision-making process.
- *The rationalised alternative*: the move is not viewed as desirable, but the older person comes to terms with it as being the only possible option.

- *The discredited option*: initial perceptions of what the move would entail become changed, e.g. the older person was under the impression that it was a temporary move but it becomes permanent.
- *The fait accompli*: the decision for the move is taken by others, without real or meaningful involvement by the older person.

Nolan and colleagues suggest that nurses are well placed to support older people and their carers when making a positive choice to enter a care home. Indeed, ensuring that people have the necessary information, in a form that they can understand, to make an informed choice is central to the NMC Code. One person's experience of this decision is shown in Box 19.3.

BOX 19.3 Estaline's story

I was 35 in 1962 when I came to England. My husband sent for me by plane. He was working at the hospital where I took a job as a ward orderly. We had family here and we came to join them. There were lots of jobs available. I stayed in the job for 24 years and then retired. My husband died 2 years ago. After an amputation due to diabetes, I came in here about a year ago. I lived in a big prefab flat in Deptford. It was a lovely little flat and I cried when I had to leave it. After this happened, I decided I would move into a home. I did not want to be dependent on my stepdaughter. I did not want 'care in the community', as they said they would send somebody sometimes, and I said, 'That won't do'. I would feel worried waiting for whoever was going to come. My family worried so much about me being alone, so it was much better all round for me to have someone to look after me. It was very hard adapting at first, but I had to do something. My family helped me to come to terms with it. I like to be with other people. I have made some new friends in here. When I was not well one day, a lot of residents came up to see me as they missed me and visited me. It has helped. It is the other residents and staff together – everybody. I have more friends here, as at home they'd no sooner looked at me than they were gone, so it is better here. I have made the right choice. I would not go back, no. My life is now different. But I am OK. I like to have some Caribbean food, but I don't get it now. In the hospital they used to send for Caribbean food for me, rice and peas or pork with nice gravy. I am waiting for a prosthesis for my stump; I hope it will be soon. I will feel much better then; it will give me more independence and I shall be able to do more. I don't want to be too dependent on the staff for my daily care needs. That is what is most important to me now.

(Estaline Banfield, care home resident, quoted in Owens and NCHRDF, 2006, p. 26, with permission from Help the Aged)

Reflection point 19.4
Which of Nolan's four types of decision do you feel most closely reflects the experiences described by Estaline Banfield in Box 19.3?

Estaline's experience most closely fits the 'rationalised alternative' described by Nolan *et al.* Although Estaline was able to reach the decision to move to a care home, she was very sad about leaving her flat and would probably have remained there for longer if community services had been available to meet her needs.

We have already touched upon a number of factors that impact upon quality of life in old age. In the next section we consider these factors in more detail.

SUMMARY

- Experiences of ageing are diverse and are linked closely to the person's ability to do the things they want to do.
- It is essential that nurses and other health care professionals take time to get to know the older person in order to appreciate what is important to them and to learn about their individual coping skills.
- Assisting older people to manage life transitions is an important function of nursing. Transitions with the potential to impact on health and well-being include retirement from paid employment, bereavement and moving accommodation.
- Careful planning and involvement in decision-making are important factors in achieving successful transitions.

Factors influencing quality of life in old age

Quality of life is notoriously difficult to define, as it pervades a range of aspects of everyday living in significant and complex ways (Reed, 2007). Other terms such as 'well-being', 'life satisfaction' and 'happiness' are often used interchangeably with 'quality of life', which makes it difficult to be clear exactly what is being referred to and how it can be supported. What creates a good quality of life is likely to be individual to each older person. However, research studies have identified a number of common factors that have been linked to perceptions of a good quality of life. Other researchers have explored perceptions of what constitutes successful aging in an attempt to access this elusive concept. For example, in a report of a survey of personal definitions of successful aging, Bowling and Dieppe (2005) note the following suggestions:

> [Successful ageing is to] go out a lot and enjoy life, take it day by day, and enjoy what you can . . . Have good health – that's more important than anything else. Keep active – while your legs are moving get out on them.
> [It's] good health. Well, if you're fit and able to do more . . . active . . . you . . . contribute to society and get actively involved. It's your outlook on life to start with. I think I have been an active person. It's your whole outlook. Do you make an effort to keep fit? I don't think about getting old. I just don't feel old and act accordingly.
>
> (Bowling and Dieppe, 2005, p. 1549)

On the basis of a systematic review of the literature on 'successful ageing', Bowling and Dieppe identified a number of theoretical definitions. These were supplemented with lay definitions from the survey of older people's views (Box 19.4).

BOX 19.4 Main constituents of successful aging

Theoretical definitions
- life expectancy;
- life satisfaction and well-being, including happiness and contentment;
- mental and psychological health and cognitive function;

BOX 19.4 (Continued)

- personal growth and learning new things;
- physical health and independent functioning;
- psychological characteristics and resources, including perceived autonomy, control, independence, adaptability, coping, self-esteem, positive outlook, goals and sense of self;
- social, community and leisure activities, integration and participation;
- social networks, support, participation and activity.

Additional lay definitions
- accomplishments;
- enjoyment of diet;
- financial security;
- neighbourhood;
- physical appearance;
- productivity and contribution to life;
- sense of humour;
- sense of purpose;
- spirituality.

Source: Bowling and Dieppe (2005, pp. 548–51).

The most common definitions of successful ageing identified in the survey are shown in Figure 19.2. The authors suggest that these findings reveal the limitations of biomedical models of health as a basis for assessing health outcomes in old age and the importance of sociopsychological models to a more comprehensive and accurate assessment.

The dominant themes within Bowling and Dieppe's definitions are roles and responsibilities, socioeconomic factors (including income, ethnicity, housing and access to services), relationships and health. We will consider each of these in more detail.

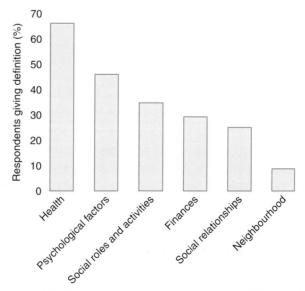

Figure 19.2 Most common definitions of successful ageing given by 854 people aged ⩾50 years in Britain. From Bowling A and Dieppe P (2005). What is successful ageing and who should define it? *British Medical Journal*, **331**, 1548–51. Reproduced with permission from the BMJ Publishing Group.

Roles and responsibilities

Within this chapter, we make the basic assumption that all older people, including those with cognitive or physical frailty, have the potential to make a contribution to the society in which they live. Older people have accumulated a lifetime of wisdom and experience, and sharing this knowledge with others can take place even in the context of severe cognitive impairment. Furthermore, many older people make a very practical contribution to the lives of others. For example, more than one-third of older people are carers to ill or disabled people, while others provide childcare for relatives who are working mothers. Research carried out on behalf of Carers UK found that more than 1.5 million people over the age of 60 years are providing unpaid care for a relative or friend (Buckner and Yeandle, 2005). More than 8000 of these carers are aged 90 years or over, predominantly husbands caring for their wives. Older people also provide substantial voluntary help to organisations that contribute to health and social care (Davis Smith and Gay, 2005; Faulkner and Davies, 2005).

Another area in which older people make a valuable contribution is in the field of paid work. Although retirement from paid work is now almost universal for workers in the developed world, there is wide variability in the age at which people retire (Marshall and Taylor, 2005). In the UK, more than one million people over the age at which they are eligible to receive the state pension are in paid employment (Equal Opportunities Commission, 2005). Flexible forms of employment such as self-employment and part-time working enable many older people to ease the transition from full-time employment to retirement (Platman, 2003). For some people, this can provide a much-needed supplement to pension income; for others, the main motivation is the sense of worth and identity gained from being employed. There are many advantages for employers in hiring older workers, including reliability, prior investment in skills and know-how, and company loyalty (Schultz, 2001). However, national (and international) trends in the employment of older workers show a decline in the economic participation of older people, and especially older men. Age discrimination within the workplace has been cited as the main reason for this (Platman and Tinker, 1998).

Socioeconomic factors

A number of socioeconomic factors influence and impact upon quality of life in old age. These include income, housing and access to services.

Income

Increasing emphasis on private and occupational pensions, coupled with the declining real value of the basic state pension, is resulting in greater income inequality in later life (Evandrou and Falkingham, 2006). As a consequence of the housing boom of the latter part of the twentieth century, many older people are financially very comfortable. However, the risk of poverty among older people in the UK is about three to four times higher than the typical risk of poverty in Europe (Burholt and Windle, 2006). Moreover, people aged 75 years and over rely more on benefits as a source of income and get a smaller proportion of their income from occupational pensions and investments than do younger pensioners. A study carried out for the Joseph Rowntree Foundation, published in 2006, used data for 987 people aged 65 years and over to compare the material resources and financial satisfaction of different groups of older people and identify the key determinants of poverty in old age (Burholt and Windle, 2006). The findings indicate that women, people living alone, people who are widowed, divorced or separated, people in poor health, people with lower education and people living in deprived neighbourhoods tend to have low levels of material resources or income in old age. Not surprisingly, findings suggest that differences in material resources and financial well-being in old age are determined by earlier life experiences, for example engagement in the labour market and subsequent ability to save and invest. This confirms the importance of a long-term view in ensuring financial security in late life.

In 2005, the charity Age Concern published research undertaken by independent experts at the London School of Hygiene and Tropical Medicine to determine what is needed to live healthily in later life and how much it costs to meet these needs (Morris *et al.*, 2005). The research found significant gaps between the minimum income for healthy living and state pensions (the gap was £17.85 a week for a couple in their seventies for example). The cost of a healthy diet for older people carrying out the recommended level of physical activity was determined to be £32.30 for a single person and £63.70 for a couple – around 30 per cent more than older people on a low income actually spend. These findings are particularly significant for nurses engaged in health promotion work with older people.

Nurses are often reluctant to discuss financial issues with older patients and their families. However, many older people are unaware of the range of benefits are available to them, and a sensitive discussion can point them in the direction of additional resources that can make a significant difference to their quality of life.

Housing

While the condition of homes in the UK continues to improve, people in vulnerable groups, including older people and people from ethnic minorities, continue to be disproportionately represented in the worst housing conditions (Department for Communities and Local Government, 2006). The effects of sub-standard housing on the health and well-being of older people have been well documented (Lawrence, 2004). For example, research indicates links between cold, damp housing and respiratory illnesses and heart disease. Heating is particularly important for older people because they often spend longer in their homes and tend to be less active. A UK study by the charity Help the Aged found that, in the poorest neighbourhoods, 22 per cent of older people have gone without fuel to make ends meet (Help the Aged, 2004). Fuel poverty is defined as the need to spend more than 10 per cent of income on energy in order to maintain an adequate standard of warmth (Help the Aged, 2004). Increases in utility costs are likely to affect older people disproportionately. In 2003, estimates suggested that there were 2 million fuel-poor households in the UK and that 49 per cent of these contained a person over the age of 60 years (DTI and DEFRA, 2005).

Ethnic groups

The inequality faced by older people from black and minority ethnic communities in the UK is significant. Older people are currently a small proportion of the black and minority ethnic communities in Britain, and there has been little research into their specific needs. Less than 5 per cent of people from black and minority ethnic communities are currently over 60 years of age, but this will increase significantly over the next 30–40 years (PRIAE, 2006). Black and minority ethnic elders in the UK experience high levels of deprivation and social exclusion (ODPM, 2005). There are variations between ethnic groups, but nonetheless there is a substantial relationship between ethnicity and a number of indicators of deprivation. For example, black and minority ethnic elders are concentrated in large urban areas, such as London and the West Midlands, which have high levels of social deprivation. They are more likely to be living in low-income households in poorer-quality, overcrowded accommodation (PRIAE, 2006).

The English House Condition Survey 2004 (Department for Communities and Local Government, 2006) shows that ethnic minority groups are disproportionately likely to live in poor-quality housing, such as the worst pre-1919 terraced housing. Ethnic minority groups also tend to live in more densely populated households compared with the majority of the population. In Pakistani and Bangladeshi households, 43 per cent had over one person per room; this contrasts markedly with older white people, who are more likely to live alone.

All of these social and economic factors have an influence on health and well-being and can put older people at risk of ill health. However, one of the most significant factors influencing quality of life in old age is the relationships that older people maintain with others, and it is to these that we now turn.

Relationships in old age

Repeated studies have found that older people nominate family relationships and contact with others as important determinants of their quality of life (Brown *et al.*, 2004). Furthermore, numerous commentators have suggested that one of the keys to successful ageing is staying connected to others (Volz, 2000; Bowling and Dieppe, 2005). Volz (2000), for example, cites a link between social support and health: older people do better if they continue to engage with life and maintain close relationships. Helping older people to develop and maintain connections with others in their community is therefore an effective nursing intervention.

The majority of older people continue to have close contact with family and friends. Data from the 2001 General Household Survey indicate that three-quarters of people aged 65 years and over see their relatives and friends weekly, and the majority see their neighbours to chat to (Victor, 2006). Families continue to be the source of a great deal of material and emotional support across generations. In a study of older Asian people in Scotland, Bowes and Dar (2000) provide evidence of extensive use of informal carers. Recurrent themes within interview studies involving residents of care homes also highlight the importance of relationships with staff, family members and other residents as crucial to their well-being (Davies and Brown-Wilson, 2007). Expert nurses working with older people are therefore likely to be much more effective if they see themselves as having a role in supporting such relationships (Nolan *et al.*, 2001).

Relationships are important to older people in a number of ways. For example, there is research to suggest that caring relationships can prevent ill health and aid recovery from illness (Murray and Fortinberry, 2004). In a study of what constitutes a 'good old age', Godfrey *et al.* (2004) found that themes of 'caring for' and 'caring about' dominated older people's stories over different parts of the life course. This was expressed in

> the importance attached to 'neighbourliness', in their descriptions of how they looked out for each other, their stories of mutual assistance in times of adversity and the reciprocal exchange of little kindnesses that were a routine part of daily life.
>
> (Godfrey *et al.*, 2004)

We will return to ideas about caring relationships later in this chapter.

So far we have considered experiences of ageing as described by older people. However, public perceptions of ageing may also contribute to these experiences, and these are considered in the next section.

Common public perceptions and images of ageing

Images of ageing are important because they shape both professional and lay conceptions of what it means to grow older and can therefore influence the treatment that older people receive. In general, there are two broad but distinct and alternative images of ageing:

- Ageing is viewed as a time of opportunities and possibilities – an active, fluid, 'positive' image of old age.

- Ageing is viewed as a time of dependence, decline and disadvantage – a more passive, inevitable, 'negative' image of old age (Martin, 2006).

Both of these depictions represent stereotypes, in that the real experiences of older people are very diverse and likely to range between these extremes.

In negative stereotypes, older people are often caricatured as frail, forgetful, shabby, out of date, and on the edge of senility and death (Featherstone and Hepworth, 2005). Images of mental and physical decline are all too common in literature and the media and reflect the myth that they are an inevitable consequence of ageing. Older people who have in some way become dependent on their carers are sometimes treated as 'having reduced claim on conventional adult status', with the result that they are treated as if they were children (Featherstone and Hepworth, 2005). Such practices are clearly in contravention of the NMC Code, which states that professional nurses must treat people as individuals and respect their dignity.

In reality, as noted already, only a minority of older people experience severe disability. Most are able to live active and fulfilling lives until they die.

Positive stereotypes of ageing also assign broad attributes to older people, for example that they are wise and experienced. Our consumer culture has produced some optimistic, even glamorous, images of ageing and later life, particularly in retirement and self-help literature (Featherstone and Hepworth, 2005). However, Holstein and Minkler (2003) suggest that positive stereotypes can also cause problems, as they imply that successful ageing is based on three attributes:

- avoidance of disease and disability;
- high levels of physical and cognitive functioning;
- active engagement with life.

Holstein and Minkler (2003) argue that using the above criteria effectively relegates large sections of the older population to the 'unsuccessful' category, which constitutes a new and dangerous form of ageism. We now consider the notion of ageism in more detail.

Ageism

A key tenet of the NMC Code is the need to avoid any kind of discrimination against those receiving care. One example of discrimination that is unfortunately still all too prevalent within health care is ageism. Bytheway (2006) defines ageism as 'a set of beliefs about how people vary biologically as a result of the ageing process'.

In a report entitled *How ageist is Britain?*, the charity Age Concern (2005) provides evidence that ageism is the most prevalent form of discrimination in Great Britain. In a nationally representative survey, 29 per cent of respondents had experienced age discrimination, and those aged 55 years and over were twice as likely to have experienced ageism than any other form of discrimination. The authors of the report pose a series of questions in order to illustrate the range and extent of age discrimination within our society, such as:

- Why are women over the age of 70 years not invited for breast cancer screening?
- Why are magistrates or jurors not allowed to serve past the age of 70 years?
- Why are nearly a third of people between 50 years and state pension age without paid work?

As mentioned previously, ageist attitudes may also impact upon older people's experiences of health care, the focus of the next section.

SUMMARY

- Quality of life in old age is notoriously difficult to define but has been associated with the notion of successful ageing.
- Factors influencing quality of life include roles and responsibilities, socioeconomic factors, relationships and health.
- Ageist attitudes are still rife within health services, and it is the professional nurse's duty to challenge such attitudes whenever they occur.

Experiences of health and illness

Until quite recently, very little was known about the health status of older people. Epidemiological studies tended to focus on younger age groups, and there was a lack of specific outcome measures to determine older people's health and well-being. However, in recent years, health in later life has become an important government priority, and there is much more interest in understanding older people's experiences of health and illness. Some of the key facts about older people's health in the UK are summarised in Box 19.5.

BOX 19.5 Some facts about the health of older people in the UK

- Women can expect to live longer than men, with life expectancy at birth in the UK in 2002 being 75.9 years for men and 80.5 years for women. However, women are also more likely to have more years in poor health: the expected length of time lived in poor health from age 65 years onwards was 4.5 years for men and 5.8 years for women.
- The proportion of older people with a long-term illness or disability that restricts their daily activities increases with age.
- Many people in older age groups still consider themselves to be in good health, even if they have a long-term illness that restricts daily activities.
- In 2003, just over a quarter of men aged 50–59 years were current smokers compared with 23 per cent of women. The likelihood of smoking falls with age, reflecting both a 'healthy survivor' effect and patterns of smoking cessation. Over half of all smokers aged 50 years and over reported wanting to give up smoking altogether.
- Older people were more likely to drink alcohol frequently than younger people, and men were more likely than women to drink. However, older people were less likely to have exceeded the recommended number of daily units in the last week compared with younger age groups.
- Inequalities in health persist into later life. In the 2001 Census, 30 per cent of people aged 50 years and over living in council rented accommodation reported a long-standing life-limiting illness and 'not good' health over the past year, compared with 22 per cent of those residing in privately rented or rent-free accommodation and just 14 per cent of owner-occupiers.
- Inequalities in health in later life are also found by socioeconomic classification, with a greater proportion of older people who worked in semi-routine and routine occupations reporting a long-standing illness that limited their activities than those who had worked in managerial and professional occupations. Among those aged 50–74 years, the gradient by occupation widened in the 60–64 years age group, after which it flattened out. This may reflect the healthy survivor effect, as those in the worst health die.
- Health also varies by ethnicity: 27 per cent of all older people aged 50–64 reported a limiting long term illness (LLTI). However, this rose to 54 per cent among elders of Bangladeshi origin and 49 per cent among those of Pakistani origin, compared with just 20 per cent of Chinese origin.

Source: Evandrou (2005). Crown copyright material is reproduced by permission of HMSO and the Queen's Printer for Scotland.

Reflection point 19.5
Consider the points in Box 19.5 and identify any implications for your work with older people.

You might have thought of the potential for health promotion with older people, particularly in light of the number of older smokers who would like help to quit. These statistics also confirm a number of high-risk groups within the older population who might benefit from more targeted interventions, including people in particular ethnic groups and people on a low income.

We will now consider strategies for promoting the health of older people in more detail.

Health promotion and older people

A common reason for not attempting health promotion with older people is the belief that it is too late and that patterns of healthy living must begin earlier in life in order to prevent problems later. Another argument is that older people are set in their ways and resistant to change. However, a growing body of research provides evidence that much can be done in later life to maximise health potential. For example, a healthy balanced diet provides a level of protection against dementia, osteoporosis and bowel cancer (Khaw, 1997). Older people may benefit from advice about alcohol consumption; however, they are more likely to drink in line with sensible drinking guidelines, as they tend to consume alcohol over a period of time, as opposed to consuming large quantities on only one or two days each week (Foster and Marriott, 2006).

Smoking remains the single greatest cause of illness and premature death in England, killing at least 85 600 people each year and accounting for one-third of all cancers (DH, 2006). In Scotland, 13 500 people die each year as a result of tobacco use (NHS Scotland and ASH Scotland, 2007). There is evidence that older people can be assisted to stop smoking even in advanced old age (Tait *et al.*, 2007). However, a qualitative study of older smokers' health beliefs found that current smokers reported many positive associations with smoking, which often prevented a smoking cessation attempt (Kerr *et al.*, 2006). The majority were aware that smoking had damaged their health, but some were not convinced of the benefits of stopping. A common view was that 'the damage was done', and therefore there was little point in attempting to stop smoking. Some of the participants reported that they had never been advised to stop smoking, and knowledge of local smoking cessation services was generally poor. The findings of this study suggest that, when helping older people to stop smoking, it is essential to take into account their health beliefs and that issues such as knowledge of smoking cessation resources are addressed.

The importance of exercise

We know that exercise can benefit health in a whole variety of situations (Warburton *et al.*, 2006). Even people with long-standing disability can preserve some independence through regular, gentle exercise. Skelton (1993) found that older women could improve the strength of their thigh muscles by approximately 25 per cent during a 12-week gentle exercise programme. Some advantages of exercise include preventing falls and osteoporosis, improving function in osteoarthritis and alleviating depression. Exercise is also associated with reduced risk for the incidence of dementia among people aged 65 years and older (Larson *et al.*, 2006). In a study of 1740 people aged over 65 years and without cognitive impairment, the incidence rate of dementia was 13.0 per 1000 person-years for participants who exercised three or more times per week compared with 19.7 per 1000 person-years for those who exercised fewer than three times per week.

In spite of the large benefit of exercise in later life, research suggests that among people over 50 years of age, only 17 per cent of women and 25 per cent of men are sufficiently active to benefit their health (Age Concern, 2006a). One initiative that attempts to rectify this situation is shown in Box 19.6.

BOX 19.6 Walking the Way to Health

The Walking the Way to Health initiative is supported by the British Heart Foundation and Natural England, with Lottery funding. There are currently around 350 health walk schemes, catering for people of all ages and abilities. The aim is to improve the health and fitness of those who currently do little exercise. Group walks and independent walking are included in walking for health schemes. Regular walks take place in town, city and rural locations at various times of the day and usually last up to an hour. You can find more information about this scheme at www.whi.org.uk.

Dog-walking is particularly good exercise as it facilitates regular routine outings into the local area and physical activity, while giving the person companionship, an added sense of security and increased independence. In interviews exploring the relationships between people and their dogs, participants said that 'by going on walks with their dogs they met other people, and that the dogs often acted as a catalyst for conversation' (McColgan, 2006).

The charity Extend provides recreational movement to music for men and women over the age of 60 years and for less able people of all ages. The charity's mission is to promote health, to increase mobility and independence, to improve strength, coordination and balance, and to counteract loneliness and isolation, thereby enhancing quality of life. Further information can be found at www.extend.org.uk. Exercise programmes such as t'ai chi have also become very popular with older people.

Promoting mental health in later life

The range of mental health problems experienced in later life is extremely wide and the extent of unmet need considerable (Box 19.7).

BOX 19.7 Mental health problems in later life

- One in four older people living in the community has symptoms of depression that are severe enough to warrant intervention.
- Only a third of older people with depression ever discuss it with their general practitioner (GP). Only half of them are diagnosed and treated, primarily with antidepressants.
- Depression is the leading risk factor for suicide. Older men and women have some of the highest suicide rates of all ages in the UK.
- Dementia costs the health and social care economy more than cancer, heart disease and stroke combined.
- Fewer than half of older people with dementia ever receive a diagnosis.
- A third of people who provide unpaid care for an older person with dementia have depression.
- Delirium or acute confusion affects up to 60 per cent of older people who have an operation.
- There are approximately 70 000 older people with schizophrenia in the UK.
- People aged 55–74 years have the highest rates of alcohol-related deaths in the UK.
- It is agreed that rates of prescription and illicit drug misuse in later life are underestimated, but few if any definitive statistics exist.

Source: NCHRDF (2007). Reproduced with permission from Age Concern.

Evidence about the factors that affect mental health and well-being has increased in recent years. We now know much more, for example, about the link between social isolation and mental illness. In 2006, the charity Age Concern, in partnership with the Mental Health Foundation, published the first report of the UK inquiry into mental health and well-being in later life (Age Concern, 2006b). This report draws on a comprehensive review of policy and literature and identifies ways to promote mental health in old age. The inquiry also invited nearly 900 older people and carers to share their views and experiences of what helps to promote well-being in later life, together with more than 150 professionals and organisations. The review identified five main areas that influence mental health for older people:

* discrimination;
* participation in meaningful activity;
* relationships;
* physical health;
* poverty (Age Concern, 2006b).

We have considered most of these issues within earlier sections of this chapter. The report provides useful evidence of the way in which psychosocial, biological and environmental factors interact to influence well-being for older people.

One project that aims to reduce social isolation among older people by involving them in stimulating leisure activities is described in Box 19.8. An evaluation of the Upstream project found improvements in mental health and social support (Greaves and Farbus, 2006), and the intervention was well received by participants.

BOX 19.8 The Upstream Healthy Living Centre

Upstream is an independent charity with a 5-year project aimed at improving the well-being and quality of life for older, more isolated, people in mid-Devon, an area of rural isolation and pockets of social deprivation. Partly funded by the Lottery and Arts Council England, Upstream engages people in stimulating creative, leisure, learning and social activities in order to improve their quality of life, restore their self-confidence, revive their passion for life, encourage independent living, overcome social exclusion, and enable people to maintain high-quality shared experiences and supportive community networks.

The Upstream Healthy Living Centre is a community-based intervention operating on an outreach basis. Mentors work closely with participants, aiming to rekindle their passion and interest in life by engaging in participant-determined programmes of creative exercise or cultural activities with an emphasis on social interaction. The intervention is tailored individually to suit each participant's own interests and passions. Activity-based interventions are provided, with visits from mentors initially on a weekly basis, and regular telephone contact, which is gradually diminished as participants become more confident and able.

More information is available at www.upstream-uk.com.

Older people's experiences of health care

Most nurses working with older people, and many patients and service users themselves, are aware that services for older people originated in the Poor Law reforms of the late 1900s. The medical specialty of geriatrics evolved in the 1930s in the context of the workhouse through the pioneering work of Dr Marjorie Warren. She recognised that many of the sick and bed-bound older occupants of the workhouse infirmaries could benefit from assessment, diagnosis and rehabilitation. Until this time, the care of sick older people was carried out mainly by unskilled nurses, who were sometimes sent to work in a workhouse as a form of punishment for misdemeanours elsewhere in the service (Nolan, 1997). Similarly, doctors who practised in the workhouses were viewed as inferior in status and skills.

The development of gerontological nursing has been located predominantly in hospital settings and has largely followed the medical model (Evers, 1981). The pioneering work of gerontological nurse Doreen Norton (Norton *et al.*, 1962) drew attention to routinised practices in the care of older people in hospital settings, with the emphasis on meeting physical needs dictated by disease processes and 'getting through the work' (Baker, 1978). Successive studies have suggested that a routinised approach to care continues to dominate in some care settings (Waters, 1994; Nolan *et al.*, 1995; Davies, 2003).

Reports by voluntary and governmental organisations have continued to identify shortfalls in providing older people with the quality of care they would like (Healthcare Commission, Audit Commission and Commission for Social Care Inspection, 2006). For example, there are ongoing concerns about the poor standards of care that older people receive when they are admitted to acute hospital wards (NHS Quality Improvement Scotland, 2005). In particular, older people and family caregivers have expressed their dissatisfaction with discharge arrangements and access to information. Although financial constraints are often a barrier to the development of services, studies have shown that older patients are often able to identify small improvements that would not be too demanding but that could make a considerable difference to the quality of care they experience (Davies *et al.*, 1999; Meyer *et al.*, 1999). The challenges of providing high-quality care to older people in a range of care environments, such as community settings, continuing care and palliative care, and to people with learning difficulties or mental health problems, have also been described (see Nolan *et al.* (2001) for a review of literature in relation to each client group).

Some of these ongoing challenges have been linked to questions about the adequacy and appropriateness of training to work with older people (Nolan *et al.*, 2002). You may find it interesting to read the following comments from qualified nurses talking about their training in the 1980s and 1990s and how they learned about older people. These quotations are taken from a major research project that set out to explore the effectiveness of nurse education in preparing nurses to work with older people and their carers (Nolan *et al.*, 2002).

> When I look back at my training I just remember how awful it was and how there was such little interest about it [nursing older people] in the training school. The wards where older people lived were no better either, rows and rows of beds and nothing much happening for most of the time. As bad as it was I just wanted to go back and improve things after I had finished my RMN . . . to try and do something better for the older people in there, if you like.
> We had very little education on mental health and older people. It was more hands on, learn as you go along. There were no real skills taught to us at all, it was all task, task, task.
> The staff were overworked, underappreciated and underpaid. Their contribution wasn't valued so consequently patient care suffered. Therapeutic touch and communication were limited by trained staff, carers just saw to their physical needs.

> (Nolan *et al.*, 2002, p. 275)

In addition to discrimination resulting from poor attitudes as a result of inadequate training, older people may also experience inequalities in health care because of rationing. According to

Ham (2004), rationing has always been part of the NHS, and the requirements of an ageing population have added to the challenge. Indeed, there is evidence to suggest that older people may be missing out on vital health and social care services because age discrimination is not being identified (Kings Fund, 2003). In England and Wales, the *National Service Framework (NSF) for Older People* (DH, 2001) requires a systematic approach to identifying and eliminating age discrimination in access to health and social care, confirming this issue as a government priority. However, a review of the impact of the NSF for Older People published in 2006 suggested that although progress has been made in reducing age discrimination, further action is required in a number of areas, one of which is tackling discrimination through ageist attitudes (Healthcare Commission, Audit Commission and Commission for Social Care Inspection, 2006). The NMC Code makes explicit that nurses must do all they can to ensure that people are not discriminated against in their care, and demonstrate a personal and professional commitment to equality and diversity.

There is no exact equivalent of the NSF for Older People in Scotland and Northern Ireland, but the documents Scottish Executive (2006, 2007) and DHSSPSNI (2004, 2005) include recommendations relating to older people and provide useful pointers to practice.

Reflection point 19.6

Can you think of examples from your own practice experience where older people have been discriminated against in terms of access to services purely on the basis of their age? What was the outcome for these people?

You might have thought about access to screening services; for example, women in the UK are currently invited to breast screening until they are 70 years old, although they can request screening every 3 years after this age. The charity Age Concern highlights concerns that some general practitioners (GPs) may not refer patients for further investigations beyond a certain age limit (Age Concern, 2007). The impact of such discrimination for older people can be profound, in terms of missing out on possibly effective treatments and the opportunity for reassurance.

Units for the care of older people have been systematically under-resourced in the health and social services. Although this does not excuse poor nursing practice, it does go some way towards explaining it. In the past, nurses who have chosen to work with older people have frequently had to deal with comments about the 'undesirable' nature of work with older people and how it might 'damage' their career prospects (Nolan *et al.*, 2002). However, some of the most pioneering nursing research in recent years has taken place in the context of services for older people. Furthermore, the context for older people's care services has changed, with a greater emphasis on services in the community and in people's own homes. This is resulting in new models and frameworks for nursing practice that place a greater emphasis on partnership working. We will now consider some of these frameworks.

Promoting person-centred and relationship-centred care

During recent years, 'person-centredness' has become one of the main ideas underpinning nursing work with older people. In a useful review of the literature on person-centredness in gerontological nursing, McCormack (2004) suggests that the capacity for reflection and free will are essential elements of personhood, but that this capacity is often impaired through illness and disability. The role of the nurse then becomes to assist the person to 'form those desires and determine possible actions as freely as if his freedom of action had not been impaired' (McCormack, 2004, p. 33). This is consistent with the advocacy role described in the NMC Code.

When working with older people, focusing on 'the person' also requires consideration of the needs of others with whom the older person is in relationship. This is recognised increasingly by researchers working in this field (Nolan *et al.*, 2006). For example, MacDonald (2002) argues that we need to develop a relational (as opposed to an individual) approach that sees human beings as belonging to a network of social relationships within which they are 'deeply interconnected and interdependent'. Clark (2002) proposes that, if we are to provide meaningful care and services to older people, we need to 'situate' an older person's individual needs within a rich matrix of relationships and sociocultural beliefs. Similarly, McCormack (2001) suggests that we need to replace an individualistic view of autonomy in later life with one based on 'interconnectedness and partnership'. These perspectives acknowledge the potential of person-centred care but call for more attention to be paid to the interdependencies that shape our lives (McCormack, 2001; Kelly *et al.*, 2005).

This new emphasis on the interpersonal and relational aspects of care has led some commentators to suggest that the idea of relationship-centred care provides a more appropriate philosophy to underpin future developments in services for older people (Nolan *et al.*, 2002, 2004, 2006). The term 'relationship-centred care' was first coined by a task force in the USA in the early 1990s. The Pew Fetzer Task Force was set up to examine ways of developing curricula across the caring disciplines that would recognise the interaction between biomedical and psychosocial aspects of health care and that would demonstrate an integrated approach. The task force concluded that the notion of relationship-centred care should underpin all health interactions, arguing that:

> relationships are critical to the care provided by nearly all practitioners and a sense of satisfaction and positive outcomes for patients and practitioners
>
> (Tresolini and Pew-Fetzer Task Force, 1994. p. 11)

> Such relationships included those between service users, practitioners and the communities in which they live and work
>
> (Tresolini and Pew-Fetzer Task Force, 1994)

More recently, researchers have applied the idea of relationship-centred care to work with older people (Nolan *et al.*, 2002, 2006). They argue that relationships are a critical component of working effectively with older people and their supporters, and that the needs of all parties must be taken into account. Although relationships are a prerequisite to effective care and teaching, there has been little formal acknowledgement of their importance and few efforts to help students and practitioners learn to develop effective relationships in health care. Nolan *et al.* (2006) suggest that interactions are at the heart of relationship-centred care and are the 'foundations' of any therapeutic or healing activity. However, nurses and other practitioners need guidance in identifying ways of interacting with older people and their families that best support relationships. With this in mind, the Senses Framework was developed. This framework is built upon many years of research in a range of care settings (Nolan, 1997; Davies *et al.*, 1999, Nolan *et al.*, 2001, 2002). The framework suggests that the best care for older people involves the creation of a set of senses or experiences for older people, for family caregivers and for staff working with them:

- *Sense of security*: of feeling safe and receiving or delivering competent and sensitive care.
- *Sense of continuity*: recognition of biography, and using the past to contextualise the present.
- Sense *of belonging*: opportunities to form meaningful relationships or feel part of a team.
- *Sense of purpose*: opportunities to engage in purposeful activities or to have a clear set of goals to aspire to.

- *Sense of achievement*: achievement meaningful or valued goals and feeling satisfied with one's efforts.
- *Sense of significance*: to feel that you matter, and that you are valued as a person (Nolan *et al.*, 2002).

Research has shown that the most supportive relationships and the best experiences of care result when older people, their families and the staff working with them are enabled to experience the senses. Furthermore, through linking the experiences of older people, their families and staff, the Senses Framework has the potential to promote understanding of the experiences of others, thus enhancing communication and the ability to work in partnership.

Reflection point 19.7
Think about an older person you have worked with recently. How could you create each of the six 'senses' for them through your nursing practice?

Some examples are shown in Table 19.1, which also suggests how the senses might be created for staff and for family members in an acute care setting. There is growing evidence of a relationship between job satisfaction for staff and the quality of care received by older patients (Redfern *et al.*, 2002). If staff work within an environment in which positive care is actively promoted, then not only is that quality of care more likely to be sustained but also job satisfaction will be enhanced.

Table 19.1 Creating the senses on an acute ward for older people

	Older people	Staff	Family members
Security	Being able to see the staff or summon help easily	Experienced staff available to support more junior staff	Approachable staff
	Knowing that they can have painkillers when they need them	Clear boundaries within which to operate	Effective communication – being kept informed
	Knowing that the ward is clean	Being able to challenge poor practice without fear of censure	Feeling safe to complain without fear of recrimination
	Being able to find their way around the ward easily	Structured mechanisms for supervision and mentorship	Knowing that the staff have the skills they need for their role.
	Knowing who everyone is. Being introduced to new members of staff.		Having regular access to senior, experienced members of staff
	Having staff check on them regularly.		
	Knowing that the staff have the skills they need for their role.		
	Having regular access to senior, experienced members of staff		
	Being given information		
Belonging	Being made to feel that they are in the right place	Being made to feel welcome as a new member of staff	Being made to feel welcome
	Being able to welcome visitors at any time	Regular meetings with colleagues	Being encouraged to take an active part in care

(Continued)

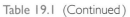

Table 19.1 (Continued)

	Older people	Staff	Family members
	Having opportunities to help other patients if they feel up to it	Being able to contribute to decision-making	Open visiting
	Having tea and coffee available for visitors	Blurring of roles	Comfortable seats for visiting
	Being able to get to know other patients		Access to beverages
Purpose	Regular discussions with staff about their treatment goals and plan of care	Regular appraisal and goal-setting for all staff	Involvement in care planning and delivery
	Having meaningful activities to pass the time	Opportunities to develop new skills	Having goals explained to them
		All staff involved in audit and practice development	Being invited to reviews
Continuity	Having the same members of staff allocated to care for them	Wards having designated therapy staff	Having the same members of staff allocated to care for them and their relative
	Being able to communicate with their families and friends	Integrated multidisciplinary documentation	Having access to care plans
		Explicit process for inducting new members of staff	
		Team nursing/named nursing as the system for organising care	
Achievement	Having regular feedback about their progress	Recognition of effort – e.g award schemes	Conflicts and concerns are addressed.
	Having their contribution to their recovery recognised and acknowledged	Designating additional responsibilities such as link nurse roles	Opportunities to evaluate their relative's progress
	Feeling that they have been able to make good relationships with ward staff and other patients	Being able to provide the best possible care	
Significance	Staff taking time to get to know me as a person	Investment in personal professional development	Being asked for their opinion and being listened to
	Feeling that staff respect my personal space and belongings	Opinions valued and listened to	Availability of service user forum
	Being able to have conversations with the staff	Adequate equipment and supplies to perform role	Having the opportunity to discuss their own needs
	Feeling that resources have been invested in making the surroundings comfortable	Work with older people is valued and recognised as important	
	Feeling that I have the same access to treatment options as a younger patient		
	Staff not using my Christian name without being invited to do so		

Adapted from Nolan *et al.* (2006), NCHRDF (2007)

Focusing on the person and their experience is becoming increasingly important in the success criteria by which all health care providers – not just older person care providers – will be judged (DH 2008).

CONCLUSION

In this chapter we have attempted to highlight some of the key factors influencing experiences of ageing in the UK. The principles exemplified within the NMC Code of treating people as individuals and respecting their dignity are particularly relevant when working with older people, because of the many threats to identity and dignity that accompany old age. Furthermore, ageist attitudes are remarkably persistent and can result in discrimination in the provision of health services. It is essential that nurses are particularly alert to ageist practices and are prepared to challenge these when they occur.

The recognition that older people now form the major proportion of users of health care services, together with the articulation of goals of care within a range of care environments, provides a clear impetus for further developing the knowledge base for practice with older people and their families, and for ensuring that nursing of older people is perceived as a positive career choice. New roles and opportunities are being created as services are reconfigured better to meet the needs of older people and their carers. Simultaneously, practice models and frameworks, such as person-centred and relationship-centred care, and the Senses Framework outlined within this chapter, are beginning to reveal the fundamentals of care for older people and are helping to define the nature of gerontological nursing. An ongoing challenge is to ensure that all older people and their family caregivers have access to the highest possible standards of care, whatever their circumstances and in whatever caring environment. As we have argued in this chapter, this will require that everyone involved in helping older people to meet their health and social care needs – staff, family members and older people – is able to participate and contribute in mutually fulfilling ways.

References

Age Concern (2005). *How Ageist is Britain?* London: Age Concern.

Age Concern (2006a). *Staying Healthy in Later Life*. London: Age Concern.

Age Concern (2006b). *Promoting Mental Health and Well-Being in Later Life*. London: Age Concern and the Mental Health Foundation.

Age Concern (2007). *Improving Services and Support for Older People with Mental Health Problems: The Second Report from the UK Inquiry into Mental Health and Well-Being in Later Life*. London: Age Concern.

Baker D (1978). Attitudes of nurses to care of the elderly. Unpublished PhD thesis. Manchester: University of Manchester.

Bowes AM and Dar N with Srivastava A (2000). *Family Support and Community Care: a study of South Asian Older People*. Edinburgh: Scottish Executive Central Research Unit.

Bowling A and Dieppe P (2005). What is successful ageing and who should define it? *British Medical Journal*, **331**, 1548–51.

Brown J, Bowling A and Flynn T (2004). Models of Quality of Life: A Taxonomy, Overview and Systematic Review of the Literature. www.agingresearch.group.shef.ac.uk/pdf/qol_review_no_tables.pdf.

Buckner L and Yeandle S (2005). *Older Carers in the UK*. London: Carers National.

Burholt V and Windle G (2006). *The Material Resources and Well-Being of Older People.* York: Joseph Rowntree Foundation.

Bytheway B (2006). Ageism. In Johnson M, with Bengtson VL, Coleman PG and Kirkwood BL (eds). *The Cambridge Handbook of Age and Ageing.* Cambridge: Cambridge University Press.

Carroll DW and Dill Linton A (2007). Age-related psychological changes. In Dill Linton A and Lach HW (eds). *Matteson and McConnell's Gerontological Nursing: Concepts and Practice*, 3rd edn. St Louis, MO: Saunders.

Cheek P, Nikpour L and Nowlin H (2005). Aging well with smart technology. *Nursing Administration Quarterly*, **29**, 329–38.

Chick N and Meleis AI (1986). Transitions: a nursing concern. In Chinn PL (ed.). *Nursing Research Methodology: Issues and Implementation.* Rockville, MD: Aspen.

Clark PG (2002). Values and voices in teaching gerontology and geriatrics. *The Gerontologist*, **42**, 297–303.

Clarke A, Hanson EJ and Ross H (2003). Seeing the person behind the patient: enhancing the care of older people using a biographical approach. *Journal of Clinical Nursing*, **12**, 697–706.

Cohen MA (2000). Bereavement groups with the elderly. *Journal of Psychotherapy in Independent Practice*, **1**, 33–41.

Davies S (2003). Creating community: the basis for caring partnerships in nursing homes. In Nolan M, Grant G, Keady J and Lundh U (eds). *Partnerships in Family Care.* Maidenhead: Open University Press.

Davies S (2007). *Exploring Ageing Study Guide*, BSC (Hons) in Nursing Studies. London: RCN Institute.

Davies S and Brown-Wilson C (2007). Creating community. In National Care Homes Research and Development Forum (NCHRDF). *My Home Life*. London: Help the Aged.

Davies S and Nolan M (2003). 'Making the best of things': relatives' experiences of decision about care-home entry. *Aging and Society*, **23**, 429–50.

Davies S, Nolan M, Brown J and Wilson F (1999). *Dignity on the Ward: Promoting Excellence in Care*. London: Help the Aged.

Davis Smith J and Gay P (2005). *Active Aging in Active Communities: Volunteering and the Transition to Retirement.* York: Joseph Rowntree Foundation.

Department for Communities and Local Government (2006). *English House Condition Survey: Annual Report 2004*. London: Department for Communities and Local Government.

Department of Health (DH) (2001). *The National Service Framework for Older People*. London: Department of Health.

Department of Health (DH) (2006). *Our Health, Our Care, Our Say: A New Direction for Community Services*. London: Department of Health.

Department of Health (DH) (2008). *High Quality Care for All: NHS Next Stage Review Final Report*. London: Department of Health.

Department of Health, Social Services and Public Safety, Northern Ireland (DHSSPSNI) (2004). A Healthier Future: A Twenty Year Vision for Health and Well-Being in Northern Ireland. www.dhsspsni.gov.uk/healthyfuture-main.pdf.

Department of Health, Social Services and Public Safety, Northern Ireland (DHSSPSNI) (2005). Realising the Vision: Nursing for Public Health – a Model for Putting Public Health into Practice. www.dhsspsni.gov.uk/nursing-for-public health.pdf#search=%22realising%20the%20vision%20DHSSPS%22.

Department of Trade and Industry (DTI) and Department for Environment Food and Rural Affairs (DEFRA) (2005). *UK Fuel Poverty Strategy: 3rd Annual Progress Report.* London: Department of Trade and Industry.

Equal Opportunities Commission (2005). Pensions Fact Sheet. www.eoc.org.uk.

Evandrou M (2005). Health and well-being. In Soule A, Baab P, Evandrou M, *et al.* (eds). *Focus on Older People.* London: The Stationery Office.

Evandrou M and Falkingham J (2006). Will the baby boomers be better-off than their parents in retirement? In Vincent J, Phillipson C and Downs M (eds) *The Futures of Old Age.* London: Sage Publications.

Evers HK (1981). Multidisciplinary teams in geriatric wards: myth or reality? *Journal of Advanced Nursing,* **6**, 205–14.

Faulkner M and Davies S (2005). Social support in the health care setting: the role of volunteers. *Health and Social Care in the Community,* **13**, 38–45.

Featherstone M and Hepworth M (2005). Images of aging: cultural representations of later life. In Johnson M, with Bengtson VL, Coleman PG and Kirkwood BL (eds). *The Cambridge Handbook of Age and Ageing.* Cambridge: Cambridge University Press.

Fisk M (1999). *Our Future Home.* London: Help the Aged.

Foster RK and Marriott HE (2006). Alcohol consumption in the new millennium: weighing up the risks and benefits for our health. *Nutrition Bulletin,* **31**, 286–331.

Froggatt K (2004). *Palliative Care in Care Homes for Older People.* London: National Council for Palliative Care.

Gallo WT, Bradley EH, Siegel M and Kasla SV (2000). Health effects of involuntary job loss among older workers: findings from the health and retirement survey. *Journals of Gerontology. Series B, Psychological Sciences and Social Sciences,* **55**, 131–40.

Godfrey M, Townsend J and Denby T (2004). *Building a Good Life for Older People in Local Communities: The Experience of Aging in Time and Place.* York: Joseph Rowntree Foundation.

Greaves CJ and Farbus L (2006). Effects of creative and social activity on the health and well-being of socially isolated older people: outcomes from a multi-method observational study. *Journal of the Royal Society for the Promotion of Health,* **126**, 134–42.

Ham C (2004). *Health Policy in Britain: Politics and Organisation of the NHS,* 5th edn. London: Macmillan.

Healthcare Commission, Audit Commission and Commission for Social Care Inspection (2006). *Living Well in Later Life: A Review of Progress against the National Service Framework for Older People.* London: Commission for Healthcare Audit and Inspection.

Help the Aged (2004). *Older and Colder – The views of older people experiencing difficulties keeping warm in winter.* London: Help the Aged.

Heywood F, Geetanjall G, Lanagan J, *et al.* (2005). *Reviewing the Disabled Living Facilities Grant Programme.* London: Office of the Deputy Prime Minister.

Holstein MB and Minkler M (2003). Self, society and the new gerontology. *Gerontologist*, **43**, 787–96.

Housing and Older People Development Group (HOPDEV) (2006). *Housing Options Advice for Older People: A Self-Training Kit for Advisers*. London: Housing and Older People Development Group.

Kalache A, Barreto SM and Keller A (2006). Global aging: the demographic revolution in all cultures and societies. In Johnson M, with Bengtson VL, Coleman PG and Kirkwood BL (eds). *The Cambridge Handbook of Age and Ageing*. Cambridge: Cambridge University Press.

Kelly TB, Tolson D, Schofield I and Booth J (2005). Describing gerontological nursing: an academic exercise or prerequisite for progress? *Journal of Clinical Nursing*, **14**, 13–23.

Kerr S, Watson H, Tolson D, Lough M and Brown M (2006). Smoking after the age of 65 years: a qualitative exploration of older current and former smokers' views on smoking, stopping smoking, and smoking cessation resources and services. *Health and Social Care in the Community*, **14**, 572–82.

Khaw KT (1997). In search of clues for a healthy old age. *Medical Research Council News*, **autumn** (75).

Kim JE and Moen P (2002). Retirement transitions: gender and psychological well-being: a life-course ecological model. *Journals of Gerontology. Series B, Psychological Sciences and Social Sciences*, **57**, 212–22.

Kings Fund (2003). *Auditing age and discrimination: a practical approach to promoting age equality in health and social care*. London: King's Fund.

Krout JA, Moen P, Holmes HH, Oggins J and Bowen N. (2002). Reasons for relocation to a continuing care retirement community. *The Journal of Applied Gerontology* **21**(2), 236–256.

Kunemund H, Kolland F (2007). Work and retirement. In Bond J, Peace S, Ditttman-Kohli F and Westerhof G (eds). *Ageing in Society*, 3rd edn. London: Sage.

Laing and Buisson (2006). *Care of Elderly People Market Survey 2006*. London: Laing & Buisson.

Larson EB, Wang L, Bowen JD, *et al*. (2006). Exercise in people aged 65 years and older is associated with lower risk for dementia. *Annals of Internal Medicine*, **144**, 73–81.

Lawrence RJ (2004). Housing, health and well-being: moving forward. *Reviews on Environmental Health*, **19**, 161–76.

Lowenstein A (2006). Global aging and challenges to families. In Johnson M, with Bengtson VL, Coleman PG and Kirkwood BL (eds). *The Cambridge Handbook of Age and Ageing*. Cambridge: Cambridge University Press.

MacDonald C (2002). Nurse autonomy as relational. *Nursing Ethics*, **9**, 194–201.

Marshall VW and Taylor P (2005). Restructuring the lifecourse: work and retirement. In Johnson M, with Bengtson VL, Coleman PG and Kirkwood BL (eds). *The Cambridge Handbook of Age and Ageing*. Cambridge: Cambridge University Press.

Martin W (2006). Age, Aging and the Body in Everyday Life. Presented at the Agenet workshop, Brave New World: Aging Research, Reading University, Reading, 3 July 2006. www.fp.rdg.ac.uk/AGEnet/PreviousMeetings/June2006/Martin.pdf.

McColgan G (2006). Walking with dogs: an alternative therapy. In Marshall M and Allan K (eds). *Dementia: Walking not Wandering – Fresh Approaches to Understanding and Practice*. London: Hawker.

McCormack B (2001). *Negotiating Partnerships with Older People: A Person-Centred Approach*. Aldershot: Ashgate.

McCormack B (2004). Person-centredness in gerontological nursing: an overview of the literature. *Journal of Clinical Nursing*, **13**, 31–8.

Meleis AI, Sawyer LM, Im E, Hilfinger Messias DK and Schumacher K (2000). Experiencing transitions: an emerging middle-range theory. *Advances in Nursing Science*, **23**, 12–28.

Meyer J, Bridges J and Spilsbury K (1999). Caring for older people in acute settings: Lessons learned from an action research study in accident and emergency. *NT Research*, **4**, 327–339.

Morris J, Dangour A, Deeming C, Fletcher A and Wilkinson P (2005). *Minimum Income for Healthy Living: Older People*. London: Age Concern England Policy Unit.

Murray B and Fortinberry A (2004). *Creating Optimism: A Proven Seven-Step Program for Overcoming Depression*. New York: McGraw-Hill.

National Care Homes Research and Development Forum (NCHRDF) (2007). *My Home Life*. London: Help the Aged.

Neimeyer RA and Werth JL (2006). The psychology of death. In Johnson M, with Bengtson VL, Coleman PG and Kirkwood BL (eds). *The Cambridge Handbook of Age and Ageing*. Cambridge: Cambridge University Press.

NHS Quality Improvement Scotland (2005). *National Overview: Older People in Acute Care*. Edinburgh: NHSQIS.

NHS Scotland and ASH Scotland (2007). An Atlas of Tobacco Smoking in Scotland: A Report Presenting Estimated Smoking Prevalence and Smoking-Attributable Deaths within Scotland. www.scotpho.org.uk/home/Publications/scotphoreports/pub_tobaccoatlas.asp.

Nursing and Midwifery Council (NMC) (2008). *The Code: Standards of Conduct, Performance and Ethics for Nurses and Midwives*. London: Nursing and Midwifery Council.

Nolan M (1997). Gerontological nursing: professional priority or eternal Cinderella? *Aging and Society*, **17**, 447–60.

Nolan M, Grant G and Nolan J (1995). Busy doing nothing: activity and interaction levels amongst differing populations of elderly patients. *Journal of Advanced Nursing*, **22**, 528–38.

Nolan M, Walker G, Nolan J, *et al.* (1996). Entry to care: positive choice or fait accompli? Developing a more proactive nursing response to the needs of older people and their carers. *Journal of Advanced Nursing*, **24**, 265–74.

Nolan M, Davies S and Grant G (2001). *Working with Older People and Their Families*. Buckingham: Open University Press.

Nolan M, Brown J, Davies S, Keady J and Nolan J (2002). Advancing Gerontological Education in Nursing: Final Report of the AGEIN Project. Report to the English National Board for Nursing, Midwifery and Health Visiting, University of Sheffield.

Nolan MR, Davies S, Brown J, Keady J and Nolan J (2004). Beyond 'person-centred' care: a new vision for gerontological nursing. *International Journal of Older People Nursing*, in association with *Journal of Clinical Nursing*, **13** supp 1, 45–53.

Nolan M, Brown J, Davies S, Nolan J and Keady J (2006). *The Senses Framework: Improving Care for Older People through a Relationship-Centred Approach*. Sheffield: University of Sheffield.

Norton D, McLaren R and Exton-Smith A (1962). *An Investigation of Geriatric Nursing Problems in Hospital*. Edinburgh: Churchill Livingstone.

Nuttman Schwartz O (2004). Like a high wave: adjustment of retirement. *Gerontologist*, **44**, 229–36.

Office of the Deputy Prime Minister (ODPM) (2005). *Housing and Black and Ethnic Communities: Review of the Evidence Base*. London: The Stationery Office.

Office for National Statistics (2004) Health expectancy: Living Longer, More Years in Poor Health. www.statistics.gov.uk/cci/nugget.asp?id=934.

O'May F (2007). Transitions into a care home. In National Care Homes Research and Development Forum (NCHRDF). *My Home Life*. London: Help the Aged.

Oswald F and Rowles GD (2006). Beyond the relocation trauma in old age: new trends in today's elders' residential decisions. In Wahl HW, Tesch-Romer C and Hoff A (eds). *New Dynamics in Old age: Environmental and Societal Perspectives*. Amityville, NY: Baywood.

Owen T and National Care Homes Research and Development Forum (NCHRDF) (2006). *My Home Life: Quality of Life in Care Homes*. London: Help the Aged.

Pinquart M (2001). Correlates of subjective health in older adults: a meta-analysis. *Psychology and Aging*, **16**, 414–26.

Platman K (2003). The self-designed career in later life: a study of older portfolio workers in the United Kingdom. *Ageing and Society*, **23**, 281–302.

Platman K and Tinker A (1998). Getting on in the BBC: a case study of older workers. *Ageing and Society*, **18**, 513–35.

Policy Research Institute on Aging and Ethnicity (PRIAE) (2006). *Developing Extra Care Housing for Black and Minority Ethnic Elders: An Overview of the Issues, Examples and Challenges*. London: Housing, Learning and Improvement Network.

Redfern S, Hannan S, Norman I and Martin F. (2002). Work satisfaction, stress, quality of care and morale of older people in a nursing home. *Health and Social Care in the Community* **10**, 512–7.

Reed J (2007). Quality of life. In National Care Homes Research and Development Forum (NCHRDF). *My Home Life*. London: Help the Aged.

Schultz JH (2001). Public policy ambiguity. In Morrow-Howell N, Hinterlong J and Sherraden M (eds). *Productive Aging: Concepts and Challenges*. Baltimore, MD: Johns Hopkins University Press.

Schumacher KL and Meleis AI (1994). Transitions: a central concept in nursing. *Image: The Journal of Nursing Scholarship*, **26**, 119–27.

Scottish Executive (2006). *Delivering Health Enabling Care: Harnessing the Nursing, Midwifery and Allied Health Professions' Contribution to Implementing Delivering for Health in Scotland*. Edinburgh: Scottish Executive.

Scottish Executive (2007). *Better Health Better Care: Action Plan*. Edinburgh: Scottish Executive.

Skelton D (1993). Muscle power and strength after strength training by women aged 75 years and over: a randomised controlled study. *Journal of Physiology*, **473**, 83.

Stuart-Hamilton I (2006). *The Psychology of Aging: An Introduction*. London: Jessica Kingsley Publishers.

Tait R, Hulse G, Waterreus A, *et al.* (2007). Effectiveness of a smoking cessation intervention in older adults. *Addiction*, **102**, 148–55.

Tresolini CP, Pew-Fetzer Task Force (1994). *Health Professions, Education and Relationship-Centred Care*. San Francisco: Pew Health Professions Commission.

Victor C (2006). Demographic and epidemiological trends in aging. In Redfern S and Ross F (eds). *Nursing Older People*. Edinburgh: Elsevier.

Volz (2000). Successful Aging: the Second 50. www.apa.org/monitor/jan00/cs.html.

Warburton D, Nicol C and Bredin S (2006). Health benefits of physical activity: the evidence. *Canadian Medical Association Journal*, **174**, 801–9.

Waters K (1994). Getting dressed in the early morning: styles of staff/patient interaction on rehabilitation wards for elderly people. *Journal of Advanced Nursing*, **19**, 239–48.

World Health Organization (WHO) (2002). *Active Aging: A Policy Framework*. Geneva: World Health Organization.

Further reading

Bengtson VL, Putney NM and Johnson ML (2005). The problem of theory in gerontology today. In Johnson M, with Bengtson VL, Coleman P and Kirkwood TB (eds). *The Cambridge Handbook of Age and Ageing*. Cambridge: Cambridge University Press.

The Cambridge Handbook of Age and Ageing is an edited textbook that has many useful contributions considering the social experiences of older people worldwide. This introductory chapter considers the role of theory and challenges to theory development in gerontology and provides an overview of selected biological, psychological and sociological theories of ageing.

Bond J, Peace S, Dittman-Kohli F and Westerhof G (eds) (2007). *Ageing in Society: European Perspectives on Gerontology*, 3rd edn. London: Sage.

The third edition of this popular text provides a comprehensive introduction to the study of ageing, exploring key theories and concepts from the behavioural and social sciences.

Clarke A and Bright L (2006). *Moving Stories: The Impact of Admission into a Care Home on Residents' Partners*. London: Relatives and Residents Association.

The Relatives and Residents Association (R&RA) is a voluntary organisation representing the interests of the residents of care homes and their families. Drawing on the experiences of callers to the R&RA telephone helpline, this report explores the emotional and practical difficulties faced by partners in this position. Further information is available at www.relres.org.

Department of Health (DH). Older people. www.dh.gov.uk/en/SocialCare/ Deliveringadultsocialcare/Olderpeople/index.htm.

Although the National Service Framework is part of English legislation, this website is a useful resource even if you work outside of England.

McCormack B (2001). *Negotiating Partnerships with Older People: A Person-Centred Approach*. Aldershot: Ashgate.

Based on the findings of a PhD study, this book explores the nature of relationships between older people and nurses in hospital settings. The focus of the book is the use of language and the way autonomy is presented through the language of health care practice. McCormack explores the many challenges in achieving person-centred care for older people and highlights strategies for creating effective and appropriate partnerships. Extracts of real-life conversations between nurses and older people taken from the research data make riveting reading and help to illustrate many of the shortfalls in current nursing practice.

National Care Homes Research and Development Forum (NCHRDF) (2007). *My Home Life: Quality of Life in Care Homes – Review of the Literature*. London: Help the Aged.
This comprehensive review of the literature was commissioned by the UK charity Help the Aged as part of a national campaign to promote quality of life in care homes. Key themes are identified, and personal accounts of care home life are included. The full report and a useful summary are accessible online at www.myhomelife.org.uk.

Nolan MR, Davies S, Brown J, Keady J and Nolan J (2004). Beyond 'person-centred' care: a new vision for gerontological nursing. *Journal of Clinical Nursing*, **13**, 45–53.
This article adopts a constructively critical look at some of the assumptions underpinning person-centredness and describes the development of the Senses Framework outlined in this chapter. A framework describing the potential dimensions of relationship-centred care is included.

Redfern S and Ross F (eds) (2005). *Nursing Older People*, 4th edn. Edinburgh: Churchill Livingstone.
This book represents a compendium of information on the nursing needs of older people and their families. Now in its fourth edition, this clear and concise text has provided many students of nursing and other disciplines with a sound grounding in the knowledge base for practice with older people across a range of care settings.

Reed J, Stanley D and Clarke C (2004). *Health, Well-Being and Older People*. Bristol: Policy Press.
This accessible text represents a collaboration between older people's groups and academics and discusses a range of issues that are important to the health of older people. Topics include attitudes and ageism, the body, the environment, family and community, sexuality and having fun. The content draws on material developed, and in some cases written, by older people.

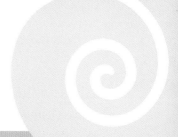

20

Care needs at home and in the community

Rosemary Cook

Introduction

This chapter looks at the determinants of individuals' care needs and the nature and characteristics of care needs at home and in the community. It explores some of the issues specifically related to delivering care to people outside of hospital settings to meet their care needs, and the implications of these for nurses working in these settings.

This chapter should be read in conjunction with Chapter 10 for a fuller understanding of the nature of health needs, and how people's desires and choices may dictate in which settings they seek health care.

Information in this chapter will help you to achieve some of the Nursing and Midwifery Council's (NMC) required standards of proficiency in the domains of professional and ethical practice, care delivery and care management (Appendix 2).

Learning objectives

After studying this chapter you should be able to:

- identify some of the influences that affect people's health and care needs;
- explain the different kinds of care needed by people living at home and in community settings;
- describe some key differences between nursing in hospitals and nursing in the home and community.

Identifying care needs

By the time an individual is admitted to hospital or attends an accident and emergency (A&E) or outpatient department, their need for care is usually already established. They may have a specific condition requiring surgery, other treatment or follow-up, or they may have a set of symptoms sufficient to convince them to seek medical care. The individual has often been referred for care by a general practitioner (GP) or other health worker, such as an NHS Direct nurse. Whether on the ward, in clinic or in a cubicle in A&E, the patient has a set of notes or a card that indicates at least in general terms what their need is. The care they subsequently receive is determined largely by the external observations of their condition made by the health professionals around them.

For the individual who is community-based in any of the settings described in Chapter 10, the decision about when to seek care is theirs. As the person is not under the hour-by-hour supervision of health workers, it is up to them to decide when they have a need for care, and when and how they will take action to have that need met.

This does not always happen at the point that health professionals would expect. Many people live at home with multiple serious illnesses, but 'manage' themselves to their own satisfaction and do not wish to be taken into hospital to have their condition 'improved'. Some prefer to trade off a shorter life at home against the chance of prolongation of life, if that involves very unpleasant treatment and long hospital stays. Sometimes people do not realise, or do not accept, that their condition is one that warrants treatment at all.

Identifying care needs involves more than simply matching components of a person's clinical condition with corrective or palliative treatments. Every individual's view of their own health, and their approach to obtaining care, is unique. It is the product of the influence of a wide range of factors in their life, which in themselves vary over a lifetime.

Reflection point 20.1

Look at Scenario 20.1. What factors will influence this individual's decision about whether, where, when and how to get health advice?

SCENARIO 20.1

Sarah is a 15-year-old girl from a traveller family. She lives in a caravan on a roadside site with three younger siblings, her parents, aunts and uncles. There are minimal services on the site, and none of the local general practices will register traveller families. Sarah's attendance record at school is patchy.

Sarah has had several attacks of abdominal pain, which she has reported to the school nurse. Her health records go back only 2 years, when her family arrived in the area. When health professionals visit her at the site, the girl is chaperoned by several members of her family.

You should have taken into account Sarah's level of understanding, her family's influence, practical considerations such as her ability to travel, and her and her family's previous experiences of health services. To meet the requirements of the NMC Code (2008) (Appendix 1), you would ensure that you found out and responded to the girl's concerns and preferences, even if they differed from her family's; presented information to her in a way that she could understand; and respected her right to confidentiality.

Determinants of care needs

The many influences on when, where and how people express the need for health care can be grouped into four categories:

- physical factors;
- cultural factors;
- environmental factors;
- mental factors.

Each of these sets of influences works differently on different individuals and adds up to a unique personal approach to care needs.

Physical factors

Physical factors include age, the illness or symptoms, genetic inheritance and lifestyle. Age may influence care needs in different ways. Young children's health is usually carefully monitored and protected by their parents or carers, so that advice or care is sought early. However, this may lead to many encounters with health professionals or services when there is little wrong with the child; visits may be labelled 'inappropriate' by health professionals, even though the relief of parental anxiety is a beneficial outcome, and the opportunity to educate the parents about normal health and signs of illness can be a valuable one. Conversely, if a parent or carer is responsible for the child's illness or injury, through abuse or neglect, then they may delay seeking help for far too long. Nurses need to be alert to both extremes and to be equally objective, professional and thorough in each case. There have been instances of missed illness in children who are presented repeatedly because health professionals have assumed that the parents were once again worrying unnecessarily; there have also been instances of children being returned to suffer badly in abusive homes because only the immediate injury was dealt with and the evidence of repeated injuries was overlooked.

For older people, concern about increasing frailty may encourage them to seek care early, or fear of going into hospital and never coming home may make them delay seeking help for illness or incapacity. Where older people are looked after by carers, anxiety, conscientiousness or a desire for respite may make the carer ask early and often for care interventions. Alternatively, fear of losing the older person to institutional care, or, where 'elder abuse' is taking place (Box 20.1), fear of discovery may make carers delay asking for health care.

BOX 20.1 Elder abuse

One definition of elder abuse is:

A single or repeated act or lack of appropriate action, occurring within any relationship where there is an expectation of trust, which causes harm or distress to an older person.

(Action on Elder Abuse, www.elderabuse.org.uk)

Elder abuse includes physical, sexual, psychological and financial abuse and neglect. It can occur in residential care, day care, nursing homes, hospitals, and in the person's own home. The abuser is often someone in a position of trust through family ties, friendship or a paid caring role. Very rarely is the abuser someone who provides a family caring role.

Other age groups have different influences on their care-seeking behaviour. Adolescents are often caught between their relative lack of knowledge of their bodies, and their self-consciousness about asking for help. They may also be concerned about seeking care without their parents' knowledge and may be particularly frightened of the effects of illness or treatment at a time when they have their lives ahead of them. People who are in employment may have to balance the need for time off work for care against their employer's attitude to sickness; alternatively, they may be keen to have a legitimate reason to be away from stressful or unpleasant work. For women of childbearing age, illness, injury and incapacity will often be seen in the context of its potential impact on their ability to have children or to care for the children or family that they have. Pregnant women have been known to refuse treatment for serious illness if the treatment might harm their unborn baby.

The nature of the illness, concern or symptoms also affects the way people determine their care needs, although not necessarily in the most obvious way. Although moderate pain might be assumed automatically to drive someone to ask for help, for another person it might bring such fear of serious disease that they attempt to ignore it. A breast lump is well known to be a potential indicator of breast cancer, and yet some women delay seeking care for a long time because they are afraid of being told they have cancer. If symptoms are considered embarrassing – for example, vaginal discharge, anal soreness or erectile dysfunction – then this may militate against seeking care.

A person's genetic inheritance can clearly affect their care needs, but it can also affect their care-seeking behaviour. A man with a family history of early male death from heart disease may well have a genetic predisposition to the condition, but, having seen his father and uncles dying from heart attacks, he may be too afraid to go for a cholesterol test in case he finds out that he has the same inherited condition. Conversely, a woman with a strong family history of breast cancer may actively seek out a test for the *BRCA1* or *BRCA2* gene in order to ask for a prophylactic mastectomy. Where an inherited condition results in learning difficulties, an individual may need extra help to understand their body, their health and their health needs, as well as the best way to get help when they need it. Some choices made as a result of genetic inheritance go against society's norms – for example, the case of two deaf parents who expressed a preference for children who had inherited their disability.

Reflection point 20.2

As a nurse, what would your attitude be to such a family if you were looking after the mother while she was pregnant and she expressed a desire for a deaf baby? Review the NMC Code to check its guidance on responding to patients' preferences.

You should have identified the clauses of the NMC Code under the heading 'Make the care of people your first concern, treating them as individuals and respecting their dignity', which require nurses to treat patients or clients as individuals, and to respond to their concerns and preferences.

Lifestyle is another physical factor that affects the way people decide and action their health needs. If a person considers that the ability to eat and drink what they want is very important to them, then they may not seek help for obesity, even if it is causing ill health, because they know that they will be advised to change their eating habits. A person addicted to alcohol, nicotine or other drugs may avoid health care because they fear blame or censure (particularly if their addiction is to illegal substances) or because they do not wish to give up their addiction; this can have serious health consequences – for example, a woman who is addicted to heroin and avoids any antenatal care endangers both herself and her baby. Alternatively, some people seek care frequently for the illnesses consequent on their lifestyle, with or without any intention of altering their lifestyle. In some cases, they may deny or hide lifestyle behaviours that they think health professionals will criticise, or they may seek help specifically to make beneficial changes to their lifestyle.

Cultural factors

Cultural factors affecting people's care needs include the following:

- *Beliefs*: these may be religious, social or simply communal. They affect when an individual decides to ask for help, who or which services are appropriate to request care from, and when care (particularly invasive intervention) should stop. The way in which death is acknowledged and the practical care of the body after death vary according to religious and cultural beliefs.
- *Community support*: this includes the amount of advice, information and practical care available informally through the community, and the ability of the individual to call on that support.
- *Community norms and expectations*: these include what is 'usually done' in a particular community – for example, whether older or frail members of the community are taken into

others' homes for care, or whether the state is expected to care for them; whether children whose parents are unable to look after them are taken in by family members or neighbours; and whether death is expected and dealt with in the home, or whether people are expected to die in hospital. The amount of crime in an area, people's expectations regarding their own safety, and people's experience of antisocial behaviour can all affect their health and their need for care.

Environmental factors

Environmental factors affecting care needs include the physical geography of the local area, family and carer availability, the industrial legacy of the area, and sudden catastrophic events.

Geography has an impact both on what people's care needs are and on how they are met. In urban areas, poor air quality, noisy or stressful surroundings, and urban poverty among some communities may adversely affect health. This may be accepted as normal by inhabitants, or it may lead to increased demand for health care – for example, for exacerbations of respiratory disease, or for mental illnesses such as anxiety or depression. The positive aspects of town and city life are that health and other services are usually readily accessible, public transport is available, amenities are close at hand, and there is the potential for meeting many different people and creating social networks. Rural environments have their positive aspects, such as better air quality, less noise and less light pollution, but they also have their own problems: health may be affected adversely by rural poverty, isolation and limited job opportunities, and rural health services are often further away and more difficult to access.

The availability of family or other carers has a direct impact on care needs. Formal services may not be called upon at all if there is help and caring in the home or may be limited to necessary interventions such as occasional consultations and the provision of specific services, for example writing prescriptions for medicines. A lack of informal carers can lead to hospital admissions, home visits and social care packages that, for another person with the same condition and a carer available, would not be needed. It is estimated that the 6 million unpaid carers in the UK save the NHS an estimated £57 billion per year (Princess Royal Trust for Carers, 2006) by the services they provide to family members, friends and neighbours in need.

The industrial legacy of an area is often reflected in the care needs of local people. Ex-mining and mill-working communities will have people suffering the characteristic illnesses associated with these industries and with specific care needs. Again, individuals' attitudes vary and determine whether they accept their illness, disability or condition as 'normal for round here' and whether they look for treatment, improvement or cure. The decline or disappearance of an industry from an area, such as the closure of coal mines in Wales, the decline of ship-building in Northern Ireland and the reduction in cod fishing from North Sea ports, has a significant impact on local communities. It can affect the mental health of all members of a family when breadwinners' jobs are lost and, if there is longer-term unemployment, then there is some evidence of an adverse effect on physical health status too (Centre for Economic Policy Research, 2006).

New catastrophic events in the local environment are another factor that clearly affect health needs. A local pollution incident, major transport accident or act of terrorism can give rise to new care needs in a large number of people over subsequent weeks and months. There may be physical illnesses caused by the nature of the event in people close enough to have been directly affected by it, and there may be mental or emotional care needs caused by people's reactions to the event, even if they were not personally involved.

Mental factors

Mental factors influence the need for care and the way people seek out care for themselves. Some of these factors include the following:

- *The individual's psychological health and strength*: determining how far they can and do care for and support themselves, and how assertive they are in asking for additional help.
- *Their mental health, illness or disability*: cognitive disorders such as dementia affect an individual's ability to cope with even minor illness that another person would manage without asking for help. Mental illness such as depression may cause the person to ignore signs and symptoms or to lack the motivation to seek help for such signs and symptoms. On the other hand, a mental illness may lead a person to seek help often and for many symptoms because they lack confidence in their own ability to cope. Stigma and discrimination in services may thwart an individual's efforts to get access to care (NIMHE, 2004). A learning disability may interfere with an individual's ability to source information about their health or to be sufficiently assertive to ensure that they are offered and receive standard services such as screening programmes that are available to others (DH, 2001).
- *Mental models of health and illness*: people's view of what constitutes 'good health', where ill health comes from and how it should be regarded, and how and when they should seek help are all influenced by their personal mental model of what it means to be healthy and how they, as individuals, should interact with services providing health care. Some people feel that anything other than full health and optimal functioning should be addressed vigorously by professionals and statutory services. Others believe that their health and well-being are in their own hands, with only minimal back-up required from external agencies, or are in the hands of a deity or fate and so can be ameliorated only partly by the intervention of health care services (Scenario 20.2).

SCENARIO 20.2

Ivan is a university-educated ex-chairman of a private company. He is an evangelical Christian who believes in divine healing. He lives with a prolapsed inguinal hernia for which he does not seek treatment because he believes that God has given him this affliction for a purpose. He is registered with a general practice surgery, but he has not attended for many years. Although a health professional would say that he has health needs that should be met, Ivan's own beliefs contradict this.

As varied as these different sets of influences are, their impact on an individual and how they recognise and express their care needs is complicated further by the way the different influences combine for any one individual.

For example, a person with a concern about their health, but living in a community that values stoicism and avoids contact with authorities, and who doesn't have use of a car and has little money, is unlikely to express that concern. Another person with the same concern, and coming from a culture in which health is much discussed and high-quality care is routinely expected, who is confident enough to arrange an appointment, and who can travel easily to the doctor's surgery, will probably have their concern addressed.

Suppose the concern described above was that many family members have died of a heart attack before the age of 60 years. The result of the different influences on the two people in this example could be an early death from heart disease for the first person, and screening, treatment and a normal lifespan for the second person. This illustrates the importance of being aware of the many factors that stand between health needs and the expression of those needs. In order to fulfil the requirement of the NMC Code that states 'you must act as an advocate for those in your care, helping them to access relevant health and social care, information and support', you need to look for and anticipate the effect of every person's unique reaction to the influences on health and care needs.

Reflection point 20.3
Look at Scenario 20.3. What actions could the nurse in this example take to ensure that he has done his best to comply with the requirement of the NMC Code cited above?

SCENARIO 20.3

A practice nurse sees 83-year-old Flora in his surgery for a 'first contact' appointment. Flora registered with the practice 4 years ago, but she has been a rare attender. After treatment for a cut on her leg, which Flora says has resulted from a fall in her kitchen at home, she is in a hurry to leave the surgery. The nurse suggests checking her blood pressure, but Flora assures the nurse that she feels fine and ends the consultation.

You should have identified actions that attempt to follow up Flora's fall by checking that it was not caused by an underlying condition that could be treated and ensuring that she has information, advice and possibly home safety equipment to avoid a similar incident in future. This would fulfil the requirements of the NMC Code. The practice nurse remains professionally accountable for their practice, as the NMC Code states that 'you are personally accountable for actions and omissions in your practice and must always be able to justify your decisions'.

The point at which an individual expresses a need for care to a nurse or other health professional is at the end point of a journey through the various physical, cultural, environmental and mental influences that is unique to the individual on each occasion. It is important for health professionals to recognise and respect the influences on that individual – which will continue to affect the negotiations about care they undertake with them – and to realise that there will be many other people who have care needs but who were prevented from expressing them somewhere along the journey.

SUMMARY

Every individual's care needs are experienced, acknowledged and expressed uniquely in response to the interaction of a wide range of internal and external influences on their life. It is, therefore, impossible to make generalised assumptions about care needs on the basis of a person's age, social circumstances or any other characteristic. Nurses are required by the NMC Code to treat each patient as an individual, and to respect and take into account their individuality, even if that means that the person refuses care that the nurse believes they need.

The nature of care needs at home and in the community

In 2002, the Department of Health (DH) published a report called *Liberating the Talents*, which described a new framework for nursing in primary care based on meeting three different kinds of care need in the community:

- *First contact care*: acute assessment, diagnosis, care, treatment and referral.
- *Continuing care*: rehabilitation, chronic disease management and delivering national service frameworks.
- *Public health*: health protection and promotion programmes that improve health and reduce inequalities.

Public health is a different kind of health need compared with those discussed earlier in the chapter. It is focused on groups and communities rather than individuals, and it aims to create the conditions to maintain the best health of the community, rather than solely to identify and treat illness in the individual (Box 20.2). Public health elicits a different kind of expression of care need from an individual, if they perceive the need at all. People may say 'I want my child to be safe from infectious diseases' or 'I don't want the food I eat to make me sick', without thinking specifically about the public health measures that will ensure these things. A full discussion of public health work is beyond the scope of this chapter, but you should be aware that it is a key element of primary care.

BOX 20.2 Public health

Ireland and Northern Ireland have produced a 'nursing vision' for public health, which has subsequently been incorporated into a strategy for public health nursing. Deliberation with groups of nurses and other public health stakeholders produced the consensus that public health is 'organised social and political effort, and health promotion for the benefit of populations, families and individuals' (Mason and Clarke, 2001; DHSSPS and DoHC, 2005).

Table 20.1 shows the kinds of practical care need that may arise under the three headings of *Liberating the Talents*. This chapter focuses mainly on care needs from the first two categories, as the specialty of public health work requires much wider consideration.

Table 20.1 The nature of care needs

	First contact care	Long-term conditions	Health promotion and public health
Information and explanation	√	√	√
Treatment and support	√	√	
Psychological support/confidence-building	√	√	√
Respite for informal carers		√	
Maintenance support		√	
Practical help/social care		√	
Interagency care coordination		√	√
Help to self-care/(re)gain independence	√	√	√

Sharing of information and explanation

The sharing of information and explanation are essential to meeting any care needs. This is more than simply naming and describing the condition in first contact care or the care of long-term conditions, and more than simply justifying a health promotion approach. Every individual has a different degree of existing knowledge and previous experience, and their need for information is affected by all the factors listed earlier. There is no single approach to sharing information that will be right for all individuals, or for all age groups, communities or groups who share a condition.

> **Reflection point 20.4**
> Think about a mother bringing her first child to the practice nurse in her GP's practice for a measles immunisation. What questions might she have for the nurse? Suppose the receptionist gives her a leaflet about measles to read in the waiting room – how well would this meet her need for information?

Your list of questions might include those about the safety and risks of the vaccine, any side effects, alternatives to the vaccine, whether her family history increases risk, what will happen afterwards, how she should look after the child in the hours following the vaccination, and the risks of not giving the vaccination. A leaflet might answer some of these questions by providing evidence-based information, but it would not be able to personalise information based on the mother's family history, previous experience, anecdotes from friends and specific anxieties.

Treatment and support

Treatment and support may be needed for many minor illnesses and injuries presenting for first contact care and for people with long-term conditions. However, treatment (in the sense of practical clinical interventions) may not always be needed, for example when a person presents asking for antibiotics for a sore throat or cough, and the health professional believes that the cause is viral and therefore not susceptible to antibiotic treatment. In such a case, more information and explanation are needed, together with skilful negotiation with the individual about the practical care and support they can give themselves, so that the person does not feel that their legitimate right to treatment has been refused.

It would be as wrong to assume that public health or health promotion work never involves treatment as it would be to assume that short- or long-term illness always requires treatment. Here there can be another difficult negotiation: to suggest to people who regard themselves as well or healthy that they need a 'treatment' that will make them feel worse (such as immunisations for travel abroad) in the interests of their longer-term health.

Psychological support

Psychological support and confidence-building are an integral part of meeting all three kinds of care need. In poor health care, the advice, information or treatment may be given but the individual is left with the impression that they are weak, vulnerable or dependent on the health system. In good health care, the necessary treatment is given along with encouragement and information to enable the person to learn something about their condition, how to prevent it, or how to care for themselves. In addition, they may be reassured that their judgement in coming for treatment was sound because they could not have helped themselves. The latter approach builds confidence, independence and a more equal relationship between individuals and professionals.

The difference between these two approaches is not necessarily in the words spoken. Either position can be conveyed through the body language, tone of voice and attitude of the health professional – and is often read very sensitively by the person receiving care.

Respite care

Respite care is generally required by people living with long-term conditions and is either for themselves (for example, if they need a complete review and simplification of a complex medication regime) or for their family or carers (if, for example, they are getting little sleep). Recognising when such a break is needed, negotiating a place for care and helping to manage the transition, both into and out of respite care, takes a particular combination of clinical and case management skills from the community nurse.

Maintenance support

Such support, which includes regular monitoring and medication management, is largely the province of people living with long-term conditions. This is one of the most rewarding kinds of nursing in primary care, since the nurse builds up a relationship with an individual and their family over the longer term, while visiting the home or seeing the individual regularly in clinic or surgery.

Practical help

Practical help and advice are needed as much by people with first contact care needs as those with longer-term conditions and those on the receiving end of health protection measures. It is not enough to put a patient's arm in a sling but then fail to tell them how to manage showering, or to give a woman contraceptive pills but not tell her what to do if she forgets to take one. People receiving care while living in the community will expect their primary care nurse to know a whole range of practical things, such as which bus goes to the hospital, where they can buy a weekly medicine dispenser, and how they can get home oxygen bottles delivered.

Coordination of care

Care coordination, or case management, is a key skill for meeting the care needs of people with long-term conditions. It often involves linking social care services with health services, arranging for a number of different professionals to provide elements of care, and finding and bringing in additional elements of care from voluntary organisations. Being able to find help for issues related to housing, income and benefits, as well as physical and emotional health care, is part of the role of the care coordinator. It is also important to be able to regularly and competently assess the individual's condition, in order to recognise when they might need care from other sectors, including inpatient care. The introduction of community matrons – community nurses with a case management role – in England (with a pilot scheme running in Wales at the time of writing) prompted the DH to issue a set of competencies that cover the different skills required for care coordination (DH, 2005).

Promotion of independence and self-care

Like giving psychological support and building confidence, promotion of independence and self-care is important in meeting all care needs. It helps the individual to take some control of their own health, reduces the impact on them of the need to seek help, and may also reduce demand on health services. If a mother with three children has to travel repeatedly to a clinic to have her child's lung capacity monitored, then it costs her a great deal in time, travel costs and lost opportunities to do other things with her children; it may also involve taking her healthy children out of school. If the mother is taught how to measure and record her child's peak flow rate, understands the condition and the implications of readings, and knows when a reading should trigger a change in medication or a call for help, then she, her family and the health service benefits.

SUMMARY

Care needs in the community are not only for a treatment-based response to a clinical condition. The nurse's actions in meeting care needs must be wide-ranging, tailored to the individual's specific situation and appropriate to the context in which the individual lives their life. A different approach is required to meet public health and health promotion needs. Whatever the individual's care needs, the nurse should always aim to work in partnership with the individual to share information, build confidence and promote self-care and independence.

Characteristics of care needs

Many of the tasks undertaken by nurses working with people at home and in their own communities will sound familiar to nurses in other settings. Giving information, monitoring conditions, managing medicines, coordinating care and providing treatments are nursing activities common to many settings. The clinical tasks involved – ranging from carrying out basic diagnostic tests to managing patients on artificial ventilation – are not unique to community settings. There are particular characteristics of nursing in primary care, however, that make it different from nursing in hospitals and that have been recognised since the very beginnings of community nursing (Box 20.3).

BOX 20.3 Early notes on the differences between hospital and community nursing

As long ago as 1943, a textbook for nurses working in the community ('Queen's Nurses', who trained at the Queen's Institute of District Nursing, now known as the Queen's Nursing Institute) stated:

The nurse will find the character of her work very different from the routine of a hospital. She is largely free to plan her rounds as she finds best for her patients and must learn to regard the family as the unit for which she is responsible and not merely the patient. This gives room for the development of initiative and resourcefulness as well as making her service not only one of comfort in the care of humanity but a part of the social and preventive schemes for the country's health.

(Queen's Institute of District Nursing, 1943)

In 1990, community nurse researchers were warning against 'the false impression that nursing in the home is nothing more than a change in practice site, requiring the same skills and skill levels as the acute care arena' (Kenyon *et al.*, 1990).

Carr (2001) talks of the 'importance of acknowledging that nursing practice in this context demands a particular "package" of interventions and approaches to care which are different to that met in the hospital setting.' She also suggests that

the difference between hospital and community may be explained by suggesting that the 'false' and 'temporary' environment of the hospital setting, imposes a change in the normal dynamics of the relationships which is not so vigorously imposed in the community settings.

(Carr, 2001)

Reflection point 20.5

Think about a particular patient you have nursed in hospital. Now imagine that you are working in a GP's surgery as a practice nurse and that the same person has an appointment to see you about their condition. What will be different about your encounter in the surgery?

You should have considered practical, emotional, physical and psychological differences as well as clinical ones.

Factors that characterise care needs outside hospitals include the following:

- *Shared responsibility*: in hospital, a lot of the responsibility for identifying and quantifying, as well as reacting to, care needs lies with the staff. Nurses are expected to take physiological measurements of the patient's condition at regular intervals, to report on their condition to nursing colleagues and medical staff, and to ensure that investigations and treatments take place at the allotted time. When the individual is home-based, the patient does many of these things themselves. A nurse practitioner may have prescribed a new inhaler for a child with asthma, but the child's parent chooses whether or not to collect the medicine from the pharmacy, and to help the child to use it as directed or even to use it at all. Only the individual and their family know whether their symptoms have worsened or improved, and only they can explain their condition to the nurse. The responsibility for reporting care needs, and then participating in the care suggested, lies largely with the individual in primary care.

- *Permission and negotiation*: Carr's (1999) research with student and qualified community nurses identified 'role negotiation' as an important facet of their practice. Whether the individual with care needs is living at home, living 'rough' on the streets, resident in a care home or serving a sentence in prison, they are in their own environment, and they can choose not to engage with a nurse at all or not to cooperate with any attempts to elicit health needs or give care. The only way to succeed in identifying and meeting care needs is to negotiate with the individual. Permission is needed to visit the person, to enter their premises, to examine them, to take samples, to give information and to undertake treatment. Negotiation is needed to persuade the individual to incorporate change, treatment or adaptation into their everyday life. Informed consent is, of course, a feature of nursing care in every setting, but it has real practical meaning when the individual has so many other options to choose from and has actively to agree to the one proposed by the nurse.

- *Episodic rather than continuous involvement*: the fact that nursing care in the community is undertaken on the basis of visits – nurse to the person's home, or person to clinic or surgery – means that there is not the continual oversight that characterises hospital care. Between visits, the individual is responsible for their own care, treatment or lifestyle activities. For the nurse, this means that it is important to be clear about how the person should care for themselves; explanations and reinforcing information need to be appropriate and understood, taking into account the patient's language, literacy and memory, and the presence or absence of family members, carers or friends who can help. Trust, negotiation and a relationship that enables questioning and discussion are essential. Practically, it helps if the nurse can be reached by telephone between visits, so that questions can be answered as soon as they arise. Otherwise, a person may be treating themselves inappropriately or ignoring key symptoms for a long time before the next visit, and their care will be compromised as a result.

- *Varying circumstances for care*: the many different care settings described in Chapter 10 illustrate how varied the physical environment for care may be. The same task of dressing a wound may need to take place in a shared bedroom, on a park bench, in a clinic treatment room or in a police cell. Such challenges highlight the importance of focusing on the essential principles for good care and the nurse–individual relationship, rather than on equipment lists and standard clinical procedures.

- *Entry into the person's world*: when a patient is in hospital, they recognise that they have entered the health professional's world. However uncooperative the patient may be, and however assiduously nurses seek informed consent for their actions on the ward, the balance of power is with the hospital staff. Outside of hospital, the individual is in their own world and, to a much greater extent, is in control of their encounters with health professionals. Nurses need to recognise that the individual shares responsibility for their care and that care plans must be negotiated rather than imposed. It also requires acceptance of the fact that other people's worlds may be radically different – even unacceptably so – compared with the nurse's own or compared with the spectrum of a particular notional 'normality'. In providing the care that every person is entitled to receive from a nurse, these differences have to be accepted and not regarded as barriers to caring.
- *Health, social and personal needs*: the artificial division that statutory services create between what are 'health needs' (to be met and funded by the health service) and 'social care needs' (to be met and funded by local authorities) does not exist in the minds or lives of people in need of care at home. For a traveller family on a temporary site, for example, the health of their children, their eating habits and their susceptibility to heart disease are connected inextricably to the need for water and sewerage services on the site, whether or not they can register with a local GP and how they are treated by the local settled community. For a person nearing the end of life and being cared for at home, their need for regular opiate analgesia and for help to wash in bed are part of the same, not different, set of care needs. The practical coordination of care from different agencies to meet these needs is one of the essential skills of community nursing.

SUMMARY

The care needs of people living at home or in other community-based settings have specific characteristics that make them different from care needs in other sectors. The relationship with the individual receiving care is fundamentally different, and the nurse needs to work in a different way, based on shared responsibility, negotiation of care, intermittent contact, and acceptance of a wide range of lifestyles and choices made by the individual. Part of the work of nursing in primary care involves joining up services that are artificially divided to ensure that the whole range of people's care needs is addressed.

Meeting care needs

The different characteristics of care needs at home mean that nurses cannot simply transfer task-based skills acquired or practised in hospital into different settings. Research on the preparation of hospital nurses to work as community matrons (with advanced clinical and case management skills) in England (Drennan *et al.*, 2005) identified a list of key factors that need to be addressed in order to deal with their transition to the new setting (Box 20.4).

In primary care, there are some important professional and practical issues that need to be understood in order to deliver appropriate care to meet people's health needs. These are:

- *Professional issues*: understanding the patient pathway; maintaining the quality of care in different settings; providing continuity of care; and communications and information-sharing.
- *Practical issues*: legal issues; travel and mobility; teamworking at a distance; isolation in practice; and personal safety and security.

> **BOX 20.4** **Making the transition from hospital to community nursing: a checklist for employers to consider for nurses who are new to primary care and working as case managers or community matrons**
>
> - Ensure that there is overt support from stakeholders in the organisation and across the local network of health and social care for both the new roles and the nurse who is new to primary care.
> - Ensure that there is a range of mechanisms for supported learning for nurses to progress from novice in primary care without compromising the patient, the care network or the nurse.
> - Ensure that the learning mechanisms address the following areas of knowledge for working in non-hospital environments:
>   - the centrality of both the patients and clients and the informal care and family networks;
>   - the service environment of working in the community and home;
>   - the physical environment of working in the community and home.
> - Recognise that nurses who will thrive in case manager roles in the community are likely to be those who build confidence in or are comfortable with uncertainty, changing priorities, decision-making, negotiation, partnership working or assertiveness.
>
> *Source*: Drennan *et al.* (2005).

Patient pathways

There is an increased focus on 'patient pathways' that bridge the traditional gap between what happens to people in their GPs' surgeries and their own homes, and what happens when they go to hospital (Figure 20.1). The primary care-based organisations that commission health care are increasingly being encouraged to commission on the basis of the whole pathway for the individual requiring care – that is, contracting for a service that deals with the individual's condition in all care settings, rather than commissioning separately for the hospital and community elements of their care. Service redesign projects are also more likely to look at the whole service to the individual, rather than at how to improve what happens in only one sector. These approaches require

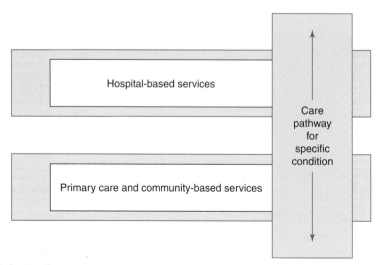

Figure 20.1 Patient pathways.

more collaboration and communication between primary and secondary care, and so they can seem difficult and slow. However, they do reflect the reality of people's lives much better than separated primary and secondary care commissioning and development. Care pathways aim to ensure that people receive a uniform quality of care for their condition, and have similar experiences, no matter who their primary care clinician is, or where or to whom they are referred for care. For the nurse, the existence of an agreed local pathway for people with a particular condition or care need helps their practice by:

- making communication easier with identified nurses based in other sectors;
- making it easier to give individuals clear and accurate information on what will happen to them in the course of their journey through the episode of care;
- clarifying the different elements that make up the package of care to be given;
- helping them to understand the nature of the condition at all stages, and the evidence-based treatment pathway for it.

Quality of care

Another professional issue that can arise in primary and community care is the need to maintain high standards of care in very diverse settings. Different degrees of hygiene, privacy, temperature, equipment, time and space are inevitable when settings vary from homes and workplaces, to schools, clinics, cells and hostels. In these circumstances, the NMC Code provides a helpful framework against which to check practice and professionalism.

Continuity of care

Where people use primary care services in their local area over a long period of time, it is possible for a nurse to provide a very valuable degree of continuity of care that is appreciated by the individual and that is rewarding to the nurse. Practice nurses provide care to individuals over the length of time that the individuals are registered with the practice, and the GP patient record (computerised or paper) makes it possible to hold a person's whole medical history in one place. School nurses, family planning nurses, nurses working in mental health, children's health nurses and nurses working in occupational health services in the community have similar opportunities to build up a relationship with an individual over time that helps them to understand and anticipate the person's health needs. Often the trust built up over time will enable the individual to talk about needs or problems that would not have been disclosed without such continuity. Disclosures of abuse are a common example. Continuity of care – both access to a continually updated care record and the same professional face – are particularly valued by people with long-term health conditions, who appreciate the fact that a regular professional carer is familiar with their history, their preferences and the idiosyncrasies of their condition.

Conversely, there are nursing roles in primary care where a single opportunity to provide health advice, information or care arises. At walk-in centres, drop-in centres, minor injury units and police custody suites, the nurse may have one brief opportunity to provide care to an individual. Here, key skills are communication and negotiation, assessment, and the clinical skills (including advanced assessment and prescribing) to deliver care on the spot.

The contrast between these two different approaches illustrates the exciting diversity of roles in primary care nursing, and the range of skills and competencies required for them.

Communication and information-sharing

The scattered physical locations for care in the community mean that communicating with colleagues is much more of a challenge than it would be on a hospital ward. The National Programme for IT (in England), being implemented by the agency Connecting for Health, aims to improve communication across care settings by, among other things, providing all professionals with shared access to a single electronic patient record and to electronically stored images and investigation results, allowing electronic booking of appointments for patients, and giving every health professional their own email address (Box 20.5). Scotland also plans to introduce electronic patient records as part of its wider strategy for future health services (Scottish Executive, 2005). In the meantime, GPs hold one set of records on each person registered with them; different community nurses often have their own records; some people hold their own records for specific purposes (such as the child health record and maternity record) or for a specific condition (typically long-term conditions such as asthma or diabetes); and the hospital has its own case notes for each inpatient. In primary care, district nurses and others who visit people at home often have to go into the GP's surgery to update the patient's record there. Some still have no regular access to a computer, and so this can be a time-consuming task.

BOX 20.5 The National Programme for IT

NHS Connecting for Health (CfH) is an agency of the Department of Health set up to deliver the National Programme for IT (NPfIT) in the NHS in England (www.connectingforhealth.nhs.uk). This programme consists of seven key elements:

- *NHS Care Records Service (CRS)*: provides an 'individual electronic NHS care record for every patient in England, securely accessible by patients and those caring for them'.
- *Choose and Book*: an electronic appointment booking service 'offering patients greater choice of hospitals or clinics and more convenience in the date and time of their appointment'.
- *Electronic Prescription Service (EPS)*: enables prescriptions to be transferred electronically from general practice to pharmacy.
- *New National Network (N3)*: 'the IT infrastructure and broadband connectivity for the NHS so patient information can be shared between organisations'.
- *Contact*: a central email and directory service for the NHS, to enable the secure transfer of patient information between staff.
- *Picture Archiving and Communication Systems (PACS)*: 'to capture, store, display and distribute static and moving digital medical images, providing clearer X-rays and scans and faster, more accurate diagnosis'.
- *IT for GPs*: including the Quality Management and Analysis System (QMAS), support for the GPs' Quality and Outcomes Framework, and a system for GP-to-GP record transfer.

Source: www.connectingforhealth.nhs.uk.

The importance of making available information on an individual's condition, care and treatment to all the health professionals who may be dealing with the person means that nurses in primary care must spend the necessary time and effort on these records. The NMC Code, in the section 'Provide a high standard of practice and care at all times', states that, as a nurse or midwife, you must:

> keep clear and accurate records of the discussions you have, the assessments you make, the treatment and medicines you give and how effective these have; complete records as soon as possible

after an event has occurred; ensure any entries you make in someone's paper records are clearly and legibly signed, dated and timed; ensure any entries you make in someone's electronic records are clearly attributable to you.

(NMC Code, 2008)

Reflection point 20.6
Think about the legal issues that might specifically affect nursing practice in primary care. What sort of areas would you need to be familiar with? Where would you get help to understand and address the issues?

Check that your list of issues includes the issues identified below. For help and information, you should have considered your employer, guidance from the NMC Code, relevant government departments and other public information sources such as the websites of national organisations.

Legal issues

Some of the legal issues that nurses working outside hospitals might need to be aware of, depending on their role, concern:

- the Human Rights Act 1998;
- rights of access to private premises such as homes and workplaces;
- the legal status of asylum-seekers, other immigrants and foreign nationals seeking health care in Britain;
- protection of vulnerable people – both adults and children;
- antidiscrimination (including disability) legislation;
- public health legislation regarding statutorily notifiable diseases, and action to be taken in the case of a public health emergency;
- health and safety legislation regarding workplaces and public places, including handling and disposal of hazardous substances and clinical waste;
- compulsory detention and treatment for people with mental disorders;
- the limits and requirements of non-medical prescribing, including private prescribing and computer-generated prescriptions;
- the legal status of street drugs and medicines, and requirements for recording and disposing of them;
- the powers of the police, coroners and other authorities;
- certification and notification of death at home;
- witnessing wills;
- medical termination of pregnancy;
- the position of nurses acting as 'good Samaritans' when required in public.

These are only some of the areas of law that can have a direct impact on the day-to-day work of nurses working in primary care. Legislation changes frequently, and a full exposition of the implications of these areas of law is beyond the scope of this chapter. However, nurses moving to work in a primary care setting should make themselves familiar with, and follow, their employing organisation's policies and procedures, which will be compliant with all relevant legislation. Where there is a temptation to overstep a legal boundary, because it seems in the patient's interest, nurses should remember that the NMC Code states specifically in the section 'Be open and honest, act with integrity and uphold the reputation of your profession' that 'you must adhere to the laws of the country in which you are practising'.

Mobility

Nurses who are based in a walk-in centre, nursing home or prison may not have to travel around as part of their working day. Many community nurses, however, visit several clinics, see people in their own homes, or cover a number of schools. In doing so, they need to take account of the time such travel will take and factor that into their daily schedule. Travel over long distances in rural areas is not necessarily slower than travel round a big city during the rush hour. Nurses who use their own cars can claim reimbursement from their employer for the costs, on the basis of a defined price per mile travelled: it is important to establish whether the employer will pay for 'actual miles' (where journeys may be longer but quicker, for example, if they avoid roadworks) or only for previously measured distances between sites. In either case, mileage must be recorded scrupulously, and not estimated, in order to avoid inaccurate claims. Some organisations carry out random diary checks to match mileage claimed against appointments on the day and may take disciplinary action if discrepancies arise.

Employers usually have an organisational policy about nurses transporting and storing patient records and clinical equipment, including dressing packs, emergency equipment, and bags containing medicines and syringes, in their cars. It is important to find out about this and to adhere to the appropriate policy. Where staff members have use of a vehicle belonging to the organisation (such as a lease car for their exclusive use or a pool car), there may be a policy about smoking in the vehicle. Other important legal issues, such as insurance and road tax, and day-to-day issues such as servicing, breakdown cover and private use, will be discussed when a lease or pool car is provided.

Using a car is not always necessary. Some nurses are able to carry out community-based jobs using public transport, and some use alternative methods such as bicycles. In one example, nurses who wanted to use bicycles for community work were initially banned from doing so by their employer on the grounds of safety and concerns about the amount of equipment they would need to carry. However, after discussions, the dispute was resolved in favour of the use of bicycles. To avoid misunderstandings and inadvertent breaches of policy that might result in disciplinary action, it is sensible to discuss the following with a new employer at the start of a placement or post, if it is going to involve peripatetic work:

- how you plan to travel between visits or sites;
- how and when you should calculate, record, claim and verify your travelling expenses for reimbursement;
- what rate of reimbursement of travel costs is offered, and what is and is not covered;
- what policies the organisation has in place relevant to your travel, including for your own health and safety, and for the protection of clinical records and equipment;
- what other equipment the employer or you should provide, such as a hands-free kit for a mobile phone.

Teamworking at a distance

The difference between working in a team in one location – whether a ward, clinic, office or care centre – and working alone for much of the day cannot be overestimated. In practical and professional terms, having a team within sight, earshot or easy walk provides another pair of hands, a word of advice, a second opinion, a different perspective or simply backup when the situation requires one of these things. From a personal point of view, a team provides company, interaction, conversation and opportunities for moments of light relief and essential moral support.

However busy the workload or dysfunctional the team, there is usually some benefit to be had from working alongside fellow team members.

In the kinds of primary care setting that involve moving between centres or people's homes, nurses work without any of these for long periods in the day. Practically, this means that they have to devise solutions themselves, or use equipment, ingenuity or negotiation with the individual or family, in order to manage situations where they might otherwise have asked colleagues to help. One advantage of this is that it encourages the involvement of the individual and their closest carers in the care provided by the professional, and so builds relationships of real partnership between them. If these solutions cannot be found or they fail, it can lead nurses to practise in a way that is risky to themselves or their patients. Nurses working alone need to be aware of this possibility and to report such situations to their employer as soon as possible.

Professionally, working alone provides the challenge of being solely responsible for the standard of your practice. With no immediate supervision or casual observance of your practice by others, maintaining standards, acting professionally and delivering the best possible care becomes a matter of personal commitment and integrity.

The sense of isolation when working in this way can be disturbing. Caring for people outside of hospitals can bring the nurse into contact with situations, conditions and people that are just as distressing or challenging as those encountered on the wards. Added to these stressors can be the very distressing circumstances in which some people live, and exposure to whole families' trauma, grief, anger or disruptive behaviour as well as the individual's. Problems with traffic, navigation, weather and other everyday irritants of a mobile role can add to the difficulties.

It is important that nurses in primary care develop the capacity for 'teamworking at a distance', actively seeking the support of their team or colleagues and building a network of personal and professional support to counteract these pressures – for example, by:

- prioritising attendance at regular team or centre meetings and protecting the time to attend;
- making time at the start or end of meetings to speak individually to others and to get to know them and their area of work;
- arranging regular clinical supervision sessions, either one-to-one or as a team (Box 20.6);
- having agreed times when team members are available to be telephoned;
- linking with other teams doing related work.

BOX 20.6 Clinical supervision

There are many definitions of clinical supervision. The following description includes all the key elements of the process of clinical supervision and its purpose:

Clinical supervision is regular, protected time for facilitated, in-depth reflection on clinical practice. It aims to enable the supervisee to achieve, sustain and creatively develop a high quality of practice through the means of focused support and development. The supervisee reflects on the part she plays as an individual in the complexities of the events and the quality of her practice. This reflection is facilitated by one or more experienced colleagues who have expertise in facilitation and the frequent, ongoing sessions are led by the supervisee's agenda. The process of clinical supervision should continue throughout the person's career, whether they remain in clinical practice or move into management, research or education.

(Bond and Holland, 1998)

Personal safety and security

It is not the case that working in primary care is necessarily more 'dangerous' than working in a hospital. However, it does present some similar and some different risks, and it is sensible to anticipate these in order to minimise them. The risks specific to work in primary care are:

- personal and professional risks of working alone;
- personal risks when travelling;
- health and safety risks when delivering care in different settings.

Working in people's homes, in isolated settings such as hostels, or simply behind closed doors in a surgery or clinic can feel more risky than being on a ward or in a residential setting where there are several other people within sight or earshot. It is important to know in advance how to avert risks and how help can be summoned, if necessary, for the nurse and the patient.

Reflection point 20.7
Try to list the risks you anticipate of working alone and what measures you might take to mitigate them.

Box 20.7 gives some examples of commonly considered risks.

BOX 20.7 Potential risks of working alone and strategies to tackle them

- *Clinical crisis requiring extra help*: mobile phones for all peripatetic staff, list of backup phone numbers, detailed information on appointment schedules (e.g. patients' addresses), good communication between staff and good record-keeping.
- *Abuse or violence from patients/clients*: training in interpersonal and negotiation skills, good record-keeping and communication by team members, choosing the environment of care where possible (e.g. clinic rather than home), setting up safety systems such as two-person visits, installing panic buttons and windows in surgery doors, and cooperation and information exchange between team members.
- *Personal risk when out and about*: adherence to local policies, taking advice from transport agencies, provision of mobile phones, sharing information about risky places, use of drivers where provided for night calls.

The keys to addressing risks, and so working without being unduly hampered by risks, are appropriate training, familiarity with the working environment, adherence to local policies designed to protect staff, and good communication and record-keeping between team members. With these in place, most potential risks can be anticipated and averted.

Risks when travelling are common to all travellers, but nurses may feel more vulnerable if they are in uniform or carrying equipment or bags that might attract thieves. Local employers' policies often specify how nurses should protect themselves, including:

- keeping bags and equipment out of sight in a car, e.g. locked in the boot;
- carrying the minimum needed for the visits/surgeries planned;
- parking in well-lit places wherever possible;
- carrying a mobile phone and appropriate emergency numbers in case of breakdown, delay or other problems;

- covering uniforms with ordinary clothing where possible;
- being accompanied by drivers when making night visits;
- alerting colleagues to potential problems and arranging joint visits where necessary;
- following the usual guidelines for safe travel issued by the police.

The health and safety risks of working in non-standard settings to deliver health care vary with every visit. The condition of the premises may present trip, slip, chemical or infection hazards. The needs of the individual requiring care may be hard to meet because of constraints of space or equipment. The presence of pets or parasites can present their own risks. Every situation needs to be assessed on every occasion, so that appropriate safety precautions can be taken, such as:

- using simple precautions, e.g. wearing protective gloves, wearing a hard hat on a building site, or asking family members to help;
- providing information to families so that they can reduce their own risks, e.g. trip hazards in the home;
- requesting extra or different equipment such as non-slip castors to stop a chair sliding when you are working with someone;
- arranging for expert help on specific issues, including a full health and safety assessment where the situation warrants it.

With care and vigilance, addressing the risks of working in a variety of environments becomes ingrained in the daily routine, but it is important not to become complacent.

SUMMARY

Meeting care needs in community settings means addressing some different issues from those encountered in hospital settings. The principle – ensuring the best possible care for the individual in need – is unchanged. It is important to recognise the potential to become isolated and unsupported in community or peripatetic practice, to make conscious efforts to maintain good team-working, and to build personal and professional support networks.

CONCLUSION

Meeting care needs in community settings is fundamentally different from meeting patients' needs in hospital settings. It offers real and exciting challenges to nurses, with the variety of non-hospital care settings providing a choice of career paths and a range of non-NHS employers. It provides the opportunity to develop new skills, work more autonomously and build different, more partnership-oriented relationships with individuals needing care.

Some primary care roles offer the chance to work with a whole family over a long period of time, taking a privileged place in their lives. Others roles test clinical skills, interpersonal skills, communication and negotiation to the limit in one-off opportunities to provide first contact care. Nursing in home and community settings requires maturity, resilience, ingenuity and flexibility and provides a rich choice of contexts for a nursing career.

Current government policies in all four countries of the UK are focused on increasing the amount of care delivered to people outside hospitals, reshaping provision to move traditionally hospital-based services into other settings, and using nurse-led health promotion and case management of long-term conditions to keep vulnerable people out of hospital. For these reasons, primary care is set to remain the fastest-developing arena for health care, and it will continue to offer an ideal learning environment for student nurses and a uniquely valuable development opportunity for newly qualified nurses.

References

Bond M and Holland S (1998). *Skills of Clinical Supervision for Nurses*. Buckingham: Open University Press.

Carr SM (1999). Experiencing practice: an exploration of the constructed meaning of nursing in the community. Unpublished PhD thesis. Newcastle: University of Northumbria at Newcastle.

Carr SM (2001). Community nursing: does the title fit the talents? *Journal of Community Nursing*, **15** (10).

Centre for Economic Policy Research (2006). Does Unemployment Damage Your Health? www.cepr.org/pubs/bulletin/meets/405.htm.

Department of Health (DH) (2001). *Valuing People: A New Strategy for Learning Disability for the 21st Century*. London: Department of Health.

Department of Health (DH) (2002). *Liberating the Talents: Helping Primary Care Trusts and Nurses to Deliver the NHS Plan*. London: Department of Health.

Department of Health (DH) (2005). *Case Management Competences Framework for the Care of People with Long-Term Conditions*. London: Department of Health.

Department of Health, Social Services and Public Safety, Northern Ireland and (DHSSPS) and Department of Health and Children (DoHC) (2005). *Nursing for Public Health: Realising the Vision – a Model for Putting Public Health into Practice*. Belfast: Department of Health, Social Services and Public Safety, Northern Ireland.

Drennan V, Goodman C and Leyshon S (2005). *Supporting Experienced Hospital Nurses to Move into Community Matron Roles*. London: Primary Care Nursing Research Unit.

Kenyon V, Smith E, Hefty L, Bell M and Maraus T (1990). Clinical competencies for community health nursing. *Public Health Nursing*, **7**, 33–9.

Mason C and Clarke J (2001). *A Nursing Vision of Public Health: All Ireland Statement on Public Health and Nursing*. Belfast and Dublin: Department of Health, Social Services and Public Safety, Northern Ireland and Department of Health and Children.

National Institute for Mental Health in England (NIMHE) (2004). *Scoping Review on Mental Health Anti Stigma and Discrimination: Current Activities and What Works*. London: Department of Health.

Nursing and Midwifery Council (NMC) (2008). *The Code: Standards of Conduct, Performance and Ethics for Nurses and Midwives*. London: Nursing and Midwifery Council.

Princess Royal Trust for Carers (2006). What Support Do You Give to Your Biggest Partner? www.carers.org/press/what-support-do-you-give-to-your-biggest-partner,33,NW.html.

Queen's Institute of District Nursing (1943). *Handbook for Queen's Nurses*. London: Faber & Faber.

Scottish Executive (2005). *Delivering for Health*. Edinburgh: Scottish Executive Health Department.

Further reading

Department of Health (DH). www.dh.gov.uk.

Department of Health (DH) (2006). *Modernising Nursing Careers*. London: Department of Health.
Published by the four UK departments of health, this UK-wide document considers the changes that have affected nursing in recent years and proposes a new approach to nursing careers, together with a number of significant workstreams to address the necessary changes to nursing pre- and post-registration education, particularly for community nurses.

Department of Health, Social Services and Public Safety, Northern Ireland (DHSSPS). www.dhsspsni.gov.uk.

Department of Health, Social Security and Public Safety in Northern Ireland (DHSSPS) (2006). *Regional Redesign of Community Nursing Project*. Belfast: Department of Health, Social Security and Public Safety in Northern Ireland.
Sets out recommendations for the future for community nursing in Northern Ireland, with specific recommendations regarding practitioners, education, organisational arrangements, the environment and support systems.

Home Office Crime Reduction. www.crimereduction.homeoffice.gov.uk.
Discusses the provisions and protections of the Human Rights Act 1998.

National Assembly for Wales (1999). *Realising the Potential: A Strategic Framework for Nursing, Midwifery and Health Visiting in Wales into the 21st Century*. Cardiff: National Assembly for Wales.
This report was followed by separate briefing papers for mental health nursing, learning disabilities nursing, midwifery, children's nursing, and nursing research and development in Wales.

NHS Primary Care Contracting. www.primarycarecontracting.nhs.uk.
Provides information on new forms of contracting for the delivery of primary medical services by non-traditional providers, e.g. nurse-led surgeries and services provided by private companies.

Nursing and Midwifery Council (NMC). www.nmc-uk.org.

Queen's Nursing Institute. www.qni.org.uk.
A charity providing project grants and professional information and support to nurses in primary and community care.

Scottish Executive Health Department. www.scotland.gov.uk.

Scottish Executive Health Department (2006). *Review of Nursing in the Community*. Edinburgh: Scottish Executive Health Department.
This proposed a radical overhaul of the different nursing roles in the community, creating one new role to combine elements of nursing care and public health.

Welsh Assembly Government Health and Social Care Department. www. wales.gov.uk.

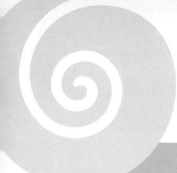

Expected and unexpected death

21

Christine Eberhardie

Introduction

In this chapter the nature and circumstances of death are discussed, along with the physical, psychosocial and ethico-legal issues that accompany expected and unexpected death. The nurse has a significant role to play in helping patients to achieve a comfortable and dignified death, wherever it takes place and within the law. The nurse also has a professional duty within the scope of the NMC Code (2008) (Appendix 1) to ensure that the health and well-being of patients and their families are protected and promoted and that their care is dignified, honest and of the highest standard from diagnosis to death.

The fact that death is a normal part of the natural process of life does not make it any easier to accept. Death is a certainty over which people have no control – apart from suicide. It is the experience of dying and the circumstances of their death that most people fear. Understanding the meaning of loss and the nature of normal grief and bereavement can help nurses to support patients and families to face death, both expected and unexpected.

Learning objectives

After studying this chapter you should be able to:
- define terms associated with expected and unexpected death;
- discuss expected death, including ethico-legal issues and coping strategies for patients and carers;
- understand the causes and consequences of unexpected death;
- recognise death and the signs of its approach;
- know the significance of the preparation of the body for disposal;
- examine the difficulties associated with violent death;
- gain an insight into transcultural issues in death and bereavement;
- identify normal and abnormal grief and be able to find sources of help from national and international voluntary, professional and statutory agencies;
- recognise signs of burnout and stress in professional colleagues.

Definitions

In the complex world of the twenty-first century, where individuals live alone, live in unmarried partnerships, have single-sex relationships or are remarried with stepchildren to consider, it is hard to find a satisfactory generic term to equate with 'spouse' or 'family'. In this chapter we use the term 'partner' to indicate the person with whom the patient has a close loving, often sexual, relationship taking on responsibilities similar to those of husband or wife. The term 'family' is used in its usual sense and includes stepchildren with whom the patient has a familial relationship.

The term 'carer' is used for those non-professionals giving regular, physical and psychosocial care to the patient and family. Finally, the term 'spiritual adviser' is used to include religious leaders as well as those giving less formal spiritual support.

Clinical death

In the days before cardiopulmonary resuscitation and mechanical ventilation, clinical death was defined as the cessation of life due to the absence of respiration and carotid pulse. Today it is more complex. Death may be clinical death, as defined above, but if the patient has been resuscitated and attached to a ventilator, then such criteria are insufficient.

Cellular death

The cells of the body die at different rates, and the rate of cellular death is important in resuscitation and transplant surgery. For example, cerebral neurones die within 3–7 minutes, but skin cells die at a slower rate.

Brain death

Earl Walker (1985), an eminent neurosurgeon in the USA in the post-war years, illustrated the complexity of defining brain stem death in his book *Cerebral Death*. There are many reasons why a patient may be in a coma and unable to breathe normally, including hypothermia and the use of sedative or anaesthetic drugs. If the patient is ventilated, they must be free from hypothermia, sedative drugs and any other natural or medical reasons in order for the diagnosis of brain death to be made and for the ventilator to be switched off. There are important legal reasons why a time of death must be established clearly in brain death, as it can affect legal procedures such as inheritance rights, criminal investigations and business contracts (Dimond, 2004). The current criteria for the diagnosis of brain death can be found in the Department of Health's Code of Practice for the Diagnosis of Brain Stem Death (DH, 1998).

Expected death

What is an expected death? Ideally, expected death is one where the patient and their partner, family and friends are given an opportunity to decide on the treatment and palliative care options, to strengthen relationships and to make arrangements for the future of loved ones. An expected death can follow a lengthy illness such as acquired immunodeficiency syndrome (AIDS), cancer, cardiac disease or degenerative neurological disease, for example motor neurone disease.

Everyone knows that they are going to die one day, but, to the person who is given a poor prognosis, death becomes a reality and a frightening unknown. The nurse has a key role in helping the patient to understand the realistic goals that they can work towards and to mourn the loss of those that will no longer be available to them. Support for the patient's partner and family is also part of the nurse's role. Expected death can give patients and those closest to them the chance to say goodbye.

Every death is unique and few are ideal, but what follows is an overview of what is considered to be a 'good' death. Costello (2006), in a study of what nurses considered to be a 'good' or 'bad' death in a hospital setting, found that it had a lot more to do with disruption to ward routine and the actual event of death than to the dying process. Preparing people for death is not about ward organisation in order to cause the least disruption. It is about dignity, privacy and support from the time that a poor prognosis is given until the end of life.

Care of the person facing death begins for many with the news that they have a life-threatening disease. The manner in which that news is given – and the relationship that the patient forms with health care professionals involved in future treatment and care – is crucial to the success of the care planned in the good times, and especially when the disease process becomes difficult.

Cecily Saunders was one of the first to talk about the concept of 'total pain', which is physical, psychological, social and spiritual pain (Saunders, 1972, 1985). Others have continued to pursue this theme in palliative care (Faull and Woof, 2002; Fisher, 2002; Kissane and Yates, 2003). In an age when medicine is more specialised, technological and pharmacological, it is important for nurses to focus on the whole person, who is more than a series of symptoms to be treated. The patient has emotional, social and spiritual needs too. Currer (2001) talks about 'social death', in which the patient becomes increasingly isolated and withdrawn from their social circle.

One of the fundamental skills of caring for the person who will die as a result of their illness is communication. Good communication skills will enable the nurse to ensure that, where humanly possible, the news is broken to the patient in a clear, unambiguous but sensitive way, ensuring privacy and dignity (Twycross, 2002; Pollard and Swift, 2003). Failure to ensure that this first step is taken can result in serious immediate consequences, as can be seen in Scenario 21.1.

SCENARIO 21.1

Maria, aged 23 years, is a ballet dancer who, 2 months before her visit to hospital, had been appointed to the corps de ballet of the national ballet of her native country. She is a practising Roman Catholic. She is delighted with her success and the possibilities that it offers for the future. Three weeks before her visit to hospital, she stumbled twice in rehearsal and she had difficulty moving her leg properly. The visit to hospital and the subsequent tests led to a diagnosis of motor neurone disease.

Maria was alone and, although her English is good, she did not understand everything the doctor said to her. She went out of the doctor's surgery with tears in her eyes. Driving back to her flat, she could focus only on the doctor's last phrase: 'You will become gradually more paralysed and there is no cure for this disease. You need to think about your future as you may not be able to dance for much longer.'

Maria drives home crying. She mounts the kerb and rolls the car over, fracturing her right clavicle and radius and suffering minor neck and head injuries.

Reflection point 21.1
- What are the losses that Maria has experienced?
- What are the responsibilities of the multiprofessional team at the hospital?
- How could the news have been broken to Maria in a more sensitive way?

Maybe you have not yet met problems such as those described for Maria, who has suddenly been faced with many losses. When thinking about the first question above, you should consider not only Maria's current physical and emotional losses but all her future losses. She faces the prospect of progressive physical deterioration, which will result in the inability to walk, speak, swallow and eventually breathe unaided. She will also face other losses, including loss of her career, status, social interaction and life itself. For each of those losses, there is some degree of mourning and bereavement.

The second question involves the part that the multiprofessional team can play in supporting Maria through this difficult time. Which members of the team would you expect to help her? You need to consider the immediate team of the general practitioner (GP) and the neurologist, and the roles that the physiotherapist, speech and language therapist, occupational therapist and nurses can play in helping Maria.

As you read further, some of the issues raised by the scenario will be addressed, but in breaking bad news there are no hard and fast rules. As you develop your therapeutic communication skills, you will grow more confident in dealing with such situations and avoid making it worse for all concerned.

Breaking bad news

Ideally, the patient's partner, family member or friend and a nurse should accompany a doctor when the news is broken of a poor prognosis. Bad news should be broken in a quiet area where the patient's privacy and dignity are respected. The patient should be prepared for the news with a phrase or 'warning' that indicates that bad news is coming (Buckman, 1988, 1992; Twycross, 2002). A warning might be 'Well, Maria, I have the results and they are not as good as I would have liked. Let us go and discuss the options available now.'

In many cases, the words are superfluous. The fact that the doctor takes the patient and partner somewhere private and sits them down with the scan results in hand is sufficient to make the patient anxious. Non-verbal communication is often stronger than words in its effect.

All the people present should be sitting at the same height, and with the doctor near to the patient so that eye contact can be maintained. Touch is a very powerful form of communication and must be used sensitively in a spontaneous rather than contrived way (Davidhizar and Giger, 1997; Randall and Wearn, 2005). Areas such as the upper arm or shoulder are less threatening than the hand or other parts of the body. Some individuals may find touch offensive if used other than for clinical examination, for personal, cultural or religious reasons. Among the personal reasons may be previous sexual assault or child abuse.

The language used to give news to the patient should be clear and without the use of euphemisms, jargon or clichés. Often doctors talk about statistics when presenting the patient with options. It is useful if the nurse is aware of these or can read exactly what options have been offered in the notes so that further questions can be answered. Importantly, no unrealistic expectations should be raised, but realistic hope should be offered based on realistic goals. It is important to retain the patient's confidence and trust (Buckman, 1988; Twycross, 2002; Randall and Wearn, 2005).

The nurse needs to listen to the patient actively. What exactly is the patient asking? What is the patient's non-verbal communication telling you? There may be long silences where information is digested, and it is important to respect that silence. Take the interview at the patient's own pace (Buckman, 1988; Randall and Wearn, 2005). This may be very challenging in a busy clinic or ward, with the workload pressures of the modern health service, but failure to do this can damage future relations and have an impact on future care. Time spent at this stage can be time saved later. Listening to the patient, carers and family will identify losses and the degree of anticipatory grief experienced by them.

Anticipatory grief

Death is preceded by a series of losses resulting from the illness or trauma, such as loss of function, body image, work, social life and financial security for patients who know they are going to die in a few weeks, months or years. This is known as 'anticipatory grief'. The person is facing not only the reality of losses as they experience them, but also the burden of imaginary losses too. The imagination can dwell on negative thoughts and move the person towards depression and, in a few cases, suicide.

Helping patients and their families to cope with emotional, social and spiritual pain requires exceptional interprofessional communications skills from the outset. If we look at the patient in Scenario 21.1 and examine all the losses that Maria faces, it is clear that she has a chronic and life-threatening illness. She will gradually experience more and more muscle weakness until eventually she will not be able to walk, speak, swallow or breathe effectively. In addition, she is going to face the fear of future emotional losses such as broken relationships, loss of her social circle, possible isolation and, above all, the loss of her dreams for the future. Maria is a practising Roman Catholic and may be asking spiritual or philosophical questions, such as 'Why me?' or 'What have I done to deserve this?' This is a question that is not exclusive to Roman Catholics or people of other religions; agnostics and atheists may also find this a time for reflection on philosophical and spiritual issues.

Maria is given the unadulterated truth while she is on her own, and she leaves the doctor's surgery in a highly emotional state preoccupied with his last phrase, which she found devastating. Even when bad news is broken in a more sympathetic manner, patients and visitors need to regain control of their emotions before they leave the hospital or clinic. Crossing roads and driving a car is dangerous when someone is totally preoccupied. Before the patient leaves the surgery, a discussion of less emotional issues can help to calm them down and refocus their thinking – for instance, asking Maria how she will get home, which route she will take and what she will do when she gets home; this uses the brain for reasoning rather than emotional activity.

Anticipatory grief can lead to a sense of hopelessness, which is a destructive emotion and can result in depression. In life-threatening illness the focus of hope changes. Herth (1992, 2000) developed the Herth Hope Index to try to measure hope. In interventional studies she found that, by using positive interventions to promote realistic hope, patients reported an increase in hope and a better quality of life.

Hope gives meaning to life, and even those who have been in extreme circumstances where they have been imprisoned and lost their freedom have found meaning in their life and something for which to hope. Victor Frankl was a qualified doctor who was deported from Vienna to concentration camps in Europe during the Second World War. His books *The Doctor and the Soul* (Frankl, 1965) and *Man's Search for Meaning* (Frankl, 1984) demonstrate the triumph of hope as a coping strategy.

An understanding of the patient's experience and the effect that reality and imagination have on that patient will help the nurse to ensure that the patient can sort out the difference between the real and the imagined, in order to work towards realistic goals and maintain realistic hope.

End-of-life decision-making

The prospect of physical disability, with or without declining mental ability, is frightening, and many people fear loss of control and independence most of all. Everyone has the right to give informed consent before treatments are given or withdrawn. As disease progresses, for example in motor neurone disease and in some cancers, such as cancers of the head and neck, decisions have to be made about withholding or withdrawing treatment. The ethical and legal issues are complex and profound and sometimes controversial (see Chapter 9).

Patients in the UK have the right to make informed decisions in the form of advanced statements or directives about their end-of-life care under the terms of the Adults with Incapacity (Scotland) Act 2000, the Mental Capacity Act 2005 (England and Wales) and its equivalent in Northern Ireland, which empower patients to make decisions about their end-of-life care while they have the mental capacity to do so. A summary of the Act can be found on the DH website (www.dh.gov.uk) and includes details of the role of advanced statements and directives that are legally binding.

A patient may wish to make a will and have their signature witnessed. The NMC Code requires nurses to maintain clear professional boundaries and to ensure that no attempt is made to abuse their position for their own ends. Therefore, nurses should not witness a patient's will, but they do have a duty to ensure that someone else who is not a beneficiary can witness it.

Palliative care

The World Health Organization (WHO) defines palliative care as:

an approach that improves the quality of life of patients and their families facing the problem associated with life-threatening illness, through the prevention and relief of suffering by means of early identification and impeccable assessment and treatment of pain and other problems, physical, psychosocial and spiritual.

(WHO, 2005)

Although palliative care was developed by the cancer hospice movement and for care of people with conditions such as motor neurone disease, it is an approach that should be applied and modified for all life-threatening diseases.

There have been two recent major initiatives in promoting effective and high-quality end-of-life care for patients who have no more than a week to live: the Liverpool Integrated Care Pathway (Ellershaw and Wilkinson, 2003; Ellershaw and Murphy, 2005) and, for people who will die in the community, the NHS Gold Standards Framework (2005). The main aims of the Liverpool Integrated Care Pathway are to promote the hospice model of palliative care in other settings.

There are seven standards within the NHS Gold Standards Framework, referred to as the '7 Cs':

* communication: to improve communication between professionals, patients and carers;
* coordination: to promote seamless care;
* control of symptoms: to ease suffering;
* continuity of care;
* continued learning for staff: to ensure high standards of care;
* carer support;
* care of the dying: to recognise the dying phase and use the Liverpool Integrated Care Pathway (Ellershaw and Wilkinson, 2003; Ellershaw and Murphy, 2005).

Reflection point 21.2
* What is expected of me when someone dies?
* How will I recognise that death is imminent?
* What do I think and feel about death?

If this is the first time that you have faced the death of someone, it is perfectly normal to be apprehensive about witnessing the last hours of a person's life, being present at the time of death and then having to handle the body. In the next section, we discuss what might happen when you face an expected death.

Recognising that death is imminent

As death approaches, the patient's symptoms change – weakness, loss of appetite, tendency to constipation, breathlessness, insomnia and confusion are all likely to be increased (Adam, 1997). All of these symptoms are part of the normal process of dying and, unless they distress the patient, do not need to be treated. The symptoms are often more distressing for those with the patient – that is, the family and the staff. For instance, the partner and family may worry that the patient is not receiving food and fluids in the last 48 hours of life, when this can be more of a burden than a comfort for the patient (Vullo-Navich *et al.*, 1998). As death approaches, the patient will grow weaker and become less responsive.

About 50 per cent of patients make a noise from an inability to clear secretions in the throat. This is often called the 'death rattle'. It can be very distressing to the patient and those by the bedside. Positioning the patient in the semi-prone position can help; in some patients, hyoscine can relieve the symptom (Twycross, 2002).

As death approaches, the patient and the family may wish to talk to their spiritual adviser, for example a chaplain, pastor, imam or rabbi. A current list of contact details of local ministers of all religions should be kept, on the ward or in the community, and it is useful to get to know the ministers before calling them in an emergency. Many families prefer to contact their personal spiritual adviser from their locality.

The role of the nurse when a person dies

When the person dies, the nurse needs to ensure that the person's body is treated with respect and dignity and that those who are with the person have some time to sit with the body in order to say their own personal farewell. A doctor should certify the death, although in some situations approved by the employing authority, a senior nurse, such as a night practitioner, might certify the death.

Last offices normally need to be carried out before the body is transferred to the mortuary. The purpose of last offices is to ensure that the body is clean and lying in a straight position and that wounds are dressed to prevent leakage and ensure that any infection is not spread to those who handle the body before burial or cremation, such as mortuary or funeral service staff. The patient's eyes and mouth should be closed and the hair combed. The removal of cannulae and feeding tubes will depend on local hospital policy and whether there is to be a coroner's investigation. If there is to be a coroner's enquiry or inquest, then the coroner's officer will give advice on the removal of tubes.

The body needs to be identified clearly with a name band and labels on the shroud and covering sheet before transfer to the mortuary. Some religions prohibit non-believers from handling the body after death. In some cases, women of childbearing age should not touch the body because if they are menstruating they may be considered 'unclean'. Hospitals and hospices usually have viewing rooms; it is important to ensure that the patient looks dignified and that only appropriate symbols of religion are on view before the family enters. This is discussed further later in the chapter.

The coroner has a legal responsibility to establish the time, place, circumstances and cause of all industrial, accidental, violent, sudden, negligent or suspicious deaths. This is discussed further in the section on unexpected death.

Bereavement, grief and mourning

Consider Scenario 21.2.

SCENARIO 21.2

John is 86 years old. He was married to Agnes for 58 years. He proudly boasted that they had never spent a night apart, except when he was called up during the Second World War and when she was in hospital having their three children. Four months ago Agnes was admitted to a nursing home. She died 3 months ago.

At Agnes's funeral he became agitated and angry. Other mourners became embarrassed and walked away from him.

John is inconsolable and wanders around the house looking for his wife. His daughter is very concerned that he is not eating and sleeping properly. She asks your advice.

Reflection point 21.3
- Is John's experience unusual or abnormal?
- What can health professionals do to help John?
- What is the purpose of mourning rituals in society?

John is bereaved. He and Agnes have been together for most of their lives and had a very happy marriage. Bereavement for John started at or before the time when Agnes went into the nursing home. The grief he felt was profound. When she died and he could no longer visit her, he felt numb, lost, alone and so sad that he could not eat or drink properly. During the funeral his feelings turned to anger and agitation, which were at odds with the expectations of others attending the funeral.

Bereavement, grief and mourning are all important aspects of dealing with loss.

When you read about bereavement, grief and mourning you will find that the words are used in different ways. What follows is a series of definitions that may help you to analyse the concepts.

Bereavement

Walter (1999) defines bereavement as 'the objective state of having lost someone or something'. Other authors limit bereavement to loss following the death of a person (Stroebe *et al.*, 1993). Bereavement can be for anything, from the loss of a relationship or a symbolic object that means a lot, such as a wedding ring, to loss of speech or loss of life. The importance and meaning of the loss will affect acceptance and recovery.

Grief

Grief is 'the emotional response to one's loss' (Stroebe *et al.*, 1993). Grief is the total experience that the individual has at the time of the loss. Earlier in this chapter, anticipatory grief was seen as a series of losses on the way to death, such as loss of health, social circle, job, hobbies and so on.

Losses do not begin with a poor prognosis. The patient and their family may have faced major life-changing losses before, such as redundancy, living with illness or loss of function, severed meaningful relationships or the need to flee a country as a refugee due to war (Parkes, 1998). The intensity of the experience depends on the circumstances of the death, and the meaning and importance that the loss has for the grieving individual. It involves a strong emotional, physical, behavioural and spiritual reaction to the loss.

All losses leave their mark, just as a deep wound leaves a scar. But, like a scar, the mark of loss can heal with time and support. Bereavement and grief are normal and do not necessitate the services of a counsellor unless the grief becomes delayed or abnormally prolonged. Abnormal grief is discussed later in this chapter.

Bereavement theory

There are several theories related to bereavement. The major categories are:

- physiological or stress theory;
- psychosocial adaptation;
- sociological.

Physiological responses

The body responds to grief as stress. The response can be seen in any acutely stressful situation, such as when receiving bad news or following a death. The throat becomes dry, with increased swallowing, faintness, lightheadedness, anorexia, sighing and insomnia. Some people complain of feeling hypersensitive, nervous and restless (Parkes, 1998). People often complain of feeling numb, cold, clammy and unable 'to take anything in'. Others pass remarks such as 'it is a dream that I hope will end soon'.

There is also heightened awareness of the senses of smell, taste, sight, hearing and touch. This stress response, or the 'alarm phase' as Parkes (1998) calls it, results in the body reacting as if survival is threatened and the endocrine and autonomic nervous system become overactive. This can lead to vivid memories of the events in the early stages of bereavement, which can affect the person's reactions later. For example, the person may continue to remember the smell of the hospital ward or the detail of what the patient or the room looked like.

The body also responds with changes to the immune system. After bereavement, the individual can be vulnerable to infections and ailments of all kinds (Gerra *et al.*, 2003).

There is also a sense of mental numbness and disbelief. The bereaved person will often talk of feeling 'woolly headed' and 'not able to think straight'. They usually experience a sense of everything being unreal or happening in slow motion. 'They were talking to me and I could not take it in' is a phrase that is often uttered. All these feelings are normal and will settle down eventually.

Another factor is that some people behave out of character and feel the need to lash out verbally or physically. Some pace up and down restlessly and cannot concentrate for long periods. Some people have a delayed response after a death – they cope well with all the necessary activities surrounding the death, such as registering the death, organising the funeral and notifying relatives, but their grief response does not come until the funeral, where they may have planned to say something about the deceased but break down in tears and cannot do so.

In nursing, it is essential to understand that grief alters behaviour. When giving bad news, it is important to ensure that the person is seated and has a drink of water available. The person in this state is unlikely to remember all that has been said to them. They may ask over and over again for the information to be repeated because they may have misheard what was said, or they may fix on one phrase or part of a phrase or a particular gesture. If we return to Scenario 21.1, Maria focused on the doctor's last phrase as she heard it.

Psychosocial adaptation theories

Psychosocial theories are often applied to the care of people who are dying and have been frequently cited in palliative care literature. Bowlby (1969, 1973, 1980) studied attachment and separation in children and formed the opinion that, throughout life, people make attachments and, when these break, it results in a feeling of insecurity and loss. Grief is the emotional and behavioural response to that loss. He described psychological phases of grief – numbness, pining, disorganisation, despair and reorganisation – in his work with Parkes (Bowlby and Parkes, 1970).

Parkes (1998) built on the work he did with Bowlby and from the experience he gained in supporting those recovering from the aftermath of the Aberfan disaster in 1966, when a slagheap slipped and engulfed a school in the small Welsh mining village of Aberfan, killing almost an entire generation of children in the close community. He also carried out research into the bereavement experience of widows and led the development of an organisation for widows called CRUSE (Parkes, 1970, 1998). He described stages of bereavement too, which he referred to as alarm, searching, mitigation, anger and guilt.

Elisabeth Kübler-Ross (1969, 1975), a Swiss psychiatrist who gained a lot of experience with East European displaced people at the end of the Second World War, developed a model for psychosocial adaptation for people who are dying. This model also has five stages: denial, bargaining, anger, despair and resignation.

Table 21.1 Normal grief

Feelings	Physical sensations	Cognitions	Behaviours
Sadness, anger	Tightness in the chest	Disbelief	Sleep disturbances
Guilt	Tightness in the throat	Confusion	Loss of appetite
Self-reproach	'Butterflies' in the stomach	Preoccupation	Absentmindedness
Anxiety	Fatigue	Sense of presence	Social withdrawal
Loneliness	Irritability	Hallucinations	Dreaming about the deceased
Fatigue	Breathlessness		Avoiding reminders of the deceased
Helplessness	Muscle weakness		Searching and calling out
Shock	Dry mouth		Sighing
Yearning	Lack of energy		Restless overactivity
Emancipation	Feeling 'unreal'		Crying
Relief			Visiting places or carrying objects reminders of the deceased
Numbness			

Source: Parkes (1998) and Worden (2003).

Patients and their families go through some or all of these stages. Sometimes a patient can go from anger to denial and back to anger in a matter of hours, and not all people die resigned to their fate. There are patterns to grief, but it is a unique and dynamic process within the individual.

Worden (2003) describes normal grief as a mixture of feelings, physical sensations, cognitions and behaviours (Table 21.1). Worden (2003) also suggests four tasks in the process of mourning:

1 Accepting the reality of the loss.
2 Working through the pain of grief.
3 Adjusting to an environment in which the deceased is missing.
4 Emotionally relocating the deceased in order to move on with life.

There are similarities in this model with those of Bowlby (1969, 1973, 1980) Parkes (1998) and Kübler-Ross (1969, 1975), but the emphasis seems to be more on recognising that the physical, mental, emotional and behavioural aspects occur in an integrated and dynamic way, rather than in a linear progression.

Sociological theories

Anthropologists and sociologists have long been interested in the cultural and social issues surrounding death. Nigel Barley, in his fascinating book on the anthropology of death and mourning, *Dancing on the Grave: Encounters with Death*, examines the meaning of life and death in different cultures, funeral rites and mourning rituals (Barley, 1995). Although the more extreme beliefs of the smaller tribes of the world may seem irrelevant in Western practice, there is a need in a multi-cultural, multi-faith society to open our minds to other cultural traditions and beliefs. The nurse is in a unique position to facilitate this by being sensitive to the need to grieve in one's own way, while ensuring that it does not disturb other patients.

As far as sociologists are concerned, there has been a considerable amount of interest in the way modern Western society regards those who are dead and bereaved. There is a resistance to the 'medicalisation' of bereavement, with its tendency to call upon counselling and therapy to treat apparently normal grief (Craib, 1999). As a result, some interesting sociological perspectives have been identified. Walter (1999) has proposed that modern society seems to abandon its dead and yet finds ways to hang on to them. He discusses the way grief is expressed in Anglo-American society, with male stoicism and restraint on the one hand and public expressions of grief, such as those shown after Princess Diana's death in 1997, on the other.

Craib (1999) reminds us of the ways in which modern society brushes bereavement aside and does not give the individual adequate amounts of time and space to mourn. Bereaved people who are at work are given a few days to bury the person who has died and then they are supposed to get back to normal as soon as possible.

Walter (1999) suggests that those who are bereaved should be encouraged to talk about the dead person and to incorporate them into their lives. With this model in mind, some people have taken to producing a biography in words and pictures for all to see or hear at a funeral service or at the post-funeral gathering. This is usually welcomed as a chance to see the dead person's whole life and not just the part each individual played in it. It can be part of the healing process for partners, family, friends and acquaintances. People who had known the dead person as an adult can explore their early life and begin to understand what made them the person they were.

Mourning

Mourning is the social expression of grief within a societal, religious or cultural context. There are different ways in which grief is expressed within a society. Mourning includes the acceptable forms of the funeral and disposal of the body, rituals, religious rites, and care of the people who are bereaved.

Mourning is both a private and a social activity, and it has several common aspects, regardless of social group, culture or religion. These common aspects include:

- rites and rituals related to the preparation of the body and its disposal;
- period of mourning;
- expression of grief and behaviour;
- food, drinking and eating;
- dress code and grooming during the mourning period.

Preparation of the body and its disposal

Nurses carrying out last offices should remain sensitive to the privacy and dignity of the deceased person and the family and also be aware of the religious and cultural beliefs of the individual. In some religions, such as Islam and Judaism, there are taboos about who can touch the body and how much preparation of the body the nurse can carry out. NHS hospital trusts in large multi-cultural, multi-faith communities have working parties involving the major religious groups in the community, in order to develop guidance for nurses and other health care professionals about what can and cannot be done by the nurse and mortuary staff.

The period of mourning varies from culture to culture. It can be strange for newcomers to Britain to learn that 3–6 days is the average amount of time allowed for compassionate leave and that, after a return to work, all is expected to return to normal.

Expression of grief and behaviour

How people express grief differs between cultural groups. Most people cry, but how they cry and where they cry differs. For instance, in Northern Europe and parts of North America, grief is usually expressed privately and in the home. Crying and sobbing are accepted, but many people remain uncomfortable if they see men crying or exhibiting uninhibited sobbing in public. However, this is changing, so that men or women can grieve in the way that is appropriate to their needs, but they should be given some privacy for this. Problems can arise if an individual is not left to work through their grief and is constantly being 'cheered up' and distracted from their grief.

In some countries, taking out anger on a tree by shaking it is acceptable. Breast-beating, shouting and wailing are commonplace in the Middle East. In some parts of Africa, people make howling sounds known as ululations (Kuipers, 1999).

Food, drinking and eating

In many cultures there is a particular role for food and drink in the mourning period. In some parts of the world, where it is customary to bury the dead within 24 hours, food must not be eaten until after the funeral. For others, a meal before the burial, as in the traditional Irish wake, or immediately after the funeral is usual. In some parts of the Indian subcontinent, it is traditional for friends and other members of the community to bring food to the grieving family, who are not expected to prepare food until after the funeral.

Dress code and grooming

In the West it has been traditional to wear black following death. In the nineteenth and early twentieth centuries, widows were expected to wear black for the rest of their lives, but this custom was relaxed after the Second World War. In some parts of Europe, however, this still applies in the older generations. In India, white is the colour of mourning.

In some parts of Africa, close members of the family in mourning, both male and female, are expected to shave their heads, but in the Hindu community it is usually only the men who do this.

What can the nurse do to help the people who are bereaved?

People who are bereaved need time and space to feel safe to express their feelings and come to terms with the situation. There are times when they need to be with people, and other times when they may prefer to be given some privacy to reflect.

Listening to bereaved people is important. They may need to talk over and over again about their loss, feelings and possible actions. Sometimes they require help to express their feelings and make sense of them. Here are some of the ways in which bereaved people can be helped by nurses and other health care professionals to express their feelings.

Performing and literary arts

Finding different ways to symbolise how a person is feeling or to find a safe outlet for strong emotions requires time, space and imagination. Creative outlets include the performing arts such as music, dance, drama and literary arts such as creative writing and reading.

Music is useful for evoking emotions and memories or changing mood. Banging a drum or dancing can be a way of releasing pent-up energy. It is sometimes helpful to ask a bereaved person to choose a piece of music or a song that expresses what they are feeling now, or to ask 'Do you find that any particular piece of music makes you feel worse or better?'

Drama therapy is mainly of use for bereaved people with relationship or emotional difficulties. Role-play is a powerful method of gaining insight into problems and acting them out, but it should be fully supported by a therapist trained to cope with the consequences of such activity.

Keeping a diary or writing poetry or stories can help bereaved people to describe events, feelings aspirations and make sense of them (Robinson, 2004). Reading is an alternative use of the literary arts, especially for those who feel inhibited by their lack of experience or who have a general shyness of writing. Finding prose or poetry that conveys one's situation or emotions can be as therapeutic as creative writing and counselling in some cases.

Visual arts and crafts

In a similar way, painting and sculpture can be therapeutic, both as an appreciation of the work of others and as an artist. However unskilled the artist, paintings can describe the emotions of those who are dying or bereaved. Bach (1991) demonstrated the importance of art in helping dying children, and this technique has been used in a wide variety of circumstances, especially in complex bereavement, such as the catastrophes of the north Sumatra earthquake and tsunami of 26 December 2004, the terrorist attack on the Twin Towers in New York on 11 September 2001 and the 7 July 2005 bombings in London.

Those who feel they cannot paint well may have craftwork skills that can be used to record their biography. One of the more personal and permanent ways to record the life of a person, apart from a written biography or photograph album, is to create a collage or embroider a sampler or biographical runner recording special events, symbols of life and achievements, with badges, logos, houses, names and dates.

When sorting out the belongings of the person who has died, choosing to keep some items and photographing other items that need to be disposed of means that memories can be kept alive without taking up too much space.

As time passes, normal bereavement becomes less acute, but significant anniversaries such as Christmas and other religious festivals, birthdays, wedding anniversaries and the day the person died revive strong memories. Events such as memorial services and formal reunions can give people a focus for reliving bereavement together and for renewing old and forming new friendships.

◎ SUMMARY

Death, both expected and unexpected, is a key part of nursing. It is an aspect of nursing that challenges our beliefs and concepts of life, respect, dignity and behaviour. Many nurses find death hard to cope with for many reasons – some reasons are personal, reflecting bereavements they have experienced, while others are practical or relate to their own fear of death or beliefs about death and its meaning. This may contribute unconsciously to a nurse's choice of specialty. It may also account for why some nurses need a break from their clinical environment.

- Death can be defined as clinical, cellular and brain death.
- Expected death brings with it fear, anxiety and uncertainty but also an opportunity to make arrangements for partners and families and to say farewell.
- Coping with expected death involves holistic, physical, psychosocial and spiritual care based on realistic goals.
- Ethico-legal issues such as informed consent and advanced directives need to be considered before the patient's condition deteriorates.
- Sensitive communication skills are crucial in helping people to come to terms with a poor prognosis.
- Grief, bereavement and mourning are a normal part of life. Nurses play a key role in enabling bereaved people to experience grief and to work their way to recovery in privacy and dignity.

Unexpected death

Much of what has been said above also applies to unexpected death, but with unexpected death there is no anticipatory grief. The world of the person who is bereaved turns chaotic and future plans are shattered. Neither the deceased nor their loved ones has time to prepare. Trauma, myocardial infarction, stroke, sudden death in epilepsy, and major disasters caused by nature or humans are among the causes of unexpected death. For the patient's partner, family and friends, grief is acute and disorienting and is often accompanied by feelings of disbelief, guilt, helplessness and anger (Parkes, 1998; Worden, 2003). A frequent phrase heard at this time is 'If only . . .' – for example, 'If only we had not argued . . .' or 'If only we had not gone by car . . .'

Parents of children of any age find it hard to come to terms with the death of a child. The natural order is that parents die before the children, and when a child dies part of the parents future dies too. Parents and grandparents alike often express their grief in terms of missed future life events, such as graduation, wedding or first grandchild.

A considerable factor in the care of the bereaved person after sudden death is the maintenance of identity, privacy and dignity for both the dead person and the family in order to prevent a stressful event becoming worse. The way in which the nurse handles the situation can have far-reaching consequences because the intensity of the immediate grief process leaves lasting memories. Nurses may come into contact with the bereaved long after the death, either as community nurses or as practice nurses. Even in hospital practice, some patients may be very anxious because they have encountered sudden death before in the same hospital.

Among the factors associated with sudden death that play a large part in the grieving process of the survivor are the following:

- the circumstances in which the death occurs;
- whether the bereaved person witnessed the death;
- whether the body is missing or disfigured;
- whether the circumstances were private or public;
- the presence or absence of the media;
- the role of the coroner and an inquest.

Sudden death at home or at work can be more difficult to cope with for some people, especially if they are the first person to find the body. If the discovery was totally unexpected, then this can result in the bereaved person being unable to enter the building again without feeling considerable distress. Equally distressing is finding a body that is disfigured or the body of a person who has been dead for some time.

If the person was taken to hospital and their condition deteriorated there, then the family may witness the resuscitation or may be sent to wait outside. Witnessed resuscitation is controversial, and there are many advantages and disadvantages to the practice. On the one hand, it is traumatic to see the patient being manhandled, hear orders being shouted and watch the defibrillator in action. Accident and emergency nurses present at witnessed resuscitation have found it stressful, not only because of concern for the family but also because of competing priorities on their time (Hallgrimsdottir, 2000). On the other hand, however, some studies show that nurses think that relatives are distressed but pleased to have seen for themselves that everything was done for the patient (Hallsgrimdottir, 2000; Kidby, 2003; Redley, *et al*., 2004).

The bereavement may be easier to bear if the circumstances of the death are private than when a death becomes very public, such as in a major incident, murder or manslaughter. People caught up in highly publicised deaths complain that their lives are taken over by the media and other intrusions.

In cases of violent death, life can be made very difficult for bereaved people if there are suspicious circumstances and media interest in the events surrounding the death. Police investigations, delays in releasing the body for burial or cremation, and failure to find a body can delay the normal grief process and cause considerable distress to the family.

The role of the nurse in unexpected death

> **Reflection point 21.4**
> Familiarise yourself with your local policy on communicating with the next of kin following an unexpected death.

Informing the next of kin

As explained in the section on expected death, the way in which the next of kin are informed of the death of an individual can affect their ability to come to terms with it. Nurses can help by ensuring that the news is broken sensitively but clearly. Ideally, nurses who have cared for the patient at the time of death should break the news (British Association of Accident and Emergency Medicine and Royal College of Nursing, 1995).

The news should be broken in an unambiguous way, avoiding euphemisms and clichés such as 'He is no longer with us' or 'She has passed away'. Bad news should be given in private, so that the next of kin and other family members can express their grief without embarrassment. Using graphic descriptions, jargon or medical terms such as 'His arm was degloved' or 'She had arrhythmia, which did not respond to cardioversion' can make the experience more distressing.

It is essential to listen carefully to what the bereaved people want to say. Some will express shock or feel a mixture of feelings such as guilt, sadness and anger, as, for example, in the case of a person who had left home after a row with their partner, driven while preoccupied and had a fatal accident. Sitting in silence with the individual is often the most helpful approach.

Although it is not helpful to the bereaved for health care professionals to be out of control of their emotions, some find comfort in the knowledge that those caring for their loved one find the occasion sad too and want to shed a tear.

Preparing the body

In the case of sudden death, the coroner's officer will need to be informed in order to establish whether a post-mortem examination is required. A death must be reported to the coroner if:

- the cause of death is unknown;
- death occurs during surgery;
- death occurs in prison;
- death occurs following an industrial disease or accident;
- the death was unnatural;
- the death was violent;
- there are suspicious circumstances (Home Office, 2002).

The nurse needs to ensure that no tubes, catheters or cannulae are removed without permission, in case there is a need for a post-mortem examination. In hospital there is a set of guidelines for carrying out last offices on a patient who is likely to be referred to the coroner. In larger hospital trusts, there is often a coroner's officer on site to answer questions and to explain the role and function of the coroner, which is to establish the identity of the person who has died, and the date, time, cause and the circumstances of the death, but not to apportion blame. The coroner can, if necessary, hold an inquest in which all the facts are put before the court and witnesses are called to establish the time, place and cause of death.

If it is established that the death was due to natural causes, the coroner will notify the registrar and the death can be registered and a funeral held. Where more investigations and post-mortem examinations need to be carried out, the body will not be released. This means that there may be a delay in being given permission to dispose of the body. Families can find this very distressing, as it delays the funeral and disrupts the grieving process. They also find attendance at a coroner's court upsetting, and it is wise to warn them that, if they do not wish to hear the detailed post-mortem report from the pathologist, they might prefer to leave the court room while this is being given.

Viewing the body

To view or not to view the body of a loved one who has died suddenly can be a difficult decision, but pressure to view should not be exerted on an individual. In some cases a body has to be viewed for identification purposes, and this can be very stressful, even if it is not a close relative who carries out this task.

Viewing the body can be calming and reassuring if the person who died looks peaceful. However, if the body is badly disfigured or damaged, and would be a shocking lasting image that the bereaved people take away, it may be necessary to find alternative methods of identification such as dental records or DNA testing. Not viewing a body can be a missed opportunity to say a final goodbye, however, and may make it more difficult for the person to grieve (Kent and McDowell, 2004).

Procedures for a person who is brought in dead

There are a number of formalities to take into account when a person is dead on admission to the accident and emergency department. The events leading up to the admission need to be recorded and the death has to be certified in the ambulance by a medical practitioner. The personal effects of the person brought in dead need to be recorded and held safely for the coroner and eventually the next of kin.

If the identity of the person cannot be established, the body must have a wristband with the hospital number, the date and time of arrival at the hospital, and the doctor who certified the death. The local hospital policy should be followed for recording the arrival of the body into the hospital and notifying the police. It is very important that this is carried out accurately and efficiently, as anxious next of kin often phone the hospital first to see whether anyone has been admitted before contacting the police.

Careful, sensitive and efficient handling of sudden death can often prevent abnormal grief from occurring. In the next section, we explore some of the different forms of abnormal grief.

Identifying abnormal grief

It is important to differentiate between normal and abnormal grief. Nurses are in a good position to pick up signs of pathological grief and to refer the patient to appropriate help.

Absent grief

Absent grief should be suspected if the bereaved person does not show signs of grieving and refuses to accept sympathy, changes the subject or leaves the room whenever death is discussed (Burnell and Burnell, 1989). The person may deny the death from the outset.

Delayed grief

Delayed grief occurs if mourning is interrupted, for example if the person has repeated losses before recovering from the earlier loss. If the grief is for someone whose body has not been found, or if the death occurred abroad and the bereaved person cannot visit the site of death or the grave, then this can lead to depression.

Inhibited grief

After a death, the bereaved person may not express any grief and may work tirelessly to organise the funeral. Frequently this form of denial or coping continues until the patient sees the coffin, when they may break down and let the tears flow. Health care professionals may experience this themselves, as others may expect them to cope with their grief and 'be strong'. This may make it difficult for such individuals to cope with their own grief.

Chronic grief

In chronic grief, the bereaved individual continues to suffer the same intensity of emotional turmoil as is normally expected in the first few weeks and months following the death. The individual may show signs of physical illness, withdrawal from social life and depression.

Mummified grief

Gorer (1965) described the phenomenon of preserving the dead person's belongings or even whole rooms in an unchanged state as 'mummification'. Perhaps the most famous example of this was Queen Victoria's reaction to the death of Prince Albert. She insisted that the room in which he died was preserved and his clothes be laid out as usual long after his death.

Such grief is more commonly seen after the death of a child, where for several years the child's room remains a shrine to the dead child, as if time has stood still (Worden, 2003).

The impact of different causes of unexpected death

Violent death

Bereavements following violent death from suicide, murder, manslaughter, war or terrorism have many features in common, as well as some that are unique. The common features are that the bereaved person has to face the horror of an unexpected death, which they may have witnessed or discovered. Feelings of anger, guilt, disbelief and fear are prevalent and acutely distressing (Riches and Dawson 1998; Armour 2002).

Accidents

Death as a result of an accident, such as a car, train or aeroplane crash, is the most common form of unexpected death. Other common causes are falls and drowning. The death may not only affect the bereaved person immediately but also distort their perception of death and bereavement later in life if not handled carefully. For example, the memory of the experience may resurface on admission to hospital or when being ushered into a waiting room or office. Such occurrences may not be part of everyday nursing, but they need to be considered if a person reacts in an unusual way.

Suicide

After a suicide, recovery for the bereaved people can be prolonged if they found the victim unexpectedly or if the circumstances were particularly distressing, such as jumping from a great height or under a moving vehicle. The bereaved people may feel guilty that they were not aware of the victim's depression and did not recognise it. If they had been trying to help the victim, then they may have a sense of failure (Royal College of Psychiatrists, 2006).

Murder and manslaughter

The most frequent complaint made by the families of those who have been victims of murder or manslaughter is that their loved one has been taken from them not only by the assailant but also by the authorities. The legal process of protecting a crime scene, post-mortem examination and criminal investigations disrupt the process of normal grief (Armour, 2002) because, in cases where the police are involved and the death is suspicious, the victim's partner may not be permitted to touch the body or even enter their house if it has been designated a crime scene. This is very intrusive and can take a long time before the body is released for burial.

The prospect of further mutilation of the deceased's body with a post-mortem examination, the distress of the coroner's inquest and the prospect of intrusive media attention make the bereavement process even more difficult.

The families often feel that the state has taken over and they resent the fact that they cannot see or touch the body. This may mean that they cannot gain comfort from smelling and holding a loved one's clothes. Their loved one is often referred to in an impersonal manner such as 'the body' or 'the deceased' or by their surname (Riches and Dawson, 1998; Victim Support, 2006). It is even worse if the person's partner or family member is under suspicion.

If the patient is brought to hospital and dies later, the hospital nursing staff may become involved in caring for the people bereaved by such loss. Nurses working in occupational health or general practice settings may find themselves coping with the delayed grief of relatives, without being fully aware of the events that caused them.

Sometimes family members turn to the local general practice, and a softer tone and understanding of what they may be suffering will be appreciated. If the investigation is prolonged, the body never found or the assailant never caught, then the individual may have prolonged grief and need counselling (Parkes, 1993). The patient may have come to the practice complaining of ailments such as headaches, lack of sleep, depression or loss of appetite.

Staff support

After any critical incident, such as a sudden death, the health care workers involved need to be supported in order that the individuals involved have a chance to share their feelings. Psychological debriefing is best offered before the end of the shift, with follow-up later if required. In most NHS trusts, a counselling service is available for the staff. Informal support between those who have shared the same experience may be all that is required.

SUMMARY

- The degree to which bereaved people recover from unexpected death depends on where the death occurs, the circumstances of the death, and whether the bereaved person witnessed the death or found the body.
- Witnessed resuscitation remains controversial, but it has helped a number of people to come to terms with the loss of the patient.

SUMMARY (Continued)

- Complicated grief can follow unexpected death, especially when the death is violent, and sensitive but efficient nursing interaction with the bereaved person can help to prevent abnormal grief.
- Staff involved in unexpected death incidents need to ensure that they have the opportunity to be debriefed and given psychological support.
- Abnormal grief needs to be treated by experienced psychologists and counsellors. Nurses need to know the sources of such counselling expertise in their area.

 CONCLUSION

In this chapter, the nature of expected and unexpected death, loss and bereavement before and after death have been discussed. It is important for nurses to understand the nature of loss and bereavement in order to improve communication and to support patients and families before, during and after death.

In addition, losses of other kinds, such as divorce, redundancy, retirement and loss of physical ability, contribute to the patient's sadness and inability to cope with new losses. Understanding accumulated loss helps nurses to support those who are bereaved.

References

Adam J (1997). ABC of palliative care. *British Medical Journal*, **315**, 1600–3.

Armour MP (2002). Experiences of co-victims of homicide: implications for research and practice. *Trauma, Violence and Abuse*, **3**, 109–24.

Bach S (1991). *Life Paints its Own Span: On the Significance of Spontaneous Paintings by Severely Ill Children*. Einsiedeln: Daimon.

Barley N (1995). *Dancing on the Grave: Encounters with Death*. London: John Murray.

Bowlby J (1969). *Attachment and Loss*. Vol. 1: Attachment. New York: Basic Books.

Bowlby J (1973). *Attachment and Loss*. Vol. 2: Separation: anxiety and anger. New York: Basic Books.

Bowlby J (1980). *Attachment and Loss*. Vol. 3: Loss, sadness and depression. New York: Basic Books.

Bowlby J and Parkes CM (1970). Separation and loss within the family. In Anthony EJ (ed.). *The Child in His Family*. New York: John Wiley & Sons.

British Association of Accident and Emergency Medicine and Royal College of Nursing (1995). *Bereavement Care in Accident and Emergency Departments*. London: Royal College of Nursing.

Buckman R (1988). *'I Don't Know What to Say'*. London: Papermac.

Buckman R (1992). *How to Break Bad News: A Practical Guide for Health Care Professionals*. Toronto: University of Toronto Press.

Burnell GM and Burnell AL (1989). *Clinical Management of Bereavement: A Handbook for Healthcare Professionals*. New York: Human Sciences Press.

Costello J (2006). Dying well: nurses' experiences of 'good and bad' deaths in hospital. *Journal of Advanced Nursing*, **54**, 594–601.

Craib I (1999). Reflections on mourning in the modern world. *International Journal of Palliative Nursing*, **5**, 87–9.

Currer C (2001). *Responding to Grief, Dying, Bereavement and Social Care*. Basingstoke: Palgrave.

Davidhizar R and Giger JN (1997). When touch is not the best approach *Journal of Clinical Nursing*, **6**, 203–6.

Department of Health (DH) (1998). *Code of Practice for the Diagnosis of Brain Stem Death*. London: Department of Health.

Dimond B (2004). The clinical definition of death and the legal implications for staff. *British Journal of Nursing*, **13**, 391–3.

Ellershaw J and Murphy D (2005). The Liverpool care Pathway (LCP). influencing the UK national agenda on care of the dying. *International Journal of Palliative Nursing*, **11**, 132–4.

Ellershaw J and Wilkinson S (eds) (2003). *Care of the Dying: A Pathway to Excellence*. Oxford: Oxford University Press.

Faull C and Woof R (2002). *Palliative Care: An Oxford Core Text*. Oxford: Oxford University Press.

Fisher M (2002). Emotional pain and eliciting concerns. In Penson J and Fisher RA (eds). *Palliative Care for People with Cancer*. London: Arnold.

Frankl V (1965). *The Doctor and the Soul: From Psychotherapy to Logotherapy*, transl. Winston R and Winston C. Harmondsworth: Penguin.

Frankl V (1984). *Man's Search for Meaning*. New York: Pocket Books.

Gerra G, Monti D, Panerai AE, *et al*. (2003). Long-term immune-endocrine effects of bereavement: relationships with anxiety levels and mood. *Psychiatry Research*, **121**, 145–58.

Gorer GD (1965). *Death, Grief and Mourning*. New York: Doubleday.

Hallgrimsdottir EM (2000). Accident and emergency nurses' perceptions and experiences of caring for families. *Journal of Clinical Nursing*, **9**, 611–19.

Herth K (1992). An abbreviated instrument to measure hope: development and psychometric evaluation. *Journal of Advanced Nursing*, **17**, 1251–9.

Herth K (2000). Enhancing hope in people with a first recurrence of cancer. *Journal of Advanced Nursing*, **32**, 1431–41.

Home Office (2002). *When Sudden Death Occurs*. London: Home Office.

Kent H and McDowell J (2004). Sudden bereavement in acute care settings. *Nursing Standard*, **19**: 38–42.

Kidby J (2003). Family-witnessed cardiopulmonary resuscitation. *Nursing Standard*, **17**, 33–6.

Kissane D and Yates P (2003). Psychological and existential distress. In O'Connor M and Aranda S (eds) *Palliative Care Nursing: A Guide to Practice*, 2nd edn. Oxford: Oxford University Press.

Kübler-Ross E (1969). *On Death and Dying*. New York: Macmillan.

Kübler-Ross (1975). *Death: The Final Stage of Growth*. Englewood Cliffs, NJ: Prentice-Hall.

Kuipers JC (1999). Ululations from the Weyewa Highlands (Sumba): simultaneity, audience response and models of cooperation. *Ethnomusicology*, **43**, 490–507.

NHS Gold Standards Framework (2005). *A Programme for Community Palliative Care*. London: NHS End of Life Care Programme.

Nursing and Midwifery Council (NMC) (2008). *The Code: Standards of Conduct, Performance and Ethics for Nurses and Midwives*. London: Nursing and Midwifery Council.

Parkes CM (1970). The first year of bereavement: a longitudinal study of the reaction of London widows to the death of their husbands. *Psychiatry*, **33**, 444.

Parkes CM (1993). Psychiatric problems following bereavement by murder or manslaughter. *British Journal of Psychiatry*, **162**, 49–54.

Parkes CM (1998). *Bereavement: Studies of Grief in Adult Life*, 3rd edn. London: Penguin.

Pollard A and Swift K (2003). Communication skills in palliative care. In O'Connor M and Aranda S (eds). *Palliative Care Nursing: A Guide to Practice*, 2nd edn. Oxford: Oxford University Press.

Randall TC and Wearn AM (2005). Receiving bad news: patients with haematological cancer reflect upon their experience. *Palliative Medicine*, **19**, 594–601.

Redley B, Botti M and Duke M (2004). Family member presence during resuscitation in the emergency department: an Australian perspective *Emergency Medicine Australasia*, **16**, 295–308.

Riches G and Dawson P (1998). Spoiled memories: problems of grief resolution in families bereaved through murder. *Mortality*, **3**, 143–59.

Robinson A (2004). A personal exploration of the power of poetry in palliative care, loss and bereavement. *International Journal of Palliative Nursing*, **10**, 32–9.

Royal College of Psychiatrists (2006). Early Grief and Mourning. www.rcpsych.ac.uk/PDF/bereavement.pdf.

Saunders C (1972). The care of the dying patient and his family. *Contact*, **38**, 12–18.

Saunders C (1985). *The Management of Terminal Illness*, 2nd edn. London: Arnold.

Stroebe MS, Stroebe W and Hansson RO (eds) (1993). *Handbook of Bereavement: Theory, Research, and Intervention*. Cambridge: Cambridge University Press.

Twycross R (2002). *Introducing Palliative Care*, 4th edn. Oxford: Radcliffe Medical Press.

Victim Support (2006). *In the Aftermath: The Support Needs of People Bereaved by Homicide – a Research Report*. London: Victim Support.

Vullo-Navich K, Smith S, Andrews M, *et al.* (1998). Comfort and incidence of abnormal sodium, BUN, creatinine and osmolality in dehydration of terminal illness. *American Journal of Hospice and Palliative Care*, **15**, 77–84.

Walker AE (1985). *Cerebral Death*. Baltimore, MD: Urban & Schwarzenberg.

Walter T (1999). *On Bereavement: The Culture of Grief*. Buckingham: Open University Press.

Worden JW (2003). *Grief Counselling and Grief Therapy*, 3rd edn. Hove: Routledge.

World Health Organization (WHO) (2005). WHO Definition of Palliative Care. www.who.int/cancer/palliative/definition/en/print.html.

Further reading

Coelho P (1998). *Veronika Decides to Die*. London: HarperCollins.

This novel illustrates a number of different thought processes experienced by people leading up to attempted suicide and gives a good insight into the mental torment of these individuals.

Compassionate Friends. www.tcf.org.uk.
Bereavement organisation for bereaved parents and siblings.

CRUSE Bereavement Care. www.crusebereavementcare.org.uk.

Department of Health (DH) (2003). *Families and Post Mortems: A Code of Practice*. London: Department of Health.
This is a useful document to read in order to understand the nature and purpose of post-mortems, and the legal and procedural issues involved for staff and families.

Diamond J (1998). *Because Cowards Get Cancer too . . .* London: Vermilion.
A moving account of a journalist's journey from diagnosis of cancer of the base of the tongue to death.

Families of Murdered Children (FOMC). www.fomc.org.uk.

Lewis CS (1961). *A Grief Observed*. London: Faber & Faber.

Mothers against Drunk Driving (MADD). www.madd.org.

Neuberger J (2004). *Dying Well: A Guide to Enabling a Good Death,* 2nd edn. Oxford: Radcliffe Medical.
Rabbi Neuberger has a wide experience of death and bereavement, both personally and professionally. This book offers some sensitive insights into the role nurses play in helping people to die comfortably.

Oswin M (1991). *Am I Allowed To Cry?* London: Souvenir Press.
A helpful book relating to bereavement in people with learning disabilities.

Parkes CM, Laungani P and Young B (eds) (1997). *Death and Bereavement Across the Cultures*. London: Routledge.
The authors contributing to this text come from a variety of different ethnic and cultural backgrounds.

Parents of Murdered Children (POMC). www.pomc.com.

RD4U (the road for you). www.rd4u.org.uk.
CRUSE bereavement care for the young.

Samaritans. www.samaritans.org.uk.

Support after Murder and Manslaughter (SAMM). www.samm.org.uk.

Victim Support. www.victimsupport.com.

PART 5

Professional support and development

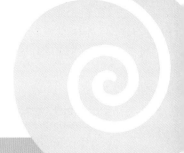

22

Supporting practitioners in giving high-quality care

John Fowler

Introduction

Supporting practitioners in giving high-quality care is an important issue for all nurses, ranging from the new student nurse to the experienced practitioner. The subject of support underpins all of the Nursing and Midwifery Council (NMC) standards of proficiency for pre-registration nursing education (NMC, 2004) (Appendix 2), and 6 of the 17 standards specifically identify the importance of supporting practitioners and the way that this influences the quality of patient care. In addition, the NMC Code (2008) (Appendix 1) identifies as one of its key components the importance of providing high standards of practice and care at all times.

This chapter presents three approaches to providing support: mentorship, preceptorship and clinical supervision. At times we ask you to reflect upon your previous experience of giving or receiving support and to identify areas of good practice or issues of concern. At other times we introduce new ideas based upon theories or current research. You are encouraged to explore how these new ideas relate to your clinical practice. Finally, there are a number of scenarios that present you with real-life situations to explore; we ask you to identify the issues within the scenarios and suggest possible ways forward.

Learning objectives

After studying this chapter you should be able to:
- understand the characteristics of professional development;
- understand the importance of learning from clinical experience;
- review a model of clinical teaching;
- compare and contrast the practices of mentorship, preceptorship and clinical supervision;
- examine the use of reflective practice.

Standards of proficiency

The six standards of proficiency (NMC, 2004), as listed below, are the six that specifically identify the importance of supporting practitioners and the ways that this influences the quality of patient care:

- Manage oneself, one's practice and that of others, in accordance with the NMC Code, recognising one's own abilities and limitations.
- Engage in, develop and disengage from therapeutic relationships through the use of appropriate communication and interpersonal skills.
- Contribute to public protection by creating and maintaining a safe environment of care through the use of quality assurance and risk management strategies.
- Delegate duties to others, as appropriate, ensuring that they are supervised and monitored.
- Demonstrate a commitment to the need for continuing professional development and personal supervision activities in order to enhance knowledge, skills, values and attitudes needed for safe and effective nursing practice.
- Enhance the professional development and safe practice of others through peer support, leadership, supervision and teaching.

These six standards of proficiency encompass a wide and quite complex range of roles and responsibilities, with the ultimate aim of ensuring safe, competent, coordinated and up-to-date practice. Read each one again and reflect on how it relates specifically to you.

Reflecting on your own experience of giving and being supported

It is very easy for the experienced nurse to forget the feelings and emotions that they had as a new student nurse entering the clinical area for the first time, or as the new staff nurse being left in charge and 'given the keys'. For most nurses, these situations contain a mixture of emotions: excitement, fear, embarrassment and pride. Having survived the experience, the nurse can then look back with a sense of achievement and accomplishment. Success in one situation gives confidence for the next and, no matter how experienced we become, there will always be new and challenging experiences.

Reflection point 22.1
Take some time to think about the first time that you had any direct contact with a patient.

- When was it?
- How did you feel before the event?
- How did you feel during the contact?
- How did you feel afterwards?
- How did the more senior nurse who was looking after you support you?

Now ask the same questions to someone with a similar amount of experience as you and compare your experiences. Finally, ask the same questions of an experienced nurse – try to find someone who registered over 10 years ago and compare their experiences with yours and those of your peers. Having done this, reflect on what has been said to you. What is common to peoples' experiences? What is valuable in terms of the support that was offered? What can you do in terms of supporting others as you become more experienced?

At this one-to-one interactional level, the support of staff focuses upon our interpersonal skills of empathy, communication, genuineness and often a sense of humour. These are crucially important and will form the underlying theme of much of this chapter. The support of staff, however, cannot be seen in isolation from the wider strategic issues that are involved in the delivery of health care. How could the senior nurse give time to the new student if the staffing levels are not adequate? Who is responsible for the student's nursing care? Being part of a team is, in itself, very supportive, but is teamwork something that just happens? These are the practical applications of the NMC's standards of practice identified at the beginning of this chapter. To help you answer these questions and examine the wider strategic issues, a research study commissioned by the English National Board for Nursing, Midwifery and Health Visiting (ENB, 1990, 1991; now defunct) identified ten key characteristics of professional development that will be used as a framework to explore these organisational issues.

Key characteristics of professional development

In 1990 the ENB (1990, 1991) undertook a research activity to identify the core elements of ongoing professional development. The report identified ten key characteristics for the development of professional practice. At that time these key characteristics formed the central structure of the ENB

Higher Award qualification and, although the ENB and Higher Award no longer exist, the ten key characteristics remain a valid framework for practice development. The characteristics are:

- accountability;
- clinical skills;
- use of research;
- teamwork;
- innovation;
- health promotion;
- staff development;
- resource management;
- quality of care;
- management of change.

Reflection point 22.2
What do these characteristics mean to you? How do you think that each of the ten key characteristics relates to supporting registered practitioners in giving high-quality care? Jot down a few ideas about what each of the characteristics might mean to you, and then compare your ideas with those below.

Accountability

There needs to be clarity about who is responsible for what. This is particularly important for the registered nurse mentoring the student nurse. It is also relevant when registered staff are under-going extended skills training or changing specialties. Who holds the authority for the action being undertaken? What degree of autonomy is there within the role? Who is responsible and accountable for the nursing care of the patient or client? Is the student aware of what is expected of them? What are the limitations of their role? These are legitimate questions when undertaking a new post or even within a span of duty.

Clinical skills

Clinical skills are usually a combination of psychomotor, cognitive and affective skills – what we do, why we do it and how we do it. It is important not to overwhelm the student with the volume or complexity of skills that they will ultimately be expected to master. However, it is also important to allow the student to participate and develop appropriate skills, under supervision. In terms of support, students will find it useful to know what they are expected to do, over what timeframe and to what degree of expertise. This is where learning objectives, opportunities and outcomes can form a supportive framework, giving guidance and promoting understanding for the clinical team.

Use of research

Supporting staff is not a precise science in which action A plus action B inevitably results in C. There is no simple formula for giving support that will work for all people in all situations. You need to develop strategies that work for you, using evidence from a wide variety of sources. Several research-based principles are described later, and the ENB's ten key characteristics are in themselves based on research undertaken with practitioners, managers, patients and a range of other stakeholders (ENB, 1990). Use the principles discussed in this chapter, review some of the papers referenced and reflect upon your own experience to develop your own way of supporting staff. Ask for, and be accepting of, feedback from your fellow students, and be willing to change and adapt your ways of working based on new and evolving ideas.

Teamwork

Working with a group of people has the potential for being a supportive, enriching experience or conversely a negative and draining one. Teamwork is the essential difference. Any new member of staff entering into an established group will very soon experience and try to make sense of the dynamics within that group. Take a few minutes to reflect on a group of staff with whom you work. Is it a positive, supportive experience? One that welcomes newcomers for the skills, experience or questions that they bring? Or is it one that has different factions, where one group does not talk to another? Where the social rules change depending on whom you are working with? Teamwork inevitably involves the multiprofessional team, and part of the responsibility of the senior members of the various disciplines is to develop positive teamwork within their own discipline and then between others.

Innovation

The provision of health care has changed, is changing and will continue to change. Certain illnesses that 10 years ago required a patient to undergo major surgery and remain hospitalised for 2 weeks are now treated by day surgery. A number of procedures that were once treated in hospitals are now treated in the community. Although the principles of care that remain at the heart of nursing remain unchanged, the ways of delivering nursing and health care are changing almost daily. Dealing positively with innovation as it affects you and your team will help others who work with you to respond in a similar way. Avoidance, negativity or denigration of new ideas will help to create a spiral of decline for both you and those who work with you. A positive and enthusiastic approach, whatever your place within the team, will support and help others as they come to terms with new ideas. Enthusiasm is not the same as unquestioning acceptance of any new idea. Enthusiasm is about openness, energy and a willingness to explore. It is infectious and supportive. Be honest with yourself – to what degree are you a positive member of your team? Give yourself a score out of 10 (0 for least and 10 for extremely positive), and then think about how you could improve that score.

Health promotion

The physical and psychological health of nursing staff can be viewed from both short- and long-term perspectives. In the short term, the senior officers have a responsibility to maintain a safe environment, to provide support and training in areas such as moving and handling, safe handling of blood and waste products, and to organise debriefing following traumatic events. Longer-term support strategies may include the provision of coffee areas away from the immediate environment, a sports and social club, and a staff support and counselling service. At a more operational level, a number of teams could organise an occasional social event in which staff have a chance to meet and relate to one another in a fun way. Encouraging and supporting staff who have chosen to stop smoking, lose weight or take some exercise can often be done by personal encouragement and peer group support. A positive approach to the health care of staff will increase their health and well-being and should indirectly influence the health and well-being of patients.

Staff development

At a formal level, staff development is about identifying a person's learning needs, helping them to form a plan of action to meet those development needs, supporting them as they develop, and then ensuring that these skills and abilities are utilised accordingly. Support will involve motivating and encouraging, but it may also require the support of money and time in order to gain appropriate clinical experience or attend suitable courses. At a more informal level, staff development is about taking an interest in what our colleagues are doing, drawing upon their experience and not resenting their development. When you are asked to give a talk or attend a meeting, then consider taking a less experienced nurse with you, or suggest to the person inviting you that this other nurse would be a very suitable person and that you would support them in their preparation for the talk or meeting. So often, we send a replacement only when we are too busy or do not want to go.

Resource management

Supporting staff takes time and money. In an outcome-driven health service with limited resources, both time and money need to be used efficiently and effectively. This means planning and management. Staff who are working longer hours and taking on extra shifts to cover for shortages will soon become demoralised and possibly ill if they feel that no one in authority knows, cares or is trying to do anything to counteract the staff shortage. Staff who feel that they will never get on a course or gain promotion because their 'face does not fit' will also become demoralised and, if opportunity allows, will probably leave the job and possibly nursing. Resource management is not about having unlimited resources. It is about fighting for resources as well as the efficient, effective and fair management of what is available. Some managers use such resources as a means of controlling staff, when actually the correct use of such resources is in enabling staff to do the job for which they are employed.

Quality of care

If all grades of staff work in a positive, supportive atmosphere, where reflection on clinical practice is encouraged, and issues of concern are voiced and discussed, then the result can only be an increase in the quality of patient care. Support that is superficial and tokenistic, at either a strategic or an operational level, will suggest to staff that this is an appropriate standard to set, not only for support of others but also for other issues such as quality of care, health and safety, patient education and infection control.

Management of change

There can be few workplaces that have not undergone significant change in the past 5 years. People vary in their reactions to change, some welcoming it, and others resisting or accepting the inevitable. Whatever people's reaction to change, everyone will experience a drain on their physical and psychological energy. Supporting people before, during and after the process of change is an important element in the management of change. Involvement, communication and ownership are important principles highlighting the way that individuals should be valued within the change process. If individuals feel valued, then they will also feel supported.

SUMMARY

Supporting staff to give high-quality care needs to be addressed at two levels: first, at the one-to-one interactional level focusing on communication, empathy and genuineness; and second, at a strategic level. The ENB's ten key characteristics are a useful way of exploring the strategic level.

Helping people learn from experience: experiential learning

Learning how to nurse has a number of parallels with learning how to swim. Unless you actually get in the water, you are not going to learn. However, if you jump in at the deep end on your first attempt, you will probably swallow considerable amounts of water before, hopefully, scrabbling to the side and vowing never to go swimming again. Likewise, if your first experience in nursing was a placement on an intensive care unit, caring for a patient with gangrenous wounds or caring for an unpredictable aggressive patient, then the experience, if not putting you off nursing altogether, would be highly traumatic.

Having established that the student nurse is in the equivalent of their 'safe depth', there are two important principles in helping someone to learn and develop nursing skills. First, they have to feel confident and safe in the clinical area and sure that, even if they did get out of their depth, there would be a 'lifeguard' on the side to pull them to safety. Second, once they have mastered some of the elements of nursing – the 'doggy paddle' equivalent – they need to learn from people who are more experienced than themselves. Steinaker and Bell (1979) identified this form of learning – learning from experience – as experiential learning and developed a taxonomy of five levels (Box 22.1).

BOX 22.1 Experiential learning taxonomy

- *Exposure*: observation, inactive participation.
- *Participation*: actively engages in activities with supervision.
- *Identification*: student performs skills competently with minimal supervision.
- *Internalisation*: student feels ownership of skill and is comfortable in its performance.
- *Dissemination*: student can transfer the skill to other areas and wishes to convey the skill to others.

Source: Steinaker and Bell (1979).

Imagine yourself as a student nurse allocated to a new placement. Initially you will feel very new. You will be exposed to a number of new staff, patients, medical conditions and the layout of the ward or community placement. There will be new or different social etiquette, rules, policies and procedures. At this initial level, the student takes on a largely inactive participation role, one of observer. As the student begins to feel more comfortable in this new environment, they will begin to participate and actively engage in the activities. At this level, the student requires close supervision and support as they develop new skills, attitudes and behaviours. With time, practice and feedback, the student moves to the third level, in which they perform these new skills competently with minimal supervision. At the fourth level, the student takes ownership of the new skills, attitudes and behaviours. They will appear at ease and comfortable with this developing role. Finally, at the fifth level, the student begins to apply and transfer these skills to new areas and begins to teach them to others. Thus, the swimmer goes from standing on the side observing others, to jumping in, getting to grips with the basics under close supervision, swimming within their own depth and swimming several lengths. If they continue to develop and learn, they may eventually become an instructor or lifeguard.

Reflection point 22.3

Think about the above example and your own level of nursing expertise: are you just learning to paddle or are you a strong swimmer? Can you swim confidently only in shallow water? How flexible are you as a nurse? Does your skill lie in only one very narrow area? Can you assess and provide holistic care for your patients? How long have you been a nurse, and how does that length of experience relate to your level of expertise?

Now put yourself in the position of the nurse's mentor. Is your role static as the student progresses, or do you need to take on different roles as the student works through these different taxonomy levels? Take time to examine Boxes 22.1 and 22.2. Think through your role as a mentor and how adaptable you are in meeting the changing needs of students.

Relationship of the mentor/supervisor to the student

At the first level (Box 22.2), that of exposure, the mentor has to take on a motivating role: to encourage the student to take an interest in the clinical area, to see the rewards and pleasures of working with this client group, and to make them feel safe. They need to encourage the student to jump in the water. At the second level, participation, the mentor acts as a catalyst, helping the student to take an active part, putting them in the right place at the right time, encouraging progress and praising the achievement of small targets – that is, encouraging the student to try different 'swimming strokes' and put their head under water. As the student develops competence in certain skills, the level of identification, the mentor needs to stand back but at the same time maintain an adequate distance in order to safeguard the student and the client. Watching the student swim a few lengths, the mentor acts as a moderator. As the student moves to the fourth level, internalisation, the mentor takes on the role of sustainer, helping the student to maintain their interest – encouraging the student to continue swimming, try different strokes, build up endurance and swim in the sea. Finally, as the student enters the level of dissemination, the role of the mentor is to give feedback and advice – to give ongoing support on how to develop their swimming in new and advanced ways, and to act as an honest critic.

BOX 22.2 Experiential learning taxonomy: mentor role and function

- *Exposure*: motivator – to encourage the student to gain an interest.
- *Participation*: catalyst – to assist and encourage the student to take an active part.
- *Identification*: moderator – to safeguard the student and client.
- *Internalisation*: sustainer – to help the student transfer the skill to other areas and remotivate if necessary.
- *Dissemination*: critic – to give feedback and advice.

Source: Steinaker and Bell (1979).

By way of a further analogy, readers who are parents will have realised that the role and skills required to parent a baby are different from those required to parent a toddler and are totally different from those required for teenagers and young adults. Also, every child is quite different in how they respond to support and guidance.

Implications

Reflection point 22.4

What are the implications of the theory of experiential learning, and the analogies to swimming and parenting, to professional development, clinical practice, supporting staff and teaching and assessing?

The implications of the experiential learning taxonomy can be summarised as follows:

- The role of the mentor/teacher encompasses different function and these change over time.
- Some people may feel more competent with one function than another.
- Learning occurs over time; it is a process, not a single action.
- The role of the student changes over time.
- Some students may be better at one stage of the process than others.
- Student and teacher are equal, but they have different roles.

Reflection point 22.5

Take some time to reflect on how the ideas contained within experiential learning relate to you.

- How do they relate to your experience of entering new clinical areas?
- How do they relate to you learning about a new clinical procedure?
- How do they relate to you as an existing or future mentor?
- How do they relate to your future professional development?
- How do they relate to the way you support staff?

Reflection point 22.6

Think through Scenarios 22.1 and 22.2 and discuss them with a colleague. If you were the mentor, how would you deal with the students in the scenarios? After you have completed this, review the reflections that follow.

SCENARIO 22.1

Jane is an 18-year-old student nurse. She is on her first clinical placement, a busy medical ward, and you are her mentor. During an initial brief assessment of her learning needs, you form an opinion of her as being very nervous, even frightened, and not really saying much. You have a busy morning in front of you, with five quite dependent patients, and two empty beds are likely to be filled by emergency admissions. Jane's placement is scheduled for 3 days a week for the next 6 weeks. She will be working with you for most, but not necessarily all, of this time.

You are busy and Jane is very nervous. How are you going to handle this first morning? How are you going to structure her 6-week placement? At this stage, what will you tell her that you are expecting from her? What will you tell her she can expect from you?

You probably have two options for Jane's first morning. Ideally, you want a relaxed morning during which you can focus on Jane's needs. However, the business of the wards prevents that. Are you going to get Jane to shadow you and possibly be overwhelmed by the speed at which you will be required to work? Or could you ask one of the more junior nurses or even a health care assistant to look after her and gently orient her to the ward, with you meeting up with her when you have dealt with the emergencies? You would need to make that decision based upon your assessment of Jane's ability to cope with pressure.

SCENARIO 22.2

Sally is 19 years old. She has previous experience as a health care assistant and this is her second clinical placement. Her first placement was in the community and now she is on a 6-week placement on a surgical ward. She works three shifts a week and you are her mentor. Following your initial meeting with Sally, you have formed an opinion that she is a very confident person, keen to undertake as many dressings and drug administration rounds as she can. You are a little concerned that she appears overconfident for her length of experience and, although not wishing to dampen her enthusiasm, feel concerned that she does not appear to appreciate her limitations.

How are you going to handle the first morning with Sally? You are busy and Sally is very keen to take an active role. How are you going to structure her 6-week placement? At this stage, what will you tell her that you are expecting from her, and what will you tell her she can expect from you?

The difficulty you have in this situation is that of balancing the acknowledgement of Sally's enthusiasm and somewhat limited experience together with your responsibility to maintain the safety of the patients in your care. You do not want to dampen Sally's enthusiasm, but also you want to make sure that her experience grows steadily and safely.

SUMMARY

People learn from practical experiences in a different way from how they learn from a textbook. Steinaker and Bell's (1979) experiential learning taxonomy is a helpful way of understanding how people learn from practical experiences.

Teaching

In a small-scale research study, the author asked a number of staff what they found most valuable and most supportive from trained staff in terms of their teaching, mentoring and support (Fowler, 1995). A considerable number of different examples were given, which could be categorised into five main areas: assessment, negotiation, listening, explaining and feedback. This work is currently being repeated, and initial analysis supports the original findings that these five areas are viewed as key characteristics of a 'good mentor':

- *Assessment of the person's previous knowledge and experience*: this was seen as important because it not only acknowledged and valued the student's previous background but also allowed the mentor to build upon the previous knowledge.
- *Being willing to negotiate regarding the process and focus of supervision/teaching*: it was not 'the teacher knows best' attitude but the recognition that both the mentor and the student had a valuable perspective on what was required. The mentor could draw upon their experience of the learning opportunities relating to their clinical area, and the experiences of past students; the student could draw upon the knowledge of their own abilities and their strengths, needs and weaknesses.
- *Listening to what the student has to say about what they learn from a specific experience*: at its simplest, this can take the form of a question and answer session, being genuinely interested in what the student has done and learned, and resisting the temptation to jump in and take over the conversation. The more advanced skills of listening will also enable the mentor to assist the student in reflecting upon clinical practice and patient interactions, encouraging a deeper understanding of events.
- *Being able to explain ideas and knowledge in an easily understandable way*: students valued both informal and formal teaching sessions, but not if the session confused them or went over

their heads. They valued someone who could explain ideas and facts to them in an easy-to-understand way.

- *Commenting on good practice, not just criticising the weak areas*: feedback is an important aspect of a nurse's professional development, particularly in relation to any specific learning outcomes. All of the NMC professionally validated courses require students to have a mentor who is responsible for giving them feedback on their developing specialist skills. If done in a positive and supportive way, then feedback can be a powerful means of identifying strengths and weaknesses and of shaping and developing advanced nursing skills. The students in this study commented that it was the combination of commenting on their good practice as well as criticising their weak areas that was important.

Reflection point 22.7

- How do these above areas relate to your own experience?
- How can you use this framework to enhance your own learning?
- How can you use this structure to enhance your own teaching?

A model of clinical teaching

For the outsider, nursing structures that encompass management, leadership and support can appear complex and confusing.

Reflection point 22.8

How do you answer the following relatively simple questions?

1 Who is your manager?
2 Who provides professional leadership?
3 Who provides advice on clinical issues?
4 Who do you turn to for career guidance?
5 Who supervises your clinical practice?
6 Who do you turn to for support following a difficult shift?

Ask these questions of four or five other nurses, ranging from a junior staff nurse to a senior nurse or clinical nurse specialist.

You will probably find that for the more junior nurse, the ward sister or equivalent combines most of those roles. However, as nurses become more experienced and specialised, no single person has the knowledge, skills, experience or authority to fulfil such roles. Here lies the somewhat confusing complexity of the management, leadership and support structures within nursing. There are a number of different ways that nurses are given support, guidance and teaching on a fairly routine basis:

- working with more experienced staff;
- in-service training sessions;
- staff handovers;
- at coffee breaks;
- debriefing following traumatic events;
- clinical supervision;
- preceptorship;

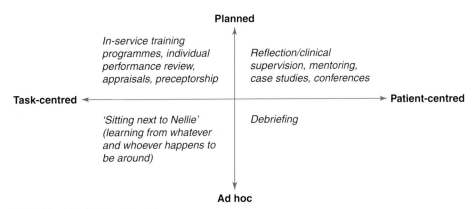

Figure 22.1 Model of clinical teaching.

- individual performance review;
- mentoring;
- reflection;
- study days;
- courses;
- talking with friends.

This is not an exhaustive list. What other forms of support, guidance and teaching have you experienced?

What structure is there to all these differing support processes? How do they all relate to one another? The model in Figure 22.1 attempts to give some meaning to these various structures by identifying two continuums, 'task-centred' versus 'patient-centred' and 'planned' versus 'ad hoc'. Task-centred events are those that focus on a particular nursing procedure, a series of skills, an aspect of physiology or psychology, or any fairly discrete body of knowledge. Patient-centred events are those that are generated by a particular patient or group of patients, such as a patient's medical condition, nursing problems, social environment or general management. Planned activities are those that are planned in advance and put in the diary. Ad hoc activities are those things that happen on the spur of the moment; they may be a response to a traumatic event or occur simply because the ward is quiet and there is time to do some teaching or sit down and discuss a particular patient. Using these two continuums, we can begin to give some structure to the support and teaching processes that exist within the structure and management of nursing.

Thus, processes that are planned and task-centred are those such as in-service training programmes, individual performance reviews, preceptorship, moving and handling study days, asthma care study days and some post-registration courses. Activities that are planned but patient-centred are those such as clinical supervision, patient handovers and case studies, reflection and possibly mentoring, although this can be task-centred depending on the style adopted. Situations that are patient-centred but ad hoc usually focus on some form of emergency or traumatic event, following which staff take time to discuss what has happened and how it was handled, and the effects that it has had on staff – that is, debriefing. Finally, there is the intersection of ad hoc and task-centred events. This is typified by the phrase 'sitting next to Nellie' – the belief that, by working alongside a more experienced person, we will pick up some useful tips and ways of working.

Reflection point 22.9

Think through each of the four approaches above and identify the strengths and weaknesses of each one. Then compare your ideas with those in Table 22.1.

Consider how each of those four approaches is or could be used in your current clinical area.

Table 22.1 Model to analyse clinical teaching

	Strength	Weakness
Planned and task-centred	Structured: allows important aspects to be highlighted, rules and guidelines can be clearly set, people generally feel comfortable with structure	Paperwork and completion of a list of learning outcomes can override the principle of what the structure was set up for
Planned and patient-centred	Patient care and associated nursing actions form the focus of development	Requires considerable skills from supervisor/mentor to use patient-centred situations in a positive way
Ad hoc and task-centred	Tends to occur because all parties want it to; therefore, it is usually relevant and positive	Important aspects may not be covered and there may be a lack of structure and depth to support or learning
Patient-centred and ad hoc	Relevant and immediate to the needs of the clinical area and of the staff	Requires considerable skill of the senior staff; events that are not stressful in themselves, but may become so over time, are often overlooked

 SUMMARY

Teaching in the clinical area can be planned and task-centred, planned and patient-centred, ad hoc and task-centred, or patient-centred and ad hoc.

Mentorship

Although the idea of experienced nurses directing less experienced nurses in their clinical work has been in existence since the days of Florence Nightingale, the idea of a mentoring relationship is a far more recent concept, appearing in the nursing literature from about 1980 onwards (Darling, 1984). Woodrow (1994) suggests that the nursing profession's sympathetic acceptance of a humanistic philosophy, in both its clinical practice and nurse education, has led to an embracing of partnership between learners and teachers, staff and patients.

The terms 'mentorship', 'preceptorship' and 'clinical supervision' have found their way into the everyday language of the clinical nurse (Burnard, 1990; Maggs, 1994; Fowler, 2005). Some people appear to use these terms interchangeably, recognising little or no difference between them. This is understandable, as they have a common theme regarding a nurturing relationship, usually between an experienced person and someone new to the situation. The term 'mentorship' is probably the most ambiguous of the three: 'Finding a definition of mentorship is not difficult. The problem lies in selecting one from the many available and widely contrasting definitions' (Earnshaw, 1995, p. 274).

Nevertheless, 'mentoring' is a frequently used term, both within and outside nursing. It is often used in everyday nursing conversation but appears to mean different things to different people.

Many of the more substantive reviews of mentoring within the nursing profession make reference to the historical derivation of the term 'mentor' from Homer's Odyssey, in which Odysseus entrusts the upbringing of his son Telemachus to Mentor, a trusted advisor and friend (Donovan, 1990; Earnshaw, 1995). Mentoring within the business and professional world often utilises a close relationship between an experienced and less experienced person to help them through a transitional period in their life or, more usually, their career. The relationship seems to vary from intense interpersonal experiences to formalised organisational programmes (May, 1982; Hagerty, 1986).

There are two distinctive ways in which the term 'mentoring' is used within nursing in the UK: one concerned with student nurses and the other with registered nurses. Originally, the ENB (1989, 1993) gave the role of mentor prominence within nurse education by stipulating that each student nurse should have a mentor throughout the clinical placements of their training. It defined this as someone who would, by example, facilitate, guide and support the learner in the development of new skills, new behaviours and new attitudes. There was a separate and more experienced person who undertook the assessing of students (ENB, 1993). Later, the ENB altered the focus regarding the supervision of students. The mentor was to take on the full responsibility for the teaching, assessing and support of the student.

> The term mentor is used to denote the role of the nurse, midwife or health visitor who facilitates learning and supervises and assesses students in the practice setting. Different professional groups use differing terminology. The term assessor is often used to denote a role similar to that of the mentor as defined in this publication.
>
> (ENB and DH, 2001)

In 2002 the ENB ceased to exist and the NMC took over the responsibility for setting training and assessment standards. However, the role and function of the mentor as defined above has remained central for student supervision standards (NMC, 2002), although refinements in terminology – currently a 'sign off mentor' – and greater definition of the role – 'one who facilitates learning, supervision and assessment' (NMC 2006d) – have been established.

For most nurse training curricula, the mentor is a clinically based nurse who mentors the student for the time that they are learning in their clinical area, normally 4–12 weeks. This means that the student will have a number of different mentors throughout their pre-registration period – one for each clinical placement and 10–15 throughout their 3 years of preparation. There are only rare examples where the same mentor is attached to a pre-registration student for all or most of their training (Morris *et al.*, 1988).

As well as the specific use of mentoring for student nurses, the term is also used for a more general relationship between registered nurses in the UK (Burnard, 1990; Maggs, 1994; Butterworth, 1998). Here, the term is not well defined and tends to have a wide usage. It ranges from a committed and intense relationship, focusing on personal and professional development of the mentee, to a general pairing of a new staff member with a more experienced one, for induction and orientation to a new area. Thus, the term 'mentor' may be used to describe any of the following:

- the supporting, facilitating and assessing role that a suitable experienced and qualified registered nurse has with a nurse in training;
- a long-term, nurturing and professional development relationship between senior and less experienced registered staff;
- someone who shows you where to hang up your coat and takes you to coffee on your first day.

Reflection point 22.10

Think back through your experience, both before and during your nursing career, and identify people who have acted as a mentor to you. Was this a formal system as occurs in some schools and colleges – sometimes called a 'buddy' or 'pairing' system – or was there someone 'older and wiser' who seemed to have time for you, someone who you respected? What was that relationship like? What did you get out of that relationship? What do you think the other person got out of it?

Mentoring relationships occur in all walks of life, sometimes spontaneously but at other times planned and organised. The nursing profession, like many other professional and business organisations, recognises the potential benefits that such a relationship offers, both to the members and to the organisation. However, trying to capture and replicate the richness of that relationship to make it available for all staff has proved difficult.

Consider Scenario 22.3:

SCENARIO 22.3

Joan, aged 32 years, has been a staff nurse for 5 years on the same ward. One year ago you were appointed as the nurse in charge of that ward. You are a similar age to Joan but have greater clinical experience. Having worked with Joan for the past year, you have developed respect for her experience in this specialty but feel she is not really achieving her potential. She does her clinical work well but never seems to volunteer for anything new and seems to avoid teaching students and new staff. She appears to be someone who would benefit from a positive, nurturing relationship with someone more experienced – a mentoring relationship.

You make a list of the various staff whom you consider may be appropriate mentors (see below). Think through each of the people listed and identify the strengths and weakness of using each one, based upon the information given. Having done that, decide who to approach to act as Joan's mentor. Finally, think through how you are going to set up this mentoring relationship and identify some key steps that you will need to make.

- *You*: you are the ward manager and have wider clinical experience; you know Joan's strengths and where she needs to develop, and you feel that you have a good working relationship.
- *Staff nurse Jenny Smith*: aged 39 years, Jenny has been on the ward for 10 years and is a very capable staff nurse. She works part-time, has two young children and has a very mature outlook on life. She is a supportive person and a good friend of Joan's.
- *Julie Brown, a clinical nurse specialist*: aged 42 years, Julie frequently comes to the ward to give advice on patient care and holds a number of informal teaching sessions with staff. She is well respected by staff and will always give advice when asked.
- *Susan Peters, a professional development officer for the trust*: aged 45 years old and with a previous clinical background in your specialty. Susan runs a 2-day counselling course for the trust and has a reputation for being a caring person.
- *Sally Walters, a ward manager within the same directorate*: Sally is the same age as you and has been a personal friend of yours for a number of years. You know that she would be very happy to take on this role as a mentor for Joan.

There are no absolute right and wrong answers to the questions in Scenario 22.3 because the real-life situation is far more complex than a short scenario can capture. The personalities of the people involved will influence your decision significantly, but the following factors would probably be important in your decision-making:

- You are an option, but probably not the first choice. You are the manager and need to make sure that you don't overload yourself with roles and responsibilities that can be delegated. Also, the role of manager is not always compatible with that of a mentor.
- Jenny Smith is an option, but the fact that Jenny is a good friend of Joan's might inhibit the mentor relationship developing, as Jenny may be worried about hurting Joan's feelings. It would depend on your assessment of Jenny's professional skills in incorporating a mentorship within a friendship – a number of excellent mentorship relationships appear to work well in this situation, but there is a real danger of it becoming a little too much of a 'cosy' relationship.
- Julie Brown appears to be the obvious choice, as it involves a well-respected professional person who has good experience and expertise, which she seems willing to share.
- Susan Peters is an option, but the danger here is that what should be a mentoring relationship could become a counselling session, which may be useful but is not the aim to the relationship.
- Sally Walters is a possibility, although the fact that it is known that you are a friend of Sally's may inhibit the confidential nature of the mentoring relations from the perspective of Joan.

SUMMARY

The term 'mentorship' is used and defined in different ways: in the business world, as a one-to-one relationship during a transitional period; for student nurses, as the person who is responsible for the teaching, supervision and assessment of the student while on a clinical placement; and as a general supportive relationship for any member of staff.

Preceptorship

Preceptorship is similar to mentoring. In the USA, the term is used to describe the support, teaching and direction that student nurses receive while on clinical placement. This includes developing a learning contract (Andrusyszyn and Maltby 1993), teaching (Williams *et al.*, 1993), clinical socialisation (Ouellet, 1993; Dibert and Goldenberg, 1995), and developing clinical competence and confidence (Myrick and Barrett 1994). In addition, it is used to describe a general orientation and teaching programme for new or junior staff (Dibert and Goldenberg, 1995; Dusmohamed and Guscott, 1998). Peutz (1985) differentiates preceptorship from mentoring in that the former has a more active teaching and supervision role.

The term 'preceptorship' was formally introduced into the UK nursing language in 1990. Its specific use arose from the UK Central Council for Nursing, Midwifery and Health Visiting (UKCC) post-registration education and practice project (PREP) (UKCC, 1990, 1994). Recommendations 1 and 2 stated that:

There should be a period of support for all newly registered practitioners to consolidate the competencies or learning outcomes achieved at registration (4.4). A preceptor should provide the support for each newly registered practitioner (4.10).

This was later expanded to include not only newly registered nurses but also those moving to an unfamiliar area, and the UKCC stated that this support should extend for a minimum of 4 months (UKCC, 1993). Although not introduced as a statutory requirement, the UKCC (1993) stated that this should be introduced as good practice. More recently, the NMC (2006a) has revised the *PREP Handbook*, and overt reference to the term or concept of preceptorship has been removed from this document. The *PREP Handbook* now reflects more specifically the requirements for periodic re-registration. However, the NMC has maintained its commitment to the original concept and usage of preceptorship, and this is detailed in its A–Z advice sheet on preceptorship (NMC, 2006b).

Preceptorship, in terms of support for newly qualified staff, has been introduced within nursing in a fairly consistent way across the UK (Ashton and Richardson, 1992; Gately, 1992; Brennan, 1993; Burke, 1994; Skyte, 1997; Fowler, 2005). It is seen as a short-lived programme (Burke, 1994), with the focus on the acquisition of knowledge and skills designed specifically to enable the newly registered nurse to work safely and effectively in a new environment. Although there is an emphasis on assessing this nurse's individual needs (Ashton and Richardson, 1992), the focus is on the programme of development and support rather than on the one-to-one relationship common to the mentor literature (Brennan, 1993).

Thus, the practice of preceptorship, as it is used within the UK, has a fairly precise and well-defined role. It is defined by the NMC (2006b) as good practice and distinguishes certain groups of staff with specific needs and then identifies a particular way of meeting those needs for an identified period of time. Guidelines on issues such as the accountability of the practitioner are also fairly well explained. Once the period of preceptorship has finished, the registered nurse is subject to whatever staff development processes are available in their place of employment. This may be a poorly structured system, or it may be a formal clinical supervision process incorporating a formalised staff development programme.

Reflection point 22.11

Talk to some of the more experienced staff you are working with and ask them about their experiences of preceptorship. Does your unit or community practice have an identified preceptorship package? If so, review it and see whether you think it is relevant and useful. What else would you add to it?

Consider Scenario 22.4:

SCENARIO 22.4

Sarah is a newly registered nurse. She is due to start work on your area in 2 weeks' time. The nurse in charge has asked you to be Sarah's preceptor. You have been qualified for just over a year and this is the first time you will have been a preceptor. There is a well-structured preceptorship pack, which contains learning outcomes and a weekly schedule.

Identify the concerns and questions that you would have at this stage in this situation. Discuss these concerns with a more experienced staff nurse in your clinical area.

- Now try and predict what Sarah's concerns and questions might be. How would you deal with these?
- When would you try and set up your first meeting with Sarah? Before she starts, or on her first day?
- How would you try to personalise the well-structured but somewhat formal preceptorship pack?
- What sort of support would you want in taking on this new role? Who would you look to for this support?

Scenario 22.4 is an example of the most common type of a preceptorship relationship: a newly qualified nurse being preceptored by someone with more experience, but not so experienced that they have forgotten what it was like to be in that situation. There are other occasions when preceptorship is required but the situation is more complicated. It is important to make sure that the person asked to be the preceptor has the experience, skills and support to take on the more complex roles.

Now consider Scenario 22.5:

SCENARIO 22.5

Peter trained as a nurse in 1988. After working as a staff nurse for a number of years, he left the profession and worked as a tour guide for an international coach holiday company. A year ago he left the coach company and worked as a care assistant in a nursing home. He then decided to return to nursing and undertook a return to practice course. This course updated him on recent developments and provided a placement for him in the community team in which he would work as a staff nurse. Following successful completion of this course and re-registration, he was offered a permanent post in the community, again in the team in which you work. The district nursing sister has asked you to be Peter's preceptor for the next 4 months.

- How are you going to assess Peter's learning needs?
- In what way is this preceptorship relationship different from that of a mentoring relationship (see above)?
- You are 15 years younger than Peter and have much less life experience than him. How will this affect the preceptorship relationship?
- For Peter's first 2 weeks in the community, he can work in a supernumerary capacity. How would you want to structure this time?
- Reflecting on the team that you are currently working on, identify, in order of priority, ten learning outcomes that you would want Peter to achieve in the first 8 weeks of his work.
- How would you organise the support and feedback you give Peter throughout this period of preceptorship?

If you feel that Scenario 22.5 is beyond your current experience and abilities, discuss it with a more experienced registered nurse on your clinical area. Have they ever experienced something similar? If so, how did they deal with the situation? How would they deal with this situation?

SUMMARY

The term 'preceptorship' is used in two main ways. In the USA, it refers to the relationship, in the clinical area, between the trained nurse and the student. It is predominantly a teaching relationship. In the UK, it refers to a supportive, teaching relationship for the newly qualified nurse.

Continuing professional development

Continuing professional development (CPD) is underpinned by a philosophy that seeks to counter the tendency to see an initial qualification as the end of a process rather than a phase of lifelong learning (Thompson, 1995). The NMC (2006a), via PREP, formally acknowledged the need for ongoing development for all nurses, midwives and health visitors following their initial registration. This was part of a move towards lifelong learning, changing ways of working and developing emphasis on CPD (Wallace, 1999). Thompson (1995) identifies three elements to CPD:

- *In-service training*: developing and strengthening links between ideas, action and practice.
- *Line management supervision*: focusing upon clinical practice and interventions.
- *Appraisal*: helping people to maintain a clear focus on what they are trying to achieve (the focus is on the positive and constructive side of appraisal).

Development reviews or appraisals were introduced into the NHS in the form of individual performance reviews (IPRs) in 1986 to apply to the new breed of 'general managers' and were intended to complete the 'pyramid of objective setting' from ministerial reviews to individual managers (Harrison *et al.*, 1989). IPRs predominated at the more senior levels of health service management and tended to have a large economy and efficiency agenda. With regard to the general manager culture in which they were introduced, short-term targets for financial savings dominated. When IPRs are used at more clinical levels, they usually involve an annual meeting with the line manager, where the interviewee makes a general review of their performance and identifies any needs that they have. They are useful in developing longer-term objectives for the individual and relating them to organisational goals (Harrison *et al.*, 1990).

Thompson (1995) sees CPD as contributing to maintaining motivation and increasing job satisfaction; he also feels that, if it involves reflective practice, then it becomes an important way of integrating theory and practice. In the early 1980s Benner researched the various levels of expertise with which nurses practised. 'From novice to expert' (Benner, 1982) became a standard text for any nurse advancing their clinical career. Based upon the work of Dreyfus and Dreyfus (1980; cited in Benner, 1982), Benner discussed five stages of proficiency, from novice, through advanced beginner, competent, proficient, to expert, and described an expert nurse thus:

> *The expert nurse with her/his enormous background of experience, has an intuitive grasp of the situation and zeros in on the accurate region of the problem without wasteful consideration of a large range of unfruitful problem situations.*

> (Benner, 1982, p. 405)

Benner was identifying that some nurses had greater skills, experience and expertise than others, a fact accepted within the nursing profession but not well documented at that time. Before 1990, a nurse in the UK, once registered, was free to practise, even following a break in service of many years, without any further training, support or assessment. PREP (UKCC, 1990; NMC, 2006a) brought in a number of changes regarding support, CPD and re-registration. As discussed above, it introduced a period of preceptorship for newly registered nurses. Also, following a break of service of more than 5 years, a nurse has to undergo a period of study and professional updating and to be eligible for periodic re-registration. In order to continue on the register, a registrant must complete a period of at least 35 hours of study every 3 years, maintain a portfolio of professional development and have practised for a minimum of 450 hours in the previous 3 years (NMC, 2006a,b).

Reflective practice

The use of reflective practice is central to much of the discussion regarding CPD. The work of Argyris and Schön (1974) has been influential in a number of professions where the interaction of theory and its application to practice settings is integral. This work prompted interest in the use of reflective practice, initially within nurse education and also in clinical nursing practice. Schön

(1987, 1991) identifies two types of reflection: reflection-on-action and reflection-in-action. The concept of reflection-on-action has been used in traditional nurse education settings, either in the clinical area or later in a classroom (McCaugherty, 1991; Fowler, 2006). Reflection-in-action occurs while the practice is being undertaken and, according to Schön, has the potential to influence its decisions and outcomes.

Reflection point 22.12
Why do you think reflection plays an important part in helping staff to give high-quality care? Have you tried formally to reflect upon your practice? How easy was this? What helped or hindered you?

Most people find that, if they do manage to reflect on their practice, then it is usually a quick review of a situation, and often when something has not gone as well as was expected. It is often quite superficial with little reference to any underpinning theory that may inform the reflection.

The use of reflective practice, particularly reflection-on-practice, was attractive to nursing because it offered a solution to the theory–practice gap that was recognised in the 1970s and 1980s (Birch, 1975; Gott, 1984). When reflection forms part of a structured learning experience, then theory and practice become more integrated, and theory informs practice and practice informs theory (Clark *et al.*, 2001; Fowler, 2006). This idea fitted with the concept of nursing as a practice-based profession and the theory of learning from experience developed by Kolb (1984) in the 1980s.

On clinical placement, the student's mentor became a key figure in helping the student to reflect on practice. The general move to develop a more questioning profession was being articulated to some extent by the emphasis on reflection on what the student saw and did. Most reviews of reflective practice acknowledge various stages of reflection (e.g. Mezirow, 1981; Schön, 1991; Johns, 1993; Fowler, 2006) and the difficulty of undertaking this process in isolation (Johns, 1993). Reflective practice was thus welcomed within the nursing profession (Snowball *et al.*, 1994; Johns, 1997; Marrow *et al.*, 1997) as a useful tool, particularly to help students integrate theory and practice. However, the use of reflection-in-practice and reflection-on-practice by experienced registered staff was not so evident. Atkins and Murphy (1993), in their review of the literature on reflection, stated that reflection must involve the self and must lead to a changed perspective. This is echoed by Snowball *et al.* (1994, p. 1235): 'It is clear in the literature that the involvement of self is a crucial element of the reflective process.'

Atkins and Murphy (1993) state that, for reflection to occur, the individual needs to be minimally defensive and be willing to work in collaboration with others. Although this openness and willingness to 'expose the self' is appropriate for some staff, it is an exercise that many people find difficult to accomplish without support and guidance from a skilled and caring person. The clinical supervision relationship offered an opportunity for reflection on clinical practice by registered nurses under the guidance of a more experienced clinician. It is here that CPD, the practice of reflection and the role of clinical supervision come together for all registered nurses (Dooher *et al.*, 2001). Before the early 1990s, implementation of reflective practice had been with student nurses or those staff on a post-registration course. It was seen as a valuable tool, it but required a structure that certainly was not present in any systematic way within the nursing profession at that time. Clinical supervision offered an infrastructure for reflection-on-practice for all registered nursing staff.

> ⊚ **SUMMARY**
>
> CPD and reflective practice are important ways of enhancing the development of high-quality care.

Clinical supervision

In 1993, the Department of Health NHS Management Executive (DH, 1993) published the strategic document *A Vision for the Future*. This aimed to give overall direction and focus to the contribution that nurses and midwives could make to the NHS. It was the first time that the term 'clinical supervision' had been used in a way that implied the introduction of a systematic structure. The document (paragraph 3.27) described clinical supervision in broad terms that included development, individual responsibility, consumer protection, self-assessment and reflection. This has been supported by the NMC, which has updated its guidance in the form of an information sheet (NMC, 2006c) with the aims of clinical supervision to:

- identify solutions to problems;
- increase understanding of professional issues;
- improve standards of patient care;
- further develop the nurse's skills and knowledge;
- enhance the nurse's understanding of their own practice.

Reflection point 22.13
Talk to some experienced nurses and ask them about their experiences of clinical supervision.

- How do their experiences of clinical supervision relate to the NMC aims identified above?
- What percentage of staff are engaged in a formal clinical supervision relationship?
- What prevents those staff who are not in clinical supervision from undertaking it?

Models of supervision

In the early 1990s, a number of accounts appeared describing how clinical supervision could work, or was working, in a variety of clinical settings. Different models of clinical supervision began to emerge. At the more humanistic end of the spectrum, Faugier (1992) described a growth and support model of the supervisory relationship. This focuses on first, and of prime importance, the relationship between the individuals. Then, using the interactions within the relationship, it focuses on the role of the supervisor to facilitate both educational and personal growth for the supervisee. At the same time, the relationship must be one that provides support for the developing clinical autonomy of the supervisee. Faugier describes many of the humanistic qualities associated with such growth and support, such as generosity, openness, humanity, sensitivity and trust. Chambers and Long (1995) identify a similar facilitative model of growth and support based on the relationship between the supervisor and supervisee. These approaches have their roots in a humanistic school of counselling (Farrington, 1995), with its focus on self-awareness and personal growth.

From a more behaviourist perspective, Nicklin (1995) argues that clinical supervision could become rhetoric, promoting the illusion of innovation without producing change. Although he supports the developmental elements, he feels that tangible outcomes are required. He proposes that clinical supervision be used to analyse issues and problems, clarify goals and identify 'strategies for goal attainment and establish an appropriate plan of action'. Nicklin (1997) developed these ideas into a six-stage process of supervision. Focusing on practice, it starts with practice analysis, problem identification, objective-setting, planning, implementation action and evaluation. Nicklin (1995) states that the process of clinical supervision should complement other managerial and professional processes and that clinical supervision should not develop as a vehicle for diluting or fragmenting managerial responsibility. This 'outcome' approach, with its focus on problem identification and problem-solving, has its roots in a behavioural school of psychology (Farrington, 1995), with the focus of supervision being on what the supervisee is doing for the client.

Principles of clinical supervision

People's experiences of clinical supervision vary widely. Three principles, however, appear to be core (Fowler, 1996) (Figure 22.2):

- at least two people meeting together for the purpose of clinical supervision;
- using reflection to focus upon clinical practice;
- meetings being structured and organised.

The purpose and function of clinical supervision can encompass one or a combination of the following (Fowler, 1995):

- a learning process;
- a supportive process;
- a monitoring process.

Senior staff who work predominantly on their own may develop clinical supervision in a way that allows them to meet in a small supportive peer group. Junior staff nurses will require a clinical supervision relationship that focuses largely on a learning, challenging process. For others, a combination of all three processes defines the purpose of clinical supervision. The more specialised the nurse, the more specific the relationship they will require. A nurse practitioner may value the opportunity to work with a medical consultant in developing a new area of practice. A ward manager may use clinical supervision to provide an opportunity to reflect on their leadership

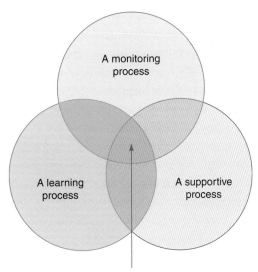

The interaction of clinical supervision

Figure 22.2 Interactive process of clinical supervision.

style with the director of nursing or with a group of peers. The important principle with clinical supervision is that it is your time to reflect upon your practice. The supervisor is there to help you do that, not to tell you what to do.

Reflection point 22.14

Think through your own experiences, if any, of clinical supervision. Write down what you consider the purpose to be. How do your experiences relate to:

- a *learning process*, which could range from a junior member of staff learning specific skills to the experienced ward sister who wants to develop research skills or financial management?
- a *support process*, which might include the discussion of difficult clinical or working conditions?
- a *monitoring process*, which could range from informal, formative feedback to formal summative assessments, with quality assurance of defined standards falling somewhere in the middle?

Once you have identified the purpose of clinical supervision for your own practice, you need to consider who should be your supervisor. This may be someone who is appointed by the ward manager, but most areas will try to match the two people together and allow the supervisee some say in who their supervisor is going to be. The general rule for the choice of appointment as supervisor is someone who is enthusiastic to take on the role and who has the appropriate experience. The more experienced and specialised you become, the harder it will be to find a more experienced supervisor.

Once you have identified your ideas as to the purpose of clinical supervision and you have an identified supervisor, you need to be clear regarding certain ground rules. These may have been well thought out within your area of work, or they may be areas that you and your supervisor need to explore in the early stages of your supervision. Consider the following:

- What is the relationship between the supervisor and supervisee, the structure of the supervisory sessions, and the issues of confidentiality and record-keeping? It is likely that there will be some hospital guidelines for some of these issues. The important principle is to relate the ground rules to the purpose of clinical supervision and to your needs. The 'contract' and 'record-keeping' for a junior staff nurse are likely to be quite different from those of an experienced ward manager or clinical specialist. However, the principles may be quite similar.
- It is important to identify the time involvement, as this will help you to set realistic targets. The manager, supervisor and supervisee should all agree the amount of time to be invested in the process. You need to identify how long and how often you are going to meet. Again, this may vary for different staff. As a general guide, more inexperienced staff will need shorter periods of supervision fairly often – maybe an hour a week; experienced staff may require a longer session, but not as often – maybe an afternoon every month.
- The supervisor, supervisee and manager all need to develop a simple agreement on what is expected of all parties involved. A danger with the implementation of clinical supervision is that there are good intentions at the planning stage but it never gets beyond two or three sessions, because the practical issues have not been thought through and planned for. If you know that your ward gets very busy at certain times of the year, then how will you safeguard clinical supervision time? What happens when someone moves wards? Do they keep their supervisor? You cannot predict all the eventualities, but try to identify common probabilities. The agreement or contract should be used to strengthen the process of clinical supervision, not to inhibit it.

Consider Scenarios 22.6 and 22.7:

> ## SCENARIO 22.6
>
> You have just taken up a new post on an acute admissions ward. You have been qualified for 6 months, and this is your second ward. There is a strong culture of clinical supervision on the ward, and the ward manager has suggested that Peter Young could be your supervisor. You have worked with Peter for a few shifts and respect his professional skills, knowledge and attitudes to work. You feel that this would be a good match, and he and you agree to meet up the following week. Peter asks you to come to that meeting with some ideas as to what you want from the clinical supervision relationship.
>
> - Identify the areas that you would like the first 3 months of clinical supervision to focus on.
> - What questions will you ask Peter regarding the structure and ground rules?

> ## SCENARIO 22.7
>
> David has been registered for 3 years. You are the F grade on the ward and have just been asked to be his clinical supervisor. You have arranged your first meeting for the following week – a 1-hour meeting at the end of the early shift.
>
> - How will you plan this first session? Consider the venue, content and focus of the session. Are you going to ask David to do any preparatory work before the meeting?
> - What are your long-term goals for clinical supervision with David? How often are you going to meet? How are you going to structure the sessions?

If clinical supervision is going to result in a warm, challenging, reflective relationship, then both the supervisor and the supervisee have to commit to the relationship. A good way of demonstrating commitment is for both parties to prepare for the session and to regard the meeting as a high priority. The supervisee needs to feel an equal partner with the supervisor. The experience and knowledge of the supervisor should lead the direction of, but not dominate, the supervision. Both people should feel equally in control of the situation and the 'agenda'; if there is something important to discuss, then you should feel free to discuss it.

The more specialist and independent the practitioner becomes, the greater is the need for a formalised system of clinical supervision. Whereas staff working in a ward team may have a number of informal opportunities for support, discussion and development, the same cannot always be said for staff working in isolated specialised posts.

SUMMARY

Clinical supervision offers a way of safeguarding and monitoring standards, development of practice and support of practitioners. It requires commitment of time, openness to reflect on practice, and maturity to admit weakness and be willing to learn new ideas and skills.

⊙ CONCLUSION

The support required by staff to enable them to give high-quality patient care must be developed at a strategic level, e.g. NMC guidance on preceptorship and clinical supervision; at an organisation level, e.g. establishing adequate staffing levels and coffee areas; and at a personal interactional level, e.g. developing listening and mentoring skills. Skills that are common to all supportive relationships are:

- assessment of the person's previous knowledge, experience and concerns;
- being willing to negotiate about the process and focus of the relationship;
- listening to what the person has to say about what they are experiencing;
- explaining ideas and knowledge in an easily understood way;
- commenting on good practice as well as exploring areas where development is needed.

At an individual level, each of us has a responsibility to support and care for colleagues with whom we have daily contact. This may take the form of formal preceptorship, mentoring or clinical supervision relationships, but it also involves informal means, such as having coffee together or organising the occasional night out to celebrate a birthday or engagement. Remember people's names and treat them as individuals: greet the pharmacist by name as they enter the ward, thank the domestic by name as they finish for the day, and leave a note for the night staff thanking them for the way that they sorted out the problem the night before. These are little things that everyone can do at no extra cost but make our working environment a much more positive place to work in. The way that we treat each other will reflect upon the way we treat our patients.

References

Andrusyszyn M and Maltby H (1993). Building on strengths through preceptorship. *Nurse Education Today*, **13**, 277–81.

Argyris C and Schön D (1974). *Theory in Practice*. San Francisco, CA: Jossey-Bass.

Ashton P and Richardson G (1992). Preceptorship and PREP. *British Journal of Nursing*, **1**, 143–6.

Atkins S and Murphy K (1993). Reflection: a review of the literature. *Journal of Advanced Nursing*, **18**, 1188–92.

Benner P (1982). From novice to expert. *American Journal of Nursing*, **82**, 402–7.

Birch J (1975). *To Nurse or Not to Nurse: An Investigation into the Cause of Withdrawal During Nurse Training*. London: Royal College of Nursing.

Brennan A (1993). Preceptorship: is it a workable concept? *Nursing Standard*, **7**, 34–6.

Burke L (1994). Preceptorship and post registration nurse education. *Nurse Education Today*, **14**, 60–6.

Burnard P (1990). The student experience: adult learning and mentorship revisited. *Nurse Education Today*, **10**, 349–54.

Butterworth A (1998). Clinical supervision as an emerging idea in nursing. In Butterworth A, Faugier J and Burnard P (eds). *Clinical Supervision and Mentorship in Nursing*. Cheltenham: Stanley Thornes.

Chambers M and Long A (1995). Supportive clinical supervision: a crucible for personal and professional change. *Journal of Psychiatric and Mental Health Nursing*, **2**, 311–16.

Clark A, Dooher J and Fowler J (2001). *The Handbook of Practice Development*. Dinton: Quay Books.

Darling L (1984). What do nurses want in a mentor? *Journal of Nursing Administration*, **14**, 42–4.

Department of Health (DH) (1993). *NHS Management Executive: A Vision for the Future – the Nursing, Midwifery and Health-Visiting Contribution to Health and Health Care*. London: HSMO.

Dibert C and Goldenberg D (1995). Preceptors' perception of benefits, rewards, supports and commitment to the preceptor role. *Journal of Advanced Nursing*, **21**, 1144–51.

Donovan J (1990). The concept and role of mentor. *Nurse Education Today*, **10**, 294–8.

Dooher J, Clark A and Fowler J (2001). *Case Studies on Practice Development*. Dinton: Quay Books.

Dusmohamed H and Guscott A (1998). Preceptorship: a model to empower nurses in rural health settings. *Continuing Nurse Education*, **29**, 154–60.

Earnshaw G (1995). Mentorship: the student's view. *Nurse Education Today*, **15**, 274–9.

English National Board for Nursing, Midwifery and Health Visiting (ENB) (1989). *Preparation of Teachers, Practitioners/Teachers, Mentors and Supervisors in the Context of Project 2000*. London: English National Board for Nursing, Midwifery and Health Visiting.

English National Board for Nursing, Midwifery and Health Visiting (ENB) (1990). *A New Structure for Professional Development: The Framework for Continuing Professional Education and the Higher Award*. London: English National Board for Nursing, Midwifery and Health Visiting.

English National Board for Nursing, Midwifery and Health Visiting (ENB) (1991). *Framework for Continuing Professional Education for Nurses, Midwives and Health Visitors*. London: English National Board for Nursing, Midwifery and Health Visiting.

English National Board for Nursing, Midwifery and Health Visiting (ENB) (1993). *Regulations and Guidelines for the Approval of Institutions and Courses*. London: English National Board for Nursing, Midwifery and Health Visiting.

English National Board for Nursing, Midwifery and Health Visiting (ENB) and Department of Health (DH) (2001). *Preparation of Mentors and Teachers: A New Framework of Guidance*. London English National Board for Nursing, Midwifery and Health Visiting and Department of Health.

Farrington A (1995). Models of clinical supervision. *British Journal of Nursing*, **4**, 876–8.

Faugier J (1992). The supervisory relationship. In Butterworth T and Faugier J (eds). *Clinical Supervision and Mentorship in Nursing*. London: Chapman & Hall.

Fowler J (1995). Nurses' perceptions of the elements of good supervision. *Nursing Times*, **91**, 33–7.

Fowler J (1996). The organisation of clinical supervision within the nursing profession. *Journal of Advanced Nursing*, **23**, 471–8.

Fowler J (ed.) (2005). *Staff Nurse Survival Guide*. Dinton: Quay Books.

Fowler J (2006). The importance of reflective practice for nurse prescribers. *Nurse Prescribing*, **4**, 103–6.

Gately E (1992). PREPP: from novice to expert. *British Journal of Nursing*, **1**, 88–91.

Gott M (1984). *Learning Nursing*. London: Royal College of Nursing.

Hagerty B (1986). A second look at mentors. *Nursing Outlook*, **34**, 16–24.

Harrison S, Hunter D, Marnoch D and Pollitt C (1989). *The Impact of General Management in the NHS*. Leeds: Nuffield Institute.

Harrison S, Hunter D, Marnoch D and Pollitt C (1990). *The Dynamics of British Health Policy*. London: Unwin Hyman.

Johns C (1993). Professional supervision. *Journal of Nursing Management*, **1**, 9–18.

Johns C (1997). Reflective practice and clinical supervision: part 1. The reflective turn. *European Nurse*, **2**, 87–97.

Kolb D (1984). *Experiential Learning: Experience as the Source of Learning and Development*. Englewood Cliffs, NJ: Prentice-Hall.

Maggs C (1994). Mentorship in nursing and midwifery education: issues for research. *Nurse Education Today*, **14**, 22–9.

Marrow C, Macauley D and Crumbie A (1997). Promoting reflective practice through structured clinical supervision. *Journal of Nursing Management*, **5**, 77–82.

May K (1982). Mentorship for scholarliness. *Nursing Outlook*, **30**, 22–6.

McCaugherty D (1991). The use of a teaching model to promote reflection and the experiential integration of theory and practice in first-year student nurses: an action research study. *Journal of Advanced Nursing*, **16**, 534–43.

Mezirow J (1981). A critical theory of adult learning and education. *Adult Education*, **32**, 3–24.

Morris N, John G and Keen T (1988). Mentors: learning the ropes. *Nursing Times*, **84**, 24–7.

Myrick F and Barrett C (1994). Selecting clinical preceptors for basic baccalaureate nursing students. *Journal of Advanced Nursing*, **19**, 194–8.

Nicklin P (1995). Super supervision. *Nursing Management*, **2**, 24–5.

Nicklin P (1997). A practice centred model of clinical supervision. *Nursing Times*, **12**, 52–4.

Nursing and Midwifery Council (NMC) (2002). *Standards for the Preparation of Teachers of Nurses, Midwives and Specialist Community Public Health Nurses*. London: Nursing and Midwifery Council.

Nursing and Midwifery Council (NMC) (2004). *Standards of Proficiency for Pre-Registration Nursing Education*. London: Nursing and Midwifery Council.

Nursing and Midwifery Council (NMC) (2006a). *The PREP Handbook Standards*. London: Nursing and Midwifery Council.

Nursing and Midwifery Council (NMC) (2006b). *Nursing and Midwifery Council Advice Sheet: Preceptorship*. London: Nursing and Midwifery Council.

Nursing and Midwifery Council (NMC) (2006c). *Nursing and Midwifery Council Advice Sheet: Clinical Supervision*. London: Nursing and Midwifery Council.

Nursing and Midwifery Council (NMC) (2006d). *Nursing and Midwifery Council Standards to Support Learning and Assessment in Practice*. London: Nursing and Midwifery Council.

Nursing and Midwifery Council (NMC) (2008). *The Code: Standards of Conduct, Performance and Ethics for Nurses and Midwives*. London: Nursing and Midwifery Council.

Ouellet L (1993). Relationship of a preceptorship experience to the views about nursing as a profession. *Nurse Education Today*, **13**, 16–23.

Peutz B (1985). Learning the ropes from a mentor. *Nursing Success Today*, **2**, 11–13.

Schön D (1987). *Educating the Reflective Practitioner*. San Francisco, CA: Jossey-Bass.

Schön D (1991). *The Reflective Practitioner*. Aldershot: Avebury.

Skyte S (1997). PREP: the key to safe practice and upholding standards. *Nursing Times Learning Curve*, **1**, 2–3.

Snowball J, Ross K and Murphy K (1994). Illuminating dissertation supervision through reflection. *Journal of Advanced Nursing*, **19**, 1234–40.

Steinaker N and Bell R (1979). *The Experiential Taxonomy*. New York: Academic Press.

Thompson N (1995). *Theory and Practice in Health and Social Welfare*. Buckingham: Open University Press.

UK Central Council for Nursing, Midwifery and Health Visiting (UKCC) (1990). *The Report of the Post-Registration Education and Practice Project (PREP)*. London: UK Central Council for Nursing, Midwifery and Health Visiting.

UK Central Council for Nursing, Midwifery and Health Visiting (UKCC) (1993). *The Council's Position Concerning a Period of Support and Preceptorship*. Registrar's letter 1/1993 Annexe One. London: UK Central Council for Nursing, Midwifery and Health Visiting.

UK Central Council for Nursing, Midwifery and Health Visiting (UKCC) (1994). *The Future of Professional Practice: The Council's Standards for Education and Practice Following Registration*. London: UK Central Council for Nursing, Midwifery and Health Visiting.

Wallace M (1999). *Lifelong Learning: PREP in Action*. Edinburgh: Churchill Livingstone.

Williams J, Baker G, Clark B, *et al.* (1993). Collaborative preceptor training: a creative approach in tough times. *Journal of Continuing Education in Nursing*, **24**, 153–7.

Woodrow P (1994). Mentorship: perceptions and pitfalls for nursing practice. *Journal of Advanced Nursing*, **19**, 812–18.

Further reading

Clark A, Dooher J and Fowler J (2001). *The Handbook of Practice Development*. Dinton: Quay Books. *This edited book is written by a variety of practitioners, managers and educators and provides a broad overview of the development of practice and quality care. It explores the various ways in which practice can develop. It looks at a number of influences, such as clinical governance, power, education, multiprofessional approaches, and the place of audit and research. It is a useful resource for the student nurse, as each chapter can be read in isolation.*

Dooher J, Clark A and Fowler J (2001). *Case Studies on Practice Development*. Dinton: Quay Books. *Written as a companion to the more traditional textbook The Handbook of Practice Development (Clark et al., 2001), this book is a collection of 23 reflective accounts of practitioners' experiences of clinical practice and practice development. It commences with accounts from student nurses through to nurse consultants and nurse practitioners. It provides useful insights into the realities of practice within a complex world of health care. This is an interesting book to read, as each person is sharing an important part of their life and work with the reader. Each chapter contains a wealth of truth and theory evolving from clinical experience.*

Fowler J (ed.) (1998). *The Handbook of Clinical Supervision: Your Questions Answered*. Dinton: Quay Books.

For the newly qualified nurse exiting their preceptorship period, clinical supervision should form an integral part of ongoing development and quality assurance. This is a particularly useful book that is designed to give the reader short precise answers to over 50 commonly asked questions on clinical supervision. Students will find it a useful resource in helping them to understand the development of clinical supervision within the nursing profession and the part that supervision has to play in their clinical practice and future professional development.

Lillyman S and Ward C (1999). *Balancing Organisational and Personal Development Needs*. Dinton: Quay Books.

This book provides an operational and strategic approach to understanding how individuals need to be supported to give high-quality care. It identifies personal, organisational, professional and governmental needs and wider issues that influence clinical, educational and professional development. It contains a number of appendixes that give useful examples of issues such as action plans from a training and development strategy and a personal profile proforma.

Nursing and Midwifery Council (NMC) (2008). *The Code: Standards of Conduct, Performance and Ethics for Nurses and Midwives*. London: Nursing and Midwifery Council.

The NMC Code is one of the most useful and important publications available. All nurses should not only read but also discuss and debate the values and standards embodied in this short publication. The purpose of the NMC Code is to inform nurses and midwives of the standard of professional conduct required of them in the exercise of their professional accountability and practice. The NMC Code also informs the public, other professionals and employers of the standard of professional conduct that they can expect of a registered practitioner.

Wallace M (1999). *Lifelong Learning: PREP in Action*. Edinburgh: Churchill Livingstone.

The concept of good-quality care based upon lifelong learning was at the heart of the UKCC's PREP project in the early 1990s. Maggy Wallace, formally the director of standards promotion for the UKCC, was the architect of the PREP proposals. She explains the context of PREP within lifelong learning, spelling out individuals' responsibilities for developing and maintaining professional expertise.

Fundamental Aspects of Nursing – various titles. Dinton: Quay Books.

This is series of textbooks written for student nurses and junior staff nurses. Each book focuses on a specific area of clinical practice and provides the reader with a wealth of information regarding procedures, roles and underpinning knowledge. These and similar texts provide junior nurses with an overview and essential underpinning knowledge on various specialties.

23

Your career: your opportunity as a professional nurse

Jane Schober

Introduction

This chapter provides a comprehensive overview of the personal and professional requirements nurses need to maintain their licence to practise. Ultimately, the purpose of fulfilling these requirements is to maintain standards that result in the delivery of optimum care standards for those needing nursing and health care. Career opportunities for nurses are also explored, as are the factors influencing career choices, career opportunities and career management.

Learning objectives

After studying this chapter you should be able to:

- state the Nursing and Midwifery Council (NMC) requirements to maintain your licence to practise nursing;
- develop and maintain your personal professional profile;
- identify and manage career opportunities;
- consider ways to manage career decisions;
- prepare for selection and job interviews;
- maintain a curriculum vitae.

Overview

When we visit and are cared for by a doctor, nurse or any member of the multiprofessional team, our expectations are that they will be competent to practise. This expectation is central to the relationship between the public and health care professionals. It is considered so important within the nursing profession that all nurses are required to meet certain criteria, which are used to monitor their licence to practise and thus their suitability to practise as a registered nurse. When nurses register with the NMC, they have successfully completed a course of study and been declared fit to practise nursing in the UK through the fulfilment of a range of practice, academic and professional requirements. As with a driving licence, a licence to practise nursing depends on nurses exercising their responsibilities in accordance with statutory, professional and employment requirements. Much of the responsibility to fulfil these requirements lies with each nurse as an accountable practitioner, but they should be supported by, for example, the existence of policies in the workplace, the NMC Code (2008) (Appendix 1) and professional standards (NMC, 2004a).

All branches of nursing have a range of roles and expectations for nurses when they register. The successful acquisition of a role, for example as a staff nurse, usually depends on a process of selection that relies on thorough preparation and self-presentation to ensure that any career development opportunity is pursued appropriately. In recent times, the demand for nursing posts has increased dramatically. No longer can it be an expectation that all qualifying nurses seeking employment in a nursing role will be successful. The market for posts is changeable, subject to health care workforce pressures and highly competitive. It is vital, therefore, that nurses are thoroughly prepared for initial posts following registration and all subsequent career moves. With these demands in mind, this chapter seeks to provide the guidance necessary for nurses to maintain their licence to practise and to support the process of career development.

NMC requirements to maintain a licence to practise nursing

Since 2000, the requirements for student nurses to enter a branch programme – and subsequently to be declared fit to practise as a registered nurse – have been described clearly (NMC, 2004a). They take the form of competencies, which are assessed theoretically and practically throughout a pre-registration study programme and address the four domains of:

- professional and ethical practice;
- care delivery;
- care management;
- personal and professional development (NMC, 2004a).

The publication of the NMC Code (Appendix 1) provides a means of linking the required standards of professional conduct with the legal requirements for nurse education charged to the NMC by the Nursing and Midwifery Order (2001) and the NMC (2004a). Hence, these form the foundation for the professional development of all nurses. Because the focus of this chapter is on maintaining a licence to practise and the management of career opportunities, the professional development and expectations of nurses are discussed and explored here.

In relation to professional development, the NMC Code states:

Keep your skills and knowledge up to date

- *You must have the knowledge and skills for safe and effective practice when working without direct supervision*
- *You must recognise and work within the limits of your competence*
- *You must keep your knowledge and skills up to date throughout your working life*
- *You must take part in appropriate learning and practice activities that maintain and develop your competence and performance.*

(NMC Code, 2008)

Reflection point 23.1

Consider this quote from the NMC Code, and make a list of how a registered nurse may work towards the achievement of each of these points. Think about the resources needed for their achievement and who could, and should, help in this process.

Before considering the resources in any detail, reflect on any pre-registration experiences relevant to this process. First, there are the competencies and outcomes relating to professional development that should be demonstrated in order to enter the branch programme. These form the basis for the teaching and learning experiences during pre-registration courses as follows:

Demonstrate responsibility for one's own learning through the development of a portfolio of practice and recognize when further learning is required:

- *identify specific learning needs and objectives*
- *begin to engage with, and interpret, the evidence-base which underpins nursing practice.*

Acknowledge the importance of seeking supervision to develop safe nursing practice.

(NMC, 2004a, p. 34)

The emphasis here is on personal learning, personal reflection and taking responsibility for this process. The development of a portfolio of practice is evidence of the student nurse's learning experience, but this occurs only with supervision and support. From the period of the common foundation programme, there are professional and personal expectations that focus on the student's learning experiences in practice and their understanding of research and theoretical evidence relating to practice. Thus, the scene is set for personal and professional development. By the end of a branch programme, the competencies demand that the responsibility for ongoing learning and continuing professional development (CPD) extends beyond personal responsibility for learning to the skills necessary to support the personal and professional development of others.

The NMC's (2004a) personal and professional development competencies for entry to the register are:

- *demonstrate a commitment to the need for CPD and personal supervision activities in order to enhance knowledge, skills, values and attitudes needed for safe and effective nursing practice:*
  - *identify one's own professional development needs by engaging in activities such as reflection in, and on, practice and lifelong learning*
  - *develop a personal development plan which takes into account personal, professional and organizational needs*
  - *share experiences with colleagues and patients and clients in order to identify the additional knowledge and skills needed to manage unfamiliar or professionally challenging situations*
  - *take action to meet any identified knowledge and skills deficit likely to affect the delivery of care within the current sphere of practice*
- *enhance the professional development and safe practice of others through peer support, leadership, supervision and teaching*
  - *contribute to creating a climate conducive to learning*
  - *contribute to the learning experiences of others by facilitating the mutual sharing of knowledge and experience*
  - *demonstrate effective leadership in the establishment of safe nursing practice.*

(NMC, 2004a, p. 34)

It is from this background that registered nurses embark on their professional careers. The personal and professional competencies are far reaching and demand that nurses have been assessed to demonstrate the necessary skills that meet these criteria before registration. This, then, is the foundation for all registered nurses. It is this combination of the adherence to the NMC Code and the fulfilment of post-registration requirements for maintaining the licence to practise nursing that emphasises the nursing profession's pledge to provide competent practice. However, this process does not occur without support and resources.

Reflection point 23.2

Look again at your resources list from Reflection point 23.1. You may find that they fall into particular categories, such as support from staff and colleagues, learning resources, financial support and study time, information and skill development, for example in relation to teaching and supervision. This is a tall order. However, it emphasises what registered nurses are responsible for within this domain and clarifies that all registered nurses have a duty and responsibility to initiate the necessary activities in order for these requirements to be met.

The NMC provides clear requirements to maintain a licence to practise, which apply to all nurses registered with the NMC. A set of post-registration and practice standards (PREP) has been designed to support this process of maintaining the best possible care for patients (NMC, 2006a) In essence, these standards support the process of updating yourself in the relevant practice area, personal reflection and decision-making, supporting practice development and the promotion of optimum care of patients. The PREP standards, which are legal requirements, are as follows:

- *The PREP (practice) standard – you must have worked in some capacity by virtue of your nursing, midwifery or specialist community public health nursing qualification during the previous 3 years for a minimum of 450 hours, or have successfully undertaken an approved return-to-practice course within the last three years.*
- *The PREP (continuing professional development) standard – you must have undertaken and recorded your continuing professional development (CPD) over the 3 years prior to the renewal of your registration. All registrants have been required to comply with this standard since April 1995. Since April 2000, registrants have needed to declare on their NOP form that they have met this requirement when they renew their registration.*

(NMC, 2006a, p. 5)

So far, elements of the NMC Code and the PREP requirements have been considered. It can be seen that they serve to protect the public by setting clear standards for practice, professional development, behaviour and decision-making. It is through the pursuit of these demands that the competencies necessary for registration may be developed further throughout a nursing career.

Returning to practice

Many nurses have a break in service of 3 years or more. Such nurses are unable to fulfil the practice standard without successfully completing a return-to-practice course. These are available across the UK and are 5 days or more in length. The courses are validated by the NMC and provide participants with input relating to health and social policy, practice-related updates and support to enhance professional development. Details of courses in Scotland, Wales and Northern Ireland are available on the NMC website and for England from NHS Careers.

The NMC requirements for renewal of registration are summarised in Box 23.1. The personal professional profile is a key tool with which each nurse can maintain details of their professional life as well as being a document that may be requested by the NMC for audit purposes.

BOX 23.1 NMC requirements for the renewal of registration

- Completion of the notification of practice form giving details of qualifications and area of practice (NPO).
- Signed declaration that the PREP requirements have been met:
  - *PREP practice standard*: must have worked for a minimum of 450 hours of practice in the 3 years before renewal or successful completion of an approved return-to-practice course during the previous 3 years.
  - *PREP continuing professional development standard*: must have undertaken and recorded CPD activity during the previous 3 years (minimum of 35 hours).
- Maintenance of a personal professional profile.
- Compliance with the NMC audit.

Maintaining a personal professional profile

For nurses who have registered in recent years, the profile has become an integral part of pre- and post-registration activities. For student nurses, the profile now serves as a means of recording learning needs and experiences and a record of the elements of evidence-based learning. In many higher education institutions, the profile forms a component of course assessment, and thus students are encouraged to use it as a basis for tutorials and dialogue with experienced nurses. The profile is a valuable means of professional support. Although the NMC competencies refer to it as a portfolio, there are marked similarities between the terms 'profile' and 'portfolio', and they are often used interchangeably. There is, therefore, a natural extension of the process of profile maintenance between the pre- and post-registration periods, making it a personal record of professional development.

For registered nurses, the profile is a record of professional development and career progression. The minimum PREP requirement is the record of evidence of any CPD activity, but it may also include:

- biographical information;
- the record of academic and professional qualifications;
- a summary of current and previous posts;
- details of relevant responsibilities and activities, e.g. management roles, interest groups, research activities and publications;
- the record of education and formal learning experiences, e.g. courses, study days and updates, conference attendance and teaching activities;
- a record of working hours during the previous 3 years;
- reflection and evaluation of performance; this may also include critical incident analysis and examples of feedback from mentors and peers;
- personal and professional objectives; this may be in the form of an action plan.

Other tips

The profile is a live document and should be kept up to date. For nurses who work closely with a preceptor or mentor, the profile is a tool that may serve to shape and prioritise dialogue relating to practice and professional and career development. It is also a useful tool to support job applications and to develop the analytical skills necessary for reflective practice.

Aim to use a clear structure and an index, and record and date all entries. The profile may be completed in the Welsh language if required. Care should be taken to ensure confidentiality, particularly if incidents or examples from practice are described and analysed. Names should always be omitted.

Lifelong learning

The links between CPD and PREP represent an important part of lifelong learning. The notion that individuals are responsible for their learning is made clear in developments such as the portfolio and the achievement of practice and CPD standards. Support for this process is essential through preceptorship, mentoring and effective role models.

SUMMARY

In order to maintain a licence to practise nursing, all registered nurses must:
- protect the public through adhering to professional standards;
- comply with the NMC Code;
- meet the PREP standards;
- maintain a personal professional profile.

Managing career opportunities

Understanding the available options for registered nurses and consideration of career opportunities serves to support the process of professional development. As nurses are personally accountable for their practice, it is essential that personal, professional and career decision-making are as effective as possible.

Regardless of the choice of branch, there is a wide range of career options for nurses. Making an informed choice, and one that will result in a positive work role, places demands on any applicant. Over the years, the job market has fluctuated greatly. The government drive to recruit more nurses has led to increases in student numbers, with resulting pressure on students when applying for their first-choice staff nurse post. Competition for many posts in acute hospitals and larger units can be great, and the way each nurse prepares for and proceeds with career choices impacts significantly on all stages of their career.

Factors affecting career choices

Initially, the pursuit of career opportunities depends on a range of factors and resources, such as:

- employment opportunities;
- educational and training opportunities;
- career guidance opportunities for nurses;
- work, personal and social needs;
- information relating to career options;
- career pathways for nurses;
- preparation for selection procedures and interviews.

Employment opportunities

Historically, most newly registered nurses have opted to apply for a band 5 or equivalent staff nurse post local to their higher education institution or elsewhere in their base country. There are many employment opportunities for nurses, depending on their qualifications, skills and experience. Box 23.2 illustrates the range of options and the potential further learning demands on

---

BOX 23.2 Key employers of nurses in the UK
- Charitable organisations, e.g. Macmillan Nurses, King's Fund
- Further education colleges
- Armed forces, e.g. army, navy, air force
- Higher education institutions (universities)
- Local authorities
- NHS trusts, including primary care trusts
- Nursing agencies
- Occupational health services
- Overseas development services, e.g. British Red Cross
- Independent health care organisations
- Pharmaceutical companies
- Professional organisations, e.g. Royal College of Nursing
- Publishing houses
- Statutory bodies, e.g. the NMC
- Trades unions.

registered nurses who have already completed at least a 3-year course of full-time study. Progress through the tiers of bands or grades in the NHS or private health sectors, or diversification into non-clinical roles, usually requires further qualifications, skills and role developments.

Knowing the employment options is crucial to any career or role development. Seeking information through advertisements is only a part of the process. If you aspire to a particular role, have ambitions and have your sights set on a particular path, then information-gathering is the essential first step. Key sources of employment information are summarised in Box 23.3. These will be complemented by knowledge of:

- qualifications and other professional requirements necessary to apply;
- required previous experience;
- terms and conditions of employment, e.g. contract and salary details;
- employment policies, e.g. family-friendly policies, health and safety policies;
- role specification for the post-holder;
- employment opportunities for the post-holder;
- details of the induction programme and staff training;
- details of staff appraisal and support networks;
- evidence of quality assurance mechanisms.

Some of this information will feature on an advertisement, but usually only key elements of the role are outlined. Later in the chapter, guidance is offered on the process of applying for a post.

BOX 23.3 Sources of employment information

- National websites, e.g. NHS, DHSSPS (Scotland), NMC, RCN, local trusts
- Human resources departments for local employment information
- Prospectuses for university details
- Specialist journals for specialist posts
- Libraries for local information
- National and local press for job advertisements
- Internal communications and newsletters
- Staff noticeboards

Educational and training opportunities for nurses

Following registration, most nurses recognise that they have reached a stage when, despite the achievements of registering as a nurse, learning is just beginning in relation to many facets of their chosen role. The generation of a personal development plan (see above) may be supported by attention to education and training opportunities. Recognition of the demands of professional nursing practice and the support needed to maintain standards of practice is manifest in the provision of the following:

- *Work-based learning*: this is characterised by opportunities to learn relevant skills and competencies in the workplace, which are assessed. Successful outcomes may result in the award of academic credits if the course or module has been approved using academic approval criteria. This scheme is supported by the Department of Health's Working Together, Learning Together recommendations (DH, 2001) for lifelong learning.
- *CPD*: this is characterised by opportunities for learning following registration (and may include work-based learning). Higher education institutions work in partnership with NHS

trusts to identify, prepare and gain approval and necessary contracts for the provision of courses. These are subject to academic and professional approval by the NMC and higher education provider. Courses are offered through modular schemes using the credit accumulation and transfer scheme (CATS), where academic credits are awarded following successful outcome at the academic level approved for the stage of the course.

Consider Scenario 23.1.

SCENARIO 23.1

Jasmine Robertson is a registered mental health nurse who has worked full-time in a community psychiatric day centre for 18 months. She has a diploma in higher education (mental health nursing). Following a performance review, she has the support of her line manager to apply for a BSc (Hons) nursing course. The purpose of this would be to facilitate her development in relation to the academic study of nursing and to undertake modules in the theory and practice of research methodology and counselling.

The achievement of a diploma level course results in the award of 120 CATS points – level 1 and 120 CATS points – level 2. The requirement of a first degree course (either a BA (Hons) or a BSc (Hons)) is the achievement of a further 120 credits at level 3 – usually the third year of a full-time 3-year degree course. CATS allows applicants to transfer previously acquired points to a course of further study that would be subject to accreditation under the accreditation of a prior achievement scheme (APA). In addition, approval of prior experiential learning (APEL) may also be assessed by the course admissions team, as this may also be counted. In Sceneario 23.1, Jasmine's academic achievement and professional experience may result in her needing to complete only the level 3 modules, which would usually be undertaken over 2 years part time or 1 year full time.

There is a wide range of modules and courses for registered nurses. They are based in higher education institutions and trusts. Your ability to undertake a course of study will usually depend on:

- relevance to you and your workplace needs;
- available funding – you may be asked to self-fund;
- the nature, content, level and availability of the course;
- the study leave approval processes.

Making the most appropriate choices relating to ongoing education may be supported by career guidance advice and information.

Career guidance opportunities for nurses

Making career choices is a complex process. Avoiding mistakes in the choice of new posts, courses of study and career changes depends on each of us being aware of the range of possibilities and options available, as well as being conversant with the necessary information and skills to succeed with, for example, an application. Historically, career guidance for nurses has been limited to national and local sources of career information and experienced nursing staff providing opportunities for nurses to explore, discuss and review their career options. Job availability remains a key factor in the process of career management. Although this cannot be underestimated, it is important that nurses aspire to their optimum potential through making effective career choices.

Work, personal and social needs

All career decisions may be influenced by personal and social factors. In recent years, changes in working patterns have become evident, in particular in relation to the increase in numbers of those working part time, returning to nursing and pursuing more flexible working practices.

Reflection point 23.3

Consider the factors important to you in a choice of job or career change. What is particularly helpful here is what motivates you. You may find the following categories helpful: work needs, personal needs, and family and social needs.

Now examine Box 23.4, which lists the factors found to be important to nurses making career choices (Schober, 1990). They influence motivation and, in particular, job satisfaction, which is central to the sense of well-being at work.

There is much discussion in the nursing and national press about the concerns over the terms and conditions of nurses in work and their pay levels. Given high house prices and the cost of living, the influence of these factors should not be underestimated. Indeed, many employers offer initiatives such as flexible working and family-friendly policies to support nurses. Nurses, however, identify other factors that emphasise the importance of job satisfaction and positive work relationships. Stechmiller and Yarandi (1992) found that the quality of supervision, promotion opportunities and the meaningfulness of work were more influential than pay and job security.

BOX 23.4 Factors affecting career choices

Work needs include:

- the need to work;
- promotion;
- motivation and opportunities to learn and develop professionally;
- interest in and commitment to the work and role;
- range of responsibility;
- dynamics of the team and management structure;
- Agenda for Change banding.

Personal needs include:

- job satisfaction;
- job security;
- status of the role;
- salary;
- reluctance to change roles;
- terms of the contract.

Family and social needs include:

- family's need for income;
- childcare availability;
- availability of accommodation;
- travelling distance from home;
- house prices;
- support of partner and family members.

Source: Schober (1990).

Schober (2000) suggests a range of factors influencing job satisfaction in a clinical post (Box 23.5). These factors may also serve to help nurses in the process of deciding their preferred clinical placement.

BOX 23.5 Factors influencing job satisfaction in a clinical post

- Factors relating to care and the patient/client group
- The clinical specialty
- The pace of work, e.g. patient turnover, day care
- Opportunities to develop the nurse–patient relationship
- Opportunities and support for learning
- Team membership and support
- Staff support network
- Style of leadership
- Staff morale
- Opportunities for professional development

Reflection point 23.4

Consider your favourite clinical placements. To what extent did the factors listed in Box 23.5 influence your choice? To confirm your choice, it may help you to place these in order of importance and compare them with your needs, as listed in Box 23.4.

You may find a pattern emerging that helps you to feel confident about what is important to you when choosing a role and, just as importantly, what you would not enjoy or would be disadvantageous to your ways of working.

Information relating to career options

Understanding what motivates nurses in work needs to be supported by sound advice and information. It is rare to find career officers or counsellors in the health services, but there are often highly motivated lecturers, managers and clinical staff willing to offer advice. The preceptorship and mentor systems are additional ways of finding support. Despite this type of networking, it is a challenge for staff to keep abreast of the career information available and necessary for sound decision-making. Information may relate to:

- current career options;
- job availability;
- career pathways;
- in-service education and training;
- courses of study;
- prerequisites to promotion and development, e.g. a teaching qualification;
- senior clinical roles, e.g. nurse specialists, nurse consultants, modern matrons and community matrons.

Career pathways for nurses

The DH (2006) is driving a key initiative to facilitate the development of nursing careers across the UK. Four key priority areas have been identified to address this. They are to:

- *Develop a competent and flexible workforce*
- *Update career pathways and career choices*

- *Prepare nurses to lead in a changed health care system*
- *Modernise the image of nursing and nursing careers.*

(DH, 2006, p. 17)

The impact of this initiative will be far reaching. The report recognises that generalist, specialist and advanced nursing roles will need to be reviewed in response to changing health care, patient needs and multiprofessional teamworking. Therefore, other major elements will be affected, namely education, training and development opportunities. Career options and opportunities will develop further as skills and competency frameworks respond to developments in patterns of care, for example caring for older people, family-centred care, integrated health and social care, and mental health care needs.

Whether a nurse opts to develop a career that includes the pursuit of promotion, working full time or working until retirement is a personal decision. Currently, more nurses appear to be opting for periodic career breaks, part-time working and flexibility to meet domestic needs. Trends in working patterns also show that more nurses are working in the private sector, and up to 47 per cent take a career break, mainly for maternity leave. With more nurses returning to practice, the expansion of community nursing roles (e.g. practice nurses), and initiatives such as the modern matron, community matron and nurse consultants, there is a wide range of available posts.

Traditionally, nurses pursued a linear clinical pathway until professional development and promotion opportunities resulted in the acceptance of a teaching, management or research role. Nowadays, the *Agenda for Change* (DH, 2005) banding structures for nurses demand the integration of these three activities with clinical responsibilities to a greater or lesser extent throughout the scheme (Box 23.6). Ultimately, this structure supports the opportunity for nurses to remain in clinical practice and to have an advancing clinical career, rather than finding promotion by opting for educational or managerial posts.

BOX 23.6 Role specifications

Band 5 specifications usually include:

- experience (usually 1 year) and satisfactory performance in the specialty;
- previous teaching experience;
- experience of supervising students or other staff;
- evidence of effective interpersonal, teamworking and communication skills;
- evidence of development of leadership skills;
- evidence of research appreciation and evidence-based practice;
- personal and professional updating and development;
- post-registration qualification in the specialty;
- teaching qualification.

Band 6 grade role specifications usually include:

- all the band 5 specifications;
- the potential to lead a team;
- experience in the specialty (usually 2 years);
- evidence of clinical and managerial skills.

BOX 23.6 (continued)

Band 7 grade role specifications usually include:

- all the band 6 specifications;
- experience in the specialty (e.g. 3–5 years);
- evidence of clinical, managerial, educational and leadership skills;
- evidence of the potential to undertake research;
- qualifications or advanced study relating to the specialty;
- the potential for innovative practice.

Band 8 role specifications usually include:

- all the band 7 specifications;
- proven leadership ability;
- evidence of relevant managerial, educational and research ability;
- potential to initiate and respond to policies, innovations and quality initiatives.

The specialist practitioner

Opportunities for nurses to undertake courses leading to specialist practitioner roles have facilitated learning relating to clinical practice, care and programme management, practice development and clinical practice leadership. Courses are available and may relate to any specialty, although the NMC (2004b, 2006b) specified standards relating to:

- specialist community public health nurses (NMC, 2004b);
- teachers of nurses, midwives and specialist community public health nurses (NMC, 2006b).

The availability of courses leading to specialist practitioner qualifications may be found on the websites of the national health departments in each of the countries in the UK. More detailed explanations of the content of courses are found in higher education institution prospectuses and websites and from senior nurses, lecturers and lecturer-practitioners in NHS trusts.

Advanced nursing practice

Over the past few years, much work has been undertaken nationally to legitimise advanced nurse practitioner (ANP) roles (NMC, 2005), with the intention that ANPs may be registered with the NMC. This process would facilitate the recognition of specialist and advanced nursing skills and confirm a framework for accepting existing practitioners on to the register. It would also promote the clarification of educational criteria for courses of preparation for the roles and criteria for approval by higher education institutions and the NMC.

The NMC (2005) suggests that:

Advanced nurse practitioners are highly skilled nurses who can:

- *Carry out physical examinations;*
- *Use their expert knowledge and clinical judgement to decide whether to refer patients for investigations and make diagnoses;*
- *Decide on and carry out treatment, including the prescribing of medicines, or refer patients to an appropriate specialist;*

- *Use their extensive practice experience to plan and provide skilled and competent care to meet patients' health and social care needs, involving other members of the health care team as appropriate;*
- *Ensure the provision of continuity of care including follow-up visits;*
- *Assess and evaluate, with patients, the effectiveness of the treatment and care provided and make changes as needed;*
- *Work independently, although often as part of a health care team that they will lead; and*
- *As a leader of the team, make sure that each patient's treatment and care is based on best practice.*

(NMC, 2005, p. 3)

Further consultations have occurred since 2005 between the DH and the NMC to pursue the debate for the registration of the ANP role and to agree standards for the preparation for this role. The NMC website contains current information regarding the progress of this work.

Career pathways in educational, managerial and research roles

So far, consideration has been given to the development of a clinical career pathway. Career pathways may also facilitate emphasis on teaching, management and research roles. Currently, one in four nurses works outside the NHS, and so it is vital that nurses are aware of the necessary information to make informed decisions at all stages.

Sources of information for these roles include the following:

- *UK websites for career information*: each UK country has a website containing information relating to roles and available courses. Some, e.g. Northern Ireland, include details of the centres offering specific courses.
- *Statutory organisations*: for example, the NMC provides details of statutory requirements for specific roles, re-registration and educational requirements for key roles, e.g. nurse teachers.
- *Professional organisations*: for example, the RCN provides details of services to members, professional guidance, and support and learning opportunities, e.g. conferences and professional forums. The *RCN Bulletin* also provides information on job opportunities.

Educational opportunities fall into different categories. Details of professional and statutory courses and continuing education are available from the NMC, Health Professionals Wales, NHS Education for Scotland and the Northern Ireland Practice and Education Council.

Open learning and additional educational opportunities are available from higher education institutions, the RCN and professional journals.

Embarking on a pathway that focuses on research, management or education demands that the applicant has undertaken appropriate academic preparation and completed necessary prerequisites for the role.

Nursing research

The expectation that research is applied in practice settings is specified at the outset of all pre-registration courses. Opportunities for nurses to participate in research processes have increased in recent years, as nurse education has become integrated within higher education institutions and more opportunities have developed for nurses to study aspects of nursing beyond diploma level. Research posts exist in a range of sectors, although mainly in university departments, specialist research centres and through specifically funded research projects. When considering a research post, there are a number of issues that influence the role:

- *Length of contract*: often of a fixed term and for a short period, e.g. 1 year, especially for research assistants.
- *Role specification*: may demand unsocial hours for gathering data.
- *Opportunities for education and training*: examine what is available and what skills are expected.
- *Resources*: consider the available resources, e.g. office accommodation, secretarial support and IT facilities.
- *Responsibilities*: there may be teaching requirements and responsibilities for disseminating research outcomes through writing papers and presenting at seminars and conferences.
- *Opportunities for promotion to senior roles, e.g. readership or professorial position*: consider the available research activity and funding, the work of the research active staff, the history of research activity within the department and the evidence of quality assessment. The research assessment exercise (RAE) ranking is a valuable measure of the quality of previous research outputs. Currently, this assessment invites academic departments to submit evidence of research activity every 4 years. The score is an indicator of quality and activity, is a useful guide for potential applicants, and influences the degree of funding that the higher education institution receives from the relevant funding body.

Whatever the research activity, whether it be as part of a clinical role, a course of study or a specific post, the potential is there to contribute to the growing body of nursing knowledge and the evidence base for practice. The use of research findings is integral to teaching and education roles.

Teaching and education

As with research, teaching and learning may be exercised at all levels of experience. Indeed, there is a professional expectation for nurses to teach others, disseminate information and promote learning within the process of patient care. Support for this begins during pre-registration programmes, although it is following registration that those intent on specific teaching roles have the opportunity to undertake them. One of the key developments in nursing in recent years has been the recognition of the value of learning in practice settings and the necessity to balance the emphasis of teaching between the theoretical perspectives necessary for academic attainment and the practice skills essential to the quality of patient interventions. The competency-based curriculum and the standards required of pre-registration programmes (NMC, 2004b) are central to this process. Subsequently, changes to the preparation of nurse teachers have facilitated educational pathways for the preparation of practice educators and for those wishing to teach in a practice environment, as well as opportunities for preparation as a lecturer to teach in an academic department in a higher education institution (NMC, 2006b).

Teaching courses are now equivalent to 1 year's full-time study and result in a recordable teaching qualification on the NMC register. Most courses are part time, which enables applicants to maintain their professional role. The courses have a range of entry requirements, including:

- a degree or equivalent qualification;
- entry on the NMC register;
- 3 years' full-time practice experience (or equivalent) with student nurses in the past 10 years;
- evidence of professional knowledge.

These courses demand study at postgraduate diploma level and may lead to a master of science degree in many institutions. Details of these courses are available from the NMC website.

Nurses embarking on this career pathway will need to consider carefully the implications of these two means, or pathways, of achieving a teaching qualification. The choice may ultimately be influenced by the nature and responsibility of their current role. The employer, therefore, may recommend that the completion of one of the pathways is essential to the professional development of the particular nurse. It would be necessary, as with many courses, for the candidate to negotiate study leave and support for funding.

Career opportunities for those willing to teach usually demand both a teaching qualification and evidence of academic attainment at master's level in a subject relevant to the post. Most practice educators are employed in the NHS, and most lecturers are employed in the higher education sector. However, the partnerships that exist to support students at pre- and post-registration levels facilitate opportunities for both parties to work closely together in order to achieve learning objectives and other educational requirements. Terms and conditions of service and role specifications differ in a number of ways, and candidates should explore these carefully.

Lecturer–practitioner roles, although not as numerous, exist to span the academic and practice-based learning environments. Most require a teaching qualification but are often limited to a fixed-term contract, which may deter some applicants. Historically, these posts have been allied more closely to the educational support of registered nurses in specialist clinical areas.

Nurse management

As with teaching, management is integral to the role of any registered nurse but will increase in complexity and emphasis as more senior roles are adopted. Nurse managers exist at all levels in the NHS and independent sectors, and significant opportunities exist for nurses to manage effectively from the point of registration, as there is immediate responsibility for the management of patient care and personal and professional development.

Beyond the initial management responsibilities required of staff nurses, for example, nurse managers who lead teams of staff and manage departments, units and significant caseloads also have responsibilities, including:

- monitoring standards of practice;
- clinical governance;
- staff recruitment and retention;
- audit of nursing and clinical services;
- managerial and clinical leadership;
- staff support and development;
- policy implementation;
- financial management.

More and more nurse managers are graduates and, in many cases, this is a prerequisite for posts with a specific practice base. It is recognised that senior managers benefit from educational opportunities that address skills such as leadership, the management of change and innovation, team-building, conflict management, project development and quality assurance systems. The development of information technology (IT) services relating to patient care management and outcomes requires ongoing updating of staff (Chapter 11).

These skills are often featured in degree courses that focus on, for example, health service management and nursing studies. Scrutiny of prospectuses and higher education websites will reveal the key features of such courses.

SUMMARY

Managing a career pathway depends on:
- acquisition of relevant information;
- scrutiny of employment opportunities;
- self-assessment of family, work and social needs;
- maximising personal and professional development opportunities;
- maintaining professional standards.

Preparation for selection procedures and interviews

Making career decisions depends on a range of factors, including those summarised above relating to the management of a career pathway. Embarking on the process of applying for a post demands additional skills. Whether a nurse is considering a first post, a new post, promotion opportunities or a complete change in a clinical area, there is a range of issues to consider. The RCN (1995) suggests that the following are important to the quality of a working environment because they support individuals at work:

- Value is given to nurses and nursing.
- Teamwork is evident.
- Staff are supported.
- Training and education opportunities are evident.
- Successes are celebrated.
- Mistakes are regarded as opportunities for learning.
- Ability is regarded as an asset rather than a threat.

In addition, employee-friendly policies facilitate a positive working environment and should be explored for their relevance to your needs as a potential employee as part of the process of seeking information about a post.

Reflection point 23.5
Consider the importance to you of the following features:

- any flexible working opportunities, e.g. school holiday contracts, flexi-time, self-rostering and special shifts;
- a workplace crèche or nursery;
- paternity, parental and adoption leave;
- emergency carer leave;
- career breaks;
- counselling and advice services;
- sabbatical leave.

These features provide nurses with a useful guide to what to expect from a working environment. They combine to make a positive workplace where the leaders encourage an approach to work in which individuals are valued, supported and praised. Dissatisfaction usually occurs when one or more of these features is absent. They may serve to help you decide whether it is opportune to consider a change of post.

Before applying for any post, a range of information is needed in order to produce an effectively planned application, including:

- location of the post;
- role description;
- terms and conditions of service;
- length of the contract;
- grade of the post;
- prerequisites, e.g. qualifications and required experience;
- care management systems;
- patient quality outcomes;
- management style in the unit;
- opportunities for support and preceptorship (as relevant to band);
- teaching and learning opportunities;
- appraisal scheme;
- closing date for applications.

The informal visit

Although not always possible, an informal visit to a new work area is invaluable. It gives you the opportunity to gain insight into the atmosphere, the environment and the attitudes of staff. More pertinently, much may be gleaned from such a visit and may convince you – or otherwise – about pursuing the application.

Writing a curriculum vitae

One of the most important documents associated with any application is your curriculum vitae (CV). Your CV is used to demonstrate to a potential employer that you have the necessary skills and experience for a post. You can submit your CV with your application form as it may include details that an application form does not request. Your CV may also be used for speculative applications and in response to an advertisement that requests you apply in writing.

There is no standard format for a CV, but the following key features should be included:

- personal details;
- qualifications and educational background;
- work and professional experience;
- professional activities;
- personal activities, e.g. voluntary work.

A suggested format is offered in Box 23.7. This may be modified depending on the post applied for and the details requested by the employer.

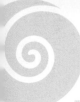

BOX 23.7 Suggested format for a curriculum vitae

Name:
Address:
Telephone number:
Email address:

NMC PIN:	**Expiry date:**
Qualifications:	Professional qualifications, with dates, should be listed. Educational awards, with dates and the college/university attended, should be given.
Previous experience:	List all previous relevant employment, with dates, and highlight your current post.
Professional activities:	These may include details of publications, in-service education, training, CPD, membership of professional groups, conferences attended and papers given, and research activities.
Personal:	You may wish to include reference to relevant details of other activities, e.g. voluntary work and committee membership, but this is not essential.

Reflection point 23.6

This is your opportunity to create or revise your own CV. Consider the format in Box 23.7 and complete the details for yourself. Aim to identify any queries or uncertainties and compare them with the following additional tips:

- Note that the request for date of birth is omitted – this is not necessary on a CV.
- Explain any gaps in your employment history, e.g. to raise a family or to undertake voluntary work.
- Use 'action words' to explain particular achievements, responsibilities and activities, e.g. 'organised', 'produced', 'implemented', 'managed' or 'developed'.
- Keep the presentation clear and well laid out, and limit the number of font styles and type faces.
- Avoid abbreviations that may not be familiar.
- Use good-quality paper.
- Enclose a covering letter with your CV. This may be used to highlight key points and their relationship to the post applied for.

Completing the application form

Application forms are central to the first stage of the selection process and are used for shortlisting suitable candidates. The form should be completed to the highest possible standard and contain relevant and factual information. Ensure that all requested information is given and, where relevant, include your CV. Application forms are usually photocopied; therefore, in order to ensure a positive presentation, type the form or use black ink unless requested to do otherwise. One of the most demanding sections on an application form is the question concerning why you are applying for this post. This is usually referred to as 'supporting information' and should be written in a way that links your skills and qualities with the skills and experience required for the post. Prepare this carefully and organise it logically. It may be useful, for example, to use the sub-headings on the role description to organise your supporting information.

The health assessment form

Usually, applicants are requested to complete a health assessment form, which is sent to the occupational health department and should remain confidential to that department. Any health-related declaration may result in being called for an interview with an occupational health nurse.

Previous convictions

If requested, you must declare any previous convictions, even those that occurred over 10 years ago. If the post requires you to work with vulnerable people, then the employer will check your police record with the Criminal Records Bureau.

Choosing referees

Usually, two referees are requested, one being your previous employer or your educational institution if you are applying for your first post after registration. Referees are asked a range of questions about the applicant and should be prepared for the task. Liaise closely with your referees; they should be fully conversant with your plans, have worked with you in a senior position or have knowledge of your professional capabilities over a period of time. Their support is essential and they should be honest enough to discuss any reservations they might have about the suitability of an application. Maintain contact with your referees and give them feedback about the outcomes of interviews, as they may be needed for a number of years in some cases.

The interview

The complexity of the interview procedure usually depends on the seniority of the post. A range of interview techniques may be used; the most common is the panel interview, where there may be two to four members present.

Preparation

Thorough preparation for the interview is essential, particularly as candidates are usually nervous and aware of the competitive nature of the event. Preparation should include:

- becoming familiar with and understanding the role specification;
- consideration of how your experience and skills link with the requirements of the role;
- being prepared to expand on any detail on your application form and CV;
- being familiar with relevant professional and practice-related initiatives;
- details of how you keep up to date with local and national initiatives and fulfil CPD and PREP requirements;
- preparing questions you expect to be asked and practising a mock interview with colleagues;
- planning the journey to the interview and working out the necessary timing;
- ensuring you are smartly dressed and well-presented.

The presentation

Many selection procedures request that the candidates prepare a presentation on a given topic, which is usually related closely to the job. The time allowed for this is usually included and is often 15–20 minutes. Aim to prepare colour acetates or a computer presentation if you have the skills and the necessary equipment is available. A brief summary of the presentation may be prepared and copied for each panel member. The presentation is usually delivered before the interview.

The interview

Panel interviews are commonly used, as they allow a range of interested parties to meet and assess the candidates. Panel members mainly include the line manager, a member of the human resources team, a representative of any associated partner organisation, and a senior member of the unit or department staff.

Panel members tend to ask the same questions of each candidate and may follow them up with secondary questions to encourage a detailed response. The areas of questioning relate to key areas and will reflect the demands of the post. They may include the following:

- *Background details*: biographical details are checked and reasons for the application are explored. Reference is made to the application form and CV.
- *Clinical and practice-related details*: clinical posts will require exploration of relevant practice-related issues, such as, reflection of skills, questioning based on problem-solving and understanding of current issues.
- *Professional issues*: professional awareness and how up to date you are may be explored. Questions that explore your professional values and commitment may also be asked.
- *Teaching and management issues*: issues such as teamworking, leadership potential, teaching and preceptorship experience may be explored.

The interview is your opportunity to communicate your qualities and skills. It is also a time for you to demonstrate your enthusiasm, commitment and professionalism. Maintain good eye contact with the questioner and other panel members, avoid rushing into a response, and try to pause and reflect on your answers. If necessary, ask the panel to clarify a question if it is not clear to you.

Following the interview

The outcome of an interview may not be communicated for anything from a number of hours to a number of days after the event. If you are offered a post, then you are in a position to discuss the start date, pay scale and any other contractual details when the contract arrives. If any aspect of the contract is unclear, seek advice from the human resources department initially. Avoid resigning from your current post until you have received the offer of the post in writing. An unsuccessful outcome is disappointing, but you should learn from any feedback about your performance, suitability for the post and advice for the future.

SUMMARY

When considering a career move:
- gather thorough information about the post;
- maintain an up-to-date CV;
- plan an informal visit;
- liaise closely with your referees;
- relate your supporting information on the application form to the role specification;
- prepare a well-presented application form;
- rehearse necessary elements of the interview;
- prepare key responses and questions.

CONCLUSION

This chapter has examined the relationship between the nurse's responsibilities for maintaining a licence to practise nursing and the associated NMC requirements. The general public expects and deserves to be cared for by competent accountable practitioners, and nurses are charged to deliver standards of care in order to meet this requirement.

Nurses need support to progress and develop their careers. Professional standards relating to re-registration, education, training and conduct exist to facilitate this process, and each nurse is responsible for the maintenance and development of professional knowledge and skills. Career opportunities are many and varied and may not always result in promotion. Successful career moves reflect not only professional development but also thorough planning, networking and professional commitment. It is hoped that the guidance offered in this chapter will help to support the process of career development and the realisation of your professional potential.

References

Department of Health (DH) (2001). *Working Together, Learning Together: A Framework for Lifelong Learning for the NHS*. London: Department of Health.

Department of Health (DH) (2005). *Agenda for Change: NHS Terms and Conditions Handbook*. London: Department of Health.

Department of Health (DH) (2006). *Modernising Nursing Careers: Setting the Direction*. London: Department of Health.

Nursing and Midwifery Council (NMC) (2004a). *Standards of Proficiency for Pre-Registration Nursing Education*. London: Nursing and Midwifery Council.

Nursing and Midwifery Council (NMC) (2004b). *Standards of Proficiency for Specialist Community Public Health Nurses*. London: Nursing and Midwifery Council.

Nursing and Midwifery Council (NMC) (2005). *Implementation of a Framework for the Standard of Post Registration Nursing*. Agendum 27.1 December 2005/c/05/160. London: Nursing and Midwifery Council.

Nursing and Midwifery Council (NMC) (2006a). *The PREP Handbook*. London: Nursing and Midwifery Council.

Nursing and Midwifery Council (NMC) (2006b). *Standards to Support Learning and Assessment in Practice*. London: Nursing and Midwifery Council.

Nursing and Midwifery Council (NMC) (2008). *The Code: Standards of Conduct, Performance and Ethics for Nurses and Midwives*. London: Nursing and Midwifery Council.

Royal College of Nursing (RCN) (1995). *A Guide to Planning Your Career*. London: Royal College of Nursing.

Schober JE (1990). Your career: making the choices. In Tschudin V and Schober JE (eds). *Managing Yourself*. London: Macmillan.

Schober JE (2000). Career opportunities for nurses working with surgical patients. In Manley K and Bellman L (eds). *Surgical Nursing Advancing Practice*. Edinburgh: Churchill Livingstone.

Stechmiller J and Yarandi H (1992). Job satisfaction among critical care nurses. *American Journal of Critical Care*, **1**, 37–44.

Further reading

Nursing and Midwifery Council (NMC) (2004). *The Standards for Specialist Community Public Health Nurse Part of the Register*. London: Nursing and Midwifery Council.
This is essential reading for all nurses considering a career or course in community public health nursing.

Nursing and Midwifery Council (NMC) (2006). *The PREP Handbook*. London: Nursing and Midwifery Council.
This document is an essential resource for ongoing education and practice for nurses, midwives and community public health nurses.

Nursing and Midwifery Council (NMC) (2006). *Standards to Support Learning and Assessment in Practice*. London: Nursing and Midwifery Council.
This document explains the standards for mentors, practice teachers, and teachers of nursing and midwifery.

Peate I (2006). *Becoming a Nurse in the 21st Century*. Chichester: John Wiley & Sons.
This is a comprehensive text that explores the four domains and the standards required for entry to the NMC register. This is essential reading for the student nurse wishing to understand the complexities of professional development.

Thomas J (2006). *Survival Guide for Ward Managers, Sisters and Charge Nurses*. Edinburgh: Churchill Livingstone.
A comprehensive guide for ward-based registered nurses. This is a very useful resource: it is rooted in practice and covers a broad range of issues, including roles and responsibilities, workload and supporting yourself and staff.

Appendix 1 The NMC Code (2008)

Reproduced with permission of the Nursing and Midwifery Council.

Standards of conduct, performance and ethics for nurses and midwives

The people in your care must be able to trust you with their health and wellbeing.
  To justify that trust, you must

- make the care of people your first concern, treating them as individuals and respecting their dignity
- work with others to protect and promote the health and wellbeing of those in your care, their families and carers, and the wider community
- provide a high standard of practice and care at all times
- be open and honest, act with integrity and uphold the reputation of your profession

As a professional, you are personally accountable for actions and omissions in your practice and must always be able to justify your decisions.

You must always act lawfully, whether those laws relate to your professional practice or personal life.

Failure to comply with this Code may bring your fitness to practise into question and endanger your registration.

This Code should be considered together with the Nursing and Midwifery Council's rules, standards, guidance and advice available from www.nmc-uk.org.

Make the care of people your first concern, treating them as individuals and respecting their dignity

Treat people as individuals

- You must treat people as individuals and respect their dignity
- You must not discriminate in any way against those in your care
- You must treat people kindly and considerately
- You must act as an advocate for those in your care, helping them to access relevant health and social care, information and support

Respect people's confidentiality

- You must respect people's right to confidentiality
- You must ensure people are informed about how and why information is shared by those who will be providing their care
- You must disclose information if you believe someone may be at risk of harm, in line with the law of the country in which you are practising

Collaborate with those in your care

- You must listen to the people in your care and respond to their concerns and preferences
- You must support people in caring for themselves to improve and maintain their health
- You must recognise and respect the contribution that people make to their own care and wellbeing
- You must make arrangements to meet people's language and communication needs
- You must share with people, in a way they can understand, the information they want or need to know about their health

Ensure you gain consent

- You must ensure that you gain consent before you begin any treatment or care
- You must respect and support people's rights to accept or decline treatment and care
- You must uphold people's rights to be fully involved in decisions about their care
- You must be aware of the legislation regarding mental capacity, ensuring that people who lack capacity remain at the centre of decision making and are fully safeguarded
- You must be able to demonstrate that you have acted in someone's best interests if you have provided care in an emergency

Maintain clear professional boundaries

- You must refuse any gifts, favours or hospitality that might be interpreted as an attempt to gain preferential treatment
- You must not ask for or accept loans from anyone in your care or anyone close to them
- You must establish and actively maintain clear sexual boundaries at all times with people in your care, their families and carers

Work with others to protect and promote the health and wellbeing of those in your care, their families and carers, and the wider community

Share information with your colleagues

- You must keep your colleagues informed when you are sharing the care of others
- You must work with colleagues to monitor the quality of your work and maintain the safety of those in your care
- You must facilitate students and others to develop their competence

Work effectively as part of a team

- You must work cooperatively within teams and respect the skills, expertise and contributions of your colleagues
- You must be willing to share your skills and experience for the benefit of your colleagues
- You must consult and take advice from colleagues when appropriate
- You must treat your colleagues fairly and without discrimination
- You must make a referral to another practitioner when it is in the best interests of someone in your care

Delegate effectively

- You must establish that anyone you delegate to is able to carry out your instructions
- You must confirm that the outcome of any delegated task meets required standards
- You must make sure that everyone you are responsible for is supervised and supported

Manage risk

- You must act without delay if you believe that you, a colleague or anyone else may be putting someone at risk
- You must inform someone in authority if you experience problems that prevent you working within this Code or other nationally agreed standards
- You must report your concerns in writing if problems in the environment of care are putting people at risk

Provide a high standard of practice and care at all times

Use the best available evidence

- You must deliver care based on the best available evidence or best practice
- You must ensure any advice you give is evidence based if you are suggesting healthcare products or services
- You must ensure that the use of complementary or alternative therapies is safe and in the best interests of those in your care

Keep your skills and knowledge up to date

- You must have the knowledge and skills for safe and effective practice when working without direct supervision
- You must recognise and work within the limits of your competence
- You must keep your knowledge and skills up to date throughout your working life
- You must take part in appropriate learning and practice activities that maintain and develop your competence and performance

Keep clear and accurate records

- You must keep clear and accurate records of the discussions you have, the assessments you make, the treatment and medicines you give and how effective these have been
- You must complete records as soon as possible after an event has occurred
- You must not tamper with original records in any way
- You must ensure any entries you make in someone's paper records are clearly and legibly signed, dated and timed
- You must ensure any entries you make in someone's electronic records are clearly attributable to you
- You must ensure all records are kept confidentially and securely

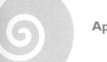

Be open and honest, act with integrity and uphold the reputation of your profession

Act with integrity

- You must demonstrate a personal and professional commitment to equality and diversity
- You must adhere to the laws of the country in which you are practising
- You must inform the NMC if you have been cautioned, charged or found guilty of a criminal offence
- You must inform any employers you work for if your fitness to practise is impaired or is called into question

Deal with problems

- You must give a constructive and honest response to anyone who complains about the care they have received
- You must not allow someone's complaint to prejudice the care you provide for them
- You must act immediately to put matters right if someone in your care has suffered harm for any reason
- You must explain fully and promptly to the person affected what has happened and the likely effects
- You must cooperate with internal and external investigations

Be impartial

- You must not abuse your privileged position for your own ends
- You must ensure that your professional judgment is not influenced by any commercial considerations

Uphold the reputation of your profession

- You must not use your professional status to promote causes that are not related to health
- You must cooperate with the media only when you can confidently protect the confidential information and dignity of those in your care
- You must uphold the reputation of your profession at all times

Information about indemnity insurance

The NMC recommends that a registered nurse, midwife or specialist community public health nurse, in advising, treating and caring for patients/clients, has professional indemnity insurance. This is in the interests of clients, patients and registrants in the event of claims of professional negligence.

Whilst employers have vicarious liability for the negligent acts and/or omissions of their employees, such cover does not normally extend to activities undertaken outside the registrant's employment. Independent practice would not be covered by vicarious liability. It is the individual registrant's responsibility to establish their insurance status and take appropriate action.

In situations where an employer does not have vicarious liability, the NMC recommends that registrants obtain adequate professional indemnity insurance. If unable to secure professional indemnity insurance, a registrant will need to demonstrate that all their clients/patients are fully informed of this fact and the implications this might have in the event of a claim for professional negligence.

Contact

Nursing and Midwifery Council
23 Portland Place
London W1B 1PZ
020 7333 9333
advice@nmc-uk.org
www.nmc-uk.org

Healthcare professionals have a shared set of values, which find their expression in this Code for nurses and midwives. These values are also reflected in the different codes of each of the UK's healthcare regulators. This Code was approved by the NMC's Council on 6 December 2007 for implementation on 1 May 2008.

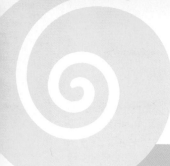

Appendix 2 Standards of education to achieve the NMC standards of proficiency

Taken from Nursing and Midwifery Council (NMC) (2004). *Standards of Proficiency for Pre-Registration Nursing Education.* London: Nursing and Midwifery Council. Reproduced with permission of the Nursing and Midwifery Council.

Introduction

This section presents the NMC standards of education to achieve the NMC standards of proficiency for nursing. These are provided for both first and second level nurses. The NMC sets the standards for pre-registration nursing programmes for the UK and, in assessing overseas nurses from outside of the European Economic Area, ensures that they have attained a comparable standard for entry to the NMC register as a nurse. There is no recognition of second level qualifications that have been gained outside of the EEA.

The standards of proficiency define the overarching principles of being able to practise as a nurse; the context in which they are achieved defines the scope of professional practice. Those undertaking education in the UK have the choice of four branch programmes, adult nursing, mental health nursing, learning disabilities nursing and children's nursing. They must achieve the NMC standards of proficiency in the context of practice in their chosen branch. The adult nursing branch must meet the requirements agreed by Member States of the European Community. Overseas nurses normally follow a programme of general nursing that is assessed on application to the NMC for its comparability to the adult nursing branch. Overseas nurses who have qualified and practised in mental health nursing, learning disabilities nursing or children's nursing are required to provide comparable evidence of achievement of proficiency in their area of practice when applying to the NMC for UK registration.

The NMC no longer approves programmes for entry to the second level of the nurses' part of the register. This level remains open only for those nurses in the UK who are already qualified and working at that level, and also for European nurses who may access it through their right to freedom of movement. The second level standards of proficiency are presented to inform employers and registrants of the standard that will have been achieved for entry to the register. The NMC expects that, through continuing professional development, second level nurses will advance their knowledge, skills and proficiency beyond that of initial registration.

All nurses on the second level of the nurses' register, who wish to do so, are able to enter a pre-registration nursing programme to enable them to become a first level nurse. They may seek appropriate accreditation of prior learning, in accordance with nursing Standards 3 and 4, to enable them to undertake a shortened programme of preparation.

First level nurses – nursing standards of education to achieve NMC standards of proficiency

Article 5(2)(a) of the Order requires the NMC to:

'establish the standards of proficiency necessary to be admitted to the different parts of the register being the standards it considers necessary for safe and effective practice under that part of the register;'

There are three parts of the register: nurses, midwives, and specialist community public health nurses. The nurses' part of the register has two sub-parts for level 1 and level 2 nurses. The nurses' part has marks to identify the branch of nursing practice in which the nurse has achieved the standards of proficiency. The NMC has previously used the term competency to describe'. . . the skills and ability to practise safely and effectively without the need for direct supervision . . .' (Fitness for practice 12, 1999). These competencies have, after consultation, been adopted as standards of proficiency by the NMC.

Article 15(1)(a) of the Order requires the Council from time to time to establish:

'Standards of education and training necessary to achieve the standards of proficiency it has established under article 5(2)' (to be admitted to the register).

The standards of education enable the NMC standards of proficiency to be achieved for entry to the nurses' part of the register. They must be achieved within the context of practice in the branch programme followed by the student. This provides comparability of proficiency at the point of entry to the register, whilst ensuring that the specific knowledge, skills and proficiencies pertaining to each field of nursing are achieved for safe and effective practice.

The pre-registration nursing programme should be designed to prepare the student to be able, on registration, to apply knowledge, understanding and skills when performing to the standards required in employment and to provide the nursing care that patients and clients require, safely and effectively, and so assume the responsibilities and accountabilities necessary for public protection.

The development of nursing programmes arises from the premise that nursing is a practice-based profession, recognising the primacy of patient and client well-being and respect for individuals, and is founded on the principles that:

- evidence should inform practice through the integration of relevant knowledge
- students are actively involved in nursing care delivery under supervision
- *The NMC code of professional conduct: standards for conduct, performance and ethics* applies to all practice interventions
- skills and knowledge are transferable
- research underpins practice
- the importance of lifelong learning and continuing professional development is recognised.

The outcomes and standards of education expressed will be achieved under the direction of a registered nurse. This support will enable the standards of proficiency to enter the register as a nurse to be achieved within the practice of the branch programme studied.

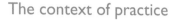

Appendix 2

The context of practice

Practice may be within one of four areas of nursing – adult, mental health, learning disabilities or children's. The NMC recognised that there was comparability between the standards of proficiency achieved by all nursing students and that it was the application of these standards to practise within different contexts of nursing that defined the scope of professional practice. The particular focus of each branch may be described as follows:

Adult nursing

This area requires the care of adults, from 18 year olds to elder people, in a variety of settings for patients with wide ranging levels of dependency. The ethos of adult nursing is patient centred and acknowledges the differing needs, values and beliefs of people from ethnically diverse communities. Nurses engage in and develop therapeutic relationships that involve patients and their carers in on-going decision-making that informs nursing care. Adult nurses have skills to meet the physical, psychological, spiritual and social needs of patients, supporting them through care pathways and working with other health and social care professionals to maximise opportunities for recovery, rehabilitation, adaptation to ongoing disease and disability, health education and health promotion. New ways of working provide enhanced opportunities for adult nurses to provide safe and effective care that meets the defined needs of this group in partnership with them. Their ability to be self-directed throughout their professional careers to support lifelong learning, in turn, contributes to continuous quality improvement in care delivery.

Mental health nursing

Mental health nurses care for people experiencing mental distress, which may have a variety of causative factors. The focus of mental health nursing is the establishment of a relationship with service users and carers to help bring about an understanding of how they might cope with their experience, thus maximising their potential for recovery. Mental health nurses use a well developed and evidence-based repertoire of interpersonal, psychosocial and other skills that are underpinned by an empathetic attitude towards the service user and the contexts within which their distress has arisen. Mental health difficulties can occur at any age and service users may be cared for in a variety of settings, including the community and their own homes. They may require care for an acute episode or ongoing support for an enduring illness. Mental health nurses work as part of multidisciplinary and multi-agency teams that seek to involve service users and their carers in all aspects of their care and treatment.

Learning disabilities nursing

The focus of learning disabilities nursing is influencing behaviours and lifestyles to enable a vulnerable client group to achieve optimum health, and to live in an inclusive society as equal citizens, and where their rights are respected. Learning disabilities nurses have the knowledge, skills, attitudes and abilities to work in partnership with people of all ages who have learning disabilities, their families and carers, to help individuals to develop individually and fulfil their potential in all aspects of their lives irrespective of their disabilities. In particular, they use expert communication skills to engage with vulnerable people and to interpret and understand behaviour to develop individual care packages. They work in a variety of residential, day and outreach service settings, adapting the level of support they provide according to the complex needs of individuals, families, carers and the settings they are in. Risk assessment and risk management are key components of their work and enable individuals to exercise their individual rights and choices. Learning disabilities nurses have a critical role in supporting the agenda for equality and equal access to all community and public services.

Children's nursing

The philosophy of children's nursing is based upon the principle of family centred care and the belief that children should be cared for by people they know and, wherever possible, within their home environment. Children's nurses understand the complex relationships between personal, socio-economic and cultural influences upon child health and child rearing practices. They develop nursing and technological competence through the application of professional knowledge, skills, values and attitudes in order to empower children and families in health decisions, promoting and providing safe, effective and informed care. Children's nurses work in a variety of settings, across and beyond traditional boundaries, and within a multi-disciplinary and multi-agency team. In particular they contribute to child protection, in collaboration with other key professionals, respecting and promoting the rights of the child.

Achieving the NMC standards of proficiency within the context of practice

The standards of proficiency provide high level outcomes that are developed as standards of education in programmes that are 50% theory and 50% practice. The NMC, through its quality assurance processes, approves the detailed programmes that demonstrate how the standards of education enable the NMC standards of proficiency to be achieved within the context of practice in each of the four branches of nursing. NMC quality assurance annual monitoring processes confirm that the standards of proficiency are being met in practice, and that the standards of education, as developed into a detailed NMC approved programme, enable acquisition of the particular knowledge, skills, values and attitudes pertaining to the area of practice. On completion of the programme, registrants, who have ensured that students have been supported and assessed in both academic and practice settings, confirm that students have met the required standards of proficiency within the practice of the particular area of nursing – adult, mental health, learning disabilities or children's.

Standards of education

The standards of education are those that have been approved to meet the previous 'competencies' for UK pre-registration nursing education. All nursing students study together for the first part of their programme, known as the Common Foundation Programme (CFP), and the standards of education include outcomes of the CFP required for entry to the second part of the programme which is called the branch programme. The standards of proficiency are reproduced in the section of outcomes of the branch programme, achievement of which allows entry to the register, in order to define the relationship between them and the standards of education necessary to achieve proficiency. The outcomes of the CFP are aligned to the requirements for entry to the register to demonstrate how proficiency is developed in particular domains of practice throughout the whole programme of education.

Format of Standard 7

The overarching standard of proficiency is presented above the standards of education, with related domains being identified. The domains may apply to one or more standards of proficiency. The outcomes to be achieved for entry to the branch programme include defined standards of education, in italics, with associated outcomes. These allow progress towards achieving the standards of proficiency that are the ultimate outcome of the whole programme. Outcomes that demonstrate achievement of these standards of proficiency are those identified for entry to the register.

Standard 7 – First level nurses – nursing standards of education to achieve the NMC standards of proficiency

Standard of proficiency for entry to the register: professional and ethical practice

Manage oneself, one's practice, and that of others, in accordance with *The NMC code of professional conduct: standards for conduct, performance and ethics*, recognising one's own abilities and limitations

Domain	Outcomes to be achieved for entry to the branch programme	Standards of proficiency for entry to the register: professional and ethical practice
Professional and ethical practice	*Discuss in an informed manner the implications of professional regulation for nursing practice* • demonstrate a basic knowledge of professional regulation and self-regulation • recognise and acknowledge the limitations of one's own abilities • recognise situations that require referral to a registered practitioner *Demonstrate an awareness of The NMC code of professional conduct: standards for conduct, performance and ethics* • commit to the principle that the primary purpose of the registered nurse is to protect and serve society • accept responsibility for one's own actions and decisions.	• practise in accordance with *The NMC code of professional conduct: standards for conduct, performance and ethics* • use professional standards of practice to self-assess performance • consult with a registered nurse when nursing care requires expertise beyond one's own current scope of competence • consult other health care professionals when individual or group needs fall outside the scope of nursing practice • identify unsafe practice and respond appropriately to ensure a safe outcome • manage the delivery of care services within the sphere of one's own accountability.

Standard of proficiency for entry to the register: professional and ethical practice

Practise in accordance with an ethical and legal framework which ensures the primacy of patient and client interest and well-being and respects confidentiality

Domain	Outcomes to be achieved for entry to the branch programme	Standards of proficiency for entry to the register: professional and ethical practice
Professional and ethical practice	*Demonstrate an awareness of, and apply ethical principles to, nursing practice* • demonstrate respect for patient and client confidentiality • identify ethical issues in day to day practice *Demonstrate an awareness of legislation relevant to nursing practice* • identify key issues in relevant legislation relating to mental health, children, data protection, manual handling, and health and safety, etc.	• demonstrate knowledge of legislation and health and social policy relevant to nursing practice • ensure the confidentiality and security of written and verbal information acquired in a professional capacity • demonstrate knowledge of contemporary ethical issues and their impact on nursing and health care • manage the complexities arising from ethical and legal dilemmas • act appropriately when seeking access to caring for patients and clients in their own homes

Standard of proficiency for entry to the register: professional and ethical practice

Practise in a fair and anti-discriminatory way, acknowledging the differences in beliefs and cultural practices of individuals or groups

Domain	Outcomes to be achieved for entry to the branch programme	Standards of proficiency for entry to the register: professional and ethical practice
Professional and ethical practice	*Demonstrate the importance of promoting equity in patient and client care by contributing to nursing care in a fair and antidiscriminatory way* • demonstrate fairness and sensitivity when responding to patients, clients and groups from diverse circumstances • recognise the needs of patients and clients whose lives are affected by disability, however manifest.	• maintain, support and acknowledge the rights of individuals or groups in the health care setting • act to ensure that the rights of individuals and groups are not compromised • respect the values, customs and beliefs of individuals and groups • provide care which demonstrates sensitivity to the diversity of patients and clients

Standard of proficiency for entry to the register: care delivery

Engage in, develop and disengage from therapeutic relationships through the use of appropriate communication and interpersonal skills

Domain	Outcomes to be achieved for entry to the branch programme	Standards of proficiency for entry to the register: care delivery
Care delivery	*Discuss methods of, barriers to, and the boundaries of, effective communication and interpersonal relationships* • recognise the effect of one's own values on interactions with patients and clients and their carers, families and friends • utilise appropriate communication skills with patients and clients • acknowledge the boundaries of a professional caring relationship *Demonstrate sensitivity when interacting with and providing information to patients and clients*	• utilise a range of effective and appropriate communication and engagement skills • maintain and, where appropriate, disengage from professional caring relationships that focus on meeting the patient's or client's needs within professional therapeutic boundaries

Standard of proficiency for entry to the register: care delivery

Create and utilise opportunities to promote the health and well-being of patients, clients and groups

Domain	Outcomes to be achieved for entry to the branch programme	Standards of proficiency for entry to the register: care delivery
Care delivery	*Contribute to enhancing the health and social well-being of patients and clients by understanding how, under the supervision of a registered practitioner, to:* • contribute to the assessment of health needs • identify opportunities for health promotion • identify networks of health and social care services	• consult with patients, clients and groups to identify their need and desire for health promotion advice • provide relevant and current health information to patients, clients and groups in a form which facilitates their understanding and acknowledges choice/individual preference • provide support and education in the development and/or maintenance of independent living skills • seek specialist/expert advice as appropriate

Standard of proficiency for entry to the register: care delivery

Undertake and document a comprehensive, systematic and accurate nursing assessment of the physical, psychological, social and spiritual needs of patients, clients and communities

Domain	Outcomes to be achieved for entry to the branch programme	Standards of proficiency for entry to the register: care delivery
Care delivery	*Contribute to the development and documentation of nursing assessments by participating in comprehensive and systematic nursing assessment of the physical, psychological, social and spiritual needs of patients and clients* • be aware of assessment strategies to guide the collection of data for assessing patients and clients and use assessment tools under guidance • discuss the prioritisation of care needs • be aware of the need to reassess patients and clients as to their needs for nursing care	• select valid and reliable assessment tools for the required purpose • systematically collect data regarding the health and functional status of individuals, clients and communities through appropriate interaction, observation and measurement • analyse and interpret data accurately to inform nursing care and take appropriate action

Standard of proficiency for entry to the register: care delivery

Formulate and document a plan of nursing care, where possible, in partnership with patients, clients, their carers and family and friends, within a framework of informed consent

Domain	Outcomes to be achieved for entry to the branch programme	Standards of proficiency for entry to the register: care delivery
Care delivery	*Contribute to the planning of nursing care, involving patients and clients and, where possible, their carers; demonstrating an understanding of helping patients and clients to make informed decisions* • identify care needs based on the assessment of a patient or client • participate in the negotiation and agreement of the care plan with the patient or client and with their carer, family or friends, as appropriate, under the supervision of a registered nurse • inform patients and clients about intended nursing actions, respecting their right to participate in decisions about their care	• establish priorities for care based on individual or group needs • develop and document a care plan to achieve optimal health, habilitation, and rehabilitation based on assessment and current nursing knowledge • identify expected outcomes, including a time frame for achivement and/or review in consultation with patients, clients, their carers and family and friends and with members of the health and social care team

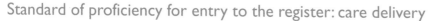

Appendix 2

Standard of proficiency for entry to the register: care delivery

Based on the best available evidence, apply knowledge and an appropriate repertoire of skills indicative of safe and effective nursing practice

Domain	Outcomes to be achieved for entry to the branch programme	Standards of proficiency for entry to the register: care delivery
Care delivery	*Contribute to the implementation of a programme of nursing care, designed and supervised by registered practitioners* • undertake activities that are consistent with the care plan and within the limits of one's own abilities. *Demonstrate evidence of a developing knowledge base which underpins safe and effecive nursing practice* • access and discuss research and other evidence in nursing and related disciplines • identify examples of the use of evidence in planned nursing interventions. *Demonstrate a range of essential nursing skills, under the supervision of a registered nurse, to meet individuals' needs, which include:* • maintaining dignity, privacy and confidentiality; effective communication and observational skills, including listening and taking physiological measurements; safety and health, including moving, and handling and infection control; essential first aid and emergency procedures; administration of medicines; emotional, physical and personal care, including meeting the need for comfort, nutrition and personal hygiene	• ensure that current research findings and other evidence are incorporated in practice • identify relevant changes in practice or new information and disseminate it to colleagues • contribute to the application of a range of interventions which support and optimise the health and well-being of patients and clients • demonstrate the safe application of the skills required to meet the needs of patients and clients within the current sphere of practice • identify and respond to patients and clients' continuing learning and care needs • engage with, and evaluate, the evidence base that underpins safe nursing practice

556

Standard of proficiency for entry to the register: care delivery

Provide a rationale for the nursing care delivered which takes account of social, cultural, spiritual, legal, political and economic influences

Domain	Outcomes to be achieved for entry to the branch programme	Standards of proficiency for entry to the register: care delivery
Care delivery		• identify, collect and evaluate information to justify the effective utilisation of resources to achieve planned outcomes of nursing care

Standard of proficiency for entry to the register: care delivery

Evaluate and document the outcomes of nursing and other interventions

Domain	Outcomes to be achieved for entry to the branch programme	Standards of proficiency for entry to the register: care delivery
Care delivery	*Contribute to the evaluation of the appropriateness of nursing care delivered* • demonstrate an awareness of the need to assess regularly a patient's or client's response to nursing interventions • provide for a supervising registered practitioner, evaluative commentary and information on nursing care based on personal observations and actions • contribute to the documentation of the outcomes of nursing interventions	• collaborate with patients and clients and, when appropriate, additional carers to review and monitor the progress of individuals or groups towards planned outcomes • analyse and revise expected outcomes, nursing interventions and priorities in accordance with changes in the individual's condition, needs or circumstances

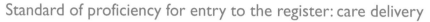

Appendix 2

Standard of proficiency for entry to the register: care delivery

Demonstrate sound clinical judgement across a range of differing professional and care delivery contexts

Domain	Outcomes to be achieved for entry to the branch programme	Standards of proficiency for entry to the register: care delivery
Care delivery	*Recognise situations in which agreed plans of nursing care no longer appear appropriate and refer these to an appropriate accountable practitioner* • demonstrate the ability to discuss and accept care decisions • accurately record observations made and communicate these to the relevant members of the health and social care team.	• use evidence based knowledge from nursing and related disciplines to select and individualise nursing interventions • demonstrate the ability to transfer skills and knowledge to a variety of circumstances and settings • recognise the need for adaptation and adapt nursing practice to meet varying and unpredictable circumstance • ensure that practice does not compromise the nurse's duty of care to individuals or the safety of the public

Standard of proficiency for entry to the register: care management

Contribute to public protection by creating and maintaining a safe environment of care through the use of quality assurance and risk management strategies

Domain	Outcomes to be achieved for entry to the branch programme	Standards of proficiency for entry to the register: care management
Care management	*Contribute to the identification of actual and potential risks to patients, clients and their carers, to oneself and to others, and participate in measures to promote and ensure health and safety* • understand and implement health and safety principles and policies • recognise and report situations that are potentially unsafe for patients, clients, oneself and others	• apply relevant principles to ensure the safe administration of therapeutic substances • use appropriate risk assessment tools to identify actual and potential risks • identify environmental hazards and eliminate and/or prevent where possible • communicate safety concerns to a relevant authority • manage risk to provide care which best meets the needs and interests of patients, clients and the public

Standard of proficiency for entry to the register: care management

Demonstrate knowledge of effective inter-professional working practices which respect and utilise the contributions of members of the health and social care team

Domain	Outcomes to be achieved for entry to the branch programme	Standards of proficiency for entry to the register: care management
Care management	*Demonstrate an understanding of the role of others by participating in inter-professional working practice* • identify the roles of the members of the health and social care team • work within the health and social care team to maintain and enhance integrated care	• establish and maintain collaborative working relationships with members of the health and social care team and others • participate with members of the health and social care team in decision-making concerning patients and clients • review and evaluate care with members of the health and social care team and others

Standard of proficiency for entry to the register: care management

Delegate duties to others, as appropriate, ensuring that they are supervised and monitored

Domain	Outcomes to be achieved for entry to the branch programme	Standards of proficiency for entry to the register: care management
Care management		• take into account the role and competence of staff when delegating work • maintain one's own accountability and responsibility when delegating aspects of care to others • demonstrate the ability to co-ordinate the delivery of nursing and health care

Standard of proficiency for entry to the register: care management

Demonstrate key skills

Domain	Outcomes to be achieved for entry to the branch programme	Standards of proficiency for entry to the register: care management
Care management	*Demonstrate literacy, numeracy and computer skills needed to record, enter, store, retrieve and organise data essential for care delivery*	• literacy – interpret and present information in a comprehensible manner • numeracy – accurately interpret numerical data and their significance for the safe delivery of care • information technology and management – interpret and utilise data and technology, taking account of legal, ethical and safety considerations, in the delivery and enhancement of care • problem-solving – demonstrate sound clinical decision-making which can be justified even when made on the basis of limited information

Standard of proficiency for entry to the register: personal and professional development

Demonstrate a commitment to the need for continuing professional development and personal supervision activities in order to enhance knowledge, skills, values and attitudes needed for safe and effective nursing practice

Domain	Outcomes to be achieved for entry to the branch programme	Standards of proficiency for entry to the register: personal and professional development
Personal and professional development	*Demonstrate responsibility for one's own learning through the development of a portfolio of practice and recognise when further learning is required* • identify specific learning needs and objectives • begin to engage with, and interpret, the evidence base which underpins nursing practice *Acknowledge the importance of seeking supervision to develop safe and effective nursing practice*	• identify one's own professional development needs by engaging in activities such as reflection in, and on, practice and lifelong learning • develop a personal development plan which takes into account personal, professional and organisational needs • share experiences with colleagues and patients and clients in order to identify the additional knowledge and skills needed to manage unfamiliar or professionally challenging situations • take action to meet any identified knowledge and skills deficit likely to affect the delivery of care within the current sphere of practice

Standard of proficiency for entry to the register: personal and professional development

Enhance the professional development and safe practice of others through peer support, leadership, supervision and teaching

Domain	Outcomes to be achieved for entry to the branch programme	Standards of proficiency for entry to the register: personal and professional development
Personal and professional development		• contribute to creating a climate conducive to learning • contribute to the learning experiences and development of others by facilitating the mutual sharing of knowledge and experience • demonstrate effective leadership in the establishment and maintenance of safe nursing practise

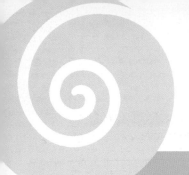

Appendix 3 An NMC guide for students of nursing and midwifery

Taken from Nursing and Midwifery Council (NMC) (2005). *An NMC Guide for Students of Nursing and Midwifery*. London: Nursing and Midwifery Council. Reproduced with the permission of the Nursing and Midwifery Council.

Protecting the public through professional standards

Welcome to your programme of nursing or midwifery education. Choosing to become a nurse of midwife is a big step, but it means that you are on the way to becoming one of the most important people in society. Patients and the public truly value the work you will be doing when you qualify.

Once you have successfully completed your programme of education, you will need to register with the Nursing and Midwifery Council (NMC) before you can practise as a nurse or midwife.

This leaflet sets out some basic information about the NMC and some guidance for the clinical experience you will undertake during your studies. It is based upon extensive consultation with individual pre-registration students of nursing and midwifery, organisations representing students and lecturers in higher education.

The leaflet should be read in conjunction with advice provided by your higher education institution.

What does the NMC do?

The NMC is the regulatory body for nursing and midwifery. Our purpose is to establish and improve standards of nursing and midwifery care in order to protect the public. These standards are set out in The NMC code of professional conduct: standards for conduct, performance and ethics, which the NMC will send to you when you first register. We urge you to get hold of a copy now. You should be able to obtain it through your university. If not, it's on our web site at www.nmc-uk.org

You may not be aware that the standards set by the NMC already apply to you. The level of entry to the programme of education that you are undertaking and the content, type and length of your programme are all part of these standards. The NMC has other key responsibilities which are to:

- maintain a register of qualified nurses and midwives
- set standards for nursing and midwifery education, performance, ethics and conduct
- provide advice and guidance on professional standards
- consider allegations of unfitness to practise due to misconduct, ill health or lack of competence.

Registration and professional accountability

When you successfully complete your course, your higher education institution will notify the NMC that you have met the required standards and that you are eligible for entry on the register. Your course director will also complete a declaration of good health and good character on your behalf. When we have received this information and you have paid your registration fee, your name will be entered on the NMC register and you will be eligible to practise as a registered practitioner. This should take a matter of days.

Registration is not simply an administrative process. The NMC's register is an instrument of public protection and anyone can check the registered status of a nurse or midwife. Registering with the NMC demonstrates that you have met the standards expected of registered nurses and midwives. It also demonstrates that you are professionally accountable at all times for your acts and omissions.

Professional accountability involves weighing up the interests of patients and clients, using your professional judgement and skills to make a decision and enabling you to account for the decision you make. On rare occasions, nurses and midwives fall short of the professional standards expected of them. The NMC investigates in the public interest any complaints made about the professional conduct or fitness to practise of registered nurses and midwives.

Throughout your career, you will need to keep up to date with developments in your area of practice. Your continuing professional development is an integral part of your professional accountability. In order to continue to practise, you will need to meet the NMC's standards for post-registration education and practice (PREP). Detailed information about PREP is available in The PREP Handbook, which you can download from the NMC web site, or obtain free of charge from our Publications Department.

You will also need to complete a notification of practice form when you renew your registration every three years and pay your annual retention fee. Practising midwives also need to complete a notification of intention to practise form annually.

Guidance on clinical experience for students

During your studentship, you will come into close contact with patients or clients. This may be through observing care being given, through helping in providing care and, later, through full participation in providing care. At all times, you should work only within your level of understanding and competence, and always under the appropriate supervision of a registered nurse or midwife, or a health professional with a registered nurse or midwife providing mentorship.

The section below provides some guidance on working with patients or clients during your studies. The principles underpinning this guidance reflect the standards that will be expected of you when you become a registered practitioner.

Your accountability

As a pre-registration student, you are not professionally accountable in the way that you will be after you come to register with the NMC. This means that you cannot be called to account for your actions and omissions by the NMC. So far as the NMC is concerned, it is the registered practitioners with whom you are working who are professionally responsible for the consequences of your actions and omissions. This is why you must always work under direct supervision. This does not mean, however, that you can never be called to account by your university or by the law for the consequences of your actions or omissions as a pre-registration student.

The wishes of patients

You must respect the wishes of patients and clients at all times. They have the right to refuse to allow you, as a student, to participate in caring for them and you should make this right clear to them when they are first given information about the care they will receive from you. You should leave if they ask you to do so. Their rights, as patients or clients, supersede at all times your rights to knowledge and experience.

Identifying yourself

You should introduce yourself accurately at all times when speaking to patients or clients either directly or by telephone. In doing so, you should make it quite clear that you are a pre-registration student and not a registered practitioner. In fact, it is a criminal offence for anyone to represent him or herself falsely and deliberately as a registered nurse or midwife.

Accepting appropriate responsibility

There may be times when you are in a position where you may not be directly accompanied by your mentor, supervisor or another registered colleague, such as emergency situations. As your skills, experience and confidence develop, you will become increasingly able to deal with these situations. However, as a student, do not participate in any procedure for which you have not been fully prepared or in which you are not adequately supervised. If such a situation arises, discuss the matter as quickly as possible with your mentor or personal tutor.

Patient confidentiality

Patients have the right to know that any private and personal information that is given in confidence will be used only for the purposes for which it was originally provided and that it will not be used for any other reason.

If you want to refer in a written assignment to some real-life situation in which you have been involved, do not provide any information that could identify a particular patient or client. Obtain access to patient records only when absolutely necessary for the care being provided. Use of these records must be closely supervised by a registered practitioner and you must follow the local policy on the handling and storage of records. Any written entry you make in a patient's or clients records must be counter-signed by a registered practitioner. You can find more advice about confidentiality in The NMC code of professional conduct: standards for conduct, performance and ethics. You should also refer to our Guidelines for records and record keeping.

Handling complaints

You will need to be aware of the local procedures for dealing with complaints by patients, clients, or their families, about the treatment or care they are receiving. If patients indicate to you that they are unhappy about their treatment or care, you should report the matter immediately to the person who is supervising your clinical experience or to another appropriate person.

What if I see something I think is wrong?

As a student, you will experience a range of different settings in your practice education placements. You will be well placed to question why something is or is not being done. In some cases, you may see a registered nurse or midwife doing something you feel is inappropriate. Although difficult, you shouldn't ignore the situation. Ask the person or someone else about it.

In some cases, you may be observing what could amount to misconduct. Whether or not this is the case, challenging experienced practitioners' ways of doing things should be encouraged. This will show you are observing and thinking, and may help a practitioner improve their own practice.

We hope that you will find these notes helpful during your programme and in understanding the important responsibilities you will later undertake as a registered nurse or midwife.

If you need to discuss any of these issues with us, please contact our professional advice service on 020 7333 6541/6550/6553, by e-mail at advice@nmc-uk.org or by fax on 020 7333 6538.

If you would like to find out more about the work of the NMC, our website at www.nmc-uk.org includes copies of all NMC publications, position statements issued by our professional advice service, and further useful information and contacts for students of nursing and midwifery.

Good luck in your programme of preparation for registration and in your future career.

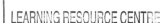

Index

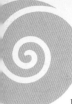

Index

blood tests, myocardial infarction
370–2
body (of dead person)
disposal 474
preparation/handling 474, 478
in unexpected death 482–3
viewing in unexpected death 493
body temperature, assessment 308
Bolam test (*Bolam v. Friern HMC* 1958)
133
books 71
boundaries, professional *see* professional
boundaries
brain death 275–6
definition 469
Branch Programme 47
breaking bad news
of terminal illness 471
of unexpected death 482
breast screening, older women 433
breathing assessment 307, 308, 309
chronic obstructive pulmonary disease
377
Briggs Report 93
Bristol Inquiry 105–6
bronchiolitis 328
bronchitis, chronic 375–81
'buddy' system 80–1, 506
*Building a Safer NHS for Patients:
Implementing an Organisation with
a Memory* 150
burns, severe, patient's personal account
4–6
bursaries 68–9

cancer, childhood 332, 339–40
adolescent 353
adolescent survivors of, late effects
services 354
capacity/competence to consent
(mental/intellectual) 185
refusal of treatment and 375
sterilisation and sexual relationships
185
car, community nurses 462
cardiology *see* heart
care (health) 247–485
care of people as first concern 98, 543
change *see* change
changing patterns 366–7
collaboration with those in your care
99–100, 544
continuity of *see* continuity
coordination *see* case management
costs for students 68
delivery *see* delivery
dispersed, IT in 227
duty of 106

evaluation 255
evidence-based *see* evidence-based care
integrated 51
key aspects 247–485
management *see* management
older people's experiences 431–3
organising 152, 252
patient-centred *see* patient-centred care
patient-controlled, IT in 227
planning *see* planning
primary, placement in 51
provision of *see* provision
provision of high standards of, at all
times 108–9
quality *see* quality
regulatory bodies in UK 95–6
secondary, placement in 51
settings of *see* settings
standards *see* standards
see also compensatory care; self-care;
services
care homes (residential and nursing),
older people in 213, 408
diabetes care 214
separation from spouse 408
Care Quality Commission 123
career 521–42
factors affecting choices 526–36
opportunities and their management
526–36
pathways 530–6
carers
care settings and views of people with
206
informal *see* carers
obtaining information from 294–5
protecting and promoting health and
well-being of 103–4, 544–5
respite care 454
stroke patients 406–7
young 352
caries prevention 199
case management (coordination of care)
combining technology and 212
in community care 454
nurses new to, employer checklist
458
catastrophic event in local environment
449
catheterisation, urinary, stroke 397
cause (aetiology) 254
caution order 140
cellular death, definition 469
Central Midwives Board 90
demise 91
Centre for the Advancement of
Interprofessional Education
(CAIPE) 56

cerebrovascular accident *see* stroke
change (in health care) 496
management 497
chaos managers 266–72
charities, employment by 222
chest infection in chronic obstructive
pulmonary disease 378
child (children) 318–46
consent 187–8
death 481
dental caries prevention 199
impact of parental ill-health on
chronic obstructive pulmonary
disease 381
stroke 401
nursing of 53, 318–46, 551
placement in 51, 53
parents/family *see* parents
see also adolescents; school
child protection 321
adolescents 358
childcare, help with 69, 74
Children Act (1989) 351
Choose and Book 460
chronic conditions *see* long-term health
conditions
chronic obstructive pulmonary disease
375–81
cigarette smoking *see* smoking
circulation, assessment 307
clients *see* patients
clinical crisis requiring extra help,
community nursing 464
clinical death, definition 468–9
clinical decision-making *see* decision-
making
clinical governance *see* governance
Clinical Governance in the New NHS
149
clinical guidelines (NICE) 153, 154
clinical judgement *see* judgement
clinical risk 161–2
clinical standards 120–1
clinical supervision *see* supervision
clinical teaching model 502–4
closed questions to patients 294
*The Code: Standards of Conduct,
Performance and Ethics for Nurses
and Midwives see* Nursing and
Midwifery Council (NMC), Code
(2008)
cognitions in bereavement 477
cognitive abilities of adolescents 352
collaboration
with professionals/colleagues 99
children's nursing 334–5
with those in your care 99–100,
544

Index

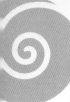

Index

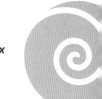

North American Nursing Diagnosis
  Association (NANDA), NANDA-I
  taxonomy of nursing diagnoses
  22, 239
Northern Ireland
  health care standards 123, 146, 154
  service commissioning responsibilities
    in 207
Norton scale 312
nosocomial infections, control *see*
  infection
now what? (in reflective practice) 131
numeracy skills, demonstrating 336
nursery children 325
Nurses, Midwives and Health Visitors
  Act (1979) 91
  1992 amendment 91, 93
Nurses Registration Act (1919) 90
nursing (general references only)
  definitions/concepts of 18–22, 52,
    92, 251, 267–8
  loving 265–89
  models of *see* models
  personal views *see* personal views
  as a profession *see* practice
  theories of *see* theory
Nursing: A Social Policy Statement 23
Nursing and Midwifery Council (NMC)
  95–102, 146
  on advanced nursing practice
    532–3
  allegation of unacceptable standard of
    a practitioner 139–40
  on clinical supervision 512
  Code (in general or unspecified)
    124–7
    domains *see* domains
    on employers 222
    importance 124
    on organising care 152
  Code (2002) xi, 95
  Code (2004) 95
  Code (2008 – *The Code: Standards of
    Conduct, Performance and Ethics
    for Nurses and Midwives*) xi, 34,
    95–102, 522, 543–7
  competencies *see* competencies
  responsibility for self-determination
    65–6
  contacting 547
  functions/purpose 562
  *Guide for Students of Nursing and
    Midwifery* 562–5
  on specialist practitioners 532
  *Standards of Proficiency for Pre-
    Registration Nursing Education see*
    standards website, and student
    support 84

Nursing and Midwifery Order (2001)
  124
'nursing as doing' model 25, 27
nursing development unit movement
  279
nursing home *see* care home
nursing minimum datasets (NMDSs)
  241–2
nutritional assessment 311

observation of patient 294
occupation *see* employment
occupational therapist 53
  stroke 400
Office of Public Sector Information 84
older people (elderly) 412–44
  abuse of 447
  care homes *see* care homes
  experiences
    of ageing 414–22
    of health and illness 428–37
  government policy 392–3
  quality of life, factors influencing
    422–8
  stroke, case study 394–408
  see also ageing
oncology *see* cancer
open questions to patients 294
Opendays.com 84
openness, maintaining 101–2, 194, 546
oral assessment 309–10
Orem's self-care model 30, 261–2,
  298–9, 302, 303
organ transplantation 190–1
An Organisation with a Memory 150
organisational standards 123
organising nursing care (health) 152,
  252
orientation phase in interpersonal
  relationships 259, 300, 301, 302,
  303
outcome (in health care)
  in children's nursing, evaluation and
    documentation 331
  evidence-based, applied to patient
    care 252
  in infection control 116–17
overdose 382–5
overseas students, coping 76–7
oxygen
  administration in chronic obstructive
    pulmonary disease 377
  assessing level of 308
    in chronic obstructive pulmonary
      disease 377

PACS (Picture Archiving and
  Communication Systems) 460

paediatrics *see* child
pain
  assessment 313–15
  total, concept of 469–70
painting, bereaved persons 480
'pairing' ('buddy') system 80–1, 506
palliative care 473
  care settings and views of people in
    206
panel interview 540
paper records 234–5
paracetamol overdose 384–5
parents and family, child's 342–3
  cultural issues 322–3
  ill parent
    adolescents caring in long-term
      conditions 352
    impact on child *see* child
  immunisation advice 453
  therapeutic relationships 323–4
  working with and involving 342–3
    in adolescence 351
participation (in experiential learning)
  498, 499
partnership, commitment to (in RCN's
  definition of nursing) 25, 34,
  251
paternalism 107
  experience, five dimensions 121
patient(s), and clients/consumers/users
  abuse or violence from, in community
    nursing 464
  assessment *see* assessment
  breaking bad news 471
  care *see* care
  clinical governance and involvement
    of 169–70
  declining health advice 15
  demographic data 241
  experience 151–4, 165–6, 169–70
    of ageing 414–22
    importance 151–5
    obtaining information on 156–9,
      165–6
  identification 240
  interactions with nurse, in the
    environment 37–8
  meaning of illness to 375
  medical record sharing with 233–4
  organisations representing 146, 368
    role in addressing concerns 140
  personal needs/task, experience of
    being asked to help with 10
  personal views of nursing 3–8, 19
  relationships (of nurse) with 176–8,
    220–1
    abuse (by nurse) 102–3, 176–7
    adolescents 354–5

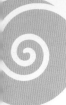

Index

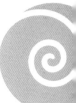